AF461861

SIGNAL TRANSDUCTION IN CANCER

Dear MyCopy Customer,

This Springer book is a monochrome print version of the eBook to which your library gives you access via SpringerLink. It is available to you at a subsidized price since your library subscribes to at least one Springer eBook subject collection.

Please note that MyCopy books are only offered to library patrons with access to at least one Springer eBook subject collection. MyCopy books are strictly for individual use only.

You may cite this book by referencing the bibliographic data and/or the DOI (Digital Object Identifier) found in the front matter. This book is an exact but monochrome copy of the print version of the eBook on SpringerLink.

Cancer Treatment and Research

Steven T. Rosen, M.D., ***Series Editor***

Goldstein, L.J., Ozols, R. F. (eds): *Anticancer Drug Resistance. Advances in Molecular and Clinical Research.* 1994. ISBN 0-7923-2836-1.
Hong, W.K., Weber, R.S. (eds): *Head and Neck Cancer. Basic and Clinical Aspects.* 1994. ISBN 0-7923-3015-3.
Thall, P.F. (ed): *Recent Advances in Clinical Trial Design and Analysis.* 1995. ISBN 0-7923-3235-0.
Buckner, C. D. (ed): *Technical and Biological Components of Marrow Transplantation.* 1995. ISBN 0-7923-3394-2.
Winter, J.N. (ed.): *Blood Stem Cell Transplantation.* 1997. ISBN 0-7923-4260-7.
Muggia, F.M. (ed): *Concepts, Mechanisms, and New Targets for Chemotherapy.* 1995. ISBN 0-7923-3525-2.
Klastersky, J. (ed): *Infectious Complications of Cancer.* 1995. ISBN 0-7923-3598-8.
Kurzrock, R., Talpaz, M. (eds): *Cytokines: Interleukins and Their Receptors.* 1995. ISBN 0-7923-3636-4.
Sugarbaker, P. (ed): *Peritoneal Carcinomatosis: Drugs and Diseases.* 1995. ISBN 0-7923-3726-3.
Sugarbaker, P. (ed): *Peritoneal Carcinomatosis: Principles of Management.* 1995. ISBN 0-7923-3727-1.
Dickson, R.B., Lippman, M.E. (eds.): *Mammary Tumor Cell Cycle, Differentiation and Metastasis.* 1995. ISBN 0-7923-3905-3.
Freireich, E.J, Kantarjian, H. (eds): *Molecular Genetics and Therapy of Leukemia.* 1995. ISBN 0-7923-3912-6.
Cabanillas, F., Rodriguez, M.A. (eds): *Advances in Lymphoma Research.* 1996. ISBN 0-7923-3929-0.
Miller, A.B. (ed.): *Advances in Cancer Screening.* 1996. ISBN 0-7923-4019-1.
Hait , W.N. (ed.): *Drug Resistance.* 1996. ISBN 0-7923-4022-1.
Pienta, K.J. (ed.): *Diagnosis and Treatment of Genitourinary Malignancies.* 1996. ISBN 0-7923-4164-3.
Arnold, A.J. (ed.): *Endocrine Neoplasms.* 1997. ISBN 0-7923-4354-9.
Pollock, R.E. (ed.): *Surgical Oncology.* 1997. ISBN 0-7923-9900-5.
Verweij, J., Pinedo, H.M., Suit, H.D. (eds): *Soft Tissue Sarcomas: Present Achievements and Future Prospects.* 1997. ISBN 0-7923-9913-7.
Walterhouse, D.O., Cohn, S. L. (eds.): *Diagnostic and Therapeutic Advances in Pediatric Oncology.* 1997. ISBN 0-7923-9978-1.
Mittal, B.B., Purdy, J.A., Ang, K.K. (eds): *Radiation Therapy.* 1998. ISBN 0-7923-9981-1.
Foon, K.A., Muss, H.B. (eds): *Biological and Hormonal Therapies of Cancer.* 1998. ISBN 0-7923-9997-8.
Ozols, R.F. (ed.): *Gynecologic Oncology.* 1998. ISBN 0-7923-8070-3.
Noskin, G. A. (ed.): *Management of Infectious Complications in Cancer Patients.* 1998. ISBN 0-7923-8150-5
Bennett, C. L. (ed): *Cancer Policy.* 1998. ISBN 0-7923-8203-X
Benson, A. B. (ed): *Gastrointestinal Oncology.* 1998. ISBN 0-7923-8205-6
Tallman, M.S. , Gordon, L.I. (eds): *Diagnostic and Therapeutic Advances in Hematologic Malignancies.* 1998. ISBN 0-7923-8206-4
von Gunten, C.F. (ed): *Palliative Care and Rehabilitation of Cancer Patients.* 1999. ISBN 0-7923-8525-X
Burt, R.K., Brush, M.M. (eds): *Advances in Allogeneic Hematopoietic Stem Cell Transplantation.* 1999. ISBN 0-7923-7714-1
Angelos, P. (ed): *Ethical Issues in Cancer Patient Care* 2000. ISBN 0-7923-7726-5
Gradishar, W.J., Wood, W.C. (eds): *Advances in Breast Cancer Management.* 2000. ISBN 0-7923-7890-3
Sparano, Joseph A. (ed): *HIV & HTLV-I Associated Malignancies.* 2001. ISBN 0-7923-7220-4.
Ettinger, David S. (ed): *Thoracic Oncology.* 2001. ISBN 0-7923-7248-4.
Bergan, Raymond C. (ed): *Cancer Chemopre*vention. 2001. ISBN 0-7923-7259-X.
Raza, A., Mundle, S.D. (eds): *Myelodysplastic Syndromes & Secondary Acute Myelogenous Leukemia* 2001. ISBN: 0-7923-7396.
Talamonti, Mark S. (ed): *Liver Directed Therapy for Primary and Metastatic Liver Tumors.* 2001. ISBN 0-7923-7523-8.
Stack, M.S., Fishman, D.A. (eds): *Ovarian Cancer.* 2001. ISBN 0-7923-7530-0.
Bashey, A., Ball, E.D. (eds): *Non-Myeloablative Allogeneic Transplantation.* 2002. ISBN 0-7923-7646-3
Leong, Stanley P.L. (ed): *Atlas of Selective Sentinel Lymphadenectomy for Melanoma, Breast Cancer and Colon Cancer.* 2002. ISBN 1-4020-7013-6
Andersson , B., Murray D. (eds): *Clinically Relevant Resistance in Cancer Chemotherapy.* 2002. ISBN 1-4020-7200-7.
Beam, C. (ed.): *Biostatistical Applications in Cancer Research.* 2002. ISBN 1-4020-7226-0.
Brockstein, B., Masters, G. (eds): *Head and Neck Cancer.* 2003. ISBN 1-4020-7336-4.
Frank, D.A. (ed.): ***Signal Transduction in Cancer.*** 2003. ISBN 1-4020-7340-2.

SIGNAL TRANSDUCTION IN CANCER

edited by

David A. Frank, MD, PhD
Dana-Farber Cancer Institute
Harvard Medical School
Boston, Massachusetts
USA

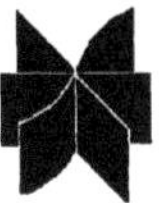

SPRINGER SCIENCE+BUSINESS MEDIA, LLC

Library of Congress Cataloging-in-Publication Data

A C.I.P. Catalogue record for this book is available
from the Library of Congress.

DOI 10.1007/978-0-306-48158-1

Copyright © 2003 by Springer Science+Business Media New York
Originally published by Kluwer Academic Publishers in 2003
MyCopy version of the original edition 2003

All rights reserved. No part of this work may be reproduced, stored in a retrieval system, or transmitted in any form or by any means, electronic, mechanical, photocopying, microfilming, recording, or otherwise, without the written permission from the Publisher, with the exception of any material supplied specifically for the purpose of being entered and executed on a computer system, for exclusive use by the purchaser of the work.

Permission for books published in Europe: permissions@wkap.nl
Permissions for books published in the United States of America: permissions@wkap.com

Printed on acid-free paper.

The Publisher offers discounts on this book for course use and bulk purchases. For further information, send email to laura.walsh@wkap.com.
www.springer.com/mycopy

CONTENTS

PREFACE

Cancer is the second leading cause of death in developed societies, and epidemiologists predict that in a few years cancer will surpass cardiovascular disease to become the leading cause of mortality. After years of growth, the rate of death from many forms of cancer seems to be leveling off. However, most human cancers remain essentially incurable once they have spread, and relatively little progress has been made in this area since the dawn of the chemotherapy era over 50 years ago.

In contrast to the slow progress in treating cancer, our understanding of the physiology of normal and neoplastic cells has increased phenomenally in recent years. This has raised the hope that we can have a clearer understanding of the molecular abnormalities which distinguish a cancer cell from its normal counterpart, resulting in the development of targeted molecular approaches which will kill tumor cells while leaving normal cells unscathed. In the end, it is this issue of "therapeutic index" that makes treating cancer so difficult with current cytotoxic agents.

In designing such sophisticated treatments for cancer, it is necessary to consider the processes which govern normal cellular physiology. After the first few cell divisions in embryogenesis, the biological program of a cell is directed by extracellular cues, such as soluble molecules (e.g., cytokines or hormones), cell-cell interactions, and cell-matrix interactions. The information triggered by these stimuli must be conveyed into the cell, to both nuclear and cytoplasmic targets, to direct the cellular response. The transmission of this information, or signal transduction, is critical to the appropriate response of a normal cell. However, these signaling pathways can often be subverted in malignancy. One of the consequences of the mutations which characterize cancer is the activation of signaling cascades leading to survival, proliferation, or pluripotentcy (blocked differentiation) of a cell which is inappropriate for its physiological circumstances.

If nothing else, the recent advances in understanding how signaling pathways control normal cellular function, and how these pathways become deranged in cancer, would make this a perfect time to review signal transduction in this context. However, in addition, we are now at the dawn of a new age in the treatment of cancer based on molecular strategies. New therapeutic approaches are targeting growth factor receptors which are over-expressed, oncogenic tyrosine kinases resulting from chromosomal translocations, or pro-survival proteins whose expression is being driven inappropriately. It seems clear that the next major advances in the therapy of cancer will arise from strategies targeting the molecular abnormalities of the tumor cells and its environs.

Thus, the goal of this volume is to explore signal transduction pathways of particular importance to human cancer. While it is impossible to be fully comprehensive in a fast-moving field which encompasses most aspects of cellular physiology, the 14 contributions in this volume were chosen to reflect major areas of signaling research. Although one cannot draw rigid boundaries as to where signaling pathways reside, the volume has been divided into four sections reflecting physiological groupings. These focus on receptors at the cell surface, intracellular signaling cascades, transcription factors functioning in the nucleus, and pathways triggering programs of cell death. These chapters provide a panoramic view of signaling pathways which control critical cellular events, and which are commonly subverted in human cancers.

Without question, the contributions in this volume reflect the state of the art of one of the most exciting areas of cell biology, biochemistry, and molecular genetics. However, "signal transduction" is no longer a topic restricted to sophisticated scientific discussions. It is on the minds of practicing oncologists around the world as a leading hope for the future of cancer therapy. As such, these 14 chapters also represent a blueprint for strategies which can be translated into the clinical arena with relatively brief development times. In this exciting era in which scientific advances and medical practice are rapidly converging, the goal of this volume is to inform and inspire scientists and physicians alike.

David A. Frank, M.D., Ph.D.
June 2002

GROWTH, SURVIVAL AND MIGRATION: THE TRK TO CANCER

JOSHUA B RUBIN & ROSALIND A SEGAL

1. INTRODUCTION

Cancers possess two cardinal features, dysregulated growth and invasiveness or the ability to metastasize. While single inherited or acquired genetic events have been identified as oncogenic, multiple events are necessary for the genesis of the cancer phenotype. Thus increased proliferation produces only a hyperplastic state while the acquisition of additional abnormalities is required for true malignancy. Activation of telomerase and survival pathways, inactivation of cell cycle checkpoints, and increased motility all contribute to the malignant phenotype (Hahn et al., 1999).

Trk is a receptor tyrosine kinase that was originally described as a transforming oncogene in colon cancer. The Trks are a family of neurotrophin receptors that are essential for the normal development and function of multiple tissues. These receptors are also activated in a broad range of cancers, where they modulate tumor growth and motility. In this chapter we will review how Trks function as critical determinants of the cancer phenotype. We will begin with a discussion of how Trks link to intracellular signaling pathways. Then we will describe the data implicating Trks as oncogenes and regulators of cancer growth and movement. Finally we will examine the efforts to develop pharmacological agents for the treatment of patients with Trk-expressing cancers.

2. TRK SIGNALING

The Trk family of receptor tyrosine kinases consists of three members- TrkA, TrkB and TrkC. These distinct gene products are single-pass transmembrane proteins that share more than 75% homology in the kinase domain, and 30-40% homology in the extracellular and transmembrane domains (Tsoulfas et al., 1993). Each Trk serves as the primary receptor for one or more neurotrophin ligands (Lamballe et al., 1991a). TrkA preferentially binds NGF (Kaplan et al., 1991; Klein et al., 1991) TrkB binds BDNF and NT4 (Squinto et al., 1991) while TrkC binds NT3 (Lamballe et al., 1991b). Given the homology between Trks, it is not surprising that there is considerable overlap in their downstream signaling activities (rev. (Kaplan and Miller, 2000; Sofroniew et al., 2001). Following ligand binding, Trks dimerize, and become catalytically active as kinases (Jing et al., 1992). All signaling events downstream of Trks are dependent upon the activation of this tyrosine kinase activity. The dimerization of the Trk kinase leads to phosphorylation of five tyrosines within the cytoplasmic domain. Three of these are in the activation loop itself, and are required for catalytic activity (Cunningham et al., 1997; Martin-Zanca et al., 1989; Segal et al., 1996). These same tyrosines additionally serve as binding sites for signal adapter proteins SH2-b and rAPS

(Qian et al., 1998). Phosphorylation of these activation loop tyrosines and thus Trk kinase activity is tightly regulated by phosphatases, such as PTP1B that have a predilection for double phospho-tyrosine sites (Zabolotny et al., 2002) like those found in this loop.

In addition to the activation loop tyrosines, the Trk intracellular domain contains two other tyrosine residues known to be phosphorylated in response to ligand binding (Loeb et al., 1994; Middlemas et al., 1994; Stephens et al., 1994). This is in contrast to the PDGF receptor where at least nine tyrosines can be phosphorylated and function in signaling (Bernard and Kazlauskas, 1999). One of these two Trk tyrosines is part of an NPXY motif that functions in binding either Frs or Shc family members (Meakin et al., 1999; Stephens et al., 1994). Intriguingly competition for binding to this site may be important in generating the differential biological responses to different neurotrophins (Meakin et al., 1999; Nakamura et al., 2002). The remaining tyrosine, Y785, is present in the carboxyterminal YILDG sequence and functions in the binding of phospholipase C-gamma (Obermeier et al., 1993a; Vetter et al., 1991).

Autophosphorylation of receptor kinases provides binding sites for linker proteins and enzymes that propagate signals for growth, survival or differentiation. Many of these signaling molecules are common to all receptor tyrosine kinases. Distinction between the receptor kinases may be determined by the extent and duration of stimulation of individual pathways, the combination of pathways activated, and the intracellular location of activated receptors. Four major pathways known to be stimulated by Trk receptors are the PI3 kinase pathway, phospholipase C- gamma, and two MAP kinase pathways- the classic Erk1/2 pathway, and the more recently understood big MAP kinase pathway- involving Erk5. The mechanisms by which these pathways are stimulated by Trk activation are reviewed below (Figure 1).

2.1 PI3 kinase

Like the insulin receptor family, Trks are very strong activators of PI3 kinases. This may reflect the ability of Trk to activate PI3 kinase via several different pathways. While the regulatory subunit was initially thought to bind directly to Trk (Obermeier et al., 1993b), more recent work indicates that the activation is more indirect. Phosphorylation at the NPXY motif leads to the phosphorylation and activation of Shc/grb2 and Gab1/2. Both Grb2 and Gab can serve as general docking sites for the regulatory subunit of PI3 kinase (Wang et al., 1995). These interactions activate the enzyme and promote its access to phospholipid substrates. Grb2 also interacts with the G-protein exchange factor, SOS, which leads to the activation of the small G-protein Ras. Activated Ras is able to directly stimulate PI3 kinase through interaction with its regulatory domain. Additionally PI3 kinase is activated downstream of Y785 phosphorylation (see below).

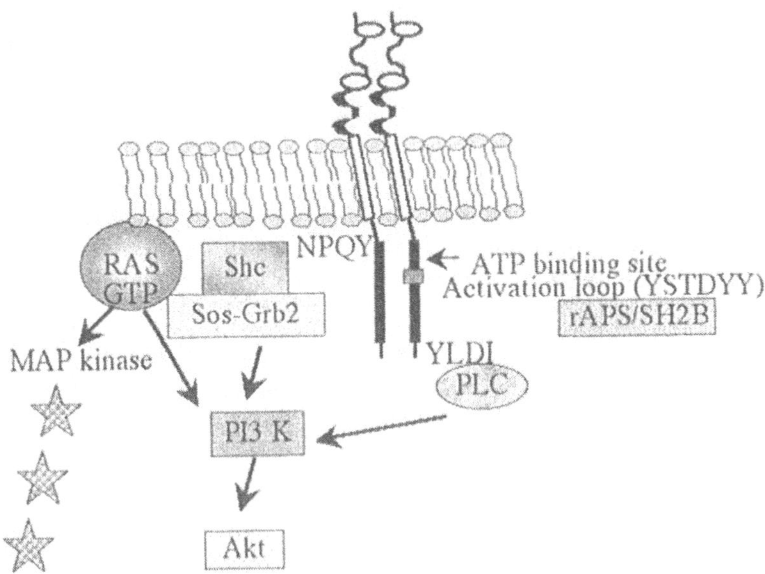

Figure 1: Trk Signaling. Trks are single transmembrane glycoproteins. Following ligand binding, the Trks dimerize, and phosphorylate their partners in trans. Phosphorylation creates binding sites for several proteins, including FRS2 or Shc, and Phospholipase C (PLC). Shc of Frs can link to the small G-protein Ras, leading to activation of the MAP kinase pathway. In addition, PI3 kinase, and the downstream protein kinase Akt/Protein kinase B, are activated by multiple pathways downstream of Trks.

PI3 kinase activity is critical for the strong pro-survival, anti-apoptotic actions of the Trk receptors (Yao and Cooper, 1995). This reflects in large part the fact that Akt/protein kinase B is potently stimulated by the lipid products of PI3 kinase (Burgering and Coffer, 1995; Dudek et al., 1997). Thus, increased PI3 kinase activity results in increased activation of Akt. Akt in turn phosphorylates and regulates a large number of substrates including the pro-apoptotic factor Bad (Datta et al., 1997), and forkhead transcription factors (Brunet et al., 1999). These substrates regulate both transcription independent, and transcription dependent increases in survival (Brunet et al., 2001). The importance of PI3 kinase pathways for promoting the unwanted survival of cancer cells is made manifest by the ability of mutations in the PI3 lipid phosphatase, PTEN, to result in tumors including brain, breast and prostate carcinomas (rev. (Di Cristofano and Pandolfi, 2000; Maehama and Dixon, 1999).

2.2 PLC-γ

Phospholipase C- γ binds directly to Trk receptors, where it is phosphorylated by the receptor kinase (Obermeier et al., 1993a; Vetter et al., 1991). The catalytically active, receptor bound form of this enzyme constitutes the most direct signaling event of Trk activation. The short pathway from Trk to PLC- γ allows this to be a very early response to Trk activation (Choi et al., 2001; Widmer et al., 1993). PLC- γ generates DAG and IP3. The IP3 lipids bind to specific receptors on internal membranes, releasing calcium from intracellular stores (Berridge, 1993). The increase in intracellular calcium together with the second messenger DAG, promotes a variety of protein kinase C activities, as well as indirectly activating PI3 kinase and MAP kinase. Thus, in developing neurons, this pathway contributes to both differentiation and survival.

2.3 MAP kinase

Many receptor tyrosine kinases stimulate proliferation by activating a kinase cascade that culminates in the activation of the MAP kinases Erk1 and 2 (rev. (Pearson et al., 2001). Like EGF-R, PDGF-R and FGF-Rs, Trks stimulate MAP kinase, by activation of the small G-protein Ras. This leads to the sequential activation of a Raf family member, Mek1/2 and finally Erk1/2. Recent studies have also identified a second MAP kinase pathway that is activated by Trks (Cavanaugh et al., 2001; Kamakura et al., 1999) (Watson et al., 2001). Like the classic MAP kinase pathway, the big MAP kinase or Erk5 pathway, remains active for a prolonged period of time following Trk stimulation (Cavanaugh et al., 2001). In response to activation both Erk1/2 and Erk5 can translocate to the nucleus (Traverse et al., 1992; Watson et al., 2001), where directly and/or indirectly they stimulate diverse transcription factors. CREB, SRF, and Elk are among the factors stimulated by Erk1/2 (Bonni et al., 1999; Gille et al., 1995). Erk5 stimulates a partially overlapping group of factors including CREB and MEF2 (Cavanaugh et al., 2001; Watson et al., 2001). Surprisingly, while the MAP kinase pathway is generally credited with stimulating proliferation, in the case of Trk signaling this does not appear to be its normal role. Instead, during neuronal development, Trk activation of Erks promotes increased differentiation and survival. This may be due in part to the sustained activation of Erks by Trks (Qiu and Green, 1992; Traverse et al., 1992) (Marshall, 1995) and the transcription of anti-apoptotic bcl family members (Bonni et al., 1999; Riccio et al., 1999).

2.4 Endocytosis and Termination of signal

Most receptor tyrosine kinases are rapidly endocytosed following ligand binding. This was initially thought to be the first step in terminating the signal, and in the downregulation of receptor. However, it has recently been appreciated that endocytosis is instead an intrinsic part of receptor signaling (McPherson et al., 2001). In the case of Trk receptors, endocytosis attenuates PI3 kinase activity but increases activation of the Erks (Howe et al., 2001; York et al., 2000; Zhang et al.,

2000). Thus Trks that fail to be endocytosed are potent stimulators of PI3 kinase-dependent survival.

2.5 Trk signaling and cancer

Which aspects of Trk signaling are most relevant for tumor biology? Activation of the receptor tyrosine kinase and its subcellular localization determine the effects of Trk signaling. Tumors are known to co-opt the activation of the receptor kinase in several different ways. Oncogenic fusion proteins containing the Trk kinase domain and sequences that promote oligomerization are present in several different cancers. These fusion proteins possess ligand-independent, constitutively active kinases that promote dysregulated tumor growth. In other instances tumor cells make both the neurotrophin ligand and Trk receptor thus generating an autocrine loop for kinase activation. This allows for a non-regulated survival signal that is only poorly amenable to changes in the environment. Trks in tumors can also be activated in a paracrine fashion by ligands produced by the normal surrounding tissue. Finally, abnormal receptor trafficking may be present in tumors and this could alter the normal balance between Trk activation of survival, differentiation and proliferative pathways. Regardless of the precise mechanism for abnormal activation of Trks, interventions that poisoned the kinase might be an efficacious means of therapy in Trk-responsive cancers.

3. TRK AS AN ONCOGENE

Trk was originally identified by Mariano Barbacid in a screen designed to identify oncogenes that contribute to cancer (Martin-Zanca et al., 1986). He created a library from a human colon cancer cell line, and screened the resultant clones for the ability to transform a fibroblastic cell line. One of the clones identified in this oncogene screen contained tropomyosin sequences fused to a novel tyrosine kinase domain which Barbacid designated Trk, for tropomyosin related kinase (Martin-Zanca et al., 1989). The tropomyosin sequences allowed for unregulated oligomerization of the fusion protein and consequent constitutive activation of the kinase domain. Consistent with this initial view of Trks as oncogenes, Barbacid and colleagues subsequently demonstrated that fibroblasts undergo transformation when the TrkA gene is expressed, and the cells are treated with NGF (Cordon-Cardo et al., 1991).

While the initial identification of TrkA came from a colon cancer cell line, it rapidly became apparent that Trk fusion genes were not a medically relevant cause of colon cancer. However, several examples were discovered in which Trk fusion genes caused papillary thyroid cancers (Bongarzone et al., 1989; Greco et al., 1992). Similar to the original Trk oncogene, these fusion genes contained the Trk kinase and a multimerization domain. TrkA fused to tropomyosin (TPM3), the TPR gene, or the TFG gene, have all been found in thyroid cancers, and are sufficient for transformation (Butti et al., 1995; Greco et al., 1995; Greco et al., 1997; Russell et al., 2000). The fusion proteins all create a cytoplasmic, multimeric tyrosine kinase, which is catalytically active at all times. The constitutive activation, and inappropriate localization of the TrkA kinase due to fusion proteins are most common in papillary thyroid cancers of younger patients. These fusion genes account for up to 20% of papillary thyroid cancers in distinct series of patients (Butti et al., 1995).

While TrkA is most commonly associated with thyroid cancers, TrkC has been found to be oncogenic in other cancers. In each case, fusion of a Trk kinase domain with the multimerizing domain of a distinct protein, leads to a constitutively active, cytoplasmic enzyme. Infantile congenital fibrosarcoma occurs in children younger than two years of age. This fibroblastic tumor has a surprisingly low incidence of metastases, and has a relatively good prognosis. In several of these patients a fusion between the ETV6/TEL gene and TrkC has been identified as the oncogenic event (Knezevich et al., 1998; Sheng et al., 2001). A similar fusion between ETV6/TEL and TrkC has been found in one example of AML (Eguchi et al., 1999). Thus, the kinase domain of TrkC, as well as TrkA, can become oncogenic when fused to a mutlimerizing gene. It is worth noting that cancers associated with oncogenic forms of Trk fusion proteins, papillary thyroid cancer and infantile congenital fibrosarcoma, are cancers that have relatively good prognoses.

3. TRKS AND THE REGULATION OF CANCER GROWTH

The regulation of cell number during development or in cancer growth reflects a balance of signals that promote proliferation or differentiation and survival or apoptosis. Neurotrophin activation of Trks helps to determine this balance during development and oncogenesis. Thus in cancer Trks can be helpful or hurtful biological modifiers and positive or negative prognostic indicators. Trk activities have been described in diverse cancers arising from many tissues including medullary thyroid carcinoma (McGregor et al., 1999), Wilms' tumor (Donovan et al., 1994; Eggert et al., 2001), glioblastoma multiforme (Singer et al., 1999), lung cancer (Ricci et al., 2001), pancreatic cancer (Schneider et al., 2001), melanoma (Innominato et al., 2001), leukemia (Eguchi et al., 1999), breast cancer (Descamps et al., 1998) and Ewing's sarcoma (Nogueira et al., 1997) (Table 1). A review of well described Trk activities in prostate cancer, medulloblastoma and neuroblastoma serves to demonstrate the range of effects Trks can have in cancer.

3.1 Prostate Cancer-Survival

Androgen-sensitive prostate cancer is a treatable disease because the cancer cells depend upon an androgen source for survival (Kyprianou et al., 1990). Androgen ablation and removal of the survival signal results in widespread apoptosis. Lethal, metastatic, prostate cancer is characterized by a dependence upon androgens and other factors for cancer cell survival. Androgen ablation results in the apoptosis of only the subset of cells that are androgen-dependent. The remainder of the cells, continue to survive through the actions of other survival factors. NGF acting through TrkA appears to be a critical survival factor for androgen- independent prostate cancer.

Normal prostate epithelium expresses TrkA, but neither TrkB nor TrkC. Normal prostatic stroma expresses NGF (Dalal and Djakiew, 1997; Guate et al., 1999; Pflug et al., 1995) establishing a paracrine relationship between normal stroma and epithelium. Acquisition of an abnormal autocrine Trk survival pathway is common in malignant prostate carcinoma: 60-70% of primary prostate cancers express TrkA, often at elevated levels. In addition, 60-70% of primary prostate cancers also exhibit abnormal expression of TrkB or TrkC. Increased TrkA and C expression is positively correlated with increasingly abnormal patterns of growth (Dionne et al., 1998; Guate et al., 1999). Consequently, as many as 80% of metastatic lesions express one or more Trks. These same malignant prostate cancers also synthesize and secrete neurotrophins that stimulate Trk signaling and downstream survival in an autocrine/paracrine fashion (Weeraratna et al., 2000).

In the normal prostate the role of NGF is unclear. Pharmacological inhibition of TrkA signaling in normal prostate has no effect on TrkA expressing prostate cells (Dionne et al., 1998). Thus while TrkA may mediate a survival signal in normal prostate, survival is not exclusively dependent upon this activity. In contrast, malignant prostate cancer can exhibit exclusive dependence on the Trk survival signal. In several studies utilizing different pharmacological agents, inhibition of Trk kinase activity and all downstream signaling resulted in dramatic growth inhibition and apoptosis of prostate cancer in vitro and in xenograft models of disease (Delsite and Djakiew, 1996; Dionne et al., 1998; George et al., 1999; Weeraratna et al., 2001). Thus prostate cancer, through the acquisition of an autocrine/paracrine neurotrophin survival signal develops a survival advantage. Clinical experience in treating androgen-independent prostate cancer suggests that this renders it relatively resistant to apoptosis inducing agents such as chemotherapy.

3.2 Medulloblastoma-Apoptosis

Neurotrophins are best known for their role in the development and functioning of the nervous system. Among the model systems that have helped illuminate the diverse functions of neurotrophins is the cerebellum. Here neurotrophins are known to regulate differentiation, apoptosis and migration of neuronal precursor cells and modulate synaptogenesis and synaptic functioning. Some of these roles are recapitulated in a tumor of cerebellar granule cells, medulloblastoma (Eberhart et al., 2001). The role of Trks in medulloblastoma first became apparent when a clear correlation between increased levels of TrkC expression and patient survival was established (Segal et al., 1994). In addition to TrkC, some medulloblastoma tumors also express TrkA and TrkB as well as NGF, BDNF and NT3 (Tajima et al., 1998). Anatomical co-localization of neurotrophin ligands and receptors does occur and suggests that autocrine/paracrine loops can exist in the case of BDNF/TrkB and NT3/TRkC (Tajima et al., 1998; Washiyama et al., 1996).

All medulloblastomas appear to express TrkC but only those with high levels of expression possess favorable biological behavior (Grotzer et al., 2000; Pomeroy et al., 2002; Segal et al., 1994). This appears to be the result of the TrkC transduction of differentiation and pro-apoptotic NT3 signals (Kim et al., 1999). In addition the co-localization of NT3 and TrkC with markers of differentiation such as neurofilament suggest that NT3 may induce neuronal differentiation of medulloblastoma (Tajima et al., 1998).

Table 1. TRK activation in human cancer.

Diagnosis	*Neurotrophin Expression*	*Trk Expression*	*Correlation with prognosis*	*Evidence for function*
Oncogenic Fusion Proteins				
Papillary Thyroid Ca		TrkA-TPM3,TPR, TFG		(Martin-Zanca et al., 1989)
Infantile Fibrosarcoma		TrkC-ETV6/TEL		(Wai et al., 2000)
AML		TrkC-ETV6/TEL		
Trk Receptors				
Prostate Cancer	NGF and/or BDNF and/or NT3	TrkA and/or TrkB, and/or TrkC	worse prognosis	(Dionne et al., 1998) (Weeraratna et al., 2000)
Medulloblastoma	NGF and/or BDNF and/or NT3	TrkA and/or TrkB and/or TrkC	better prognosis	(Kim et al., 1999) (Grotzer et al., 2000)
Neuroblastoma	BDNF	TrkA TrkB TrkC	better prognosis worse prognosis better prognosis	(Matsushima and Bogenmann, 1993) (Middlemas et al., 1999) (Yamashiro et al., 1997)
Malignant Melanoma	NGF and/or BDNF and/or NT3	TrkB	worse prognosis	
Pancreatic Cancer	BDNF and/or NT3	TrkA and/or TrkB and/or TrkC	worse prognosis	(Sakamoto et al., 2001) (Miknyoczki et al., 1999)
Medullary Thyroid Ca		TrkB TrkC	hyperplasia worse prognosis	(McGregor et al., 1999)
Wilms' Tumor	BDNF	TrkA and/or TrkB and/or TrkC	TrkB a/w better outcome Co-expression of BDNF and TrkB a/w worse outcome	
Breast Cancer	NGF	TrkA		
PNET		TrkA and/or TrkB and/or TrkC	TrkA a/w differentiated tumors TrkB & TrkC a/w undifferentiated tumors	

The relationship between Trk signaling and the regulation of apoptosis in medulloblastoma is further supported by in vitro work with medulloblastoma cell lines engineered to express TrkA. In the absence of TrkA expression NGF has no effect on the survival of these cell lines. However, when TrkA is introduced, NGF induces apoptosis of transfected cells in a cell-cycle dependent manner (Muragaki et al., 1997). This effect is dependent upon receptor auto-phosphorylation and may involve the activation of a novel Ras and/or Raf signaling pathway (Chou et al., 2000). Thus medulloblastoma behavior can be regulated by Trk mediated differentiation and apoptotic signals. The positive effect of Trk expression in medulloblastoma is in stark contrast to the negative effect of Trk expression seen in prostate cancer.

3.3 Neuroblastoma-Survival, Differentiation and Apoptosis

The pleiotrophic nature of neurotrophin signaling in cancer is most clearly evident in neuroblastoma. Neuroblastoma arises from a neural crest lineage that is destined for adrenal medullary or sympathetic neuron differentiation. Differentiation of this lineage is regulated by neurotrophins during development, and neuroblastoma continues to exhibit significant responsiveness to neurotrophin modulation of survival and differentiation. Prognosis in neuroblastoma can be closely correlated with a number of negative biological markers including, amplification of n-myc (Brodeur et al., 1984), near diploid or tetraploid DNA (Look et al., 1991), deletion of chromosome 1p (Caron et al., 1996) and gain of chromosome 17q (Bown et al., 1999). Conversely, a strong positive biological marker associated with good prognosis is expression of TrkA (Azar et al., 1994; Brodeur et al., 1997b; Matsunaga et al., 1998; Nakagawara et al., 1993; Tanaka et al., 1998). Furthermore, expression of TrkC (Svensson et al., 1997; Yamashiro et al., 1997) and truncated forms of TrkB (Brodeur et al., 1997b) are also associated with a good prognosis. In contrast, full length TrkB (Brodeur et al., 1997b) (Nakagawara et al., 1994) or truncated TrkC (Svensson et al., 1997) are associated with a poor outcome.

The effects of neurotrophins and Trks in neuroblastoma have been extensively studied in primary cultures and transfected neuroblastoma cell lines. The clinical correlation between Trk expression and neuroblastoma biology is consistent with their observed in vitro actions. Primary cultures of neuroblastoma derived from low stage disease were induced to differentiate in response to NGF or NT3. Differentiation was accompanied by increased survival and decreased proliferation, and correlated with the level of TrkA expression (Svensson et al., 1997). These same cells did not respond to BDNF. Thus high levels of TrkA or C expression may have a positive impact on clinical outcome through the mediation of survival and differentiation signals.

Transfection of TrkA (Lavenius et al., 1995; Lucarelli et al., 1997; Matsushima and Bogenmann, 1993; Nakagawara and Brodeur, 1997) and TrkC (Yamashiro et al., 1997) into neuroblastoma cell lines further supports a role for Trks in growth inhibition through enhanced induction of differentiation. Similarly, NGF treatment of PC12 cells is a potent stimulus for differentiation whose effect is correlated with decreased proliferation (Greene and Kaplan, 1995). For these tumors, differentiation towards a neuronal phenotype is correlated with a strong anti-proliferative effect.

The relative importance of different downstream events to TrkA induced survival and differentiation has been studied in neuroblastoma cell lines engineered to express high levels of TrkA. The growth inhibitory effect of TrkA expression appeared to be dependent upon the activation of PLC-γ through the phosphorylation of TrkA tyrosine 785. The differentiating effects of TrkA exhibited both Ras-dependent and Ras-independent components but were not dependent upon PI3-kinase activation (Eggert et al., 2000a)

It would thus appear that in neuroblastoma, the differentiating effect of Trks is a greater determinant of their net effect on growth than their activity as a survival factor. This is in contrast to the situation in prostate cancer where survival is not accompanied by differentiating activity. Therefore, the net result of neurotrophin action in neuroblastoma is the promotion of tumor growth through enhanced survival and proliferation.

While TrkB expression in neuroblastoma correlates with poor prognosis it is not clear whether or nor TrkB is an independent, negative biological modifier in neuroblastoma. TrkB expression is associated with other negative biological modifiers such as n-myc amplification (Brodeur et al., 1997a; Nakagawara et al., 1994). In vitro studies however, have demonstrated that TrkB activation can protect cells from apoptotic responses to DNA damage following chemotherapy or gamma radiation (Middlemas et al., 1999a; Middlemas et al., 1999b). In addition, transfection of neuroblastoma cell lines with TrkB can increase their growth rate (Eggert et al., 2000b) and invasiveness (Matsumoto et al., 1995). Overall, these in vitro studies suggest a possible independent role for TrkB in the determination of advanced stage neuroblastoma behavior as a survival stimulus (Sugimoto et al., 2001). Unlike NGF, BDNF is frequently expressed by neuroblastomas with unfavorable biology. Thus autocrine/paracrine stimulation of proliferative and anti-apoptotic responses may occur in these poor prognosis tumors.

3.4 Summary

Tumor growth and progression reflects a balance among signals that regulate proliferation, differentiation and survival. Neurotrophins, acting through Trks are key regulators of differentiation and survival during development and thereby contribute to the normal regulation of tissue growth. Trks as part of autocrine/paracrine neurotrophin loops or independently, maintain these signaling properties in a wide range of tumor types and consequently can function to regulate tumor growth in either positive, or negative ways.

4. TRKS AND METASTATIC DISEASE

During development of the nervous system neurotrophins can regulate the migration of neuronal precursor cells through the activation of high affinity Trk receptors. NGF activation of TrkA appears to be important for the motility of embryonic spinal cord neuroblasts (Behar et al., 1994a; Behar et al., 1994b) and during cerebellar development TrkB activation by BDNF increases the motogenicitiy of and serves as a chemotactic factor for granule cell precursors (Borghesani et al., 2002). In addition microglia (Gilad and Gilad, 1995) and macrophages (Kobayashi and Mizisin, 2001) exhibit chemotactic responses to NGF and NGF or NT3 respectively.

Neurotrophins also induce the migration of cancer cells by activating Trks and by activating a second receptor, a member of the Fas receptor family, p75NTR. The activation of p75 appears to be important in the invasiveness of melanoma through the upregulation of secreted heparanase and the degradation of extracellular matrix (Herrmann et al., 1993; Innominato et al., 2001; Marchetti et al., 1996; Marchetti et al., 1993; Marchetti and Nicolson, 1997). This activity may be essential for the development of CNS metastatic lesions in melanoma (Menter et al., 1994; Menter et al., 1995).

In a similar fashion, activation of Trks has been suggested to play an important role in the perineural invasiveness of pancreatic cancer. Normal pancreatic islet and ductal cells express TrkA and TrkC (Sakamoto et al., 2001). Increased expression of Trks was associated with increased tumor size and perineural invasion (Sakamoto et al., 2001). In addition dose dependent movement of tumor cells in response to BDNF and NT3 could be demonstrated in vitro (Miknyoczki et al., 1999c). That this was mediated through Trks and important to tumor cell movement was established by inhibition of xenograft invasiveness with an inhibitor of Trk tyrosine kinase CEP-701 (Miknyoczki et al., 1999a; Miknyoczki et al., 1999b). Thus tumor cell expression of Trks could increase the baseline motor activity of cancer cells, making them more responsive to migratory cues from normal sources of neurotrophins, such as nervous tissue.

5. TRKS AS THERAPEUTIC TARGETS

All Trk mediated events commence with the activation of the Trk tyrosine kinase. Therefore blocking this enzymatic activity could inhibit all Trk responses. This could be of great advantage in the treatment of malignant prostate cancer or advanced stage neuroblastoma. Several drugs are known to inhibit Trk kinase activity. The family of indolocarbazoles, including the naturally occurring parent compound K252a (Koizumi et al., 1988) and its synthetic analogues CEP-701, CEP-751 (Camoratto et al., 1997) and CEP-2563 (Ruggeri et al., 1999) are competitive antagonists for ATP binding and function as inhibitors of protein kinase C, Trk, Flk 1 and PDGFR receptor kinases (George et al., 1999). In addition monoamine-activated α 2-macroglobulin functions as a pan-Trk inhibitor (Hu and Koo, 1998; Koo et al., 1994) and endocannabinoids (Melck et al., 2000) can promote the downregulation of TrkA and thus decrease its activity.

In vitro studies with these inhibitory compounds demonstrate that blockade of the Trk kinase can decrease the growth rate of tumor cells (Delsite and Djakiew, 1996). Xenograft models of prostate (George et al., 1999; Weeraratna et al., 2001) and pancreatic cancer (Miknyoczki et al., 1999a) and neuroblastoma (Evans et al., 2001) suggest that Trk inhibition can both increase the rate of apoptosis and decrease metastatic spread. These studies not only confirm the importance of Trk signaling in cancer growth and spread but also suggest that inhibition of Trk activity is a viable candidate therapeutic target. A phase I clinical trial of CEP-2563 has been conducted and indicates that the drug was well tolerated (Bhargava et al., 1998). A phase II study to examine efficacy is planned.

6. CONCLUSIONS

Trk signaling is of widespread importance during development as it regulates the differentiation, survival and migration of multiple cell types. Similar functions for Trks can be found in a wide variety of cancers. These activities not only determine the biology of these cancers but also offer a potentially unique target for the control of cancer cell growth and motility through the inhibition of the Trk kinase.

7. ACKNOWLEDGEMENTS

This work was supported by grants from the NIH (NS37757 to R. A. S. and HD 01393 to J. B. R.), Barr Program to R.A.S.

Joshua B. Rubin & Rosalind A. Segal
Department of Pediatric Oncology
Dana Farber Cancer Institute
Department of Neurobiology
Harvard Medical School
Boston, Massachusetts

8. REFERENCES

Azar, C. G., Scavarda, N. J., Nakagawara, A. and Brodeur, G. M. (1994). Expression and function of the nerve growth factor receptor (TRK-A) in human neuroblastoma cell lines. *Prog Clin Biol Res* 385, 169-75.

Behar, T. N., Schaffner, A. E., Colton, C. A., Somogyi, R., Olah, Z., Lehel, C. and Barker, J. L. (1994a). GABA-induced chemokinesis and NGF-induced chemotaxis of embryonic spinal cord neurons. *J Neurosci* 14, 29-38.

Behar, T. N., Schaffner, A. E., Tran, H. T. and Barker, J. L. (1994b). Correlation of gp140trk expression and NGF-induced neuroblast chemotaxis in the embryonic rat spinal cord. *Brain Res* 664, 155-66.

Bernard, A. and Kazlauskas, A. (1999). Phosphospecific antibodies reveal temporal regulation of platelet- derived growth factor beta receptor signaling. *Exp Cell Res* 253, 704-12.

Berridge, M. (1993). Inositol triphosphate and calcium signaling. *Nature* 361, 315-325.

Bhargava, P., Marcshall, J., Dahut, W., Rizvi, N., Dordal, E., Samara, E., El-Shoubagy, T., Ness, E., Bischoff, J. and Hawkins, M. (1998). Phase I study of CEP-2563 dihydrochloride in patients with advanced cancer. *Annal of Oncology* 9, A424.

Bongarzone, I., Pierotti, M. A., Monzini, N., Mondellini, P., Manenti, G., Donghi, R., Pilotti, S., Grieco, M., Santoro, M., Fusco, A. et al. (1989). High frequency of activation of tyrosine kinase oncogenes in human papillary thyroid carcinoma. *Oncogene* 4, 1457-62.

Bonni, A., Brunet, A., West, A., Datta, S., Takasu, M. and Greenberg, M. (1999). Cell survival promoted by the Ras-MAPK signaling pathway by transcription-dependent and -independent mechanisms. *Science* 286, 1358-62.

Borghesani, P. R., Peyrin, J. M., Klein, R., Rubin, J., Carter, A. R., Schwartz, P. M., Luster, A., Corfas, G. and Segal, R. A. (2002). BDNF stimulates migration of cerebellar granule cells. *Development* 129, 1435-42.

Bown, N., Cotterill, S., Lastowska, M., O'Neill, S., Pearson, A. D., Plantaz, D., Meddeb, M., Danglot, G., Brinkschmidt, C., Christiansen, H. et al. (1999). Gain of chromosome arm 17q and adverse outcome in patients with neuroblastoma. *N Engl J Med* 340, 1954-61.

Brodeur, G. M., Maris, J. M., Yamashiro, D. J., Hogarty, M. D. and White, P. S. (1997a). Biology and genetics of human neuroblastomas. *J Pediatr Hematol Oncol* 19, 93-101.

Brodeur, G. M., Nakagawara, A., Yamashiro, D. J., Ikegaki, N., Liu, X. G., Azar, C. G., Lee, C. P. and Evans, A. E. (1997b). Expression of TrkA, TrkB and TrkC in human neuroblastomas. *J Neurooncol* 31, 49-55.
Brodeur, G. M., Seeger, R. C., Schwab, M., Varmus, H. E. and Bishop, J. M. (1984). Amplification of N-myc in untreated human neuroblastomas correlates with advanced disease stage. *Science* 224, 1121-4.
Brunet, A., Bonni, A., Zigmond, M. J., Lin, M. Z., Juo, P., Hu, L. S., Anderson, M. J., Arden, K. C., Blenis, J. and Greenberg, M. E. (1999). Akt promotes cell survival by phosphorylating and inhibiting a Forkhead transcription factor. *Cell* 96, 857-68.
Brunet, A., Datta, S. R. and Greenberg, M. E. (2001). Transcription-dependent and -independent control of neuronal survival by the PI3K-Akt signaling pathway. *Curr Opin Neurobiol* 11, 297-305.
Burgering, B. and Coffer, P. (1995). Protein kinase B (Akt) in phosphatidylinositol-3-OH kinase signal transduction. *Nature* 376, 599-602.
Butti, M. G., Bongarzone, I., Ferraresi, G., Mondellini, P., Borrello, M. G. and Pierotti, M. A. (1995). A sequence analysis of the genomic regions involved in the rearrangements between TPM3 and NTRK1 genes producing TRK oncogenes in papillary thyroid carcinomas. *Genomics* 28, 15-24.
Camoratto, A. M., Jani, J. P., Angeles, T. S., Maroney, A. C., Sanders, C. Y., Murakata, C., Neff, N. T., Vaught, J. L., Isaacs, J. T. and Dionne, C. A. (1997). CEP-751 inhibits TRK receptor tyrosine kinase activity in vitro OFF exhibits anti-tumor activity. *Int J Cancer* 72, 673-9.
Caron, H., van Sluis, P., de Kraker, J., Bokkerink, J., Egeler, M., Laureys, G., Slater, R., Westerveld, A., Voute, P. A. and Versteeg, R. (1996). Allelic loss of chromosome 1p as a predictor of unfavorable outcome in patients with neuroblastoma. *N Engl J Med* 334, 225-30.
Cavanaugh, J. E., Ham, J., Hetman, M., Poser, S., Yan, C. and Xia, Z. (2001). Differential Regulation of Mitogen-Activated Protein Kinases ERK1/2 and ERK5 by Neurotrophins, Neuronal Activity, and cAMP in Neurons. *J Neurosci* 21, 434-443.
Choi, D. Y., Toledo-Aral, J. J., Segal, R. and Halegoua, S. (2001). Sustained signaling by phospholipase C-gamma mediates nerve growth factor-triggered gene expression. *Mol Cell Biol* 21, 2695-705.
Chou, T. T., Trojanowski, J. Q. and Lee, V. M. (2000). A novel apoptotic pathway induced by nerve growth factor-mediated TrkA activation in medulloblastoma. *J Biol Chem* 275, 565-70.
Cordon-Cardo, C., Tapley, P., Jing, S., Nanduri, V., O'Rourke, E., Lamballe, F., Kovary, K., Klein, R., Jones, K. R., Reichardt, L. F. et al. (1991). The trk tyrosine protein kinase mediates the mitogenic properties of nerve growth factor and NT3. *Cell* 66, 173-183.
Cunningham, M. E., Stephens, R. M., Kaplan, D. R. and Greene, L. A. (1997). Autophosphorylation of activation loop tyrosines regulates signaling by the TRK nerve growth factor receptor. *J Biol Chem* 272, 10957-67.
Dalal, R. and Djakiew, D. (1997). Molecular characterization of neurotrophin expression and the corresponding tropomyosin receptor kinases (trks) in epithelial and stromal cells of the human prostate. *Mol Cell Endocrinol* 134, 15-22.
Datta, S. R., Dudek, H., Tao, X., Masters, S., Fu, H., Gotoh, Y. and Greenberg, M. E. (1997). Akt phosphorylation of BAD couples survival signals to the cell- intrinsic death machinery. *Cell* 91, 231-41.
Delsite, R. and Djakiew, D. (1996). Anti-proliferative effect of the kinase inhibitor K252a on human prostatic carcinoma cell lines. *J Androl* 17, 481-90.
Descamps, S., Lebourhis, X., Delehedde, M., Boilly, B. and Hondermarck, H. (1998). Nerve growth factor is mitogenic for cancerous but not normal human breast epithelial cells. *J Biol Chem* 273, 16659-62.
Di Cristofano, A. and Pandolfi, P. P. (2000). The multiple roles of PTEN in tumor suppression. *Cell* 100, 387-90.
Dionne, C. A., Camoratto, A. M., Jani, J. P., Emerson, E., Neff, N., Vaught, J. L., Murakata, C., Djakiew, D., Lamb, J., Bova, S. et al. (1998). Cell cycle-independent death of prostate adenocarcinoma is induced by the trk tyrosine kinase inhibitor CEP-751 (KT6587). *Clin Cancer Res* 4, 1887-98.
Donovan, M. J., Hempstead, B., Huber, L. J., Kaplan, D., Tsoulfas, P., Chao, M., Parada, L. and Schofield, D. (1994). Identification of the neurotrophin receptors p75 and trk in a series of Wilms' tumors. *Am J Pathol* 145, 792-801.
Dudek, H., Datta, S. R., Franke, T. F., Birnbaum, M. J., Yao, R., Cooper, G. M., Segal, R. A., Kaplan, D. R. and Greenberg, M. E. (1997). Regulation of neuronal survival by the serine-threonine protein kinase Akt [see comments]. *Science* 275, 661-5.

Eberhart, C. G., Kaufman, W. E., Tihan, T. and Burger, P. C. (2001). Apoptosis, neuronal maturation, and neurotrophin expression within medulloblastoma nodules. *J Neuropathol Exp Neurol* 60, 462-9.

Eggert, A., Grotzer, M. A., Zhao, H., Brodeur, G. M. and Evans, A. E. (2001). [Expression of the neurotrophin-receptor TrkB predicts outcome in nephroblastomas: results of a pilot-study]. *Klin Padiatr* 213, 191-6.

Eggert, A., Ikegaki, N., Liu, X., Chou, T. T., Lee, V. M., Trojanowski, J. Q. and Brodeur, G. M. (2000a). Molecular dissection of TrkA signal transduction pathways mediating differentiation in human neuroblastoma cells. *Oncogene* 19, 2043-51.

Eggert, A., Ikegaki, N., Liu, X. G. and Brodeur, G. M. (2000b). Prognostic and biological role of neurotrophin-receptor TrkA and TrkB in neuroblastoma. *Klin Padiatr* 212, 200-5.

Eguchi, M., Eguchi-Ishimae, M., Tojo, A., Morishita, K., Suzuki, K., Sato, Y., Kudoh, S., Tanaka, K., Setoyama, M., Nagamura, F. et al. (1999). Fusion of ETV6 to neurotrophin-3 receptor TRKC in acute myeloid leukemia with t(12;15)(p13;q25). *Blood* 93, 1355-63.

Evans, A. E., Kisselbach, K. D., Liu, X., Eggert, A., Ikegaki, N., Camoratto, A. M., Dionne, C. and Brodeur, G. M. (2001). Effect of CEP-751 (KT-6587) on neuroblastoma xenografts expressing TrkB. *Med Pediatr Oncol* 36, 181-4.

George, D. J., Dionne, C. A., Jani, J., Angeles, T., Murakata, C., Lamb, J. and Isaacs, J. T. (1999). Sustained in vivo regression of Dunning H rat prostate cancers treated with combinations of androgen ablation and Trk tyrosine kinase inhibitors, CEP-751 (KT-6587) or CEP-701 (KT-5555). *Cancer Res* 59, 2395-401.

Gilad, G. M. and Gilad, V. H. (1995). Chemotaxis and accumulation of nerve growth factor by microglia and macrophages. *J Neurosci Res* 41, 594-602.

Gille, H., Kortenjann, M., Thomae, O., Moomaw, C., Slaughter, C., Cobb, M. H. and Shaw, P. E. (1995). ERK phosphorylation potentiates Elk-1-mediated ternary complex formation and transactivation. *Embo J* 14, 951-62.

Greco, A., Mariani, C., Miranda, C., Lupas, A., Pagliardini, S., Pomati, M. and Pierotti, M. A. (1995). The DNA rearrangement that generates the TRK-T3 oncogene involves a novel gene on chromosome 3 whose product has a potential coiled-coil domain. *Mol Cell Biol* 15, 6118-27.

Greco, A., Miranda, C., Pagliardini, S., Fusetti, L., Bongarzone, I. and Pierotti, M. A. (1997). Chromosome 1 rearrangements involving the genes TPR and NTRK1 produce structurally different thyroid-specific TRK oncogenes. *Genes Chromosomes Cancer* 19, 112-23.

Greco, A., Pierotti, M. A., Bongarzone, I., Pagliardini, S., Lanzi, C. and Della Porta, G. (1992). TRK-T1 is a novel oncogene formed by the fusion of TPR and TRK genes in human papillary thyroid carcinomas. *Oncogene* 7, 237-42.

Greene, L. A. and Kaplan, D. R. (1995). Early events in neurotrophin signalling via Trk and p75 receptors. *Curr Opin Neurobiol* 5, 579-87.

Grotzer, M. A., Janss, A. J., Phillips, P. C. and Trojanowski, J. Q. (2000). Neurotrophin receptor TrkC predicts good clinical outcome in medulloblastoma and other primitive neuroectodermal brain tumors. *Klin Padiatr* 212, 196-9.

Guate, J. L., Fernandez, N., Lanzas, J. M., Escaf, S. and Vega, J. A. (1999). Expression of p75(LNGFR) and Trk neurotrophin receptors in normal and neoplastic human prostate. *BJU Int* 84, 495-502.

Hahn, W. C., Counter, C. M., Lundberg, A. S., Beijersbergen, R. L., Brooks, M. W. and Weinberg, R. A. (1999). Creation of human tumour cells with defined genetic elements. *Nature* 400, 464-8.

Herrmann, J. L., Menter, D. G., Hamada, J., Marchetti, D., Nakajima, M. and Nicolson, G. L. (1993). Mediation of NGF-stimulated extracellular matrix invasion by the human melanoma low-affinity p75 neurotrophin receptor: melanoma p75 functions independently of trkA. *Mol Biol Cell* 4, 1205-16.

Howe, C. L., Valletta, J. S., Rusnak, A. S. and Mobley, W. C. (2001). NGF Signaling from Clathrin-Coated Vesicles. Evidence that Signaling Endosomes Serve as a Platform for the Ras-MAPK Pathway. *Neuron* 32, 801-814.

Hu, Y. Q. and Koo, P. H. (1998). Inhibition of phosphorylation of TrkB and TrkC and their signal transduction by alpha2-macroglobulin. *J Neurochem* 71, 213-20.

Innominato, P. F., Libbrecht, L. and van den Oord, J. J. (2001). Expression of neurotrophins and their receptors in pigment cell lesions of the skin. *J Pathol* 194, 95-100.

Jing, S., Tapley, P. and Barbacid, M. (1992). Nerve growth factor mediates signal transduction through trk homodimer receptors. *Neuron* 9, 1067-1079.

Kamakura, S., Moriguchi, T. and Nishida, E. (1999). Activation of the protein kinase ERK5/BMK1 by receptor tyrosine kinases. Identification and characterization of a signaling pathway to the nucleus. *J Biol Chem* 274, 26563-71.

Kaplan, D. R., Hempstead, B. L., Martin-Zanca, D., Chao, M. V. and Parada, L. F. (1991). The trk proto-oncogene product : A signal transducing receptor for nerve growth factor. *Science* 252, 558-561.

Kaplan, D. R. and Miller, F. D. (2000). Neurotrophin signal transduction in the nervous system. *Curr Opin Neurobiol* 10, 381-91.

Kim, J. Y., Sutton, M. E., Lu, D. J., Cho, T. A., Goumnerova, L. C., Goritchenko, L., Kaufman, J. R., Lam, K. K., Billet, A. L., Tarbell, N. J. et al. (1999). Activation of neurotrophin-3 receptor TrkC induces apoptosis in medulloblastomas. *Cancer Res* 59, 711-9.

Klein, R., Jing, S. Q., Nanduri, V., O'Rourke, E. and Barbacid, M. (1991). The trk proto-oncogene encodes a receptor for nerve growth factor. *Cell* 65, 189-97.

Knezevich, S. R., McFadden, D. E., Tao, W., Lim, J. F. and Sorensen, P. H. (1998). A novel ETV6-NTRK3 gene fusion in congenital fibrosarcoma. *Nat Genet* 18, 184-7.

Kobayashi, H. and Mizisin, A. P. (2001). Nerve growth factor and neurotrophin-3 promote chemotaxis of mouse macrophages in vitro. *Neurosci Lett* 305, 157-60.

Koizumi, S., Contreras, M. L., Matsuda, Y., Hama, T., Lazarovici, P. and Guroff, G. (1988). K-252a: a specific inhibitor of the action of nerve growth factor on PC 12 cells. *J Neurosci* 8, 715-21.

Koo, P. H., Liebl, D. J., Qiu, W. S., Hu, Y. Q. and Dluzen, D. E. (1994). Monoamine-activated alpha 2-macroglobulin inhibits neurite outgrowth, survival, choline acetyltransferase, and dopamine concentration of neurons by blocking neurotrophin-receptor (trk) phosphorylation and signal transduction. *Ann N Y Acad Sci* 737, 460-4.

Kyprianou, N., English, H. F. and Isaacs, J. T. (1990). Programmed cell death during regression of PC-82 human prostate cancer following androgen ablation. *Cancer Res* 50, 3748-53.

Lamballe, F., Klein, R. and Barbacid, M. (1991a). The trk family of oncogenes and neurotrophin receptors. *Princess Takamatsu Symp* 22, 153-70.

Lamballe, F., Klein, R. and Barbacid, M. (1991b). TrkC, a new member of the trk family of tyrosine protein kinases, is a receptor for neurotrophin 3. *Cell* 66, 967-979.

Lavenius, E., Gestblom, C., Johansson, I., Nanberg, E. and Pahlman, S. (1995). Transfection of TRK-A into human neuroblastoma cells restores their ability to differentiate in response to nerve growth factor. *Cell Growth Differ* 6, 727-36.

Loeb, D. M., Stephens, R. M., Copeland, T., Kaplan, D. R. and Greene, L. A. (1994). A Trk nerve growth factor (NGF) receptor point mutation affecting interaction with phospholipase C-gamma 1 abolishes NGF-promoted peripherin induction but not neurite outgrowth. *J Biol Chem* 269, 8901-10.

Look, A. T., Hayes, F. A., Shuster, J. J., Douglass, E. C., Castleberry, R. P., Bowman, L. C., Smith, E. I. and Brodeur, G. M. (1991). Clinical relevance of tumor cell ploidy and N-myc gene amplification in childhood neuroblastoma: a Pediatric Oncology Group study. *J Clin Oncol* 9, 581-91.

Lucarelli, E., Kaplan, D. and Thiele, C. J. (1997). Activation of trk-A but not trk-B signal transduction pathway inhibits growth of neuroblastoma cells. *Eur J Cancer* 33, 2068-70.

Maehama, T. and Dixon, J. E. (1999). PTEN: a tumour suppressor that functions as a phospholipid phosphatase. *Trends Cell Biol* 9, 125-8.

Marchetti, D., McQuillan, D. J., Spohn, W. C., Carson, D. D. and Nicolson, G. L. (1996). Neurotrophin stimulation of human melanoma cell invasion: selected enhancement of heparanase activity and heparanase degradation of specific heparan sulfate subpopulations. *Cancer Res* 56, 2856-63.

Marchetti, D., Menter, D., Jin, L., Nakajima, M. and Nicolson, G. L. (1993). Nerve growth factor effects on human and mouse melanoma cell invasion and heparanase production. *Int J Cancer* 55, 692-9.

Marchetti, D. and Nicolson, G. L. (1997). Neurotrophin stimulation of human melanoma cell invasion: selected enhancement of heparanase activity and heparanase degradation of specific heparan sulfate subpopulations. *Adv Enzyme Regul* 37, 111-34.

Marshall, C. J. (1995). Specificity of receptor tyrosine kinase signaling: transient versus sustained extracellular signal-regulated kinase activation. *Cell* 80, 179-85.

Martin-Zanca, D., Hughes, S. H. and Barbacid, M. (1986). A human oncogene formed by the fusion of truncated tropomyosin and protein tyrosine kinase sequences. *Nature* 319, 743-748.

Martin-Zanca, D., Oskam, R., Mitra, G., Copeland, T. and Barbacid, M. (1989). Molecular and biochemical characterization of the human trk proto-oncogene. *Mol. and Cell. Biol.* 9, 24-33.

Matsumoto, K., Wada, R. K., Yamashiro, J. M., Kaplan, D. R. and Thiele, C. J. (1995). Expression of brain-derived neurotrophic factor and p145TrkB affects survival, differentiation, and invasiveness of human neuroblastoma cells. *Cancer Res* 55, 1798-806.
Matsunaga, T., Shirasawa, H., Enomoto, H., Yoshida, H., Iwai, J., Tanabe, M., Kawamura, K., Etoh, T. and Ohnuma, N. (1998). Neuronal src and trk a protooncogene expression in neuroblastomas and patient prognosis. *Int J Cancer* 79, 226-31.
Matsushima, H. and Bogenmann, E. (1993). Expression of trkA cDNA in neuroblastomas mediates differentiation in vitro and in vivo. *Mol Cell Biol* 13, 7447-56.
McGregor, L. M., McCune, B. K., Graff, J. R., McDowell, P. R., Romans, K. E., Yancopoulos, G. D., Ball, D. W., Baylin, S. B. and Nelkin, B. D. (1999). Roles of trk family neurotrophin receptors in medullary thyroid carcinoma development and progression. *Proc Natl Acad Sci U S A* 96, 4540-5.
McPherson, P. S., Kay, B. K. and Hussain, N. K. (2001). Signaling on the endocytic pathway. *Traffic* 2, 375-84.
Meakin, S. O., MacDonald, J. I., Gryz, E. A., Kubu, C. J. and Verdi, J. M. (1999). The signaling adapter FRS-2 competes with Shc for binding to the nerve growth factor receptor TrkA. A model for discriminating proliferation and differentiation. *J Biol Chem* 274, 9861-70.
Melck, D., De Petrocellis, L., Orlando, P., Bisogno, T., Laezza, C., Bifulco, M. and Di Marzo, V. (2000). Suppression of nerve growth factor Trk receptors and prolactin receptors by endocannabinoids leads to inhibition of human breast and prostate cancer cell proliferation. *Endocrinology* 141, 118-26.
Menter, D. G., Herrmann, J. L., Marchetti, D. and Nicolson, G. L. (1994). Involvement of neurotrophins and growth factors in brain metastasis formation. *Invasion Metastasis* 14, 372-84.
Menter, D. G., Herrmann, J. L. and Nicolson, G. L. (1995). The role of trophic factors and autocrine/paracrine growth factors in brain metastasis. *Clin Exp Metastasis* 13, 67-88.
Middlemas, D. S., Kihl, B. K. and Moody, N. M. (1999a). Brain derived neurotrophic factor protects human neuroblastoma cells from DNA damaging agents. *J Neurooncol* 45, 27-36.
Middlemas, D. S., Kihl, B. K., Zhou, J. and Zhu, X. (1999b). Brain-derived neurotrophic factor promotes survival and chemoprotection of human neuroblastoma cells. *J Biol Chem* 274, 16451-60.
Middlemas, D. S., Meisenhelder, J. and Hunter, T. (1994). Identification of TrkB autophosphorylation sites and evidence that phospholipase C-gamma-1 is a substrate of the TrkB receptor [Review]. *Journal of Biological Chemistry* 269, 5458-5466.
Miknyoczki, S. J., Chang, H., Klein-Szanto, A., Dionne, C. A. and Ruggeri, B. A. (1999a). The Trk tyrosine kinase inhibitor CEP-701 (KT-5555) exhibits significant antitumor efficacy in preclinical xenograft models of human pancreatic ductal adenocarcinoma. *Clin Cancer Res* 5, 2205-12.
Miknyoczki, S. J., Dionne, C. A., Klein-Szanto, A. J. and Ruggeri, B. A. (1999b). The novel Trk receptor tyrosine kinase inhibitor CEP-701 (KT-5555) exhibits antitumor efficacy against human pancreatic carcinoma (Panc1) xenograft growth and in vivo invasiveness. *Ann N Y Acad Sci* 880, 252-62.
Miknyoczki, S. J., Lang, D., Huang, L., Klein-Szanto, A. J., Dionne, C. A. and Ruggeri, B. A. (1999c). Neurotrophins and Trk receptors in human pancreatic ductal adenocarcinoma: expression patterns and effects on in vitro invasive behavior. *Int J Cancer* 81, 417-27.
Muragaki, Y., Chou, T. T., Kaplan, D. R., Trojanowski, J. Q. and Lee, V. M. (1997). Nerve growth factor induces apoptosis in human medulloblastoma cell lines that express TrkA receptors. *J Neurosci* 17, 530-42.
Nakagawara, A., Arima-Nakagawara, M., Scavarda, N. J., Azar, C. G., Cantor, A. B. and Brodeur, G. M. (1993). Association between high levels of expression of the TRK gene and favorable outcome in human neuroblastoma. *N Engl J Med* 328, 847-54.
Nakagawara, A., Azar, C. G., Scavarda, N. J. and Brodeur, G. M. (1994). Expression and function of TRK-B and BDNF in human neuroblastomas. *Mol Cell Biol* 14, 759-67.
Nakagawara, A. and Brodeur, G. M. (1997). Role of neurotrophins and their receptors in human neuroblastomas: a primary culture study. *Eur J Cancer* 33, 2050-3.
Nakamura, T., Komiya, M., Gotoh, N., Koizumi, S., Shibuya, M. and Mori, N. (2002). Discrimination between phosphotyrosine-mediated signaling properties of conventional and neuronal Shc adapter molecules. *Oncogene* 21, 22-31.
Nogueira, E., Navarro, S., Pellin, A. and Llombart-Bosch, A. (1997). Activation of TRK genes in Ewing's sarcoma. Trk A receptor expression linked to neural differentiation. *Diagn Mol Pathol* 6, 10-6.
Obermeier, A., Halfter, H., Wiesmuller, K. H., Jung, G., Schlessinger, J. and Ullrich, A. (1993a). Tyrosine 785 is a major determinant of Trk--substrate interaction. *EMBO Journal* 12, 933-41.

Obermeier, A., Lammers, R., Wiesmuller, K. H., Jung, G., Schlessinger, J. and Ullrich, A. (1993b). Identification of Trk binding sites for SHC and phosphatidylinositol 3'-kinase and formation of a multimeric signaling complex. *Journal of Biological Chemistry* 268, 22963-6.
Pearson, G., Robinson, F., Beers Gibson, T., Xu, B., Karandikar, M., Berman, K. and Cobb, M. H. (2001). Mitogen-activated protein (map) kinase pathways: regulation and physiological functions. *Endocr Rev* 22, 153-83.
Pflug, B. R., Dionne, C., Kaplan, D. R., Lynch, J. and Djakiew, D. (1995). Expression of a Trk high affinity nerve growth factor receptor in the human prostate. *Endocrinology* 136, 262-8.
Pomeroy, S. L., Tamayo, P., Gaasenbeek, M., Sturla, L. M., Angelo, M., McLaughlin, M. E., Kim, J. Y., Goumnerova, L. C., Black, P. M., Lau, C. et al. (2002). Prediction of central nervous system embryonal tumour outcome based on gene expression. *Nature* 415, 436-42.
Qian, X., Riccio, A., Zhang, Y. and Ginty, D. (1998). Identification and characterization of novel substrates of Trk receptors in developing neurons. *Neuron* 21, 1017-1029
Qiu, M. and Green, S. (1992). PC12 cell neuronal differentiation is associated with prolonged p21 ras activity and consequent prolonged ERK activity. *Neuron* 9, 705-717.
Ricci, A., Greco, S., Mariotta, S., Felici, L., Bronzetti, E., Cavazzana, A., Cardillo, G., Amenta, F., Bisetti, A. and Barbolini, G. (2001). Neurotrophins and neurotrophin receptors in human lung cancer. *Am J Respir Cell Mol Biol* 25, 439-46.
Riccio, A., Ahn, S., Davenport, C., Blendy, J. and Ginty, D. (1999). Mediation by a CREB family transcription factor of NGF-dependent survival of sympathetic neurons. *Science* 286, 2358-61.
Ruggeri, B. A., Miknyoczki, S. J., Singh, J. and Hudkins, R. L. (1999). Role of neurotrophin-trk interactions in oncology: the anti-tumor efficacy of potent and selective trk tyrosine kinase inhibitors in pre- clinical tumor models. *Curr Med Chem* 6, 845-57
Russell, J. P., Powell, D. J., Cunnane, M., Greco, A., Portella, G., Santoro, M., Fusco, A. and Rothstein, J. L. (2000). The TRK-T1 fusion protein induces neoplastic transformation of thyroid epithelium. *Oncogene* 19, 5729-35.
Sakamoto, Y., Kitajima, Y., Edakuni, G., Sasatomi, E., Mori, M., Kitahara, K. and Miyazaki, K. (2001). Expression of Trk tyrosine kinase receptor is a biologic marker for cell proliferation and perineural invasion of human pancreatic ductal adenocarcinoma. *Oncol Rep* 8, 477-84.
Schneider, M. B., Standop, J., Ulrich, A., Wittel, U., Friess, H., Andren-Sandberg, A. and Pour, P. M. (2001). Expression of nerve growth factors in pancreatic neural tissue and pancreatic cancer. *J Histochem Cytochem* 49, 1205-10.
Segal, R. A., Bhattacharyya, A., Rua, L. A., Alberta, J. A., Stephens, R. M., Kaplan, D. R. and Stiles, C. D. (1996). Differential utilization of Trk autophosphorylation sites. *J Biol Chem* 271, 20175-81.
Segal, R. A., Goumnerova, L. C., Kwon, Y. K., Stiles, C. D. and Pomeroy, S. L. (1994). Expression of the neurotrophin receptor TrkC is linked to a favorable outcome in medulloblastoma. *Proc Natl Acad Sci U S A* 91, 12867-71.
Sheng, W. Q., Hisaoka, M., Okamoto, S., Tanaka, A., Meis-Kindblom, J. M., Kindblom, L. G., Ishida, T., Nojima, T. and Hashimoto, H. (2001). Congenital-infantile fibrosarcoma. A clinicopathologic study of 10 cases and molecular detection of the ETV6-NTRK3 fusion transcripts using paraffin-embedded tissues. *Am J Clin Pathol* 115, 348-55.
Singer, H. S., Hansen, B., Martinie, D. and Karp, C. L. (1999). Mitogenesis in glioblastoma multiforme cell lines: a role for NGF and its TrkA receptors. *J Neurooncol* 45, 1-8.
Sofroniew, M. V., Howe, C. L. and Mobley, W. C. (2001). Nerve growth factor signaling, neuroprotection, and neural repair. *Annu Rev Neurosci* 24, 1217-81.
Squinto, S. P., Snitt, T. N., Aldrich, T. H., Davis, S., Bianco, S. M., Radjewski, C., Glass, D. F., Masiakowski, P., Furth, M. E., Valenzuela, D. M. et al. (1991). trkB encodes a functional receptor for brain-derived neurotrophic factor and neurotrophin 3 but not nerve growth factor. *Cell* 65, 1-20.
Stephens, R. M., Loeb, D. M., Copeland, T. D., Pawson, T., Greene, L. A. and Kaplan, D. R. (1994). Trk receptors use redundant signal transduction pathways involving SHC and PLC-gamma 1 to mediate NGF responses. *Neuron* 12, 691-705.
Sugimoto, T., Kuroda, H., Horii, Y., Moritake, H., Tanaka, T. and Hattori, S. (2001). Signal transduction pathways through TRK-A and TRK-B receptors in human neuroblastoma cells. *Jpn J Cancer Res* 92, 152-60
Svensson, T., Ryden, M., Schilling, F. H., Dominici, C., Sehgal, R., Ibanez, C. F. and Kogner, P. (1997). Coexpression of mRNA for the full-length neurotrophin receptor trk-C and trk-A in favourable neuroblastoma. *Eur J Cancer* 33, 2058-63.

Tajima, Y., Molina, R. P., Jr., Rorke, L. B., Kaplan, D. R., Radeke, M., Feinstein, S. C., Lee, V. M. and Trojanowski, J. Q. (1998). Neurotrophins and neuronal versus glial differentiation in medulloblastomas and other pediatric brain tumors. *Acta Neuropathol (Berl)* 95, 325-32.

Tanaka, T., Sugimoto, T. and Sawada, T. (1998). Prognostic discrimination among neuroblastomas according to Ha-ras/trk A gene expression: a comparison of the profiles of neuroblastomas detected clinically and those detected through mass screening. *Cancer* 83, 1626-33

Traverse, S., Gomez, N., Paterson, H., Marshall, C. and Cohen, P. (1992). Sustained activation of the mitogen-activated protein (MAP) kinase cascade may be required for differentiation of PC12 cells. Comparison of the effects of nerve growth factor and epidermal growth factor. *Biochemical Journal* 288, 351-5.

Tsoulfas, P., Soppet, D., Escandon, E., Tessarollo, L., Mendoza-Ramirez, J.-L., Rosenthal, A., Nikolics, K. and Parada, L. F. (1993). The rat trkC encodes multiple neurogenic receptors that exhibit differential response to Neurotrophin-3 in PC12 cells. *Neuron* 10, 975-990.

Vetter, M. L., Martin-Zanca, D., Parada, L. F., Bishop, J. M. and D.R.Kaplan. (1991). Nerve growth factor rapidly stimulates tyrosine phosphorylation of phospholipaseC by a kinase activity associated with the product of the trk protooncogene. *Proc. Nat. Acad. Sci. USA* 88, 5650-5654.

Wang, J., Auger, K., Jarvis, L., Shi, Y. and Roberts, T. (1995). Direct association of Grb2 with the p85 subunit of phosphatidylinositol 3-kinase. *J Biol Chem* 270, 12774-12780.

Washiyama, K., Muragaki, Y., Rorke, L. B., Lee, V. M., Feinstein, S. C., Radeke, M. J., Blumberg, D., Kaplan, D. R. and Trojanowski, J. Q. (1996). Neurotrophin and neurotrophin receptor proteins in medulloblastomas and other primitive neuroectodermal tumors of the pediatric central nervous system. *Am J Pathol* 148, 929-40.

Watson, F. L., Heerssen, H. M., Bhattacharyya, A., Klesse, L., Lin, M. Z. and Segal, R. A. (2001). Neurotrophins use the Erk5 pathway to mediate a retrograde survival response. *Nat Neurosci* 4, 981-8.

Weeraratna, A. T., Arnold, J. T., George, D. J., DeMarzo, A. and Isaacs, J. T. (2000). Rational basis for Trk inhibition therapy for prostate cancer. *Prostate* 45, 140-8.

Weeraratna, A. T., Dalrymple, S. L., Lamb, J. C., Denmeade, S. R., Miknyoczki, S., Dionne, C. A. and Isaacs, J. T. (2001). Pan-trk inhibition decreases metastasis and enhances host survival in experimental models as a result of its selective induction of apoptosis of prostate cancer cells. *Clin Cancer Res* 7, 2237-45.

Widmer, H. R., Kaplan, D. R., Rabin, S. J., Beck, K. D., Hefti, F. and Knusel, B. (1993). Rapid phosphorylation of phospholipase C gamma 1 by brain-derived neurotrophic factor and neurotrophin-3 in cultures of embryonic rat cortical neurons. *J Neurochem* 60, 2111-23.

Yamashiro, D. J., Liu, X. G., Lee, C. P., Nakagawara, A., Ikegaki, N., McGregor, L. M., Baylin, S. B. and Brodeur, G. M. (1997). Expression and function of Trk-C in favourable human neuroblastomas. *Eur J Cancer* 33, 2054-7.

Yao, R. and Cooper, G. (1995). Requirement for phosphatidylinositol-3 kinase in the prevention of apoptosis by nerve growth factor. *Science* 267, 2003-2006.

York, R. D., Molliver, D. C., Grewal, S. S., Stenberg, P. E., McCleskey, E. W. and Stork, P. J. (2000). Role of phosphoinositide 3-kinase and endocytosis in nerve growth factor-induced extracellular signal-regulated kinase activation via Ras and Rap1. *Mol Cell Biol* 20, 8069-83.

Zabolotny, J. M., Bence-Hanulec, K. K., Stricker-Krongrad, A., Haj, F., Wang, Y., Minokoshi, Y., Kim, Y. B., Elmquist, J. K., Tartaglia, L. A., Kahn, B. B. et al. (2002). PTP1B Regulates Leptin Signal Transduction In Vivo. *Dev Cell* 2, 489-95.

Zhang, Y., Moheban, D., Conway, B., Bhattacharyya, A. and Segal, R. (2000). Cell surface Trk receptors mediate NGF-induced survival while internalized receptors regulate NGF-induced differentiation. *J Neurosci* 20, 5671-8.

THE ROLE OF GROWTH FACTOR SIGNALING IN MALIGNANCY

ROY S. HERBST, AMIR ONN, & JOHN MENDELSOHN

1. GROWTH FACTOR OVERVIEW

Growth factors and their receptors are the core components of signal transduction pathways. Growth factors are proteins that bind to receptors on the cell surface and stimulate various cellular functions, including growth and differentiation. Some growth factors stimulate a wide variety of cell types, while others are specific for a given cell type. When these growth-regulating polypeptides bind to their cognate receptors, they induce cell growth or differentiation through receptor stimulation and initiation of the signal transduction cascade or modulation in normal tissues. A number of growth factors have been studied in a great detail, including epidermal growth factor (EGF), platelet-derived growth factors (PDGF), vascular endothelial growth factor (VEGF), transforming growth factors (TGF), fibroblast growth factors (FGF), insulin-like growth factors (IGF), hepatocyte growth factor (HGF), erythropoietin, and nerve growth factor (NGF).

Under certain conditions, growth factors can promote malignancy. In a variety of human cancers, modification of growth factor production, receptor expression, and alterations in the intracellular mitogenic signals play a critical role in directing normal tissues to become cancerous (Aaronson, 1991). In many types of cancers, growth factors or their receptors are aberrantly expressed. This chapter focuses primarily on EGF, PDGF, VEGF, TGFs, FGF, IGF, and their receptors and role in human malignancies. These growth factors are involved in cell proliferation and differentiation in various cell types. The growth factors that stimulate hematopoietic cells and lymphocytes will not be covered. Numerous molecular therapies targeted at aberrant growth factor signaling are being investigated, with some agents in the late stages of clinical testing. Targeted therapies may provide an important therapeutic option for patients with tumors that are often considered incurable using traditional cytotoxic approaches. (Schiller et al., 2002)

1.1. Growth Factor Receptor Molecular Structure

Growth factor receptors are categorized based on their primary signal transduction mechanisms. Types of receptors include ligand-gated ion-channels, GTPase (G-protein)-linked receptors, and protein kinase-linked receptors. Protein kinase-linked receptors have intrinsic tyrosine kinase or serine/threonine kinase activity and are linked to cytosolic kinases (reviewed in Mendelsohn, Baird, Fan, & Markowitz, 2001).

The majority of growth factors exert their effects through binding to receptors with an intrinsic tyrosine kinase (RTKs). These transmembrane receptors are composed of extracellular ligand binding, transmembrane, and cytoplasmic tyrosine kinase domains.

The extracellular domains of these receptors contain cysteine moieties that fold into tertiary structures and form either immunoglobulin (Ig)-like domains (loop structures) created by disulfide bonds between cysteine moieties, or cysteine-rich domains that exist as a complex structure resulting from formation of closely positioned disulfide bonds. Both of these structures create pockets that allow growth factors to bind to the receptor with high affinity (Ullrich & Schlessinger, 1990).

Tyrosine kinase transmembrane receptors have been divided into several classes or families based on their extracellular domain structure. Examples of these receptors include the following: the EGF receptors (EGFR), PDGF receptors (PDGFR), VEGF receptors (VEGFR), FGF receptors (FGFR), and the IGF receptors (IGFR). Most transmembrane tyrosine kinase receptors are monomeric. Upon ligand binding, the monomeric receptors undergo dimerization. However, the members of the IGFR exist as homodimers of cysteine-rich peptides that are linked by disulfide bounds. Following ligand binding, transphosphorylation of specific tyrosine residues occurs on the cytoplasmic portions of the receptors. PDGFR and FGFR have Ig-like structures as their extracellular domains, while the EGF receptor family members have a cysteine-rich extracellular domain (Ullrich & Schlessinger, 1990).

The TGF-β receptors possess serine/threonine kinase activity (Massague, 1998). Like RTKs, these receptors are transmembrane proteins consisting of extracellular (ligand-binding), transmembrane, and intracellular kinase domains. When the heterodimeric TGF-β receptor complex is activated via ligand binding, it induces a potent antiproliferative activity in many cell types (Massague, 1990). The mechanisms of cellular responses to the receptor serine/threonine kinases are not as well understood as those of the RTKs.

Growth factor binding to the extracellular domain of the receptors leads to activation of transcription factors and, eventually, production of protein molecules that control cell functions.

1.2. Ligands of Tyrosine Kinase Receptors and Signal Transduction Pathways

Tyrosine kinase receptors and their cognate ligands contain complementary domains created by particular amino acid sequences that render their receptor-ligand relationship unique. Binding of the ligand to the receptor and subsequent receptor oligomerization brings the kinase domains of the 2 receptor chains closer to each other, activating the intrinsic tyrosine kinase, which transphosphorylates tyrosine residues on the receptors and on signaling molecules in the cytosol. (Figure 1) Substrates in the cytosol containing Scr-homology-2 (SH2) domains bind to the activated receptors at docking sites that consist of a phosphotyrosine residue and a specific sequence of amino acids in close proximity on the receptor. Thus, receptor phosphorylation both stimulates kinase activity and allows binding of downstream-signaling molecules. SH2 domains are present in a diverse range of eukaryotic proteins, including many proteins involved in signal transduction (Pawson, 1995).

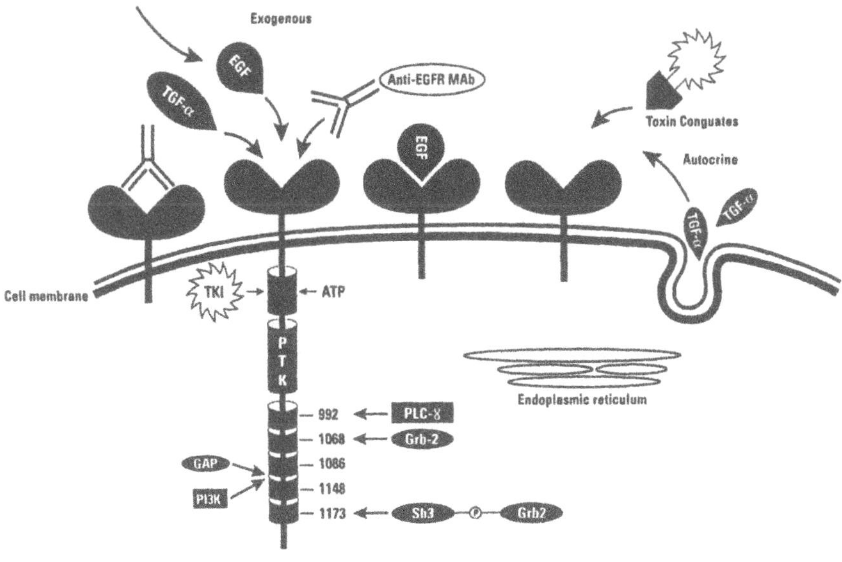

Figure 1. Using the epidermal growth factor receptor as an example, this figure illustrates the mechanisms by which growth factors and their receptors transduce extracellular signals into intracellular processes, in particular, migration, angiogenesis, gene transcription, cell cycle progression, survival, and proliferation. In addition, some mechanisms by which signal transduction can be blocked are depicted.

SH2 domains are stretches of 100 amino acids with highly conserved residues that create binding compartments for molecules containing phosphotyrosine residues. The molecules containing SH2 domains are involved in tyrosine phosphorylation and dephosphorylation, phospholipid metabolism, activation of Ras-like GTPases, gene expression, protein trafficking, and cytoskeletal architecture (Pawson, 1995). SH2 is also a component of adapter proteins, for instance Grb-2, which serve to link activated receptors to specific enzymes.

Many adapter proteins also contain SH3 domains, composed of up to 75 amino acids, which are responsible for protein-protein interactions. The SH3 segments of adapter molecules that also contain SH2 domains are able to connect tyrosine-phosphorylated receptors to downstream effector proteins, achieving signal transduction (Pawson, 1995). Important signal transduction pathways and proteins involved in growth factor signaling, including phosphatidylinositol 3-kinase (PI3K) dependent pathways, Ras proteins, and Janus kinase (Jak) signaling molecules, are described in detail elsewhere in this volume.

1.3. Receptor and Ligand Modulation

Receptor activation is achieved by very low concentrations of growth factors and is short lived. Once the growth factor binds to its receptor, the growth factor-receptor complex is internalized into endosomes within less than 1 hour (Carpenter, 1987). While in the endosomes, the binding equilibrium is shifted due to decreased pH leading to ligand release. The separated ligand and receptor are transported to lysosomes and are catabolized. Some of the free receptors may be recycled and transported to the cell surface, where they are used for further activation before they are catabolized in the lysosomes.

Activation of a particular signal pathway is achieved within seconds of the binding of the growth factor to its receptor. Shortly after activation by a growth factor, receptor internalization and degradation occurs, and signal transduction terminates. In order to achieve a prolonged receptor-mediated signal, new receptors and growth factors must be produced (Carpenter, 1987).

1.4. The Role of Growth Factors in Cell Cycle Progression

One of the most important roles of growth factors is stimulating quiescent (G_0 phase) cells into active traversal of the cell cycle and cell division. In this regard, growth factors are divided into 2 groups: competence factors, such as EGF, FGF, and PDGF; and progression factors, including insulin and IGF. Quiescent cells are initially advanced into the G_1 phase under the influence of competence factors and then become committed to DNA synthesis (S phase) by progression factors (Pledger, Stiles, Antoniades, & Scher, 1977). The stimulatory effects of growth factors must be present throughout this transitional process, which takes several hours, and if the signal is disrupted before the cell becomes committed to DNA synthesis, the cell will retreat to the G_0 phase (Figure 2).

At a critical point in the cell cycle, the restriction point, the cell is committed to progress into the S phase (Pardee, 1989). This point of the cell cycle occurs at the G_1 checkpoint, which is controlled by the level of phosphorylation of the retinoblastoma (Rb) protein. There are several factors affecting the level of phosphorylation of Rb proteins, including cyclins, cyclin-dependent kinases (CDKs), and the CDK inhibitors. For instance, elevated cyclin D levels shorten the duration of the G_1 phase and reduce the dependency of the cell on exogenous growth factors (Sherr, 1996; Sherr & Roberts, 1995).

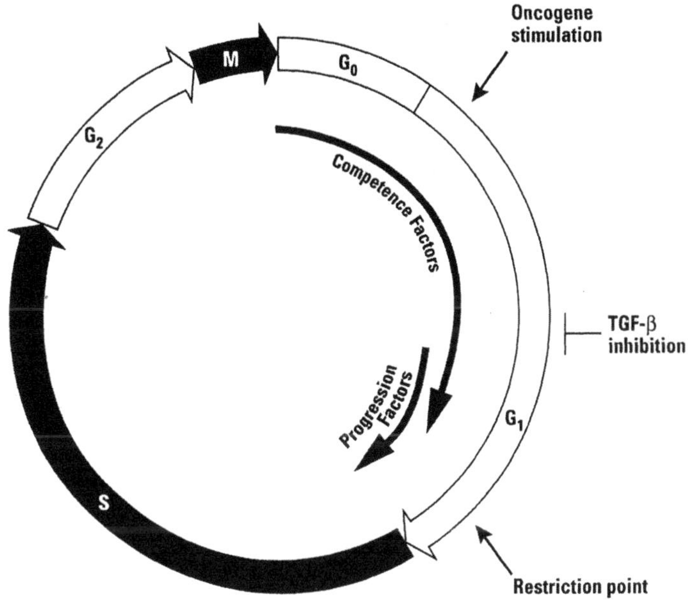

Figure 2. This diagram illustrates the various points at which growth factors regulate cell cycle progression. The competence factors, EGF, PDGF, and FGF are important early in G_1, while the progression factors are more important in late G_1. In addition, the inhibitory effects of TGF-β are illustrated.

1.5. Growth Factors and Their Receptors

1.5.1. The Epidermal-related Growth Factors

There are several ligands that can bind to the EGFR: EGF, TGF-α, amphiregulin (AR), heparin-binding EGF-like growth factor (HB-EGF), cripto, vaccinia virus growth factor (VVGF), betacellulin (BTC), tomoregulin, neuregulin, and epiregulin (EPR). (Ciccodicola et al., 1989; Derynck, 1988; Higashiyama, Abraham, Miller, Fiddes, & Klagsbrun, 1991; Laurence & Gusterson, 1990; Normanno, Bianco, De Luca, & Salomon, 2001; Reisner, 1985; Shoyab, Plowman, McDonald, Bradley, & Todaro, 1989; Toyoda et al., 1995) EGF and TGF-α are believed to be the most important and widely expressed endogenous ligands.

EGF is synthesized as a large 1217-amino acid transmembrane precursor, which initially is anchored to the cell surface. It has biological activity, since it can stimulate EGFR located on the same cell or nearby cells. Subsequently, an extracellular portion of this protein is cleaved to release a 53-amino acid molecule, which has biological activity (Carpenter & Cohen, 1990; Normanno et al., 2001). EGF has important effects on cell growth, differentiation, and survival. EGF is produced primarily in the submandibular salivary glands, Brunner's glands in the small intestine, and the kidney (Kajikawa et al., 1991).

TGF-α is synthesized in many cell types and was first isolated from the culture medium of an oncogenically transformed cell line (de Larco & Todaro, 1978). TGF-α is synthesized as a precursor protein and, after 2 sequential endoproteolytic cleavages, forms a 50-amino acid single polypeptide chain that shares 42% homology with EGF (Dunn, Hesse, & Black, 2000; Massague & Pandiella, 1993). TGF-α is present in regenerating epithelial cells and cells of many other normal and malignant adult tissues as well (Yasui et al., 1992).

1.5.2. Epidermal Growth Factor (erb-B) Receptor Family

The EGFR family of RTKs consists of 4 related receptors: EGFR/HER1 (c-*erb*-B1), HER2 (c-*erb*-B2), HER3 (c-*erb*-B3), and HER4 (c-*erb*-B4). (Figure 3) These receptors are functional as homodimers or heterodimers of combinations of receptors and have different affinities to various growth factors.

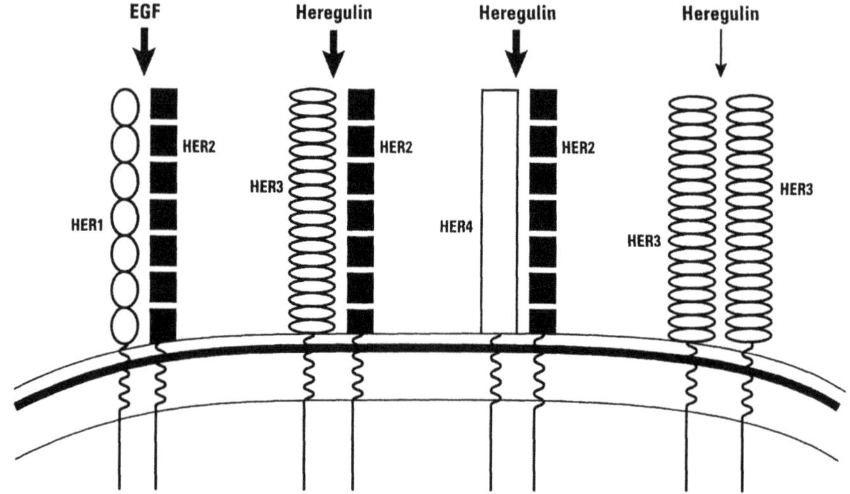

Figure 3. EGF receptors are commonly expressed on most epithelial and mesenchymal cells and are responsible for cell proliferation and differentiation. EGF binds with higher affinity to heterodimers of receptors that contain HER2 than to any other EGF pairs. Similarly, one of the HER3 and HER4 ligands, heregulin, binds preferentially to heterodimers of HER3 and HER2 than to homodimers of HER3 (Pinkas-Kramarski et al., 1996; Sliwkowski, 1994) (Larger arrows indicate higher affinity).

1.5.3. Vascular Endothelial Growth Factor

VEGF, also known as vascular permeability factor (VPF), is a heparin-binding glycoprotein that is secreted as a homodimeric protein. Currently, there are 6 related proteins identified as vascular endothelial growth factors: VEGF-A, placenta growth factor (PIGF), VEGF-B, VEGF-C, VEGF-D, and VEGF-E. VEGF-A (generally known as VEGF) is the most potent angiogenic isoform. Alternative splicing of mRNA in the process of VEGF production creates various isoforms composed of 205-, 189-, 165-, 145-, and 121-amino acid residues (Gerwins, Sköldenberg, & Claesson-Welsh, 2000; Kerbel, 2000). Several studies have indicated that the different VEGF isoforms have distinct functions. For instance, in animal models lacking certain VEGF isoforms ($VEGF_{165}$ and $VEGF_{189}$), myocardial angiogenesis is impaired and ischemic cardiomyopathy has resulted. (Carmeliet 1999 VEGF-A has potent mitogenic effects, specifically on vascular endothelial cells (angiogenesis), and is one of the most important growth and survival factors for the endothelium (Ferrara, 1999; Houck, Leung, Rowland, Winer, & Ferrara, 1992; Park, Keller, & Ferrara, 1993). Additionally, VEGF causes vasodilatation partly through stimulation of nitric oxide synthase in endothelial cells (Yang et al., 1996) VEGF can also stimulate cell migration and inhibit apoptosis (programmed cell death) (Alon et al., 1995).

Inactivation of any of 4 of these growth factors (VEGF-A, PIGF, VEGF-B, and VEGF-E) influences vascular endothelial cells, while others, VEGF-C and -D, act on lymphatic endothelial cells. (Gerwins et al., 2000) VEGF-B is likely to be involved in vasculogenesis and activation of invasive enzymes on endothelial cells (Aase, 1999; Olofsson et al., 1998). VEGF-C has been linked to lymph angiogenesis and, recently, to tumor angiogenesis (Lymboussaki et al., 1998; Salven et al., 1998; Tsurusaki et al., 1999; Veikkola & Alitalo, 1999).

The family of VEGFR includes 3 structurally related tyrosine kinase receptors, VEGFR-1 (flt-1), VEGFR-2 (KDR/flk-1), and VEGFR-3 (flt-4). These receptors are almost exclusively expressed on endothelial cells. Like VEGF isoforms, the receptor types have different roles in the angiogenesis process. VEGFR-2 expression is crucial in the differentiation of angioblasts into endothelial cells (Shalaby et al., 1995); VEGFR-1 gene disruption results in abnormal vessel morphogenesis (Fong, Rossant, Gertsenstein, & Breitman, 1995); and inactivation of VEGFR-3 leads to defective lumen formation in large vessels (Dumont et al., 1998).

1.5.4. Platelet-derived Growth Factor (PDGF)

PDGF is a potent mitogenic growth factor for cells of mesenchymal origin that express high levels of PDGFR. PDGFs are dimers of disulfide-bound polypeptide chains, A and B, creating 3 biologically active isomers of PDGF (AA, AB, and BB) (Inui, Kitami, Tani, Kondo, & Inagami, 1994). Additional two novel members of this growth factor family were recently identified, i.e., PDGF-C and

PDGF-D (Heldin, Eriksson, & Östman, 2002). PDGF isoforms stimulate and inhibit cellular activities in diverse ways, depending on the cell type, thus generating a tremendous range of possibilities for biological responses. In vascular smooth muscle cells, PDGF-AA increases protein synthesis (hypertrophy) while PDGF-BB initiates mitosis (hyperplasia) (Inui et al., 1994). In fibroblasts, however, PDGF-AA inhibits chemotaxis, while PDGF-BB stimulates chemotactic activities (Siegbahn, Hammacher, Westermark, & Heldin, 1990). In general, the biological activities of PDGF include migration, proliferation, contraction, inhibition of gap junctional communications, cytokine production, and lipoprotein uptake. Collectively, these activities promote wound healing in adults and the formation of blood vessels, kidney glomeruli, and lung alveoli in embryos. PDGFs are ligands for two receptors, PDGFR α and β, which are primarily localized on connective tissue, smooth muscle, and vascular endothelial cells and are not normally expressed on epithelial cells (Beitz, Kim, Calabresi, & Frackelton, 1991; Westermark & Sorg, 1993).

1.5.5. Fibroblast Growth Factor (FGF)

FGFs and their signaling pathways play significant roles in the normal development of embryonic cells and in wound healing by regulating cell growth and differentiation. Twenty FGFs have been identified (FGF1–FGF20). This family of polypeptide growth factors stimulates proliferative, chemotactic, and angiogenic activities primarily in cells of mesodermal origin; however, they also have effects on cells derived from the ectoderm and endoderm (Basilico & Moscatelli, 1992). The members of this family of growth factors are classified as FGFs solely on the basis of their structural similarities and not on their biological activities. For instance, FGF-7 does not stimulate fibroblasts (Powers, McLeskey, Wellstein, 2000).

FGFs exert their mitogenic and angiogenic effects in target cells by signaling through cell-surface tyrosine kinase receptors. In order to affect differing cells as extensively as FGFs do, the signaling system requires a variety of receptors. There are 4 distinct genes that encode for FGFR, designated as FGFR1 (Flg), FGFR2 (Bek), FGFR3, and FGFR4. The diverse collection of FGFRs is produced through alternate splicing of the same gene or analogous splicing of different genes (Powers et al., 2000). The various isoforms of FGFRs bind to FGF ligands with differing affinities. (Ornitz 1992) Similarly, different FGFRs may have different signaling roles, evident by the involvement of FGFR1, more than the other receptors in the FGFR family, in malignancies and cell transformation (reviewed in Mendelsohn et al., 2001).

1.5.6. Transforming Growth Factor-β

The TGF group includes TGF-α and -β, which are structurally unrelated and bind to a completely different family of receptors (Dunn, Heese, & Black, 2000). TGF-α binds to EGF receptors and acts similarly to EGF, as described above.

Members of the TGF-β superfamily signal through a single common receptor complex that is a heteromeric serine/threonine kinase receptor. Mammalian TGF-β exists in 3 isoforms: TGF-β1, TGF-β2, and TGF-β3 (Massague, 1990). The various TGF-β isoforms share many biological activities and their actions on cells are qualitatively similar in most cases. These isoforms are involved in embryogenesis, cell proliferation, tissue repair, hematopoiesis, and regulation of the immune response (Kulkarni et al., 1993; Massague, 1990; Shull et al., 1992).

The TGF-β heteromeric receptor complex contains type I (RI) and type II (RII) subunits. Additionally, subunit RIII has been identified but has no signaling domain and serves as an auxiliary unit in presenting TGF-β2 to the RI and RII components. TGF-β inhibits proliferation in a number of normal cell types, with several proposed mechanisms, and it antagonizes mitogenic effects of several growth factors, including PDGF, EGF, and FGF2 (Hunter, Sporn, & Davies, 1993). The chemical and structural changes in the receptor after TGF-β binds to it, lead to phosphorylation of a number of downstream effectors, including Smad proteins. After phosphorylation by the TGF-β receptor, Smad2 and Smad3 form heterodimers with Smad4 and translocate to the nucleus to activate gene expression. Increased expression of several cyclin-dependent kinase inhibitors, including $P21^{WAF1/CIP1}$, $P27^{KIP1}$ and $P15^{INK4B}$, has been observed after TGF-β receptor activation (Rich, Zhang, Datto, Bigner, & Wang, 1999). Expression of these proteins has been shown to be associated with decreased activity of Cdk2 followed by hypophosphorylation of Rb, and, therefore G_1 cell cycle arrest (Platten, Wick, & Weller, 2001).

1.5.7. Insulin-like Growth Factor

Insulin, IGF-I, and IGF-II are the members of this peptide-based family of growth-stimulating molecules, with a 50% similarity at the structural level (Daughaday & Rotwein, 1989). IGF-I and -II are produced mainly by the liver, the major source of endocrine IGFs (Werner & Rotwein, 2000), and insulin is produced by the β-cells in the islets of Langerhans. Six IGF binding proteins (IGFBPs), IGFBP-related proteins, and IGFBP-proteases modulate the activity of the IGFs by altering their available free fraction since IGFBPs have a higher affinity (2- to 50-fold) to IGFs than do IGF receptors (reviewed in Mendelsohn et al., 2001).

The circulating growth hormone level in the body controls IGF-I release patterns; therefore, IGF-I gene expression and blood levels are increased by 10- to 100-fold between birth and adulthood (Roberts et al., 1986). Increased levels of circulating IGF-II are detected in adults compared to those in children. Since multiple studies have demonstrated that many tissue cells are capable of producing IGFs regardless of development stage, it is believed that IGFs have local (autocrine and paracrine) activities in addition to their endocrine actions (Adamo, Ben-Hur, Roberts, & LeRoith, 1991; D'Ercole, Applewhite, & Underwood, 1980).

Insulin regulates metabolic functions primarily by affecting cells in liver, muscle, and adipose tissues (Kahn, 1985). In contrast, IGF-I and -II modulate the growth and differentiation of cells in almost every tissue in the body (Daughaday & Rotwein, 1989). IGF-I regulates several cellular activities, including cell proliferation, differentiation, and apoptosis; IGF-I acts as a potent mitogen for a variety of cell types stimulating cyclin D1 expression, which, in turn stimulates cell cycle progression from G_1 to S phase (Dufourny et al., 1997; Furlanetto, Harwell, & Frick, 1994). IGF-I also inhibits apoptosis by stimulating expression of Bcl protein and suppressing expression of Bax (Minshall et al., 1997; Parrizas & LeRoith, 1997; Wang, Ma, Markovich, Lee, & Wang, 1998). IGF-II also has mitogenic and antiapoptotic activities and regulates cellular proliferation and differentiation.

The IGF receptors include insulin, IGF-I, and IGF-II receptors. IGF-I and insulin receptors are structurally similar; however, the IGF-II receptor is a mannose 6-phosphate receptor, and its cellular actions are not understood. IGF-I receptors are expressed on actively proliferating cells, whereas insulin receptors are mainly present on highly differentiated, noncycling cells, including hepatocytes and adipocytes (O'Dell, 1998).

2. THE ROLE OF GROWTH FACTORS AND THEIR RECEPTORS IN PROMOTING MALIGNANCY

Research conducted over the last several decades has vastly improved understanding of the molecular basis for cancer, particularly with respect to growth factor-mediated processes. In addition to regulating normal cellular functions, namely cell cycle progression, survival, and angiogenesis, growth factors can contribute to malignant transformation when their signaling pathways become dysregulated. Dysregulation can occur at various stages during growth factor signal transduction: specifically, growth factor production, receptor expression, or along signaling pathways (Aaronson, 1991). In the early 1980s, researchers discovered the link between oncogenes (genes causing cellular transformation), growth factors, and malignant transformation. The product encoded by the retroviral oncogene, v-*sis*, was found to be structurally similar to the B-chain of PDGF (Doolittle et al., 1983; Waterfield et al., 1983), and the *erb*-B oncogene was found to encode a truncated form of the EGFR (Downward et al., 1984). These findings led to subsequent discoveries that many oncogenes are related to proto-oncogenes (normal genes) that encode for growth factors or their receptors (Table 1).

Transformed cells can become autonomous and proceed through the cell cycle, proliferating and differentiating in the absence of an external source of growth factors (Barnes & Sato, 1980; de Larco & Todaro, 1978; Kaplan, Anderson, & Ozanne, 1982). de Larco's historical paper (1978) described the autocrine production of a growth factor by tumor cells with resultant EGF receptor stimulation. Subsequent studies provided evidence for autocrine secretion of growth factors by many tumor cells (reviewed in Sporn & Roberts, 1985). Such autocrine secretion can enhance growth factor signaling in the absence of receptor overexpression. Additional mechanisms by which malignant cells grow in the absence of or with decreased levels of growth factors include alterations in growth factor receptor expression or function, or activation of the signaling pathways in the absence of ligand-receptor binding (Goustin, Leof, Shipley, & Moses, 1986). For example, enhanced growth factor receptor expression on tumor cells enhances the cells' sensitivity to growth factors, thus diminishing growth factor requirements (Ennis, Lippman, & Dickson, 1991).

Growth factors regulate the signaling pathways that ultimately control the cell cycle. Growth factors promote cell survival via activation of three signaling pathways, the PI3K/AKT pathway, the ras/MAPK pathway, and the Jak/STAT pathway (Figure 4) (reviewed in Talapatra & Thompson, 2001). Loss of regulation at any of these steps, the growth factors, their receptors, or their signaling pathways, can contribute to malignant transformation and cell survival. Relevant preclinical and clinical evidence for a variety of growth factors and their role in malignancy are presented.

Table 1. Oncogenes related to proto-oncogenes that encode growth factors or growth factor receptors

Oncogene	*Proto-oncogene*	*Original Source*
v-*sis*	PDGF, β chain	Simian retrovirus
v-*erb*-B	EGF receptor	Avian retrovirus
neu	*HER2* receptor	Rat neuroblastoma
v-*fms*	*Csf*-1 receptor	Feline retrovirus
v-*ros*	Insulin receptor, β chain	Avian retrovirus
met	Hepatocyte growth factor receptor	Human osteosarcoma
k-*fgf/hst*	FGF-4	Human stomach cancer, Kaposi's sarcoma
int-2	FGF-3	Murine mammary tumors
trk family	NGF receptor family	Human colon carcinoma
v-*kit*	*Kit* ligand receptor	Feline retrovirus
v-*sea*	Related to insulin receptor	Avian erythroblastosis/ sarcoma virus
v-*erb*-A	Thyroid hormone receptor	Avian retrovirus

PDGF indicates platelet-derived growth factor; EGF, epidermal growth factor; FGF, fibroblast growth factor; NGF, nerve growth factor.
Table adapted from Mendelsohn et al., 2001.

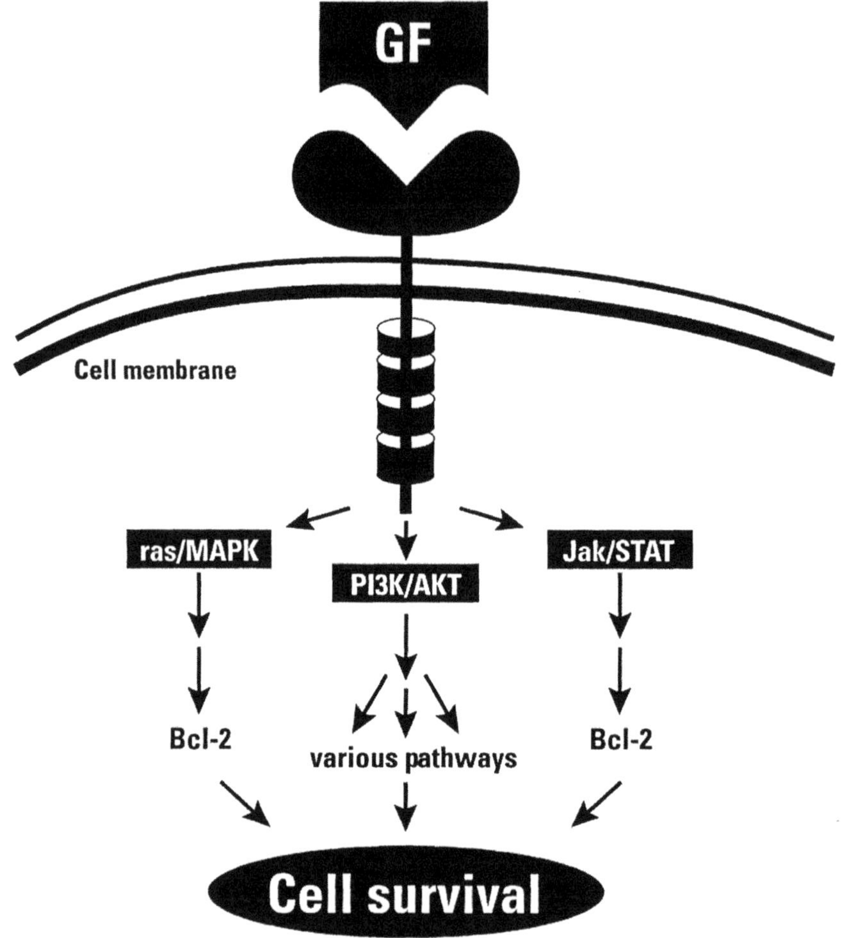

Figure 4. The 3 signaling pathways, PI3K/AKT, ras/MAPK, and Jak/STAT; pathways through which growth factors promote cell survival.

2.1. Epidermal Growth Factor Receptor Family

The role of the EGFR family of RTKs and their ligands in promoting human cancers has been studied extensively. There is clearly a correlation between aberrant EGFR signaling and malignancy. EGF and TGF-α are the primary mediators of EGFR-mediated activities.

2.1.1. Epidermal Growth Factor Receptor

Enhanced EGFR expression has been documented in a variety of tumors, including colon, squamous cell carcinoma of the head and neck (SCCHN), pancreatic , non–small cell lung cancer (NSCLC), breast, renal cell, ovarian, bladder, and gliomas (Salomon, Brandt, Ciardiello, & Normanno, 1995; Uegaki, 1997; Chow 1997). For some tumors, such as colorectal carcinoma and squamous cell carcinoma of the head and neck, the vast majority are EGFR-positive.

Alterations in EGFR expression or function can occur via enhanced ligand production, increased receptor gene transcription or amplification, or receptor mutations resulting in constitutive activation of tyrosine kinase (Chu et al., 1997; Ennis et al., 1991). Three EGFR mutations known to alter receptor function or activity have been identified, EGFRvI (Bigner et al., 1990), EGFRvII (Humphrey et al., 1991), and EGFRvIII. EGFRvIII, the most common variant, is expressed only on malignant cells and has been documented in a variety of tumor types, including gliomas, and prostate, breast, ovarian, and non–small cell lung cancers. (Garcia de Pallazzo et al., 1993; Moscatello et al., 1995; Wikstrand et al., 1995) The EGFRvIII possesses a constitutively activated tyrosine kinase and functions independent of ligands; in fact, it is unable to bind ligands or undergo dimerization (Chu et al., 1997). Furthermore, EGFRvIII has been shown to transform NIH3T3 cells (Moscatello et al., 1996).

Most recently, the existence of interreceptor communication and interconnected signaling networks has been identified. For example, EGFR and HER2 are involved in transducing signals by G-protein-coupled receptors (GPCRs), cytokines, RTKs, and integrins, and other stimulatory signaling pathways. This type of receptor activity has been linked to gene transcription and proliferation (reviewed in Prenzel, Fischer, Streit, Hart, & Ullrich, 2001). The HER-2 receptor has no known ligand, and is activated by heterodimerization with ligand-activated EGFR or HER-3.

2.1.2. Epidermal Growth Factor

The proliferative effects of EGF were demonstrated when EGF genes introduced into EGFR-positive NIH3T3 mouse fibroblasts resulted in cellular transformation and proliferation (Riedel, Massoglia, Schlessinger, & Ullrich, 1988). EGF has been implicated in a variety of tumorigenic mechanisms, including inhibition of apoptosis, promotion of angiogenesis, and enhanced motility and metastasis of cancer cells. Activation of the EGFR pathway can prolong survival. In a number of tumor cell lines with enhanced EGFR expression, the presence of EGF resulted in antiapoptotic activities and enhanced survival (Rodeck et al., 1997). EGF has been shown to protect breast adenocarcinoma cells against Fas-induced apoptosis (Gibson, Tu, Oyer, Anderson, & Johnson, 1999). EGF is mitogenic for endothelial cells *in vitro,* and, while it is not the most important growth factor affecting angiogenesis, it does activate angiogenic activities *in vivo* (Schreiber, Winkler, & Derynck, 1986) EGF enhances motility and metastatic potential in HER2-overexpressing breast cancer cells (Watabe et al., 1998). When the renal adenocarcinoma cell line, A704, was stimulated with EGF, the *in vitro* invasiveness, tumor cell motility, and matrix metalloproteinase (MMP-9) production were significantly increased, while cellular adhesion was significantly diminished, thus demonstrating a role in enhancing metastatic potential (Price, Wilson, & Haites, 1996). Additionally, EGF induced transfected breast cancer cells to migrate through an artificial membrane (Verbeek, Adriaansen-Slot, Vroom, Beckers, & Rijksen, 1998), increased the motility of squamous cell carcinoma cell lines (Shibata et al., 1996), and enhanced the invasiveness of glioma cells (Engebraaten, 1993).

2.1.3. Transforming Growth Factor-α

A variety of solid tumors, including gliomas, and kidney and lung tumors, were shown to secrete TGF-α. (Nickell, Halper, & Moses, 1983) The correlation between enhanced TGF-α activity, cellular proliferation, and neoplastic transformation has been documented in a number of studies in transgenic mice (Jhappan et al., 1990; Sandgren, Luetteke, Palmiter, Brinster, & Lee, 1990; Smith, Sharp, Kordon, Jhappan, & Merlino, 1995). Smith et al. demonstrated that enhanced TGF-α expression conferred a growth advantage in hyperplastic tissue and tumors, and that the tumorigenic ability of TGF-α arises from its stimulation of epithelial cell proliferation and its effects on prolonged cell survival. For example, TGF-α overexpression in transgenic mice resulted in mammary gland alveoli and terminal duct hyperplasia (Matsui, Halter, Holt, Hogan, & Coffey, 1990). Morphologic abnormalities in the mammary tissue included lobular hyperplasia, cystic hyperplasia, adenoma, and adenocarcinoma. Like EGF, TGF-α exhibits angiogenic activities; however, it is more potent (Schreiber et al., 1986). TGF-α has been shown to stimulate VEGF expression (Dvorak, Brown, Detmar, & Dvorak, 1995). In addition, expression of TGF-α on the endothelium of specimens from invasive breast cancer samples was positively correlated with microvessel density (MVD) (de Jong, van Diest, van der Valk, & Baak, 1997). Furthermore, co-expression of TGF-α and EGFR yielded a stronger positive correlation with MVD than did either TGF-α or EGFR alone, suggesting potential autocrine and paracrine loops for stimulation of angiogenesis. When a transfected malignant glioma cell line, U-1242 MG, was exposed to TGF-α, cellular motility was enhanced, as evidenced by cell scattering and increased phagokinetic track area (El-Obeid et al., 1997).

2.1.4. HER2

HER2 can be overexpressed on epithelial tumor cells, including breast, non–small cell lung, prostate, ovarian, bladder, and pancreatic carcinomas, and Wilm's tumor (Agus, Bunn, Franklin, Garcia, & Ozols, 2000; Menard, 2001). The correlation between HER2 gene amplification and its overexpression in breast cancer is undisputed. In a landmark study, Slamon et al. (1987) demonstrated that the HER2/*neu* oncogene was amplified from 2- to greater than 20-fold in 30% of breast cancers. HER2/*neu* gene amplification is associated with a more aggressive form of breast cancer characterized by significantly diminished disease-free and overall survival rates. A variety of studies using transfected cells improved understanding of HER2/*neu* signal transduction and confirmed the transforming capability of HER2/*neu* (Dougall et al., 1994). Transgenic mice carrying an activated c-*neu* oncogene controlled by the mouse mammary tumor virus (MMTV) developed mammary adenocarcinomas (Bouchard, Lamarre, Tremblay, & Jolicoeur, 1989; Muller, Sinn, Pattengale, Wallace, & Leder, 1988). While malignant transformation occurred in mammary tissue, expression of the c-*neu* transgene in the parotid gland or epididymis resulted in benign hypertrophy and hyperplasia that did not undergo malignant transformation (Muller et al., 1988).

2.1.5. HER3 and HER4

The roles of HER3 and HER4 in human cancers are not as well described as for EGFR and HER2. A product of *erb*-b3 expression is the $p180^{erbB3}$ protein, which can be overexpressed in a variety of cancers, including breast, ovarian, cervix, pancreas, stomach, colon, and prostate (reviewed in Mendelsohn et al., 2001). Data have shown that the tyrosine kinase domain of ErbB-3 is homologous to those of the EGFR and HER2, with 64% and 67% homology, respectively (Kraus, Issing, Miki, Popescu, & Aaronson, 1989). Despite the high degree of homology, the differences in the ErbB-3 tyrosine kinase amino acid sequence result in an impaired tyrosine kinase activity that is substantially lower than for EGFR or HER2 (Guy, Platko, Cantley, Cerione, & Carraway, 1994). When NIH3T3 cells were transfected with EGFR, HER2, HER3, and HER4 receptors alone and in varying combinations, results showed that cells expressing only HER3 or HER4 resulted in mitogenesis but not transformation in the presence of Neu differentiation factor (NDF) (Zhang et al., 1996). This growth factor is also known as heregulin, especially when its activities outside the nervous system are focused upon. However, when EGFR or HER2 was co-expressed with HER3 or HER4, NDF-induced transformation of the NIH3T3 cells occurred. Co-expression of HER2 and HER3 resulted in transformation of NIH3T3 cells when neither gene alone resulted in transformation (Alimandi et al., 1995). Synergy between the 2 receptors was achieved via receptor heterodimerization and enhanced tyrosine phosphorylation of HER3. Receptor interactions, EGFR or HER2 with HER3, may be important in conferring the ability to transform cells and result in malignancy (Pinkas-Kramarski et al., 1996), HER3 signaling functions are constitutively activated in some breast cancer cell lines, thus providing further evidence for a role in the pathogenesis of malignancies (Kraus, Fedi, Starks, Muraro, & Aaronson, 1993). The role of HER4 in tumorigenesis has not been elucidated.

2.2. Growth Factors with Angiogenic Properties

It has become increasingly clear that angiogenesis contributes to tumor growth, invasiveness, and metastatic spread (Fidler & Ellis, 1994; Folkman, 1996). Growth factors promote angiogenesis in tumors by a variety of mechanisms, including enhanced expression of VEGF receptors, paracrine secretion of growth factors by tumor cells, and autocrine secretion of angiogenic growth factors by tumor-associated endothelial cells (Gasparini, 1999).

2.2.1. Vascular Endothelial Growth Factor (VEGF)

VEGF, expressed by many cancers, is one of the most important growth factors known to mediate angiogenesis (Dvorak et al., 1995; Senger et al., 1993). VEGF promotes tumor growth in a number of ways, including enhanced endothelial cell proliferation, increased vascular permeability, and promotion of protein extravasation (Poon, Fan, & Wong, 2001). Several studies have demonstrated that VEGF confers survival on endothelial cells in newly formed tumor vessels (Benjamin, Golijanin, Itin, Pode, & Keshet, 1999; Benjamin & Keshet, 1997). Tumor cell VEGF production is induced in response to hypoxia (Shweiki, Itin, Soffer, & Keshet, 1992). Furthermore, paracrine production of VEGF by tumor cells can further contribute to angiogenesis. VEGF expression can be mediated by a variety of factors. For example, VEGF production is upregulated by oncogenes such as *ras,* (Rak et al., 1995) a mutated form of the p53 tumor suppressor gene (Kieser, Weich, Brandner, Marme, & Kolch, 1994), and activated EGF and HER2 receptors (Petit et al., 1997).

2.2.2. Platelet-derived Growth Factor (PDGF)

Aberrant PDGF activity is implicated in the pathogenesis of a variety of solid tumors, including glioblastoma, prostate, sarcoma, and breast and may exert its effects through both autocrine and paracrine stimulation (George, 2001; Heldin & Westermark, 1999). PDGF can promote tumor growth in a variety of ways. Studies evaluating the effects of PDGF-AA and PDGF-BB found that PDGF-BB possessed a greater transforming potential (Beckmann et al., 1988) and was more effective in inducing angiogenic responses and stimulating endothelial cell chemotaxis (Risau et al., 1992). PDGF has been shown to induce VEGF expression in endothelial cells expressing βPDGFR (Wang, Huang, Kazlauskas, & Cavenee, 1999). PDGF-BB has also been shown to promote endothelial cell proliferation and differentiation (Battegay 1994). In a study by Forsberg, Valyi-Nagy, Heldin, Helyn & Westermark (1993), PDGF-BB stimulated tumor connective tissue stroma development that was rich in newly formed blood vessels. The importance of PDGF in blood vessel and connective tissue formation was highlighted in several studies of knockout mice that failed to develop fully in the absence of normal PDGF signaling (Bostrom et al., 1996; Leveen et al., 1994; Soriano, 1994). Co-expression of PDGF and PDGFR in human glioma and meningioma cell lines suggests that autocrine stimulation by PDGF may be important in cellular transformation and tumorigenesis (Maxwell, Galanopoulos, Hedley-Whyte, Black, & Antoniades, 1990; Westermark, Heldin, & Nister, 1995).

2.2.3. Fibroblast Growth Factor (FGF)

FGFs are also implicated in angiogenesis, with FGF2 being the most important. FGF2 (basic or bFGF) was the first pro-angiogenic factor, discovered in the mid-1980s (Shing et al., 1984). VEGF and FGF2 have synergistic effects on inducing angiogenesis both *in vitro* and *in vivo* (Asahara et al., 1995; Goto, Goto, Weindel, & Folkman, 1993; Pepper, Ferrera, Orci, & Montesano, 1992). FGF2 also enhanced VEGF secretion by the U-105 MG glioma cell line (Tsai, Goldman, & Gillespie, 1995).

In addition to their angiogenic effects, FGFs exert mitogenic and antiapoptotic activities upon tumor cells (reviewed in Powers et al., 2000). There is evidence to suggest a role for FGF1 and FGF2 in the modulation of cellular adhesion, differentiation, and invasion, as seen in a study of several human pancreatic adenocarcinoma cell lines (El-Hariry, Pignatelli, & Lemoine, 2001). FGFs and their receptors appear to be involved in the pathogenesis of human cancers through a variety of effects. FGFs can mediate both endothelial cell growth and chemotaxis (Aigner et al., 2001).

Dysregulation of FGF activities can occur owing to elevated FGF levels and/or activity, or by increased expression of their receptors in tumor cells. Greater than 90% of human gliomas express FGF1 and FGF2 messenger ribonucleic acid (mRNA), with the level of FGF2 expression positively correlated with the degree of malignancy (Stefanik, Rizkalla, Soi, Goldblatt, & Rizkalla, 1991; Takahashi et al., 1990). Additional studies demonstrated FGF2 production by glioma tumor cells, providing evidence for promotion of tumorigenesis in an autocrine manner (Takahashi et al., 1992). Four mechanisms resulting in aberrant FGFR signaling have been identified: inappropriate expression, point mutations, splice variations, and genomic alterations; however, not all of these alterations have a proven role in promoting human cancers (Powers et al., 2000). Alterations in FGFR overexpression or signaling have been detected in a variety of cancers, including pancreatic (Wagner, Lopez, Cahn, & Korc, 1998), thyroid (Onose, Emoto, Sugihara, Shimizu, & Wakabayashi, 1999), prostate (Giri, Ropiquet, & Ittmann, 1999), multiple myeloma (Plowright et al., 2000), breast (Tannheimer, Rehemtulla, & Ethier, 2000), glioblastoma (Morrison et al., 1994), astrocytoma (Yamaguchi, Saya, Bruner, & Morrison, 1994), malignant melanoma (Ahmed et al., 1997), and salivary gland (Myoken et al., 1996). Several FGFR gene chromosomal rearrangements resulting in enhanced FGFR activity have been identified: one in a rat osteosarcoma cell line and another in a human myeloma cell line. (Lorenzi, Horii, Yamanaka, Sakaguchi, & Miki, 1996; Otsuki et al., 1999)

2.3. *Transforming Growth Factor-β Pathway*

TGF-β normally inhibits the proliferation of most cell types, but in tumor cells this effect is often bypassed (Massague, 1990). In addition, TGF-β possesses angiogenic and immunosuppressive effects, such as inhibition of tumoricidal natural and lymphocyte-activated killer cells (Gold 1999). TGF-β has also been shown to promote tumor cell invasion and metastasis by autocrine stimulation (Dumont & Arteaga, 2000; Roman, Saha, & Beauchamp, 2001). Taken together, these effects confer a survival advantage for tumor cells (Platten et al., 2001).

Dysregulation of TGF-β signaling resulting in oncogenesis can occur owing to alterations at the level of the receptor, the signal transduction pathway, or the cell cycle proteins (Gold, 1999). Many human cancer cell lines, including retinoblastoma, squamous cell, endometrial, breast, bladder, small-cell lung, gastric, colon, and lymphomas, develop resistance to the antiproliferative effects normally associated with TGF-β (Filmus & Kerbel, 1993; reviewed in Mendelsohn et al., 2001). TGF-β overexpression is associated with a loss in the inhibitory effects generally mediated by TGF-β, and this typically occurs in the late stages of carcinogenesis (Gold 1999; Haddow, Fowlis, Parkinson, Akhurst, & Balmain, 1991 Rossmanith & Schulte-Hermann, 2001).

Downregulation or loss of function of the TGF-β receptors also has been shown to contribute to cancer development. A number of studies have demonstrated that genetic mutations of TGF-β RII are present in various cancers and that such mutations confer a growth advantage and allow cells to escape from the antiproliferative effects of TGF-β (Markowitz et al., 1995; Myeroff et al., 1995; Parsons et al., 1995). In neoplastic breast samples, diminished TGF-β RII expression was correlated with resistance to inhibition, proliferation, or tumor progression, and a significant inverse correlation between diminished TGF-β RII expression and tumor grade and mitotic count was observed (Gobbi et al., 2000).

Dysregulation of TGF-β signal transduction can occur owing to alterations in Smad proteins, the downstream mediators of the action of TGF-β receptor signals (Rooke & Crosier, 2001). A number of studies have identified cancers that express mutations in Smad genes , which alter TGF-β signaling (Eppert et al., 1996; Howe et al., 1998; Riggins et al., 1996). These results suggest that Smad genes may be tumor suppressors important in regulating the antiproliferative effects of TGF-β (Eppert et al., 1996). Loss of functional Smad proteins has been correlated with carcinogenesis.

2.4. Insulin-like Growth Factor

Elevated levels of IGF-I and IGF-II and overexpression of the IGF-I-R are observed in most tumors and transformed cell lines (Baserga, Porcu, Rubini, & Sell, 1994; Baserga, Sell, Porcu, & Rubini, 1994; Werner & LeRoith, 1996). Studies in transgenic mice have demonstrated the carcinogenic potential of IGF-I and IGF-II (Bates et al., 1995; Bol, Kiguchi, Gimenez-Conti, Rupp, & DiGiovanni, 1997; Rogler et al., 1994). IGF-II overexpression induced the development of mammary tumors that expressed elevated levels of IGF-II mRNA (Bates et al., 1995). Furthermore, the incidence of tumor development in transgenic mice with persistently elevated levels of serum IGF-II was greater than in controls (Rogler et al., 1994). Hepatocellular carcinomas, lymphomas, squamous cell carcinomas, sarcomas, and thyroid carcinomas were observed in the transgenic mice. The authors speculated that given the long latency period and the variety of tumor types, IGF-II may promote tumor progression by both autocrine and endocrine stimulation. In comparison to control mice, mice overexpressing IGF-I demonstrated hyperplasia, spontaneous tumor development, faster onset to tumor development, and increased incidence of tumors (Bol et al., 1997).

The IGF-I-R has a variety of functions that are important in the development of human cancers. It has been shown to mediate cellular proliferation in vivo and in vitro, to establish and maintain the transformed phenotype, and to protect cells from apoptosis (Rubin & Baserga, 1995). In vitro studies have shown antiapoptotic effects of IGFs and IGF-I-R, which confer increased cell survival (Baserga, 1995). IGF-I-R protects cells from apoptosis via three signaling pathways, each of which results in phosphorylation of Bad, a member of the Bcl-2 family of proteins. This includes activation of the phosphoinositide 3-kinase (PI3-K), Akt/protein kinase B path; activation through the mitogen-activated protein kinase (MAPK) path; and activation and mitochondrial translocation of Raf-1 (Peruzzi et al., 1999). In vivo studies have also demonstrated that the anti-apoptotic effects of the IGF-I-R, which lead to increased cell survival, are independent of its mitogenic activity (Resnicoff, Burgaud, Rotman, Abraham, & Baserga, 1995; Sell, Baserga, & Rubin, 1995).

A number of factors have been shown to regulate the expression of the IGF-I-R and its ligands, including growth factors (e.g., PDGF, FGF2, EGF), steroid hormones (e.g., estradiol and progesterone), oncogenes (e.g., SV40 T antigen, hepatitis B virus X [HBx] protein, and c-myb), and tumor suppressor genes (e.g., WT1, p53, and RB) (Baserga, Porcu et al., 1994; Baserga, Sell et al., 1994; Werner & LeRoith, 2000). The authors theorize that these factors may promote the growth and transformation of cells by directly or indirectly activating the IGF autocrine loop.

3. CLINICAL IMPLICATIONS: TARGETING GROWTH FACTOR SIGNAL TRANSDUCTION

Given the effects of growth factors on processes such as proliferation, differentiation, survival, apoptosis, angiogenesis, invasion, and metastasis, it is clear that aberrant growth factor signaling is a major factor in malignant transformation. Targeting growth factors at the molecular level and disrupting aberrant signaling pathways presents a rational and unique approach to anticancer treatment, particularly for cancers for which only limited treatment options are available. Traditional chemotherapeutic and radiation approaches used for late-stage cancers typically provide modest benefit, often limited to short-term palliation. In addition to the efficacy limitations associated with chemotherapy and radiation, their toxicity profiles often limit administration at the dose and/or schedule necessary for tumor eradication. The field of molecular targeting of various aspects of the growth factor signaling pathways has grown tremendously over the past few decades, and promising preclinical and clinical results have been achieved in a variety of human cancers.

3.1. Prognostic Value of Growth Factor and Receptor Expression in Malignancy

With the identification of the role of growth factor signaling in malignancy, researchers began investigating the prognostic value of growth factor and growth factor receptor expression in a variety of tumors. While some conflicting data exist, even within the same tumor type, a large body of evidence suggests that expression of growth factor receptors and/or their ligands in various tumors may provide invaluable information in cancer management, not only with respect to diagnosis, but also regarding prognosis and response to therapy. Many studies have demonstrated a positive correlation between growth factor or growth factor receptor expression and a poor prognosis; examples are presented in Table 2.

3.2. Growth Factor Signaling Pathways as Therapeutic Targets

Biological therapy specifically targeted to growth factor signaling pathways presents a unique, rational approach to the treatment and management of cancer.

Table 2. Prognostic value of growth factor and receptor expression

Growth Factor or Receptor	*Tumor Type*	*Observation*	*Reference*
EGFR	NSCLC	Diminished overall survival, enhanced invasiveness, poor differentiation, high growth rate	(Pavelic, Banjac, Pavelic, & Spaventi, 1993; Veale, Kerr, Gibson, Kelly, & Harris, 1993; Volm, Rittgen, & Drings, 1998)
	SCCHN	Diminished relapse-free survival and overall survival, increased tumor size, advanced stage	(Grandis et al., 1998; Maurizi et al., 1996; Santini et al., 1991)
	Breast	Diminished relapse-free survival and overall survival short-term (1-4 years)	(Klijn, Berns, Schmitz, & Foekens, 1992)
	Bladder	Increased risk of and diminished time to recurrence and progression	(Neal et al., 1990; Turkeri, Erton, Cevik, & Akdas, 1998)
	Ovarian	Diminished progressive-free period and overall survival, resistance to chemotherapy	(Bartlett et al., 1996; Fischer-Colbrie et al., 1997)
	Colorectal	Poor prognosis	(Mayer et al., 1993)
HER2	Breast	Diminished time to disease relapse and overall survival	(Harris, Nicholson, Sainsbury, Wright, & Farndon, 1992; Slamon et al., 1987)

VEGF	Various (breast, lung, colorectal, gastric, pancreatic, hepatocellular, prostate, bladder, ovarian, head and neck, osteosarcoma, melanoma, leukemia)	Tumor progression, advanced tumor stage, diminished survival	(Reviewed in Poon et al., 2001)
PDGF	Various (lung, gastric, breast, pulmonary adenocarcinoma, epithelial ovarian)	Poor prognosis, advanced stage, nodal metastasis, diminished survival, decreased response to chemotherapy	(Henriksen et al, 1993; Kawai, Hiroi, & Torikata, 1997; Nakamura, Katano, Fujimoto, & Morisaki 1997; Seymour & Bezwoda, 1994; Takanami, Imamura, Yamamoto, & Kodaira, 1995)
TGF-β	NSCLC	Lymph node metastasis, advanced stage	(Hasegawa et al., 2001)
	Prostate	Poor prognosis	(Wikstrom, Damber, & Bergh, 2001)
	Gastric	Depth of invasion, advanced stage	(Saito et al., 1999)

Based upon the impressive anti-tumor activities observed in extensive preclinical testing utilizing in both *in vitro* and *in vivo* models, many agents aimed at blocking growth factor-mediated pathways are in clinical testing for a variety of tumor types. Clinical results for those agents furthest along in testing are presented below in some detail. Some other agents in preclinical or early clinical testing are listed in Table 3.

Table 3. Agents targeting growth factor signaling pathways: preclinical and early clinical testing

Target	*Type*	*Example(s)*	*Reference*
EGFR	Humanized IgG_1 Mab	h-R3	(Morales et al., 2000)
	Murine MAb	EMD55900	(Faillot et al., 1996)
	Rat MAb	ICR-62	Modjtahedi et al., 1996)
	Bispecific antibody (EGFR X FcγRI)	H22-EGF, MDX-447	(Goldstein, Graziano, Sundarapandiyan, Somasundaram, & Deo, 1997; Wallace et al., 2000)
	EGFR conjugates	Anti-EGFR MAb fused to *Pseudomonas exotoxin* A, gelonin, or recombinant ricin A	(Engebraaten, Sivam, Juell, & Fodstad, 2000)
	Antisense therapy		
EGF	EGF conjugate	EGF fused to genistein or *Pseudomonas exotoxin*	(Saito, Mitsui, & Mizuno, 2000)
TGF-α	TGF-α conjugate	TGF-α fused to saporin or *Pseudomonas exotoxin* A	(Baldwin, Kobrin, Tran, Pastan, & Korc, 1996)
	Antisense therapy		
HER2	Bispecific antibody (HER2 X FcγRI)	MDX-H210	(James et al., 2001)
	HER2 oncogenic protein vaccine		(Esserman et al., 1999)
	DNA immunization		
	Gene therapy	Adenovirus 5 E1A gene	(Ueno, Yu, & Hung, 2001)
	Antisense therapy		
IGF	GHRH antagonist		
	IGF-competitor	Suramin	(Benini et al., 2001)
	Antisense therapy		
IGF-IR	Mab	AlphaIR3	(Benini et al., 2001)

3.2.1 Epidermal Growth Factor Receptor

A variety of approaches to block the EGFR-mediated signaling pathways are undergoing clinical evaluation, including use of anti-EGFR monoclonal antibodies (MAbs), tyrosine kinase inhibitors (TKIs), ligand-toxin conjugates, immunoconjugates, and antisense oligonucleotides. The anti-EGFR MAbs and TKIs are the most promising, and thus far are furthest along in clinical testing, with phase III trials underway in a variety of cancers. Data suggest that EGFR blocking agents can exert their greatest therapeutic benefit when first administered with cytotoxic therapy in order to enhance initial response rates (Mendelsohn & Baselga, 2000), and then given as maintenance in order to prevent disease progression or recurrence (Slichenmyer & Fry, 2001).

Anti-Epidermal Growth Factor Receptor Monoclonal Antibodies. IMC-C225 (Erbitux™, cetuximab), a human:murine chimeric anti-EGFR IgG_1 MAb with a binding affinity greater than or equal to that of natural ligands (Fan, Masui, Altas, & Mendelsohn, 1993; Goldstein, Prewett, Zuklys, Rockwell, & Mendelsohn, 1995; Wu et al., 1996), was the first EGF receptor inhibitor discovered (Kawamoto et al., 1983; Kawamoto et al., 1984; Masui et al., 1984) and is the MAb furthest along in clinical evaluation. IMC-C225 has been studied in cultures and xenographs of colorectal, squamous cell head and neck, non–small cell lung, pancreatic, renal cell, prostate, and breast tumor cells, primarily in combination with chemotherapy or radiation (Baselga et al., 1993; Fan, Baselga, Masui, & Mendelsohn, 1993; Mendelsohn, 2000). IMC-C225 exerts its antitumor effects via multiple proposed mechanisms of action, including inhibition of cell cycle progression, promotion of apoptosis, inhibition of angiogenesis and metastasis, and immunologic effects (Herbst, Kim, & Harari, 2001; Mendelsohn, 2000). There are extensive data to confirm enhanced antitumor activity in numerous tumor types when IMC-C225 is combined with various chemotherapeutic agents or radiation (Herbst, Tran et al., 2001). Results of a pivotal phase II trial in which 121 patients with refractory colorectal carcinoma received IMC-C225 in combination with irinotecan yielded a 22.5% partial response for a median duration of 84 days in patients who had progressed on an irinotecan-containing regimen (Saltz et al., 2001). Additionally, in a phase II study of IMC-C225 monotherapy for chemotherapy-refractory colorectal carcinoma, 11% of patients achieved a partial response (Saltz et al., 2002). With a median follow-up of 4 months, the median survival had not been reached. In another phase II study, patients with recurrent SCCHN received 2 cycles of a cisplatin-containing regimen, and those who demonstrated progressive or stable disease went on to receive IMC-C225 and cisplatin. (Hong et al., 2001) Patients who demonstrated stable disease (n=38) after the initial cisplatin-containing regimen achieved a 21% objective response rate (1 complete response and 7 partial response). Results from a third phase II trial, evaluating IMC-C225 in combination with gemcitabine in patients with previously untreated advanced pancreatic cancer, showed a 12% partial response rate after two courses of therapy. Additionally, 39% of the patients had stable disease or a minor response. This clinical trial showed that median time to progression (TTP) improved when compared to previous phase III trial results of gemcitabine monotherapy when patients received IMC-C225 in combination with gemcitabine (Abbruzzese et al., 2001; Burris et al., 1997). In a phase II trial of IMC-C225 in combination with radiation for advanced SCCHN, 13 of 15 patients achieved a complete response (Bonner, 2000). A phase III trial has completed accrual. The most clinically significant adverse events in the IMC-C225 trials were an acne-like rash and an allergic reaction. While the majority of patients develop an acne-like rash at the target dose, it is generally mild (grade 1 or 2), is not dose limiting, and typically resolves completely within 4–8 weeks after therapy has been discontinued (Herbst, Kim et al., 2001). The incidence of grade 3–4 allergic reactions is small (4%), and a number of patients were successfully rechallenged by administration of prophylactic antihistamines and by slowing the infusion rate (Cohen, Falcey, Paulter, Fetzer, & Waksal, 2000). Over 900 patients have received IMC-C225, and clinical experience confirms the favorable toxicity profile of this agent in combination with cytotoxic therapy (Cohen et al., 2000). These studies document the clinical activity for combination therapy with IMC-C225 in various tumors and the ability to safely administer IMC-C225 in combination with cytotoxic therapies.

ABX-EGF, a human IgG_2 MAb that binds to the EGFR with high affinity (5×10^{11} M), completely eradicated well-established A431 xenografts and significantly prolonged tumor inhibition, suggesting its potential as single-agent therapy for EGFR-positive solid tumors (Yang et al., 1999; Yang et al., 2000; Yang, Jia, Corvalan, Wang, & Davis, 2001). An assessment of the efficacy of ABX-EGF monotherapy requires additional clinical testing. A phase I study evaluating the safety of ABX-EGF monotherapy in various advanced cancers (renal, prostate, pancreatic, non–small cell lung, and esophageal) revealed the appearance of grades 1 and 3 cutaneous toxicity that completely resolved within 4 weeks (Figlin et al., 2001). Human anti-human antibodies (HAHA) were not detected in any patients. One patient achieved disease stabilization for a period of 6 months, and additional dose levels are being explored.

Tyrosine Kinase Inhibitors (TKIs). TKIs are small molecular weight inhibitors that target the intracellular tyrosine kinase by inhibiting receptor autophosphorylation and subsequent signal transduction. TKIs compete with the ATP binding site and inhibit tyrosine trans-phosphorylation (Raymond, Faivre, & Armand, 2000). Given the nature of TKI activity, TKIs may be able to inhibit EGFR signaling that is activated independent of ligand binding. The clinical utility of TKIs was initially hampered by their lack of potency and specificity; however, recent TKIs demonstrate increased potency and relative EGFR specificity as well as promising antitumor activity. TKIs fall into 4 main chemical classes as shown in Table 4.

Table 4. Epidermal growth factor receptor tyrosine kinase inhibitors

Class	*Example*	*Reversible/Irreversible*
Dianilinophthalimide	CGP 54211	Reversible
	CGP 53353	Reversible
Pyridopyrimidine	PK 158780	Reversible
	PD 165557 (PD 158780 analog)	Reversible
4-(phenylamino)pyr-rolopyrimidine	CPG 59326	Reversible
	PKI 166	Reversible
Quinazoline	PD 153035	Reversible
	PD 168393 (PD 153035 analog)	Irreversible
	PD 160678 (PD 153035 analog)	Irreversible
	CP 358774 (OSI-774)	Reversible
	ZD 1839	Reversible
	PD 183805 (CI-1033)	Irreversible
	EKB-569	Irreversible

Data from Fry (2000) and Ciardiello et al. (2000).

The dianilinophthalimides and pyridopyrimidines are not selective for the EGFR. It is primarily the anilinoquinazolines that have demonstrated improvements in potency, specificity for the EGFR tyrosine kinase, and in vitro and in vivo efficacy (Fry, 2000). While 2 TKIs, ZD-1839 (Iressa™) and OSI-774 (Tarceva™, formerly CP-358,774), have entered into phase II/III testing, the majority are in the early phases of preclinical and clinical testing. TKIs are administered orally, making long-term therapy convenient.

ZD-1839 potently inhibits the EGFR, with minimal activity demonstrated against other tyrosine kinases including HER2, KDR, c-flt, or serine/threonine kinases (Woodburn, Kendrew, & Fennell, 2000). Mechanisms for antitumor activities include inhibition of EGFR autophosphorylation and reduction in c-Fos mRNA, a downstream biomarker for EGFR tyrosine kinase activation (Woodburn, Barker, 1996; Woodburn et al., 2000), delay of cell cycle progression via dysregulation of cyclin-dependent kinase 2 (CDK2), upregulation of the CDK inhibitor, $p27^{Kip1}$ (Budillon et al., 2000), and inhibition of angiogenesis (Ciardiello et al., 2001). Antitumor effects may also be attributed to inhibition of autocrine and paracrine growth factor production (Ciardiello et al., 2001). In vitro and in vivo studies have confirmed its antitumor activity against various tumor types (reviewed in Baselga & Averbuch, 2000). ZD-1839 demonstrates dose- and time-dependent growth inhibition of various cell lines and cytostatic dose-dependent inhibition of tumor growth in xenograft models (Ciardiello et al., 2001). The antitumor effects of ZD-1839 are potentiated when it is administered in combination with various chemotherapeutic agents (Ciardiello et al., 2000). When cancer cells were exposed to ZD-1839 alone, reversible cytostatic antiproliferative effects and increased apoptosis were noted; however, when cells were treated with ZD-1839 in combination with a cytotoxic agent, a dose-dependent supra-additive increase in growth inhibition and markedly enhanced anti-apoptotic effects were observed. Combination therapy was associated with a significantly prolonged survival in xenografted mice ($p \leq 0.05$). Antitumor activity is achieved regardless of the EGFR expression level (Sirotnak, Zakowsky, Miller, Scher, & Kris, 2000). Additionally, there is evidence to suggest that ZD-1839 may have potential applications in cancer prevention (Chan et al., 2000). Phase I evaluation of two administration schedules, intermittent (daily for 14 days every 28 days) and continuous (daily), demonstrated that ZD-1839 exhibited predictable pharmacokinetics and was well tolerated. (Baselga & Averbuch, 2000; Ranson et al., 2002; Nakagawa et al., 2000) The most frequent adverse events included mild (grades 1–2) skin changes (characterized as an acne-like rash) and diarrhea. More severe adverse events were rare and were generally attributed to disease progression. The preliminary results of these three phase I trials of ZD-1839 alone demonstrated encouraging antitumor activity in a variety of tumors, with particularly favorable results achieved in patients with non–small cell lung cancer. The activity of 2 dose levels of ZD-1839 for advanced NSCLC was assessed in 2 phase II trials, IDEAL 1, which included patients who had failed 1 or 2 platinum-based chemotherapy regimens, and IDEAL 2, for patients who had failed 2 or more prior platinum- and docetaxel-based chemotherapy regimens. In IDEAL 1, the objective tumor response rates were 18.4% and 19.0% for the 250 mg/day and 500 mg/day groups, respectively (Fukuoka et al., 2002). The tumor response rates were lower in IDEAL 2, 11.8% and 8.8% for the 250 mg/day and 500 mg/day groups respectively (Kris et al., 2002). In patients with non–small cell lung cancer, improvements in disease status were correlated with improved quality-of-life scores and disease-related symptoms (Baselga & Averbuch, 2000). Additional data confirm PR, SD, and minor responses in some patients (Baselga & Averbuch, 2000; Ransonet al., 2002; Goss et al., 2001). Early results are available for ZD-1839 in combination with chemotherapy. Preliminary efficacy results for 25 previously untreated advanced non–small cell lung cancer patients who received ZD-1839 in combination with carboplatin and paclitaxel included 7 PR and 10 SD (Miller et al., 2001). The combination was well tolerated and ZD-1839 did not exacerbate the toxicity associated with carboplatin or paclitaxel. The efficacy of ZD-1839 in combination with 5-fluorouracil and leucovorin for patients with advanced colorectal cancer was demonstrated in a small number of patients (Hammond et al., 2001). Of 17 patients treated, 1 achieved a complete response (CR) and 4 achieved a PR (3 confirmed) without evidence of cumulative toxicity. Preliminary results from a phase I/II study of ZD-1839 monotherapy for patients with advanced or metastatic colorectal carcinoma indicated that while 4 of 27 patients demonstrated radiological evidence of tumor shrinkage, no responses were observed (Goss et al., 2002). Numerous preclinical and clinical studies are underway to further define the antitumor activities and clinical benefit associated with ZD-1839 administration. In addition to these clinical studies, a phase II multicenter trial conducted by Baselga et al. (2001) evaluated safety and efficacy of ZD-1839 in 210 patients with non–small cell lung cancer who had failed 1 or 2 previous chemotherapy regimens. Patients received either 250 mg/day or 500 mg/day ZD-1839 and demonstrated 18.7% overall relapse rate (RR), 52.9% disease control rate, and 84 days median progression-free survival. During this study, fewer patients who received 250 mg/day experienced grade 3 or 4 adverse events (32%) than those who received 500 mg/day (51%). Severe adverse events included grade 3 diarrhea and grade 3/4 rash. Approximately 10% of the patients receiving 500 mg/day withdrew from the study owing to drug-related adverse events, compared to 2% of those receiving 250 mg/day. The investigators concluded that ZD-1839 250 mg/day provided equal efficacy and was better tolerated than 500 mg/day.

OSI-774 is a potent, specific, reversible TKI. Assays of isolated kinases and whole cells demonstrated selectivity for the EGFR tyrosine kinase relative to other kinases (Moyer et al., 1997). OSI-774 completely blocked EGF-induced EGFR autophosphorylation, inhibited proliferation of tumor cells in cell culture, blocked cell cycle progression by arresting cells in the G_1 phase, resulted in accumulation of $p27^{Kip1}$ and unphosphorylated retinoblastoma protein, which may contribute to inhibition of cell cycle progression, and induced apoptosis in some cell lines (Hidalgo et al., 2001; Moyer et al., 1997). OSI-774 administered to athymic mice exhibited dose-related antitumor activity against HN5 xenografts (Pollack et al., 1999). Tumor volumes were significantly reduced during treatment; however, tumors began to enlarge after treatment was discontinued, albeit at a slower rate than in controls. Furthermore, cisplatin administered in combination with OSI-774 resulted in additive antitumor effects without exacerbation of cisplatin-induced toxicity. Phase I analyses revealed that OSI-774 exhibited a dose-dependent pharmacokinetic profile and was well tolerated; cutaneous toxicity (characterized as acneiform rashes), mucositis, diarrhea, fatigue, headache, and nausea were cited as the most common side effects (Hidalgo et al., 2001; Karp et al., 1999; Rowinsky et al., 2001; Siu et al., 1999). One study utilized positron emission tomography (PET) with ^{18}fluorodeoxyglucose to visually detect antitumor activity (Hammond et al., 2000). PET scans demonstrated a marked reduction in uptake of the tracer several weeks before radiologic imaging confirmed tumor reduction. Preliminary data from phase II studies revealed encouraging antitumor activity for OSI-774 as a single agent. Of 56 patients with stage IIIB/IV or recurrent metastatic non–small cell lung cancer, 7 achieved a PR (6 confirmed) and 19 demonstrated SD (Perez-Soler et al., 2001). Interestingly, all 6 patients with a confirmed response developed a cutaneous rash. Responses were independent of the level of EGFR expression. In 30 evaluable patients with advanced, refractory ovarian carcinoma, 3 achieved a PR and 3 SD (Finkler et al., 2001). OSI-774 also demonstrated activity in advanced SCCHN, with 10 of 78 evaluable patients achieving a PR and 23 SD (Senzer et al., 2001). In all 3 studies, the most prominent toxicities were a mild acneiform rash, noted in the majority of patients, and diarrhea. Additional reversible TKIs in early preclinical testing include PD158780, CGP 59326A, PD153035, PKI 166 (formerly CGP75166), and GW2016.

Two irreversible TKIs under evaluation are CI-033 and EKB-569. CI-1033, a pan-erbB TKI, is highly specific for EGFR, HER2, HER3, and HER4 and does not inhibit the TK activity of other receptors, even at high concentrations (Slichenmyer,

Elliot, & Fry, 2001). CI-1033 resulted in significant suppression of tumor growth in xenograft models (Slichenmyer et al., 2001). *In vitro* data suggest synergistic antitumor activities when it is administered in combination with cytotoxic agents. For example, when administered with gemcitabine, there was an increase in the apoptotic fraction with activation of p38 and suppression of Akt and MAPK activation (Nelson & Fry, 2001); synergistic antiproliferative effects when administered with an active metabolite of irinotecan (Erlichman et al., 2001); and synergistic inhibition with cisplatin (Gieseg, de Bock, Ferguson, & Denny, 2001). Preliminary phase I results in patients with advanced solid tumors showed achievement of PR and SD by a number of patients with the primary toxicities of mild (grade 1–2) acneiform rash, reversible grade 3 thrombocytopenia, diarrhea, and vomiting (Garrison et al., 2001; Shin et al., 2001). EKB-569 is a potent inhibitor of the EGFR TK and receptor autophosphorylation (Greenberger et al., 2000). In $APC^{Min/+}$ mice, a murine model of human familial adenomatous polyposis (FAP), EKB-569 in combination with sulindac provided protection from intestinal neoplasia (Torrance et al., 2000).

3.2.2. HER2

Like EGFR, there are a variety of anti-HER2 approaches undergoing preclinical and clinical testing, including anti-HER2 MAbs, bispecific MAbs, antisense strategies, and anti-HER2 immunization modalities.

Anti-HER2 Monoclonal Antibodies. A highly specific murine anti-HER2 MAb, termed 4D5, binds to the extracellular domain of HER2 and inhibits proliferation of HER2-overexpressing cells but does not inhibit proliferation of cells with low HER2 expression (Sarup et al., 1991). Binding of 4D5 resulted in agonist activities, downregulation of HER2, stimulation of receptor internalization, and HER2 phosphorylation. With extended exposure, 4D5 downregulated signaling pathways and inhibited cell proliferation of SK-BR-3 human breast carcinoma cells. In another study utilizing the SK-BR-3 cell line, 4D5 resulted in a dose-dependent decrease in VEGF expression, thus suggesting antiangiogenic activity (Petit et al., 1997). In addition, 4D5 enhanced tumor necrosis factor alpha (TNF-α) sensitivity in cells that overexpress HER2, prevented colony formation of NIH3T3 cells transformed by expression of HER2 and inhibited the growth of HER2-overexpressing xenografts (Hudziak et al., 1989, Shepard et al., 1991). Given the antitumor activities of this murine MAb, a recombinant humanized IgG_1 MAb, rhu4D5, or trastuzumab (Herceptin®), was developed (Carter et al., 1992). While rhu4D5 demonstrated cytostatic inhibition of growth when administered alone (Pietras, Pegram, Finn, Maneval, & Slamon, 1998), synergistic antitumor effects have been achieved when it was administered in combination with cisplatin, carboplatin, docetaxel, and ionizing radiation; and additive effects are seen with doxorubicin, cyclophosphamide, methotrexate, and paclitaxel (reviewed in Slamon, Leyland-Jones et al., 2001). Phase II trials evaluating the efficacy of trastuzumab alone in women with HER2-overexpressing advanced metastatic breast cancer showed objective response rates

(CP + PR) of 11.6% to 15% (Baselga et al., 1996; Cobleigh et al., 1999; Baselga et al., 1999). The most common adverse events were mild to moderate infusion-associated fever and/or chills, which primarily occurred during the first infusion; and a clinically significant adverse event was cardiac dysfunction, noted in less than 5% of patients. Phase II trials of trastuzumab in combination with docetaxel (Kuzur, 2000), cisplatin (Pegram et al., 1998), taxotere plus carboplatin (Slamon, Patel et al., 2001), and paclitaxel (Seidman et al., 2000) showed improved efficacy, evidenced by objective tumor responses, time to progression, and survival data. There was no evidence of exacerbation of toxicity for combination therapy. Results of the pivotal phase III trial showed that trastuzumab improved the clinical benefit of first-line chemotherapy (doxorubicin or epirubicin plus cyclophosphamide or paclitaxel) in women with metastatic breast cancer that overexpresses HER2 (Slamon, Leyland-Jones et al., 2001). The combined overall results comparing chemotherapy plus trastuzumab (n=235) versus either type of chemotherapy alone (n=234) showed superior outcomes for combination therapy in terms of response rate (50% vs. 32%, $p<0.001$), duration of response (9.1 vs. 6.1 mo., $p<0.001$), time to progression (TTP) (7.4 vs. 4.6 mo., $p<0.001$), time to treatment failure (6.9 vs. 4.5 mo., $p<0.001$), and median survival (25.1 vs. 20.3 mo., $p=0.046$). New York Heart Association class III or IV cardiac toxicity was observed in 27% of the patients receiving trastuzumab, cyclophosphamide, and an anthracycline. Although this side effect was potentially severe, the symptoms generally improved with standard medical management. In addition, anaphylaxis is a rare but serious side effect that must be watched for. Trastuzumab, in combination with chemotherapy, is effective and approved for the treatment of metastatic breast cancer that overexpresses HER2 (Slamon, Leyland-Jones et al., 2001).

Given the expression of HER2 in numerous epithelial malignancies and preclinical evidence suggesting activity in other cell lines, such as ovarian, gastric, and non–small cell lung (Scholl, Beuzeboc, & Pouillart, 2001), trials are either in progress or planned to evaluate the efficacy of trastuzumab in cancers including lung, prostate, ovarian, bladder. Preclinical studies demonstrating synergistic antitumor activity (Agus et al., 2000) provided a basis for evaluating trastuzumab in combination with various chemotherapeutic agents for other cancers, including colorectal, non–small cell lung, and prostate.

3.2.3. Angiogenesis Inhibitors

A series of major discoveries, many of them conducted by Judah Folkman and his colleagues, have shown that tumors can be treated chronically with antiangiogenic drugs to induce prolonged dormancy (Folkman, 1971). Many molecules have been developed to block different steps in the process of angiogenesis. With respect to how they function, the angiogenesis inhibitors can be divided into 2 types: direct and indirect angiogenesis inhibitors. Figure 5 illustrates some examples of these agents and their targets. Angiogenesis is a complex process, and there are numerous possibilities for development of agents targeting this process. In this chapter, we focus on the most promising molecules targeting angiogenesis in an attempt to treat cancer.

Endostatin. Recombinant human endostatin (rHE) is a 20 kDa C-terminal fragment of collagen XVIII, which is capable of inhibiting endothelial cell proliferation in vitro and angiogenesis in a chicken chorioallantoic membrane assay. Endostatin specifically inhibits endothelial proliferation and potently inhibits angiogenesis and tumor growth by binding to glypicans (Gpcs) (Karihaloo et al., 2001). Glypicans are a family of glycosylphosphatidylinositol (GPI)-anchored heparan sulfate proteoglycans that play a possible role in the control of cell growth and division. Endostatin has also been shown to stop the growth of metastases originating from Lewis lung carcinoma (LLC), melanoma, and fibrosarcomas (Dhanabal et al., 1999; O'Reilly et al., 1997). This agent has been shown to induce endothelial cell apoptosis and tumor regression in preclinical models. Several phase I trials have been conducted to investigate the

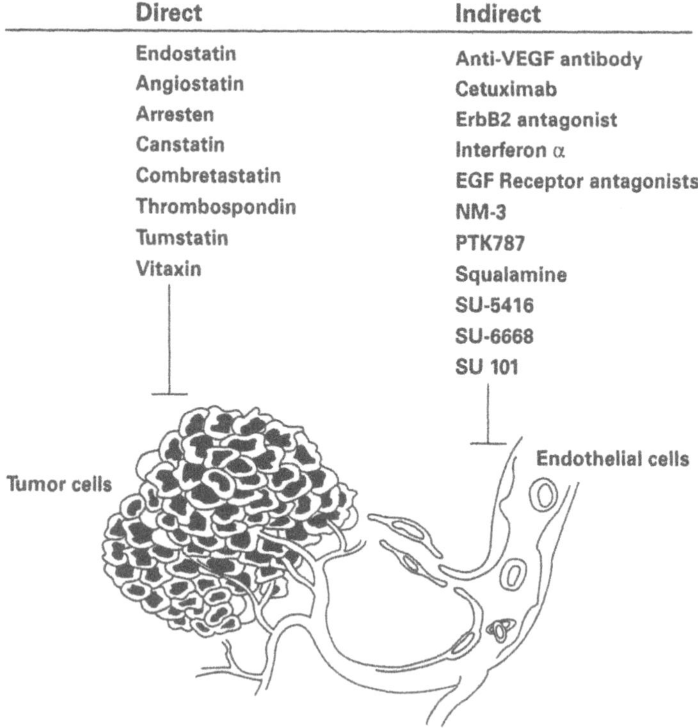

Figure 5. Examples of direct and indirect angiogenesis inhibitors: Most of the agents employed to inhibit oncogene products are considered indirect angiogenesis inhibitors. Direct angiogenesis inhibitors specifically target endothelial cells. Data from Cristofanilli, Charnsangavej, & Hortobagyi (2002).

safety, biologic and anti-tumor activity of endostatin in patients with refractory solid malignancies. In a study conducted by Eder et al. (2001) on 19 patients with refractory solid tumors, urinary VEGF and bFGF levels showed a decrease at Day 29 in 2 of 6 patients at <60 mg/m^2 and 7 of 9 patients at doses >60 mg/m^2. No dose-response effect was seen on endothelial cell proliferation in vitro, but a trend toward tumor cell death in 5 patients with stable disease was observed. During this study, grade 1 rash occurred in 3 patients in a treatment duration of up to 12 cycles.

Twenty-two patients were treated with endostatin (15–300 mg/m^2) 20-minute IV infusion during a study conducted by Herbst, Tran et al. (2001). Patients were evaluated for tumor blood flow and for evidence of endothelial cell apoptosis (ECA). Endostatin-induced apoptosis was shown to be dose dependent, and, at the 56th day of drug administration, tumor blood flow decreased significantly. During this phase I study, no grade 3–4 toxicities were observed with daily doses of up to 300 mg/m^2.

Angiostatin. Recombinant human angiostatin (rhA) is a 38-kDa fragment of plasminogen (O'Reilly et al., 1994). rhA exerts its antiangiogenic activity by binding to the α subunit of ATP synthase on the surface of endothelial cells and inducing apoptosis (Wahl et al., 2001). Systemic administration of human or recombinant human angiostatin inhibits growth of human and murine primary carcinoma in mice, without detectable toxicity or resistance (O'Reilly, Holmgren, Chen, & Folkman, 1996; Sim et al., 1997). Phase I studies are being conducted to evaluate the safety and efficacy of this agent in clinical settings for cancer treatment. When increasing daily doses (15–240 mg/m^2) of angiostatin was administered intravenously (over 20 minutes) to 15 patients, no dose-limiting toxicity was observed; adverse events included port infection in 2 patients and a transient, localized maculo-papular skin rash in 4 patients that did not progress while on therapy. Antibody titer against rhA was positive in 1 of 15 and 2 of 15 patients for IgG and IgM, respectively, with no correlation with skin rash. Seven of 10 patients had a decrease in urine bFGF levels of between 15% and 92%; 5 of 10 patients had a decrease in urine VEGF levels of between 30% and 64% (DeMoraes et al., 2001). Additional clinical trials are under way to establish the safety and efficacy of angiostatin in cancer treatment.

TNP-470. TNP-470, a synthetic derivative of fumagillin, was shown to have potent antiangiogenic activity and low toxicity in animal studies (Ingber et al., 1990; Kusaka 1991). The activity of TNP-470 is mediated via inhibition of the enzyme methionine aminopeptidase-2, which appears to be an important step in the angiogenesis pathway. Preclinical studies have shown that this agent inhibits *in vivo* growth of solid tumors and prevents their metastasis, including human neuroblastoma tumor cells (Hama, Shimizu, Hosaka, Sugenoya, & Usuda, 1997; Singh et al., 1997; Shusterman et al., 2001). Understanding of the mode of action through which TNP-470 exerts its antiangiogenic activity is expanding. TNP-470 induces p53 activation through a unique mechanism in endothelial cells, which leads to $p21^{CIP/WAF}$ expression and subsequent growth arrest (Yeh, Mohan, & Crews, 2000).

TNP-470 has proceeded to clinical development for cancer as an antiangiogenic agent. It is currently in phase I/II trials and being evaluated in patients with Kaposi's sarcoma, renal cell carcinoma, and brain, breast, cervical, and prostate cancer. In early clinical reports, TNP-470 was tolerated up to 177 mg/m^2 given IV, with neurotoxic effects (fatigue, vertigo, ataxia, and loss of concentration) being the principal dose-limiting toxicity (DLT) (Kruger & Figg, 2000). This agent has been investigated with paclitaxel in patients with advanced solid tumors, with favorable results (Baidas et al., 2000; Herbst et al., 2000). Herbst et al. investigated the combination of TNP-470 with paclitaxel in 32 patients with metastatic cancer who had received no more than 1 prior regimen of paclitaxel. The study consisted of 2 dose-escalation arms: fixed-dose TNP-470 (60 mg/m^2) with escalating doses of paclitaxel, and fixed paclitaxel (225 mg/m^2) with escalating TNP-470. During this study, the maximal dose of TNP-470 (60 mg/m^2) and paclitaxel (225 mg/m^2) was achieved without development of dose-limiting toxicity. A small number of patients had slightly more motor coordination problems; however, paclitaxel appeared to add minimal neurocognitive toxicity. Five of 15 evaluated patients (33%) with non–squamous cell lung cancer (NSCLC) showed a PR to this combination therapy. The median survival for the small subgroup of mostly pretreated patients with metastatic NSCLC was more than 14 months. The investigators concluded that TNP-470 in combination with paclitaxel is well tolerated and may be useful in the treatment of advanced NSCLC (Herbst et al., 2000).

Squalamine. Squalamine is a natural aminosterol and a novel antiangiogenic agent originally isolated from the dogfish shark, *Squalus acanthias*. The mechanism of action of this novel agent is not completely understood; however, it is postulated that squalamine acts directly on the activated endothelial cells after intracellular uptake and selectively inhibits the sodium-hydrogen antiporter exchanger (NHE3) (Akhter et al., 1999) Squalamine does not exert cytotoxic effects *in vitro;* however, it inhibits cell growth in mice bearing established xenographs. Similarly, when used alone, squalamine had no effect on tumor vascularization in the human lung tumor cells; however, the combination of squalamine and cisplatin reduced the number of vessels by approximately 25% (Bhargava et al., 2001; Schiller & Bittner, 1999; Schiller et al., 2001).

A phase IIa clinical trial is in progress to investigate the safety and efficacy of this novel agent in treatment of chemotherapy-naïve stage IIIB and IV NSCLC patients. In this trial, 18 patients were treated with squalamine following a carboplatin and paclitaxel (225 mg/m^2) regimen. There were 5 partial responses (27%) and no complete responses among these 18 patients. Survival data are not yet available; however, median TTP in this study was 3.8 months. Grade 4 neutropenia occurred in 7 patients (39%) and was associated with fever in 1 patient. Other grade 4 adverse events were hyponatremia (2 patients), liver transaminase elevation (1 patient), and anemia (1 patient); grade 3 adverse events occurred in 16 patients (89%) (Schiller et al., 2001).

Carboxyamidotriazole (CAI). Carboxyamidotriazole (CAI), an inhibitor of Ca^{++}-mediated signal transduction (Hupe, Behrens, & Boltz, 1990), inhibits angiogenesis *in vitro* and *in vivo* and downregulates matrix metalloproteinase-2 *in vitro*. It is proposed that this agent exerts its antiproliferative activity by inhibition of downstream phosphorylation events involving phospholipase-Cγ (Hupe et al., 1991). *In vitro* studies have shown that this agent inhibits proliferation and invasive characteristics of several tumor cell lines, including prostate, glioblastoma, and breast (Jacobs et al., 1997; Lambert, Somers, Kohn, & Perry, 1997; Wasilenko et al., 1996) CAI is under investigation in several types of relapsed solid tumors.

After 6 weeks of oral CAI (100 mg/kg) there was no significant change in stage or grade of tumor in a rat bladder cancer model. However, significant apoptosis and diminished tumor proliferation rate were observed (Perabo et al., 2000).

CAI in combination with paclitaxel in 39 patients with solid relapsed tumors yielded 3 partial responses and 2 minor responses without evidence of additive or cumulative toxicity; grade 3 non-hematological toxicities were rare (Kohn et al., 2001).

Thalidomide. Thalidomide suppresses levels of several cytokines, angiogenic and growth factors, including TNF-α, bFGF, VEGF, and interleukin-6 (IL-6). The resulting antiangiogenic, immunomodulatory, and growth-suppressive effects form the rationale for investigating thalidomide in the treatment of solid tumors malignancies, including metastatic renal cell carcinoma (MRCC) and metastatic squamous cell carcinoma of the head and neck (Stebbing et al., 2001; Tseng et al., 2001; Vuky et al., 2001). Thalidomide has antiangiogenic effects in preclinical models as well as a significant antitumor effect in hematologic tumors such as multiple myeloma (Deckers et al., 2001; Tosi et al., 2002). The exact mechanism by which thalidomide exerts its antiangiogenesis is not known; however, apoptosis, chromatin condensation, and nuclear DNA fragmentation were observed in a human multiple myeloma cell line (RPMI 8226) (Park, Kim, Kim, & Chung, 2001).

When thalidomide was administered as a single agent to 21 patients with recurrent or metastatic squamous cell carcinoma of the head and neck, it did not appear to have single-agent antitumor activity (Tseng et al., 2001). In this study, patients eventually developed progressive disease, and median TTP was 50 days, with a median overall survival of 194 days, similar to the progression and survival times reported with other agents for this patient group. Thalidomide was generally well tolerated, with few patients experiencing grades 3 or 4 toxicities. However, when continuous low-dose thalidomide (100 mg oral daily dose) was investigated in 66 patients with a variety of advanced malignancies, 3 of 18 patients with renal cancer showed partial responses and 3 additional patients experienced disease stabilization for up to 6 months (Eisen et al., 2000). The potential effect of thalidomide on progression-free survival of patients with advanced renal cell carcinoma is currently being investigated in an ECOG phase III randomized trial of interferon-α with and without thalidomide (Vuky et al., 2001).

3.2.4. Vascular Endothelial Growth Factor

Since VEGFs and their receptors are among the most substantial mediators of angiogenesis, different strategies have been designed to inhibit VEGF functions in an attempt to control tumor growth. These include use of specific VEGF antibodies, coupling of a toxin to VEGF itself, blocking the interaction of VEGF with its receptors, and use of purified soluble VEGF receptors. Here we review the most clinically significant anti-VEGF molecules developed to date.

Bevacizumab (rhuMAb VEGF): an Anti-VEGF Monoclonal Antibody. Bevacizumab is an experimental rhuMAb composed of human IgG_1 framework regions and antigen-binding regions from a murine monoclonal antibody (Presta et al., 1997). rhuMAb VEGF has a high affinity (10-10M) for VEGF and induces a complete blockade of its activities (Sledge et al., 2000). rhuMAb VEGF was first developed to block the effects of VEGF in the treatment of solid tumors and has been under intense investigation for treating various types of cancers, including breast, colorectal, prostate, and non–squamous cell lung cancers, both as a single agent and in combination with chemotherapeutic agents.

Based on the initial studies, after multiple IV infusions of bevacizumab (0.1–10 mg/kg) over 4 to 24 weeks as a single agent or in combination with antineoplastic agents, a long terminal half-life of 18.6 days was observed in subjects (Hsei et al., 2001). In a phase II trial, 35 women with relapsed metastatic breast cancer were treated with either 3 mg/kg (18 pts.) or 10 mg/kg (17 pts.) rhuMAb VEGF every 14 days for up to 13 injections. rhuMAb VEGF was well tolerated and there were no fatal adverse events related to these regimens. One subject discontinued rhuMAb VEGF therapy after developing malignant hypertension and nephrotic syndrome shortly after starting rhuMAb VEGF therapy. One other subject suffered a serious adverse event of hypertension that the investigator assessed as possibly related to rhuMAb VEGF therapy. One subject in each dose group experienced a PR (objective response)., and a complete response was seen in 1 patient receiving 10 mg/kg of rhuMAb VEGF. Additionally, 2 patients in the high-dose cohort experienced regression of metastatic nodules. The results of this study demonstrated that rhuMAb VEGF was generally well tolerated and had activity in metastatic breast cancer.

Another phase II study showed promising results in 104 metastatic colorectal cancer patients treated with rhuMAb VEGF (5 or 10 mg/kg) in combination with 5-fluorouracil/leucovorin (5-FU/LV). These patients demonstrated higher response rates when treated with higher doses of rhuMAb VEGF in combination with 5-FU/LV. Response rates were 20% (5-FU/LV alone), 34% (5-FU/LV and 5 mg/kg rhuMAb VEGF), and 38% (5-FU/LV and 10 mg/kg rhuMAb VEGF). This study also demonstrated that the TTP was increased when 5-FU/LV plus rhuMAb VEGF were used (TTP=5.2 months [5-FU/LV alone], 9.2 months [5-FU/LV and 5 mg/kg rhuMAb VEGF], and 7.2 months [5-FU/LV and 10 mg/kg rhuMAb VEGF]) (Bergsland et al., 2000).

Among advanced non–squamous cell lung cancer patients being treated with 15 mg/kg rhuMAb VEGF in addition to carboplatin/paclitaxel (CP), a significant benefit was observed in objective response rate, TTP, and, specifically, in mean survival time. However, life-threatening hemorrhage was observed in 6 of 66 rhuMAb VEGF-treated patients, with 4 deaths. The overall analysis of the data showed that rhuMAb VEGF therapy may prolong survival in this group of patients (Johnson et al., 2001).

SU6668 and SU5416: Anti-VEGF Small Molecules. SU6668 and SU5416 are recently discovered TKIs being investigated for efficacy against various solid tumors, including colorectal, breast, renal, and NSCLC. Administration of either of these molecules in a colon cancer hepatic metastasis model inhibited metastases, microvessel formation, and cell proliferation, while increasing tumor cell and endothelial cell apoptosis (Ellis, Takahashi, Liu, & Shaheen, 2000).

SU6668 is a new small molecule TKI that acts on the VEGF (Flk-1), PDGF (PDGFR-β), and FGF1 (FGFR1) receptors. Oral administration of this molecule in athymic mice resulted in significant growth inhibition in a diverse panel of human tumor xenographs of glioma, melanoma, lung, colon, and ovarian carcinomas (Laird et al., 2000).

Clinical trials began in 2001. In a phase I trial, 56 patients were treated with 100–2400 mg/m^2/day oral SU6668. Mild to moderate side effects included nausea, diarrhea, fatigue, and dyspnea. During this study, 12 patients received 200 or 800 mg/m^2 BD of active drug. When high doses of the drug were administered, patients developed intolerable pain, and prolonged exposure time above the desired target level was observed. There were minor declines in tumor markers and softening of palpable tumors in isolated patients. Formal assessments and full patient evaluations are not available at this point (Rosen et al., 2001).

Unlike SU6668, SU5416 is a specific VEGF inhibitor and exerts its antiangiogenic effects through Flk-1 inhibition. SU5416 demonstrates broad anti-tumor efficacy in subcutaneously implanted xenographs of tumor cells in athymic mice. SU5416 is under investigation for efficacy and safety alone and in combination with antineoplastic agents for a variety of malignancy types, including metastatic colorectal cancer, inflammatory breast cancer, AIDS-related Kaposi's sarcoma, malignant mesothelioma, and melanoma.

Based on human pharmacokinetics and pharmacodynamics studies, a dose of 145 mg/m^2 resulted in systemic exposure comparable to what was required in animals to produce effective tumor growth inhibition (Cropp, Rosen, Mulay, Langecker, & Hannah, 1999). In a phase I/II study, 8 patients with MCRC received either 85 or 245 mg/m^2 SU5416 twice weekly in addition to full-dose irinotecan/5-FU/LV. None of the patients on low-dose SU5416 developed dose-limiting toxicity, while 1 patient in the high-dose group developed neutropenic fever. Grade 3 nausea/vomiting, fatigue, and headache were among the severe side effects, regardless of dose. The effects on tumor blood flow are yet to be determined. These preliminary results suggest that the addition of SU5416 to conventional regimens used to treat colorectal carcinomas is safe and may be further tested clinically (Rothenberg et al., 2001). At this time, all trials investigating this agent are closed.

3.2.5. Platelet-derived Growth Factor

Imatinib Mesylate (STI 571). STI 571 has been shown to inhibit PDGFR, c-abl, bcr-abl oncogene, and c-KIT, in *in vitro* and *in vivo* studies. It does not inhibit other tyrosine kinase members (Buchdunger et al., 1996; Druker & Lydon, 2000; Druker et al., 1996; Okuda, Weisberg, Gilliland, & Griffin, 2001). STI 571, imatinib (Gleevec™), was approved by the USFDA in May 2001 for treatment of chronic myeloid leukemia (CML) due to its effects on Bcr-Abl tyrosine kinase, the constitutive tyrosine kinase activity created by the Philadelphia chromosome translocation abnormality in CML. After 1 month of imatinib treatment, 88% of chronic phase CML patients had a complete hematologic response and 49% had a major cytogenic response (Gleevec Package Insert, 2001).

Currently, STI 571 is being investigated in diseases in which other STI 571-target kinases are activated, such as gastrointestinal sarcoma (c-KIT), glioblastomas (PDGFR-β), SCLC (c-KIT), dermatofibrosarcoma protuberans (DFSP), and giant cell fibroblastoma (GCF) (Sjoblom et al., 2001). Sjoblom et al. demonstrated that treatment of DFSP-bearing mice with STI 571 reduced tumor growth predominantly through induction of tumor cell apoptosis. Recently, targeted clinical trials are being conducted to investigate the effects of this novel agent on solid tumors, including unresectable or metastatic gastrointestinal stromal tumors (GISTs) expressing c-KIT. Administration of 400 or 600 mg oral STI 571 in 35 patients induced symptom reduction in 89% of the patients with GISTs. Partial response was seen after 1 to 3 months of therapy in 19 patients (54%) and stable disease was seen in 12 (34%) of evaluated patients. During this study, grade 3–4 toxicities were seen in 9 (26%) of the patients, and consisted mainly of hemorrhage, abdominal pain, and abnormal electrolytes (Blanke et al., 2001).

LY 294002. Phosphatidylinositol 3-kinase (PI3k) is an enzyme implicated in growth factor signal transduction by associating with receptor and nonreceptor tyrosine kinases, including the platelet-derived growth factor receptor and the EGFR family. LY 294002 acts in vivo as a highly selective inhibitor of phosphatidylinositol 3-kinase (PI3k) (Vlahos, Matter, Hui, & Brown, 1994). To date, there have been no clinical studies conducted to show the benefits of using this compound to treat cancer.

Leflunomide (SU 101). SU 101 inhibits PDGF-mediated signaling events, including receptor tyrosine phosphorylation, DNA synthesis, cell cycle progression, and cell proliferation. SU 101 inhibited PDGF-stimulated tyrosine phosphorylation of PDGFR-β in rat glioma cells. This small molecule is known to prevent tumor growth and induce long-term survival in animals implanted with 7TD1 (murine B-cell hybridoma) tumor cells (Shawver et al., 1997). It is being investigated for activity in patients with advanced solid tumors, including SCLC, ovarian cancer, malignant glioma, and prostate cancer.

Phase I trials in patients with advanced prostate cancer demonstrated significant prostate-specific antigen (PSA) declines (43%–93%) in 3 of 5 patients receiving SU 101. Mild to moderate nausea, vomiting, anorexia, and fever were observed (Eckhardt et al., 1999). During a phase II trial, 44 patients with hormone refractory prostate cancer received 400 mg/m^2 weekly. Three of 39 patients with available PSA showed >50% decline compare to baseline, 1 patient had a PR, and 9 patients reported significant pain reduction. PDGFR expression was decreased in 80% of the metastases and 88% of the primary prostate cancers (Ko et al., 1999). Additional clinical investigations are underway to evaluate the efficacy and safety of this novel agent in various solid tumors.

Growth Factor Binder (GFB)-111. GFB-111 is a novel molecule designed to bind to PDGF. GFB-111 targets the regions of PDGF (loops I and II) that are involved in binding to its receptor and thus selectively blocks PDGF-induced receptor tyrosine kinase phosphorylation and MAP kinase activation. In addition to its effects on PDGF, GFB-111 at higher concentrations could block VEGF binding to Flk-1 on endothelial cells and inhibit angiogenesis (Blaskovich, 2000). During the initial evaluation of GFB-111, it was demonstrated that this molecule is capable of inhibiting the growth of human giloblastoma and human lung adenocarcinoma tumor cells implanted subcutaneously in nude mice. This growth inhibition was dose-dependent and attributed to angiogenesis inhibition by GFB-111.

3.2.6. Insulin-like Growth Factor

A variety of potential anti-IGF treatment strategies include growth hormone-releasing hormone (GHRH) antagonists, anti-IGF receptor MAbs, ligand analogs, and antisense approaches, all of which are in the early stages of testing.

4. CONCLUSION

Targeting growth factor-mediated signaling offers a paradigm for treating cancer. While past efforts focused on the effects of cytotoxic therapies with chemotherapy and radiation therapy, the future looks towards the integration of molecular targeted therapies into current treatment modalities. Given the primarily cytostatic nature of growth factor–targeted biological therapy, its role is likely to be administration in combination with cytotoxic therapy for tumor eradication, and in exploring advantages to administering these agents as maintenance therapy in order to obtain tumor growth inhibition (Thompson et al., 1997). The safety profiles of these biological agents allows for combination therapy with chemotherapy and/or radiation therapy, which means that multiple mechanisms of antitumor activity are possible. As early as the 1970s, Judah Folkman theorized that antiangiogenic agents could be used for chronic therapy (Folkman, 1971). It has been theorized that multiple biological therapies aimed against various targets could be combined for maximal anti-tumor effect (Herbst, Kim et al., 2001). However, the possibility of delayed toxicity with long-term administration exists and the long-term toxicity profiles of these agents are yet to be investigated.

There are a number of challenges and unanswered questions. The immediate anti-tumor effects of biologic therapies targeting growth factor pathways may be difficult to ascertain given their cytostatic activity (Owa, Yoshino, Yoshimatsu, & Nagasu, 2001; Rewcastle et al., 1998; Thompson et al., 1997). While chemotherapy and radiation generally result in rapid cytotoxic effects that can be measured by reduced tumor size and volume, biologic therapies targeting growth factor signals may not result in obvious tumor regression until prolonged treatment has been given (Weber et al., 2001). This may necessitate novel approaches to evaluate antitumor response; for example, imaging studies, such as computed tomography, magnetic resonance imaging, and ultrasound, and scintigraphic techniques, may be beneficial in evaluating the impact of antiangiogenic therapy on vascular permeability and tumor blood flow. (Weber 2001) Furthermore, while the efficacy of cytotoxic therapy has typically has been measured by tumor regression, re-evaluation of primary efficacy endpoints may be necessary to fully determine the clinical benefit of these agents. Other factors to consider are unanticipated effects of inhibition of enzymes or signaling pathways not originally targeted. In some cases, these can be beneficial; blockade of EGF receptors results in decreased angiogenesis, decreased matastatic capability, and increased apoptosis, in addition to cell cycle arrest (Mendelsohn, 2000) The field of growth factor signaling in malignancy continues to expand. Clinical results from a number of agents are anticipated to lead to changes in the approach to cancer management.

Roy S. Herbst and Amir Onn
The University of Texas M. D. Anderson Cancer Center
Thoracic and Head and Neck Oncology
Houston, TX

John Mendelsohn
The University of Texas M. D. Anderson Cancer Center
Experimental Therapeutics

Dr. Mendelsohn is a board member of and holds stock options in ImClone Systems Incorporated.

5. REFERENCES

Aaronson, S. A. (1991). Growth factors and cancer. *Science, 254* (5035), 1146-1153.

Aase K, Lymboussaki A, Kaipainen A, Olofsson B, Alitalo K, Eriksson U. (1999). Localization of VEGF-B in the mouse embryo suggests a paracrine role of the growth factor in the developing vasculature. *Developmental Dynamics; 215* (1), 12-25

Abbruzzese, J. L., Rosenberg, A., Xiong, Q., LoBuglio, A., Schmidt, W., Wolff, R., et al. (2001). Phase II study of anti-epidermal growth factor receptor (EGFR) antibody Cetuximab (IMC-C225) in combination with gemcitabine in patients with advanced pancreatic cancer. *Proceeding of the American Society of Clinical Oncology, 20*, Abstract 518

Adamo, M. L., Ben-Hur, H., Roberts, C. T., Jr., & LeRoith, D. (1991). Regulation of start site usage in the leader exons of the rat insulin-like growth factor-I gene by development, fasting, and diabetes. *Molecular Endocrinology, 5* (11), 1677-1686
Agus, D. B., Bunn, P. A. Jr., Franklin, W., Garcia, M., & Ozols, R. F. (2000). HER-2/neu as a therapeutic target in non-small cell lung cancer, prostate cancer, and ovarian cancer. *Seminars in Oncology, 27* (6 Suppl 11), 92-100
Ahmed, N. U., Ueda, M., Ito, A., Ohashi, A., Funasaka, Y., & Ichihashi, M. (1997). Expression of fibroblast growth factor receptors in naevus-cell naevus and malignant melanoma. *Melanoma Research, 7* (4), 299-305.
Aigner,A., Butscheid, M., Kunkel, P., Krause, E., Lamszus, K., Wellstein, A., et al. (2001). An FGF-binding protein (FGF-BP) exerts its biological function by parallel paracrine stimulation of tumor cell and endothelial cell proliferation though FGF-2 release. *International Journal of Cancer, 92* (4), 510-517
Akhter, S., Nath, S. K., Tse, C. M., Williams, J., Zasloff, M., & Donowitz M. (1999). Squalamine, a novel cationic steroid, specifically inhibits the brush-border Na+/H+ exchanger isoform NHE3. *The American Journal of Physiology, 276* (1 Pt 1), C136-C144
Alimandi, M., Romano, A., Curia, M. C., Muraro, R., Fedi, P., Aaronson, S. A., et al. (1995). Cooperative signaling of ErbB3 and ErbB2 in neoplastic transformation and human mammary carcinomas. *Oncogene, 10* (9), 1813-1821.
Alon, T., Hemo, I., Itin, A., Pe'er, J., Stone, J., & Keshet, E. (1995). Vascular endothelial growth factor acts as a survival factor for newly formed retinal vessels and has implications for retinopathy of prematurity. *Nature Medicine, 1* (10), 1024-1028.
Asahara, T., Bauters, C., Zheng, L. P., Takeshita, S., Bunting, S., Ferrara, N., et al. (1995). Synergistic effect of vascular endothelial growth factor and basic fibroblast growth factor on angiogenesis in vivo. *Circulation, 92* (9 Suppl), II365-371.
Baidas, S., Bhargava, P., Isaacs, C., Rizvi, N., Trocky, N., Pipkin, T., et al. (2000). Phase I Study of the Combination of TNP-470 and Paclitaxel in Patients with Advanced Cancer. *Proceedings of the American Society of Clinical Oncology, 19,* Abstract 800.
Baldwin, R. L., Kobrin, M. S., Tran, T., Pastan, I., & Korc, M. (1996). Cytotoxic effects of TGF-alpha-Pseudomonas exotoxin A fusion protein in human pancreatic carcinoma cells. *Pancreas, 13* (1), 16-21.
Barnes, D., & Sato, G. (1980). Serum-free cell culture: a unifying approach. *Cell, 22* (3), 649-655.
Bartlett, J. M., Langdon, S. P., Simpson, B. J., Stewart, M., Katsaros, D., Sismondi, P., et al. (1996). The prognostic value of epidermal growth factor receptor mRNA expression in primary ovarian cancer. *British Journal of Cancer, 73* (3), 301–306.
Baselga, J., & Averbuch, S.D. (2000). ZD1839 ('Iressa') as an anticancer agent. *Drugs, 60* (Suppl 1), 33-40.
Baselga, J., Norton, L., Masui, H., Pandiella, A., Coplan, K., Miller, W.H., Jr., Mendelsohn, J. (1993) Antitumor effects of doxorubicin in combination with anti-epidermal growth factor receptor monoclonal antibodies. *Journal of the National Cancer Institute, 85*(16), 1327-1333.
Baselga, J., Tripathy, D., Mendelsohn, J., Baughman, S., Benz, C. C., Dantis, L., et al. (1996). Phase II study of weekly intravenous recombinant humanized anti-p185HER2 monoclonal antibody in patients with HER2/neu-overexpressing metastatic breast cancer. *Journal of Clinical Oncology, 14* (3), 737-744.
Baselga, J., Tripathy, D., Mendelsohn, J., Baughman, S., Benz, C.C., Dantis, L., et al. (1999). Phase II study of weekly intravenous trastuzumab (Herceptin) in patients with HER2/neu-overexpressing metastatic breast cancer. *Seminars in Oncology, 26*(4 Suppl 12), 78-83.
Baselga, J., Yano, S., Giaccone, G., Nakagawa, K., Tamura, T., Douillard, J., et al. (2001). Initial results from phase II trial of ZD1839 (Iressa) as second- and third-line monotherapy for patients with advanced non-small-cell lung cancer (IDEAL 1). *Proceedings of the American Association for Cancer Research- National Cancer Institute-European Organization for Research and Treatment of Cancer International Conference,* Abstract 630A.
Baserga, R. (1995). The insulin-like growth factor I receptor: A key to tumor growth? *Cancer Research, 55,* 249-252.
Baserga, R., Porcu, P., Rubini, M., & Sell, C. (1994). Cell cycle control by the IGF-1 receptor and its ligands. In D. LeRoith & M. K. Raizada (Eds.), *Current Directions in Insulin-Like Growth Factor Research* (pp.105-112). New York: Plenum Press.
Baserga, R., Sell, C., Porcu, P., & Rubini, M. (1994). The role of the IGF-I receptor in the growth and transformation of mammalian cells. *Cell Proliferation, 27* (2), 63-71.
Basilico, C., & Moscatelli, D. (1992). The FGF family of growth factors and oncogenes. *Advances in Cancer Research, 59,* 115-165.
Bates, P., Fisher, R., Ward, A., Richardson, L., Hill, D. J., & Graham, C. F. (1995). Mammary cancer in transgenic mice expressing insulin-like growth factor II (IGF-II). *British Journal of Cancer, 72(5),* 1189-1193.
Battegay, E. J., Rupp, J., Iruela-Arispe, L., Sage, E. H., & Pech, M. (1994). PDGF-BB modulates endothelial proliferation and angiogenesis in vitro via PDGF beta-receptors. *The Journal of Cell Biology, 125(4),* 917-928.

Beckmann, M. P., Betsholtz, C., Heldin, C. H., Westermark, B., Di Marci, E., Di Fiore, P. P., et al. (1988). Comparison of the biological properties and transforming potential of human PDGF-A and PDGF-B chains. *Science, 241(4871),* 1346-1349.

Beitz, J. G., Kim, I. S., Calabresi, P., & Frackelton, A. R., Jr. (1991). Human microvascular endothelial cells express receptors for platelet-derived growth factor. *Proceedings of the National Academy of Sciences USA, 88* (5), 2021-2025.

Benini, S., Manara, M. C., Baldini, N., Cerisano, V., Massimo, S., Mercuri, M., et al. (2001). Inhibition of insulin-like growth factor I receptor increases the antitumor activity of doxorubicin and vincristine against Ewing's sarcoma cells. *Clinical Cancer Research, 7* (6), 1790-1797.

Benjamin, L. E., Golijanin, D., Itin, A., Pode, D., & Keshet, E. (1999). Selective ablation of immature blood vessels in established human tumors follows vascular endothelial growth factor withdrawal. *The Journal of Clinical Investigation, 103* (2), 159-165.

Benjamin, L. E., & Keshet, E. (1997). Conditional switching of vascular endothelial growth factor (VEGF) expression in tumors: induction of endothelial cell shedding and regression of hemangioblastoma-like vessels by VEGF withdrawal. *Proceedings of the National Academy of Sciences USA, 94* (16), 8761-8766.

Bergsland, E., Hurwitz, H., Fehrenbacher, L., Meropol, N. J., Novotny, W. F. F., Gaudreault, J., et al. (2000). A randomized phase II trial comparing rhuMAb VEGF (recombinant humanized monoclonal antibody to vascular endothelial cell growth factor) plus 5-fluorouracil/leucovorin (FU/LV) to FU/LV alone in patients with metastatic colorectal cancer. *Proceedings of the American Society of Clinical Oncology, 19,* Abstract 939.

Bhargava, P., Marshall, J. L., Dahut, W., Rizvi, N., Trocky, N., Williams, J. I., et al. (2001). A phase I and pharmacokinetic study of squalamine, a novel antiangiogenic agent, in patients with advanced cancers. *Clinical Cancer Research, 7* (12), 3912-3919.

Bigner, S. H., Humphrey, P. A., Wong, A. J., Vogelstein, B., Mark, J., Friedman, H. S., et al. (1990). Characterization of the epidermal growth factor receptor in human glioma cell lines and xenografts. *Cancer Research, 50* (24), 8017-8022.

Blanke, C. D., von Mehren M., Joensuu, H., Roberts, P. J., Eisenberg, B., Heinrich, M., et al. (2001). Evaluation of the safety and efficacy of an oral molecularly-targeted therapy, STI 571, in patients (pts) with unresectable or metastatic gastrointestinal stromal tumors (GISTS) expressing C-KIT (CD117). *Proceedings of the American Society of Clinical Oncology, 20,* Abstract 1.

Blaskovich MA, Lin Q, Delarue FL, Sun J, Park HS, Coppola D, et al. (2000). Design of GFB-111, a platelet-derived growth factor binding molecule with antiangiogenic and anticancer activity against human tumors in mice. *Nature Biotechnology, 18* (10):1065-1070.

Bol, D. K., Kiguchi, K., Gimenez-Conti, I., Rupp, T., & DiGiovanni, J. (1997). Overexpression of insulin-like growth factor-1 induces hyperplasia, dermal abnormalities, and spontaneous tumor formation in transgenic mice. *Oncogene, 14* (14), 1725-1734.

Bonner, J. A., Ezekiel, M. P., Robert, F., Meredith, R., F., Spencer, S. A., & Waksal, H. W. (2000). Continued reponse following treatment with IMC-C225, an EGFr MoAb, combined with RT in advanced head and neck malignancies. *Proceedings of the American Society of Clinical Oncology,* 19, Abstract 5F.

Bostrom, H., Willetts, K., Pekny, M., Leveen, P., Lindahl, P., Hedstrand, H., et al. (1996). PDGF-A signaling is a critical event in lung alveolar myofibroblast development and alveogenesis. *Cell, 85* (6), 863-873.

Bouchard, L., Lamarre, L., Tremblay, P. J., & Jolicoeur, P. (1989). Stochastic appearance of mammary tumors in transgenic mice carrying the MMTV/c-neu oncogene. *Cell, 57* (6), 931-936.

Buchdunger, E., Zimmermann, J., Mett, H., Meyer, T., Müller, M., Druker, B. J., et al. (1996). Inhibition of the Abl protein-tyrosine kinase in vitro and in vivo by a 2-phenylaminopyrimidine derivative. *Cancer Research, 56* (1), 100-104.

Budillon, A., DiGennaro, E., Barbarino, M., Bruzzese, F., DeLorenzo, S., Pepe, S., et al. (2000). ZD1839, an epidermal growth factor receptor tyrosine kinase inhibitor, upregulates $p27^{Kip1}$ inducing G1 arrest and enhancing the antitumor effect of interferon α. *Proceedings of the American Association for Cancer Research, 41,* Abstract 4910.

Burris, H. A., 3rd, Moore, M. J., Andersen, J., Green, M. R., Rothenberg, M. L., Modiano, M. R., et al. (1997). Improvements in survival and clinical benefit with gemcitabine as first-line therapy for patients with advanced pancreas cancer: a randomized trial. *Journal of Clinical Oncology, 15* (16), 2403-2413.

Carmeliet, P., Ng, Y. S., Nuyens, D., Theilmeier, G., Brusselmans, K., Cornelissen, I., et al. (1999). Impaired myocardial angiogenesis and ischemic cardiomyopathy in mice lacking the vascular endothelial growth factor isoforms VEGF164 and VEGF188. *Nature Medicine, 5* (5), 495-502.

Carpenter G. (1987). Receptors for epidermal growth factor and other polypeptide mitogens. *Annual Review of Biochemistry, 56,* 881-914.

Carpenter, G., & Cohen, S. (1990). Epidermal growth factor. *The Journal of Biological Chemistry, 265* (14), 7709-7712.

Carter, P., Presta, L., Gorman, C. M., Ridgway, J. B., Henner, D., Wong, W. L., et al. (1992). Humanization of an anti-p185HER2 antibody for human cancer therapy. *Proceedings of the National Academy of Sciences USA, 89* (10), 4285-4289.

Chan, K. C., Knox, F., Woodburn, J. R., Slamon, D., Potten, C. S., & Bundred, N. J. (2000). EGFR tyrosine kinase inhibition decreases epithelial proliferation in DCIS of the breast, whereas c-erbB2 blockade does not. *Proceedings of the American Association for Cancer Research, 41,* Abstract 3074.

Chow, N.-H., Liu, H.-S., Lee, E. I. C., Chang, C.-J., Chan, S.-H., Cheng, H.-L., et al. (1997). Significance of urinary epidermal growth factor and its receptor expression in human bladder cancer. *Anticancer Research, 17,* 1293-1296.

Chu, C. T., Everiss, K. D., Wikstrand, C. J., Batras, S. K., Kung, H. J., & Bigner, D. D. (1997). Receptor dimerization is not a factor in the signaling activity of a transforming variant epidermal growth factor (EGFRvIII). *The Biochemical Journal, 324* (Pt 3), 855–861.

Ciardiello, F. (2000). Epidermal growth factor receptor tyrosine kinase inhibitors as anticancer agents. *Drugs, 60* (Suppl 1), 25-32.

Ciardiello, F., Caputo, R., Bianco, R., Damiano, V., Fontanini, G., Cuccato, S., et al. (2001). Inhibition of growth factor production and angiogenesis in human cancer cells by ZD1839 (Iressa), a selective epidermal growth factor receptor tyrosine kinase inhibitor. *Clinical Cancer Research, 7* (5), 1459-1465.

Ciardiello, F., Caputo, R., Bianco, R., Damiano, V., Pomatico, G., DePlacido, S., et. al. (2000). Antitumor effect and potentiation of cytotoxic drugs activity in human cancer cells by ZD-1839 (Iressa), an epidermal growth factor receptor-selective tyrosine kinase inhibitor. *Clinical Cancer Research, 6* (5), 2053-2063

Ciccodicola, A., Dono, R., Obici, S., Simeone, A., Zollo, M., & Persico, M. G. (1989). Molecular characterization of a gene of the 'EGF family' expressed in undifferentiated human NTERA2 teratocarcinoma cells. *The EMBO Journal, 8* (7), 1987-1991.

Cobleigh, M. A., Vogel, C. L., Tripathy, D., Robert, N. J., Scholl, S., Fehrenbacher, L., et al. (1999). Mutinational study of the efficacy and safety of humanized anti-HER2 monoclonal antibody in women who have HER2-overexpressing metastatic breast cancer that has progressed after chemotherapy for metastatic disease. *Journal of Clinical Oncology, 17* (9), 2639-2648.

Cohen, R. B., Falcey, J. W., Paulter, V. J., Fetzer, K. M., & Waksal, H. W. (2000). Safety profile of the monoclonal antibody (MoAb) IMC-C225, an anti-epidermal growth factor receptor (EGFr) used in the treatment of EGFr-positive tumors. *Proceedings of the American Society of Clinical Oncology, 19,* Abstract 1862.

Cristofanilli, M., Charnsangavej, C., & Hortobagyi, G.N. (2002). Angiogenesis modulation in cancer research: novel clinical approaches. *Nature Reviews Drug Discovery, 1,* 415-426.

Cropp, G., Rosen, L., Mulay, M., Langecker, P., & Hannah, A. (1999). Pharmacokinetics and Pharmacodynamics of SU5416 in a Phase I, Dose Escalating Trial in Patients with Advanced Malignancies. *Proceedings of the American Society of Clinical Oncology, 18,* Abstract 619.

Daughaday, W. H., & Rotwein, P. (1989). Insulin-like growth factors I and II. Peptide, messenger ribonucleic acid and gene structures, serum, and tissue concentrations. *Endocrine Reviews, 10* (1), 68-91.

Deckers, M., van der Pluijm, G., Dooijewaard, S., Kroon, M., van Hinsbergh, V., Papapoulos, S., et al. (2001). Effect of angiogenic and antiangiogenic compounds on the outgrowth of capillary structures from fetal mouse bone explants. *Laboratory Investigation, 81* (1), 5-15.

de Jong, J. S., Van Diest, P. J., Van Der Valk, P., & Baak, J. P. A. (1997). Expression of growth factors, growth-inhibiting factors, and their receptors in invasive breast cancer. II: Correlations with proliferation and angiogenesis. *Journal of Pathology, 184,* 53-57.

de Larco, J. E., & Todaro, G. J. (1978). Growth factors from murine sarcoma virus-transformed cells. *Proceedings of the National Academy of Sciences USA, 75* (8), 4001-4005.

DeMoraes, E. D., Fogler, W. E., Grant, D., Wahl, M., Leeper, D., et al. (2001). Recombinant human angiostatin (rhA): a phase I clinical trial assessing safety, pharmacokinetics (PK) and pharmacodynamics (PD). *Proceedings of the American Association for Cancer Research,* Abstract 10.

D'Ercole, A. J., Applewhite, G. T., & Underwood, L. E. (1980). Evidence that somatomedin is synthesized by multiple tissues in the fetus. *Developmental Biology, 75* (2), 315-328.

Derynck, R. (1988). Transforming growth factor alpha. *Cell, 54* (5), 593-595.

Dhanabal, M., Ramchandran, R., Volk, R., Stillman, I. E., Lombardo, M., Iruela-Arispe, M. L., et al. (1999). Endostatin: yeast production, mutants, and antitumor effect in renal cell carcinoma. *Cancer Research, 59* (1), 189-197.

Doolittle, R. F., Hunkapiller, M. W., Hood, L. E., Devare, S. G., Robbins, K. C., Aaronson, S. A., et al. (1983). Simian sarcoma virus one gene, v-sis, is derived from the gene (or genes) encoding a platelet-derived growth factor. *Science, 221* (4607), 275-277.

Dougall, W. C., Qian, X., Peterson, N. C., Miller, M. J., Samanta, A., & Greene, M. I. (1994). The neu-oncogene: signal transduction pathways, transformation mechanisms and evolving therapies. *Oncogene, 9* (8), 2109-2123.

Downward, J., Yarden, Y., Mayes, E., Scrace, G., Totty, N., Stockwell, P., et al. (1984). Close similarity of epidermal growth factor receptor and v-erb-B oncogene protein sequences. *Nature, 307* (5951), 521-527.

Druker, B. J., & Lydon, N. B. (2000). Lessons learned from the development of an abl tyrosine kinase inhibitor for chronic myelogenous leukemia. *The Journal of Clinical Investigation, 105* (1), 3-7.
Druker, B. J., Tamura, S., Buchdunger, E., Ohno, S., Segal, G. M., Fanning, S., et al. (1996). Effects of a selective inhibitor of the Abl tyrosine kinase on the growth of Bcr-Abl positive cells. *Nature Medicine, 2* (5), 561-566.
Dufourny, B., Alblas, J., van Teeffelen, H. A., van Schaik, F. M., van der Burg, B., Steenbergh, P. H., et al. (1997). Mitogenic signaling of insulin-like growth factor I in MCF-7 human breast cancer cells requires phosphatidylinositol 3-kinase and is independent of mitogen-activated protein kinase. *The Journal of Biological Chemistry, 272* (49), 31163-31171.
Dumont, N, & Arteaga, C. L. (2000). Transforming growth factor-beta and breast cancer: tumor promoting effects of transforming growth factor-beta. *Breast Cancer Research, 2* (2), 125-132.
Dumont, D. J., Jussila, L., Taipale, J., Lymboussaki, A., Mustonen, T., Pajusola, K., et al. (1998). Cardiovascular failure in mouse embryos deficient in VEGF receptor-3. *Science, 282* (5390), 946-949.
Dunn, I. F., Heese, O., & Black, P. M. (2000). Growth factors in glioma angiogenesis: FGFs, PDGF, EGF, and TGFs. *Journal of Neuro-oncology, 50* (1-2), 121-137.
Dvorak, H. F., Brown, L. F., Detmar, M., & Dvorak A. M. (1995). Vascular permeability factor/vascular endothelial growth factor, microvascular hyperpermeability, and angiogenesis. *American Journal of Pathology, 146* (5), 1029-1039.
Eckhardt, S. G., Rizzo, J., Sweeney, K. R., Cropp, G., Baker, S. D., Kraynak, M. A., et al. (1999). Phase I and pharmacologic study of the tyrosine kinase inhibitor SU101 in patients with advanced solid tumors. *Journal of Clinical Oncology, 17(4),* 1095-1104.
Eder, J. P., Clark, J. W., Supko, J. G., Shulman, L. N., Garcia-Carbonero, R., Roper, K., et al. (2001). A phase I pharmacokinetic and pharmacodynamic trial of recombinant human endostatin. *Proceedings of the American Society of Clinical Oncology, 20,* Abstract 275.
Eisen, T., Boshoff, C., Mak, I., Sapunar, F., Vaughan, M. M., Pyle, L., et al. (2000). Continuous low dose thalidomide: a phase II study in advanced melanoma, renal cell, ovarian and breast cancer. *British Journal of Cancer, 82* (4), 812-817.
El-Hariry, I., Pignatelli, M., Lemoine, N. R. (2001). FGF-1 and FGF-2 modulate the E-cadherin/catenin system in pancreatic adenocarcinoma cell lines. *British Journal of Cancer, 84* (12), 1656-1663.
Ellis, L. M., Takahashi, Y., Liu, W., & Shaheen, R. M. (2000). Vascular endothelial growth factor in human colon cancer: biology and therapeutic implications. *Oncologist, 5* (Suppl 1), 11-15.
El-Obeid, A., Bongcam-Rudloff, E., Sorby, M., Ostman, A., Nister, M., & Westermark, B. (1997). Cell scattering and migration induced by autocrine transforming growth factor alpha in human glioma cells in vitro. *Cancer Research, 57* (24), 5598-5604.
Engebraaten, O., Bjerkvig, R., Pedersen, P. H., & Laerum, O. D. (1993). Effects of EGF, bFGF, NGF and PDGF (bb) on cell proliferative, migratory and invasive capacities of human brain-tumour biopsies *in vitro. International Journal of Cancer, 53* (2), 209-214.
Engebraaten, O., Sivam, G., Juell, S., & Fodstad, O. (2000). Systemic immunotoxin treatment inhibits formation of human breast cancer metastasis and tumor growth in nude rats. *International Journal of Cancer, 88* (6), 970-976.
Ennis, B. W., Lippman, M. E., & Dickson, R. B. (1991). The EGF receptor system as a target for antitumor therapy. *Cancer Investigation, 9* (5), 553-562.
Eppert, K., Scherer, S. W., Ozcelik, H., Pirone, R., Hoodless, P., Kim, H., et al. (1996). MADR2 maps to 18q21 and encodes a TGFbeta-regulated MAD-related protein that is functionally mutated in colorectal carcinoma. *Cell, 86* (4), 543-552.
Erlichman, C., Boerner, S. A., Hallgren, C. G., Spieker, R., Wang, X. Y., James, C. D., et al. (2001). The HER tyrosine kinase inhibitor CI1033 enhances cytotoxicity of 7-ethyl-10-hydroxycamptothecin and topotecan by inhibiting breast cancer resistance protein-mediated drug efflux. *Cancer Research, 61* (2), 739-748.
Esserman, L. J., Lopez, T., Montes, R., Bald, L. N., Fendly, B. M., & Campbell, M. J. (1999). Vaccination with the extracellular domain of p185neu prevents mammary tumor development in neu transgenic mice. *Cancer Immunology, Immunotherapy, 47* (6), 337-342.
Faillot, T., Magdelenat, H., Mady, E., Stasiecki, P., Fohanno, D., Gropp, P., et al. (1996). A phase I study of an anti-epidermal growth factor receptor monoclonal antibody for the treatment of malignant gliomas. *Neurosurgery, 39* (3), 478-483.
Fan, Z., Baselga, J., Masui, H., & Mendelsohn, J (1993). Antitumor effect of anti-epidermal growth factor receptor monoclonal antibodies plus cis-diamminedichloroplatinum on well established A431 cell xenografts. *Cancer Research, 53*(19), 4637-4642.
Fan, Z., Masui, H., Altas, I., & Mendelsohn, J. (1993). Blockade of epidermal growth factor receptor function by bivalent and monovalent fragments of 225 anti-epidermal growth factor receptor monoclonal antibodies. *Cancer Research, 33,* 4322-4328.
Ferrara, N. (1999). Vascular endothelial growth factor: molecular and biological aspects. *Current Topics in Microbiology and Immunology, 237,* 1-30.
Fidler, I. J., Ellis, L. M. (1994). The implications of angiogenesis for the biology and therapy of cancer metastasis. *Cell, 79* (2), 185-188.

Figlin, R. A., Belldegrun, A., Lohner, M. E., Roskos, O., Yang, X-D., Schwab, G., et al. (2001). ABX-EGF: a fully human anti-EGF receptor antibody in patients with advanced cancer. *Proceedings of the American Society of Clinical Oncology, 20,* Abstract 1102.
Filmus, J., & Kerbel, R.S. (1993). Development of resistance mechanisms to the growth-inhibitory effects of transforming growth factor-beta during tumor progression. *Current Opinion in Oncology, 5* (1), 123-129.
Finkler, N., Gordon, A., Crozier, M., Edwards, R., Figueroa, J., Garcia, A., et. al. (2001). Phase 2 evaluation of OSI-774, a potent oral antagonist of the EGFR-TK in patients with advanced ovarian carcinoma. *Proceedings of the American Society of Clinical Oncology, 20,* Abstract 831.
Fischer-Colbrie, J., Witt, A., Heinzl, H., Speiser, P., Czerwenka, K., Sevelda, P., et al. (1997). EGFR and steroid receptors in ovarian carcinoma: Comparison with prognostic parameters and outcome of patients. *Anticancer Research, 17* (18), 613–619.
Folkman, J. (1971). Tumor angiogenesis: therapeutic implications. *New England Journal of Medicine, 285* (21), 1182-1186.
Folkman, J. (1996). Angiogenesis and metastatic growth. *Advances in Oncology, 12* (3), 3-7.
Fong, G. H., Rossant, J., Gertsenstein, M., & Breitman, M. L. (1995). Role of the Flt-1 receptor tyrosine kinase in regulating the assembly of vascular endothelium. *Nature, 376* (6535), 66-70.
Forsberg, K., Valyi-Nagy, I., Heldin, C-H., Herlyn, M., & Westermark, B. (1993). Platelet-derived growth factor (PDGF) in oncogenesis: Development of a vascular connective tissue stroma in xenotransplanted human melanoma producing PDGF-BB. *Proceedings of the National Academy of Sciences USA, 90* (2), 393-397.
Fry, D. W. (2000). Site-directed irreversible inhibitors of the erbB family of receptor tyrosine kinases as novel chemotherapeutic agents for cancer. *Anti-Cancer Drug Design, 15* (1), 3-16.
Fukuoka M., Yano, S., Giaccone, G., Tamura, T., Nakagawa K., Douillard J-Y, et al. (2002). Final results from a phase II trial of ZD1839 ("Iressa") for patients with advanced non-small-cell lung cancer (IDEAL 1). *Proceedings of the American Society of Clinical Oncology, 21,* Abstract 1188.
Furlanetto, R. W., Harwell, S. E., & Frick, K. K. (1994). Insulin-like growth factor-I induces cyclin-D1 expression in MG63 human osteosarcoma cells in vitro. *Molecular Endocrinology (Baltimore, Md), 8* (4), 510-517.
Garcia de Palazzo, I. E., Adams, G. P., Sundareshan, P., Wong, A .J., Testa, J. R., Bigner, D. D., et al. (1993). Expression of mutated epidermal growth factor receptor by non-small cell lung carcinomas. *Cancer Research, 53* (14), 3217-3220.
Garrison, M. A., Tolcher, A., McCreery, H., Rowinsky, E. K., Schott, A., Mace, J., et al. (2001). A phase I and pharmacokinetic study of CI-1033, a pan-ErbB tyrosine kinase inhibitor, given orally on days 1, 8, and 15 every 28 days to patients with solid tumors. *Proceedings of the American Society of Clinical Oncology, 20,* Abstract 283.
Gasparini, G. (1999). The rationale and future potential of angiogenesis inhibitors in neoplasia. *Drugs, 58* (1), 17-38.
George, D. (2001). Platelet derived growth factor receptors: A therapeutic target in solid tumors. *Seminars in Oncology, 28* (5 Suppl 17), 27-33.
Gerwins, P., Sköldenberg, E., & Claesson-Welsh, L. (2000). Function of fibroblast growth factors and vascular endothelial growth factors and their receptors in angiogenesis. *Critical Reviews in Oncology/Hematology, 34* (3), 185-194.
Gibson, S., Tu, S., Oyer, R., Anderson, S. M., & Johnson, G. L. (1999). Epidermal growth factor protects epithelial cells against Fas-induced apoptosis. Requirement for Akt activation. *The Journal of Biological Chemistry, 274* (25), 17612-17618.
Gieseg, M. A., de Bock, C., Ferguson, L. R., & Denny, W. A. (2001). Evidence for epidermal growth factor receptor-enhanced chemosensitivity in combinations of cisplatin and the new irreversible tyrosine kinase inhibitor CI-1033. *Anticancer Drugs, 12* (8), 683-690.
Giri, D., Ropiquet, F., & Ittmann, M. (1999). Alterations in expression of basic fibroblast growth factor (FGF) 2 and its receptor FGFR-1 in human prostate cancer. *Clinical Cancer Research, 5* (5), 1063-1071.
Gleevec™ [Package Insert]. (2001). East Hanover, NJ: Novartis Pharmaceuticals Corporation.
Gobbi, H., Arteaga, C. L., Jensen, R. A., Simpson, J. F., Dupont, W. D., Olson, S. J., et al. (2000). Loss of expression of transforming growth factor beta type II receptor correlates with high tumor grade in human breast in-situ and invasive carcinomas. *Histopathology, 36* (2), 168-177.
Gold, L. I. (1999). The role for transforming growth factor-beta (TGF-beta) in human cancer. *Critical Reviews in Oncogenesis, 10* (4), 303-360.
Goldstein, J., Graziano, R. F., Sundarapandiyan, K., Somasundaram, C., & Deo, Y. M. (1997). Cytolytic and cytostatic properties of an anti-human Fc gammaRI (CD64) x epidermal growth factor bispecific fusion protein. *Journal of Immunology, 158* (2), 872-879.
Goldstein, N. I., Prewett, M., Zuklys, K., Rockwell, P., & Mendelsohn, J. (1995). Biological efficacy of a chimeric antibody to the epidermal growth factor receptor in a human tumor xenograft model. *Clinical Cancer Research, 1* (11), 1311–1318.
Goss, G. D., Hirte, H., Lorimer, I., Miller, W., Stewart, D. J., Batish, G., et al. (2001). Final results of the dose escalation phase of a phase I pharmacokinetics (PK), pharmacodynamic (PD) and

biological activity of ZD1839; NCIC CTG Ind. 122. *Proceedings of the American Society of Clinical Oncology, 20,* Abstract 335.

Goss, G.D., Stewart D.J., Hirte, H., Miller, W., Major, P., Batist, G., et al. (2002). Initial results of part 2 of a phase I/II pharmacokinetics (PK), pharmacodynamic (PD) and biological activity study of ZD1839 (Iressa): NCIC CTG IND.122. *Proceedings of the American Society of Clinical Oncology, 21,* Abstract 59.

Goto, F., Goto, K., Weindel, K., & Folkman, J. (1993). Synergistic effects of vascular endothelial growth factor and basic fibroblast growth factor on the proliferation and cord formation of bovine capillary endothelial cells within collagen gels. *Laboratory Investigation, 69* (5), 508-517.

Goustin, A. S., Leof, E. B., Shipley, G. D., & Moses, H. L. (1986). Growth factors and cancer. *Cancer Research, 46* (3), 1015-1029.

Grandis, J. R., Melhem, M. F., Gooding, W. E., Day, R., Holst, V. A., Wagener, M. M., et al. (1998). Levels of TGF-alpha and EGFR protein in head and neck squamous cell carcinoma and patient survival. *Journal of the National Cancer Institute, 90* (11), 824-832.

Greenberger, L. M., Discafani, C., Wang, Y.-F., Tsou, H.-R., Overbeek, E. G., Nilakantan, R., et al. (2000). EKB-569: a new irreversible inhibitor of EGFR tyrosine kinase for the treatment of cancer. *Clinical Cancer Research, 6* (Suppl), Abstract 388, 4544s.

Guy, P. M., Platko, J. V., Cantley, L. C., Cerione, R. A., & Carraway, K. L. (1994). Insect cell-expressed $p180^{erbB3}$ possesses an impaired tyrosine kinase activity. *Proceedings of the National Academy of Sciences USA, 91* (17), 8132-8136.

Haddow, S., Fowlis, D. J., Parkinson, K., Akhurst, R. J., & Balmain, A. (1991). Loss of growth control by TGF-beta occurs at a late stage of mouse skin carcinogenesis and is independent of ras gene activation. *Oncogene, 6* (8), 1465-1470.

Hama, Y., Shimizu, T., Hosaka, S., Sugenoya, A., & Usuda, N. (1997). Therapeutic efficacy of the angiogenesis inhibitor O-(chloroacetyl-carbamoyl) fumagillol (TNP-470; AGM-1470) for human anaplastic thyroid carcinoma in nude mice. *Experimental and Toxicologic Pathology, 49* (3-4), 239-247.

Hammond, L. A., Denis, L. J., Salman, U. A., Chintapall, K., Hidalgo, M., Jeraback, P., et al. (2000) ^{18}FGD-PET evaluation of patients treated with the epidermal growth factor (EGFR) tyrosine kinase (TK) inhibitor, CP-358,774. *Clinical Cancer Research, 6* (Suppl), Abstract 385, 4543s.

Hammond, L. A., Figueroa, J., Schwartzberg, L., Ochoa, L., Hidalgo, M., Olivo, N., et al. (2001). Feasibility and pharmacokinetic (PK) trial of ZK1839 (Iressa™), an epidermal growth factor receptor tyrosine kinase inhibitor (EGFR-TKI), in combination with 5-fluorouracil (5-FU) and leucovorin (LV) in patients with advanced colorectal cancer. *Proceedings of the American Society of Clinical Oncology, 20,* Abstract 544.

Harris, A. L., Nicholson, S., Sainsbury, R., Wright, C., & Farndon, J. (1992). Epidermal growth factor receptor and other oncogenes as prognostic markers. *Journal of the National Cancer Institute Monograph, (11),* 181-187.

Hasegawa, Y., Takanashi, S., Kanehira, Y., Tsushima, T., Imai, T., & Okumura, K. (2001). Transforming growth factor-beta1 level correlates with angiogenesis, tumor progression, and prognosis in patients with nonsmall cell lung carcinoma. *Cancer, 91* (5), 964-971.

Heldin, C. H., Eriksson, U., Östman, A. (2002). New members of the platelet-derived growth factor family of mitogens. *Archives of Biochemistry and Biophyssics, 398* (2), 284-290.

Heldin, C. H., & Westermark, B. (1999). Mechanism of action and in vivo role of platelet-derived growth factor. *Physiological Reviews, 79* (4), 1283-1316.

Henriksen, R., Funa, K., Wilander, E., Backstrom, T., Ridderheim, M., & Oberg, L. (1993). Expression and prognostic significance of platelet-derived growth factor and its receptors in epithelial ovarian neoplasms. *Cancer Research, 53* (19), 4550-4554.

Herbst, R. S., Kim, E. S., & Harari, P. M. (2001). IMC-C225, an anti-epidermal growth factor receptor monoclonal antibody, for treatment of head and neck cancer. *Expert Opinion on Biological Therapy, 1* (4), 719-732.

Herbst, R. S., Tran, H. T., Madden, T. L., Khuri, F. R., Meyers, C. A., Shin, D. M., et al. (2000). Phase I Study of the Angiogenesis Inhibitor TNP-470 (T) in Combination with Paclitaxel (P) in Patients with Solid Tumors. *Proceedings of the American Society of Clinical Oncology, 19,* Abstract 707.

Herbst, R. S., Tran, H. T., Mullani, N. A., Charnsangavej, C., Madden, T. L., Hess, K. R., et al. (2001). Phase I Clinical Trial of Recombinant Human Endostatin (rHE) in Patients (Pts) with Solid Tumors: Pharmacokinetic (PK), Safety and Efficacy Analysis Using Surrogate Endpoints of Tissue and Radiologic Response. *Proceedings of the American Society of Clinical Oncology, 20,* Abstract 9.

Hidalgo, M., Siu, L. L., Nemunaitis, J., Rizzo, J., Hammond, L. A., Takimoto, C., et al. (2001). Phase I and pharmacologic study of OSI-774, an epidermal growth factor receptor tyrosine kinase inhibitor, in patients with advanced solid malignancies. *Journal of Clinical Oncology, 19* (13), 3267-3279.

Higashiyama, S., Abraham, J. A., Miller, J., Fiddes, J. C., & Klagsbrun, M. (1991). A heparin-binding growth factor secreted by macrophage-like cells that is related to EGF. *Science, 251* (4996), 936-939.

Hong, W. K., Arquette, M., Nabell, L., Needle, M. N., Waksal, H. W., & Herbst R. S. (2001). Efficacy and safety of the anti-epidermal growth factor antibody (EGFR) IMC-C225, in combination with cisplatin in patients with recurrent squamous cell carcinoma of the head and neck (SCCHN) refractory to cisplatin containing chemotherapy. *Proceedings of the American Society of Clinical Oncology, 20,* Abstract 895.

Houck, K. A., Leung, D. W., Rowland, A. M., Winer, J., & Ferrara, N. (1992). Dual regulation of vascular endothelial growth factor bioavailability by genetic and proteolytic mechanisms. *The Journal of Biological Chemistry, 267* (36), 26031-26037.

Howe, J. R., Roth, S., Ringold, J. C., Summers, R. W., Jarvinen, H. J., Sistonen, P., et al. (1998). Mutations in the SMAD/DPC4 gene in juvenile polyposis. *Science, 280* (5366), 1086-1088.

Hsei, V. C., Novotny, W. F., Margolin, K., Gordon, M., Small, E. J., Griffing, S., et al. (2001). Population Pharmacokinetic (PK) Analysis of Bevacizumab (BV) in Cancer Subjects. *Proceedings of the American Society of Clinical Oncology, 20,* Abstract 272.

Hudziak, R. M., Lewis, G. D., Winget, M., Fendly, B. M., Shepard, H. M., & Ullrich, A. (1989). p185HER2 monoclonal antibody has antiproliferative effects in vitro and sensitizes human breast tumors to tumor necrosis factor. *Molecular and Cellular Biology, 9* (3), 1165-1172.

Humphrey, P. A., Gangarosa, L. M., Wong, A. J., Archer, G. E., Lund-Johansen, M., Bjerkvig, R., et al. (1991). Deletion-mutant epidermal growth factor receptor in human gliomas: effects of type II mutation on receptor function. *Biochemical and Biophysical Research Communications, 178* (3), 1413-1420.

Hunter, K. E., Sporn, M. B., & Davies, A. M. (1993). Transforming growth factor-betas inhibit mitogen-stimulated proliferation of astrocytes. *Glia, 7* (3), 203-211.

Hupe, D. J., Behrens, N. D., & Boltz, R. (1990). Anti-proliferative activity of L-651,582 correlates with calcium-mediated regulation of nucleotide metabolism at phosphoribosyl pyrophosphate synthetase. *Journal of Cellular Physiology, 144* (3), 457-466.

Hupe, D. J., Boltz, R., Cohen, C. J., Felix, J., Ham, E., Miller, D., et al. (1991). The inhibition of receptor-mediated and voltage-dependent calcium entry by the antiproliferative L-651,582. *The Journal of Biological Chemistry, 266* (16), 10136-10142.

Ingber, D., Fujita, T., Kishimoto, S., Sudo, K., Kanamaru, T., Brem, H., et al. (1990). Synthetic analogues of fumagillin that inhibit angiogenesis and suppress tumour growth. *Nature 348* (6301), 555-557.

Inui, H., Kitami, Y., Tani, M., Kondo, T., & Inagami, T. (1994). Differences in signal transduction between platelet-derived growth factor (PDGF) alpha and beta receptors in vascular smooth muscle cells. PDGF-BB is a potent mitogen, but PDGF-AA promotes only protein synthesis without activation of DNA synthesis. *The Journal of Biological Chemistry, 269* (48), 30546-30552.

Jacobs, W., Mikkelsen, T., Smith, R., Nelson, K., Rosenblum, M. L., & Kohn, E. C. (1997). Inhibitory effects of CAI in glioblastoma growth and invasion. *Journal of Neuro-oncology, 32* (2), 93-101.

James, N. D., Atherton, P. J., Jones, J., Howie, A. J., Tchekmedyian, S., & Curnow, R. T. (2001). A phase II study of the bispecific antibody MDX-H210 (anti-HER2 x CD64) with GM-CSF in HER2+ advanced prostate cancer. *British Journal of Cancer, 85* (2), 152-156.

Jhappan, C., Stahle, D., Harkins, R. N., Fausto, N., Smith, G. H., & Merlino, G. T. (1990). TGF alpha overexpression in transgenic mice induced liver neoplasia and abnormal development of the mammary gland and pancreas. *Cell, 61* (6), 1137-1146.

Johnson, D. H., DeVore, R., Kabbinavar, F., Herbst, R., Holmgren, E., Novotny, W., et al. (2001). Carboplatin (C) + Paclitaxel (T) + RhuMab-VEGF (AVF) May Prolong Survival in Advanced Non-Squamous Lung Cancer. *Proceedings of the American Association for Cancer Research, 20,* Abstract 1256.

Kahn, C. R. (1985). The molecular mechanism of insulin action. *Annu Rev Med, 36,* 429-451.

Kajikawa, K., Yasui, W., Sumiyoshi, H., Yoshida, K., Nakayama, H., Ayhan, A., et al. (1991). Expression of epidermal growth factor in human tissues. Immunohistochemical and biochemical analysis. *Virchows Archive A: Pathological Anatomy and Histopathology, 418* (1), 27-32.

Kaplan, P. L., Anderson, M., & Ozanne, B. (1982). Transforming growth factor(s) production enables cells to grow in the absence of serum: an autocrine system. *Proceedings of the National Academy of Sciences USA, 79* (2), 485-489.

Karihaloo, A., Karumanchi, S. A., Barasch, J., Jha, V., Nickel, C. H., Yang, J., et al. (2001). Endostatin regulates branching morphogenesis of renal epithelial cells and ureteric bud. *Proceedings of the National Academy of Sciences USA, 98* (22), 12509-12514.

Karp, D. D., Silberman, S. L., Csudae, R., Wirth, F., Gaynes, L., Posner, G., et al. (1999). Phase I dose escalation study of epidermal growth factor receptor (EGFR) tyrosine kinase (TK) inhibitor CP-358,774 in patients with advanced solid tumors. *Proceedings of the American Society of Clinical Oncology, 18,* Abstract 1499.

Kawai, T., Hiroi, S., & Torikata, C. (1997). Expression in lung carcinomas of platelet-derived growth factor and its receptors. *Laboratory Investigation, 77* (5), 431-436.

Kawamoto, T., Mendelsohn, J., Le, A., Sato, G.H., Lazar, C.S., Gill, G.N. (1984). Relation of epidermal growth factor receptor concentration to growth of human epidermoid carcinoma A431 cells. *The Journal of Biological Chemistry, 259*(12), 7761-7766.

Kawamoto, T., Sato, J.D., Le, A., Polikoff, J., Sato, G.H., Mendelsohn. J. (1983). Growth stimulation of A431 cells by epidermal growth factor: identification of high-affinity receptors for epidermal growth factor by an anti-receptor monoclonal antibody. *Proceedings of the National Academy of Sciences USA, 80*(5), 1337-1341.

Kerbel, R. S. (2000). Tumor angiogenesis: past, present and the near future. *Carcinogenesis, 21* (3), 505-515.

Kieser, A., Weich, H. A., Brandner, G., Marme, D., & Kolch, W. (1994). Mutant p53 potentiates protein kinase C induction of vascular endothelial growth factor expression. *Oncogene, 9* (3), 963-969.

Klijn, J. G., Berns, P. M., Schmitz, P.I., & Foekens, J. A. (1992). The clinical significance of epidermal growth factor receptor (EGF-R) in human breast cancer: a review on 5232 patients. *Endocrine Reviews, 13* (1), 3-17.

Ko YJ, Chachoua A, Small E, Reese D, Kabbinavar F, Taneja S,et al. (1999). Phase II Study of SU101 in Patients with PSA-Positive Prostate Cancer. *Proceedings of the American Society of Clinical Oncology, 1999, 18,* Abstract 1220.

Kohn, E. C., Reed, E., Sarosy, G. A., Minasian, L., Bauer, K. S., Bostick-Bruton, F., et al. (2001). A phase I trial of carboxyamidotriazole and paclitaxel for relapsed solid tumors: potential efficacy of the combination and demonstration of pharmacokinetic interaction. *Clinical Cancer Research, 7* (6), 1600-1609.

Kraus, M. H., Fedi, P., Starks, V., Muraro, R., & Aaronson, S. A. (1993). Demonstration of ligand-dependent signaling by the *erb*B-3 tyrosine kinase and its constitutive activation in human breast tumor cells. *Proceedings of the National Academy of Sciences USA, 90* (7), 2900-2904.

Kraus, M. H., Issing, W., Miki, T., Popescu, N. C., & Aaronson, S. A. (1989). Isolation and characterization of ERBB3, a third member of the ERBB/epidermal growth factor receptor family: evidence for overexpression in a subset of human mammary tumors. *Proceedings of the National Academy of Sciences USA, 86* (23), 9193-9197.

Kris, M.G., Natale, R.B., Herbst, R.S., Lynch Jr., T.J., Prager, D., Belani, C.P., et al. (2002). A phase II trial of ZD1839 ("Iressa") in advanced non-small cell lung cancer (NSCLC) patients who had failed platinum- and docetaxel-based regimens (IDEAL 2). *Proceedings of the American Society of Clinical Oncology, 21,* Abstract 1166.

Kruger, E. A., & Figg, W. D. (2000). TNP-470: an angiogenesis inhibitor in clinical development for cancer. *Expert Opinion on Investigational Drugs, 9* (6), 1383-1396.

Kulkarni, A. B., Huh, C. G., Becker, D., Geiser, A., Lyght, M., Flanders, K. C., et al. (1993). Transforming growth factor beta 1 null mutation in mice causes excessive inflammatory response and early death. *Proceedings of the National Academy of Sciences USA, 90* (2), 770-774.

Kusaka, M., Sudo, K., Fujita, T., Marui, S., Itoh, F., Ingber, D., et al. (1991). Potent anti-angiogenic action of AGM-1470: comparison to the fumagillin parent. *Biochemical and Biophysical Research Communications, 174* (3), 1070-1076.

Kuzur, M. E., Albain, K. S., Huntington, M. O., Jones, S. F., Hainsworth, J. D., Greco, F. A., et al. (2000). A phase II trial of docetaxel and Herceptin in metastatic breast cancer patients overexpressing HER-2. *Proceedings of the American Society of Clinical Oncology, 19,* Abstract 512.

Laird, A. D., Vajkoczy, P., Shawver, L. K., Thurnher, A., Liang, C., Mohammadi, M., et al. (2000). SU6668 is a potent antiangiogenic and antitumor agent that induces regression of established tumors. *Cancer Research, 60* (15), 4152-4160.

Lambert, P. A., Somers, K. D., Kohn, E. C., & Perry, R. R. (1997). Antiproliferative and antiinvasive effects of carboxyamido-triazole on breast cancer cell lines. *Surgery, 122* (2), 372-379.

Laurence, D. J., & Gusterson, B. A. (1990). The epidermal growth factor. A review of structural and functional relationships in the normal organism and in cancer cells. *Tumour Biology (Basel), 11* (5), 229-261.

Leveen, P., Pekny, M., Gebre-Medhin, S., Swolin, B., Larsson, E., & Betsholtz, C. (1994). Mice deficient for PDGF B show renal, cardiovascular, and hematological abnormalities. *Genes and Development, 8* (16), 1875-1887.

Lorenzi, M. V., Horii, Y., Yamanaka, R., Sakaguchi, K., & Miki, T. (1996). FRAG1, a gene that potently activates fibroblast growth factor receptor by C-terminal fusion through chromosomal arrangement. *Proceedings of the National Academy of Sciences USA, 1996, 93* (17), 8956-8961.

Lymboussaki, A., Partanen, T. A., Olofsson, B., Thomas-Crusells, J., Fletcher, C. D., de Waal, R. M., et al. (1998). Expression of the vascular endothelial growth factor C receptor VEGFR-3 in lymphatic endothelium of the skin and in vascular tumors. *American Journal of Pathology, 153* (2), 395-403.

Markowitz, S., Wang, J., Myeroff, L., Parsons, R., Sun, L., Lutterbaugh, J., et al. (1995). Inactivation of the type II TGF-beta receptor in colon cancer cells with microsatellite instability. *Science, 268* (5215), 1336-1338.

Massague, J. (1990). The transforming growth factor-beta family. *Annual Review of Cell Biology, 6,* 597-641.

Massague, J. (1998). TGF-beta signal transduction. *Annual Review of Biochemistry, 67,* 753-791.

Massague, J., & Pandiella, A. (1993). Membrane-anchored growth factors. *Annual Review of Biochemistry, 62,* 515-541.

Masui, H., Kawamoto, T., Sato, J.D., Wolf, B., Sato, G., Mendelsohn, J. (1984). Growth inhibition of human tumor cells in athymic mice by anti-epidermal growth factor receptor monoclonal antibodies. *Cancer Research, 44*(3), 1002-1007.

Matsui, Y., Halter, S. A., Holt, J. T., Hogan, B. L., & Coffey, R. J. (1990). Development of mammary hyperplasia and neoplasia in MMTV-TGF alpha transgenic mice. *Cell, 61* (6), 1147-1155.
Maurizi, M., Almadori, G., Ferrandina, G., Distefano, M., Romanini, M. E., Cadoni, G., et al. (1996). Prognostic significance of epidermal growth factor receptor in laryngeal squamous cell carcinoma. *British Journal of Cancer, 74* (8), 1253-1257.
Maxwell, M., Galanopoulos, T., Hedley-Whyte, E. T., Black, P. M., & Antoniades, H. N. (1990). Human meningiomas co-express platelet-derived growth factor (PDGF) and PDGF-receptor genes and their protein products. *International Journal of Cancer, 46* (1), 16-21.
Mayer, A., Takimoto, M., Fritz, E., Schellander, G., Kofler, K., & Ludwig, H. (1993). The prognostic significance of proliferating cell nuclear antigen, epidermal growth factor receptor, and *mdr* gene expression in colorectal cancer. *Cancer, 71* (8), 2454–2460.
Ménard, S., Casalini, P., Campiglio, M., Pupa, S., Agresti, R., & Tagliabue, E. (2001). HER2 overexpression in various tumor types, focusing on its relationship to the development of invasive breast cancer. *Annals of Oncology, 12* (Suppl1), S15-S19.
Mendelsohn, J. (2000). Blockade of receptors for growth factors: an anticancer therapy—The Fourth Annual Joseph H. Burchenal American Association for Cancer Research Clinical Research Award Lecture. *Clinical Cancer Research, 6,* 747-753.
Mendelsohn, J., Baird, A., Fan, Z., & Markowitz, S. D. (2001). Growth factors and their receptors in epithelial malignancies. In J. Mendelsohn, P. M. Howley, M. A. Israel, L. A. Liotta (2nd Ed.), *The molecular basis of cancer* (pp.137-161). Philadelphia, Penn: W.B. Saunders Co.
Mendelsohn, J., & Baselga, J. (2000). The EGF receptor family as targets for cancer therapy. *Oncogene, 19,* 6550-6565.
Miller, V. A., Johnson, D., Heelan, R. T., Pizzo, B. A., Perez, W. J., Bass, A., et al. (2001). A pilot trial demonstrates the safety of ZD1839 ('Iressa'), an oral epidermal growth factor receptor tyrosine kinase inhibitor (EGFR-TKI), in combination with carboplatin (C) and paclitaxel (P) in previously untreated advanced non-small cell lung cancer (NSCLC). *Proceedings of the American Society of Clinical Oncology, 20,* Abstract 1301.
Minshall, C., Arkins, S., Straza, J., Conners, J., Dantzer, R., Freund, G. G., et al. (1997). IL-4 and insulin-like growth factor-I inhibit the decline in Bcl-2 and promote the survival of IL-3-deprived myeloid progenitors. *Journal of Immunology, 159* (3), 1225-1232.
Modjtahedi, H., Hickish, T., Nicolson, M., Moore, J., Styles, J., Eccles, S., et al. (1996). Phase I trial and tumour localisation of the anti-EGFR monoclonal antibody ICR62 in head and neck or lung cancer. *British Journal of Cancer, 73* (2), 228-235.
Morales, A. A., Duconge, J., Alvarez-Ruiz, D., Becquer-Viart, M. L., Nunez-Gandolff, G., Fernandez, E., et al. (2000). Humanized versus murine anti-human epidermal growth factor receptor monoclonal antibodies for immunoscintigraphic studies. *Nuclear Medicine and Biology, 27* (2), 199-206.
Morrison, R. S., Yamaguchi, F., Bruner, J. M., Tang, M., McKeehan, W., & Berger, M. S. (1994). Fibroblast growth factor receptor gene expression and immunoreactivity are elevated in human glioblastoma multiforme. *Cancer Research, 54* (10), 2794-2799.
Moscatello, D. K., Holgado-Madruga, M., Godwin, A. K., Ramirez, G., Gunn, G., Zoltick, P. W., et al. (1995). Frequent expression of a mutant epidermal growth factor receptor in multiple human tumors. *Cancer Research, 55* (23), 5536-5539.
Moscatello, D. K., Montgomery, R. B., Sundareshan, P., McDanel, H., Wong, M. Y., & Wong, A. J. (1996). Transformational and altered signal transduction by a naturally occurring mutant EGF receptor. *Oncogene, 13* (1), 85-96.
Moyer, J. D., Barbacci, E. G., Iwata, K. K., Arnold, L., Boman, B., Cunningham, A., et al. (1997). Induction of apoptosis and cell cycle arrest by CP-358,774, an inhibitor of epidermal growth factor receptor tyrosine kinase. *Cancer Research, 57* (21), 4838-4848.
Muller, W. J., Sinn, E., Pattengale, P. K., Wallace, R., & Leder, P. (1988). Single-step induction of mammary adenocarcinoma in transgenic mice bearing the activated c-neu oncogene. *Cell, 54* (1), 105-115.
Myeroff, L. L., Parsons, R., Kim, S. J., Hedrick, L., Cho, K. R., Orth, K., et al. (1995). A transforming growth factor beta receptor type II gene mutation common in colon and gastric but rare in endometrial cancers with microsatellite instability. *Cancer Research, 55* (23), 5545-5547.
Myoken, Y., Myoken, Y., Okamoto, T., Sato, J. D., Kan, M., McKeehan, W. L., et al. (1996). Immunohistochemical study of overexpression of fibroblast growth factor-1 (FGF-1), FGF-2, and FGF receptor-1 in human malignant salivary gland tumors. *The Journal of Pathology, 178* (4), 429-436.
Nakagawa, K., Yamamoto, N., Kudoh, S., Negoro, S., Takeda, K., Tamura, T., et. al. (2000). A phase I intermittent dose-escalation trial of ZD1839 (Iressa) in Japanese patients with solid malignant tumours. *Proceedings of the American Society of Clinical Oncology, 19,* Abstract 711.
Nakamura, M., Katano, M., Fujimoto, K., & Morisaki, T. (1997). A new prognostic strategy for gastric carcinoma: mRNA expression of tumor growth-related factors in endoscopic biopsy specimens. *Annals of Surgery, 226* (1), 35-42.
Neal, D. E., Sharples, L., Smith, K., Fennelly, J., Hall, R. R., & Harris, A. L. (1990). The epidermal growth factor receptor and the prognosis of bladder cancer. *Cancer, 65* (7), 1619-1625.

Nelson, J. M., & Fry, D. W. (2001). Akt, MAPK (Erk1/2), and p38 act in concert to promote apoptosis in response to ErbB receptor family inhibition. *The Journal of Biological Chemistry, 276* (18), 14842-14847.

Nickell, K. A., Halper, J., & Moses, H. L. (1983). Transforming growth factors in solid human malignant neoplasms. *Cancer Research, 43* (5), 1966-1971.

Normanno, N., Bianco, C., De Luca, A., & Salomon, D. S. (2001). The role of EGF-related peptides in tumor growth. *Frontiers in Bioscience, 6,* D685-707.

O'Dell SD, Day IN. (1998). Insulin-like growth factor II (IGF-II). *International Journal of Biochemistry and Cell Biology 1998, 30* (7), 767-771.

Okuda, K., Weisberg, E., Gilliland, D. G., & Griffin, J. D. (2001). ARG tyrosine kinase activity is inhibited by STI571. *Blood, 97* (8), 2440-2448.

Olofsson, B., Korpelainen, E., Pepper, M. S., Mandriota, S. J., Aase, K., Kumar, V., et al. (1998). Vascular endothelial growth factor B (VEGF-B) binds to VEGF receptor-1 and regulates plasminogen activator activity in endothelial cells. *Proceedings of the National Academy of Sciences USA, 95* (20), 11709-11714.

Onose, H., Emoto, N., Sugihara, H., Shimizu, K., & Wakabayashi, I. (1999). Overexpression of fibroblast growth factor receptor 3 in a human thyroid carcinoma cell line results in overgrowth of the confluent cultures. *European Journal of Endocrinology, 140* (2), 169-173.

O'Reilly, M. S., Boehm, T., Shing, Y., Fukai, N., Vasios, G., Lane, W. S., et al. (1997) Endostatin: an endogenous inhibitor of angiogenesis and tumor growth. *Cell, 88(2),* 277-285.

O'Reilly, M. S., Holmgren, L., Chen, C., & Folkman, J. (1996). Angiostatin induces and sustains dormancy of human primary tumors in mice. *Nature Medicine, 2* (6), 689-692.

O'Reilly, M. S., Holmgren, L., Shing, Y., Chen, C., Rosenthal, R. A., Moses, M., et al. (1994). Angiostatin: a novel angiogenesis inhibitor that mediates the suppression of metastases by a Lewis lung carcinoma. *Cell, 79* (2), 315-328.

Ornitz, D. M., & Leder, P. (1992). Ligand specificity and heparin dependence of fibroblast growth factor receptors 1 and 3. *The Journal of Biological Chemistry, 267* (23), 16305-16311.

Otsuki, T., Yamada, O., Yata, K., Sakaguchi, H., Kurebayashi, J., Nakazawa, N., et al. (1999). Expression of fibroblast growth factor and FGF-receptor family genes in human myeloma cells, including lines possessing t(4:14)(q16.3;q32.3) and FGFR3 translocation. *International Journal of Oncology, 15* (6), 1205-1212.

Owa, T., Yoshino, H., Yoshimatsu, K., & Nagasu, T. (2001). Cell cycle regulation in the g1 phase: a promising target for the development of new chemotherapeutic anticancer agents. *Current Medicinal Chemistry, 8* (12), 1487-1503.

Pardee, A. B. (1989). G_1 events and regulation of cell proliferation. *Science 246* (4930), 603-608.

Park, J. E., Keller, G. A., & Ferrara, N. (1993). The vascular endothelial growth factor (VEGF) isoforms: differential deposition into the subepithelial extracellular matrix and bioactivity of extracellular matrix-bound VEGF. *Molecular Biology of the Cell, 4* (12), 1317-1326.

Park, Y. H., Kim, S. A., Kim, C. J., & Chung, J. H. (2001). Mechanism of the Effect of Thalidomide on Human Multiple Myeloma Cells. *Proceedings of the American Society of Clinical Oncology, 20,* Abstract 2685.

Parrizas, M., & LeRoith, D. (1997). Insulin-like growth factor-1 inhibition of apoptosis is associated with increased expression of the bcl-xL gene product. *Endocrinology, 138* (3), 1355-1358.

Parsons, R., Myeroff, L. L., Liu, B., Willson, J. K., Markowitz, S. D., Kinzler, K. W., et al. (1995). Microsatellite instability and mutations of the transforming growth factor beta type II receptor gene in colorectal cancer. *Cancer Research, 55* (23), 5548-5550.

Pavelic, K., Banjac, Z., Pavelic, J., & Spaventi, S. (1993). Evidence for a role of EGF receptor in the progression of human lung carcinoma. *Anticancer Research, 13* (4), 1133-1138.

Pawson, T. (1995). Protein modules and signalling networks. *Nature, 373* (6515), 573-580.

Pegram, M. D., Lipton, A., Hayes, D. F., Weber, B. L., Baselga, J. M., Tripathy, D., et al. (1998). Phase II study of receptor-enhanced chemosensitivity using recombinant humanized anti-p185HER2/neu monoclonal antibody plus cisplatin in patients with HER2/neu-overexpressing metastatic breast cancer refractory to chemotherapy treatment. *Journal of Clinical Oncology, 16* (8), 2659-2671.

Pepper, M. S., Ferrara, N., Orci, L., & Montesano, R. (1992). Potent synergism between vascular endothelial growth factor and basic fibroblast growth factor in the induction of angiogenesis in vitro. *Biochemical and Biophysical Research Communications, 189* (2), 824-831.

Perabo, F. G., Demant, A. W., Wardelmann, E., Sitzia, M., Wirger, A., Albers, P., et al. (2000). Apoptosis induction and inhibition of proliferation in rat bladder cancer by carboxyamidotriazole (CAI). *Proceedings of the American Society of Clinical Oncology, 2000, 19,* Abstract 1433.

Perez-Soler, R., Chachoua, A., Huberman, M., Karp, D., Rigas, J., Hammond, L., et. al. (2001). A phase II trial of the epidermal growth factor receptor (EGFR) tyrosine kinase inhibitor OSI-774, following platinum-based chemotherapy, in patients (pts) with advanced, EGFR-expressing, non-small cell lung cancer (NSCLC). *Proceedings of the American Society of Clinical Oncology, 20,* Abstract 1235.

Peruzzi, F., Prisco, M., Dews, M., Salomoni, P., Grassilli, E., Romano, G., et al. (1999). Multiple signaling pathways of the insulin-like growth factor 1 receptor in protection from apoptosis. *Molecular and Cellular Biology, 19* (10), 7203-7215.

Petit, A. M., Rak, J., Hung, M. C., Rockwell, P., Goldstein, N., Fendly, B., et al. (1997). Neutralizing antibodies against epidermal growth factor and ErbB-2/neu receptor tyrosine kinases down-regulate vascular endothelial growth factor production by tumor cells in vitro and in vivo: angiogenic implications for signal transduction therapy of solid tumors. *American Journal of Pathology, 151* (6), 1523-1530.

Pietras, R. J., Pegram, M. D., Finn, R. S., Maneval, D. A., & Slamon, D. J. (1998). Remission of human breast cancer xenografts on therapy with humanized monoclonal antibody to HER-2 receptor and DNA-reactive drugs. *Oncogene, 17* (17), 2235-2249.

Pinkas-Kramarski, R., Soussan, L., Waterman, H., Levkowitz, G., Alroy, I., Klapper, et al. (1996). Diversification of Neu differentiation factor and epidermal growth factor signaling by combinatorial receptor interactions. *The EMBO Journal, 15(10),* 2452-2467.

Platten, M., Wick, W., & Weller, M. (2001). Malignant glioma biology: role for TGF-β in growth, motility, angiogenesis, and immune escape. *Microscopy Research and Technique, 52(4),* 401-410.

Pledger, W. J., Stiles, C. D., Antoniades, H. N., & Scher, C. D. (1977). Induction of DNA synthesis in BALB/c 3T3 cells by serum components: reevaluation of the commitment process. *Proceedings of the National Academy of Sciences USA, 74* (10), 4481-4485.

Plowright, E. E., Li, Z., Bergsagel, P. L., Chesi, M., Barber, D. L., Branch, D. R., et al. (2000). Ectopic expression of fibroblast growth factor receptor 3 promotes myeloma cell proliferation and prevents apoptosis. *Blood, 95* (3), 992-998.

Pollack, V. A., Savage, D. M., Baker, D. A., Tsaparikos, K. E., Sloan, D. E., Moyer, J. D., et al. (1999). Inhibition of epidermal growth factor receptor-associated tyrosine phosphorylation in human carcinomas with CP-358,774: dynamics of receptor inhibition in situ and antitumor effects in athymic mice. *The Journal of Pharmacology and Experimental Therapeutics, 291* (2), 739-748.

Poon, R. T., Fan, S. T., & Wong, J. (2001). Clinical implications of circulating angiogenic factors in cancer patients. *Journal of Clinical Oncology, 19* (4), 1207-1225.

Powers, C. J., McLeskey, S. W., & Wellstein, A. (2000). Fibroblast growth factors, their receptors and signaling. *Endocrine-Related Cancer, 7* (3), 165-197.

Prenzel, N., Fischer, O. M., Streit, S., Hart, S., & Ullrich, A. (2001). The epidermal growth factor receptor family as a central element for cellular signal transduction and diversification. *Endocrine-Related Cancer, 8* (1), 11-31.

Presta, L. G., Chen, H., O'Connor, S. J., Chisholm, V., Meng, Y. G., Krummen, L., et al. (1997). Humanization of an anti-vascular endothelial growth factor monoclonal antibody for the therapy of solid tumors and other disorders. *Cancer Research, 57* (20), 4593-4599.

Price, J. T., Wilson, H. M., & Haites, N. E. (1996). Epidermal growth factor (EGF) increases the *in vitro* invasion, motility and adhesion interactions of the primary renal carcinoma cell line, A704. *European Journal of Cancer, 32A* (11), 1977-1982.

Rak, J., Mitsuhashi, Y., Bayko, L., Filmus, J., Shirasawa, S., Sasazuki, T., et al. (1995). Mutant ras oncogenes upregulate VEGF/VPF expression: implications for induction and inhibition of tumor angiogenesis. *Cancer Research, 55* (20), 4575-4580.

Ranson, M., Hammond, L.A., Ferry, D., Kris, M., Tullo, A., Murray, P.I., et al. (2002). ZD1839, a selective oral epidermal growth factor receptor-tyrosine kinase inhibitor, is well tolerated and active in patients with solid, malignant tumors: results of a phase I trial. *Journal of Clinical Oncology, 20* (9), 2240-50.

Raymond, E., Faivre, S., & Armand, J. P. (2000). Epidermal growth factor receptor tyrosine kinase as a trarget for anticancer therapy. *Drugs, 60* (Suppl 1), 15-23.

Reisner, A. H. (1985). Similarity between the vaccinia virus 19K early protein and epidermal growth factor. *Nature, 313* (6005), 801-803.

Resnicoff, M., Burgaud, J. L., Rotman, H. L., Abraham, D., & Baserga, R. (1995). Correlation between apoptosis, tumorigenesis, and levels of insulin-like growth factor I receptors. *Cancer Research, 55* (17), 3739-3741.

Rewcastle, G. W., Murray, D. K., Elliott, W. L., Fry, D. W., Howard, C. T., Nelson, J. M., et al. (1998). Tyrosine kinase inhibitors. 14. Structure-activity relationships for methylamino-substituted derivates of 4-[(3-bromophenyl)amino]-6-(methylamino)-pyrido[3,4-d] Pyrimidine (PD 158780), a potent and specific inhibitor of the tyrosine kinase activity of receptors for the EGF family of growth factors. *Journal of Medicinal Chemistry, 41* (5), 742-751.

Rich, J. N., Zhang, M., Datto, M. B., Bigner, D. D., & Wang, X. F. (1999). Transforming growth factor-beta-mediated p15(INK4B) induction and growth inhibition in astrocytes is SMAD3-dependent and a pathway prominently altered in human glioma cell lines. *The Journal of Biological Chemistry, 274* (49), 35053-35058.

Riedel, H., Massoglia, S., Schlessinger, J., & Ullrich, A. (1988). Ligand activation of overexpressed epidermal growth factor receptor transforms NIH 3T3 mouse fibroblasts. *Proceedings of the National Academy of Sciences USA, 85* (5), 1477-1481.

Riggins, G. J., Thiagalingam, S., Rozenblum, E., Weinstein, C. L., Kern, S. E., Hamilton, S. R., et al. (1996). Mad-related genes in the human. *Nature Genetics, 13* (3), 347-349.

Risau, W., Drexler, H., Mironov, V., Smits, A., Siegbahn, A., Funa, K., et al. (1992). Platelet-derived growth factor is angiogenic in vivo. *Growth Factors, 7* (4), 261-266.

Roberts, C. T. Jr., Brown, A. L., Graham, D. E., Seelig, S., Berry, S., Gabbay, K. H., et al. (1986). Growth hormone regulates the abundance of insulin-like growth factor I RNA in adult rat liver. *The Journal of Biological Chemistry, 261* (22), 10025-10028.

Rodeck, U., Jost, M., Kari, C., Shih, D. T., Lavker, R. M., Ewert, D. L., et al. (1997). EGF-R dependent regulation of keratinocyte survival. *Journal of Cell Science, 110* (Pt 2), 113-121.

Rogler, C. E., Yang, D., Rossetti, L., Donohoe, J., Alt, E., Chang, C. J., et al. (1994). Altered body composition and increased frequency of diverse malignancies in insulin-like growth factor-II transgenic mice. *The Journal of Biological Chemistry, 269* (19), 13779-13784.

Roman, C., Saha, D., & Beauchamp, R. (2001). TGF-beta and colorectal carcinogenesis. *Microscopy Research and Technique, 52* (4), 450-457.

Rooke, H. M., & Crosier, K. E. (2001). The smad proteins and TGFbeta signaling: Uncovering a pathway critical in cancer. *Pathology, 33* (1), 73-84.

Rosen, L. S., Rosen, P. J., Kabbinavar, F., Mulay, M., Mickey, J., Hernandez, L., et al. (2001). Phase I experience with SU6668, a novel multiple receptor tyrosine kinase inhibitor in patients with advanced malignancies. *Proceedings of the American Society of Clinical Oncology, 20,* Abstract 383.

Rossmanith, W., & Schulte-Hermann, R. (2001). Biology of transforming growth factor beta in hepatocarcinogenesis. *Microscopy Research and Technique, 52* (4), 430-436.

Rothenberg, M. L., Berlin, J. D., Cropp, G. F., Fleischer, A. C., Schumaker, R. D., Hande, K. R., et al. (2001). Phase I/II study of SU5416 in combination with irinotecan/5-FU/LV (IFL) in patients with metastatic colorectal cancer. *Proceedings of the Amercan Society of Clinical Oncology, 20,* Abstract 298.

Rowinsky, E. K., Hammond, L., Siu, L., Jerabek, P., Rizzo, J., Denis, L., et al. (2001). Dose-schedule-finding, pharmacokinetic (PK), biologic, and functional imaging studies of OSI-774, a selective epidermal growth factor receptor (EGFR) tyrosine kinase (TK) inhibitor. *Proceedings of the American Society of Clinical Oncology, 20,* Abstract 5.

Rubin, R., & Baserga, R. (1995). Insulin-like growth factor-I receptor. Its role in cell proliferation, apoptosis, and tumorigenicity. *Laboratory Investigation, 73* (3), 311-331.

Saito, H., Tsujitani, S., Oka, S., Kondo, A., Ikeguchi, M., Maeta, M., et al. (1999). The expression of transforming growth factor-beta1 is significantly correlated with the expression of vascular endothelial growth factor and poor prognosis of patients with advanced gastric carcinoma. *Cancer, 86* (8), 1455-1462.

Saito, M., Mitsui, T., & Mizuno, T. (2000). Genistein represses the induction of prostatic buds by testosterone. *Journal de la Societe de Biologie, 194* (2), 95-97.

Salomon, D. S., Brandt R., Ciardiello, F., & Normanno, N. (1995). Epidermal growth factor-related peptides and their receptors in human malignancies. *Critical Reviews in Oncology/Hematology, 19* (3), 183-232.

Saltz, L., Hochster, H., Tchekmeydian, N. S., Rubin, M., Waksal, H., Needle, M. N., et al. (2001). Acne-like rash predicts response in patients treated with cetuximab (IMC-C225) plus irinotecan (CPT-11) is active in CPT-11-refractory colorectal cancer (CRC) that expresses epidermal growth factor receptor (EGFR). Poster presented at the 2001 American Association for Cancer Research (AACR)-NationalCancer Institute (NCI)-European Organization for Research and Treatment of Cancer (EORTC) International Conference, Miami, Fla.

Saltz, L., Meropol N.J., Loehrer, P.J., Waksal H., Needle, M.N., Mayer, R.J. (2002) Single agent IMC-C225 (Erbitux™) has activity in CPT-11-refractory colorectal cancer (CRC) that expressed epidermal growth factor receptor (EGFR). *Proceedings of the American Society of Clinical Oncology, 21* Abstract 504.

Salven, P., Lymboussaki, A., Heikkila, P., Jaaskela-Saari, H., Enholm, B., Aase, K., et al. (1998). Vascular endothelial growth factors VEGF-B and VEGF-C are expressed in human tumors. *American Journal of Pathology, 153* (1), 103-108.

Sandgren, E. P., Luetteke, N. C., Palmiter, R. D., Brinster, R. L., & Lee, D. C. (1990). Overexpression of TGF alpha in transgenic mice: induction of epithelial hyperplasia, pancreatic metaplasia, and carcinoma of the breast. *Cell, 61* (6), 1121-1135.

Santini, J., Formento, J. L., Francoual, M., Milano, G., Schneider, M., Dassonville, O., et al. (1991). Characterization, quantification, and potential clinical value of the epidermal growth factor receptor in head and neck squamous cell carcinomas. *Head & Neck, 13* (2), 132-139.

Sarup, J. C., Johnson, R. M., King, K. L., Fendly, B. M., Lipari, M. T., Napier, M. A., et al. (1991). Characterization of an anti-p185HER2 monoclonal antibody that stimulates receptor function and inhibits tumor cell growth. *Growth Regulation, 1* (2), 72-82.

Schiller, J. H., & Bittner, G. (1999). Potentiation of platinum antitumor effects in human lung tumor xenografts by the angiogenesis inhibitor squalamine: effects on tumor neovascularization. *Clinical Cancer Research, 5* (12), 4287-4294.

Schiller, J. H., Hammond, L. A., Carbone, D. P., Hong, W. K., Holroyd, K., Williams, J. I., et al. (2001). Phase 2A Trial of Squalamine for Treatment of Advanced Non-Small Cell Lung Cancer. *Proceedings of the American Society of Clinical Oncology, 20,* Abstract 1353.

Schiller, J. H., Harrington, D., Belani, C. P., Langer, C., Sandler, A., Krook, J., et al. (2002). Comparison of four chemotherapy regimens for advanced non-small-cell lung cancer. *New England Journal of Medicine, 346* (2), 92-98.
Scholl, S., Beuzeboc, P., & Pouillart, P. (2001). Targeting HER2 in other tumor types. *Annals of Oncology, 12* (Suppl 1), S81-87.
Schreiber, A. B., Winkler, M. E., & Derynck, R. (1986). Transforming growth factor-α: a more potent angiogenic mediator than epidermal growth factor. *Science, 232* (4755), 1250-1253.
Seidman, A. D., Fornier, M., Esteva, F., Tan, L., Kaptain, S., Bach, A., et al. (2000). Final report: weekly (W) Herceptin (H) and Taxol (T) for metastatic breast cancer (MBC): analysis of efficacy by HER2 immunophenotype [immunohistochemistry (IHC)] and gene amplification [fluorescent in-situ hybridization (FISH)]. *Proceedings of the American Society of Clinical Oncology, 19,* Abstract 319.
Sell, C., Baserga, R., & Rubin, R. (1995). Insulin-like growth factor I (IGF-I) and the IGF-I receptor prevent etoposide-induced apoptosis. *Cancer Research, 55* (2), 303-306.
Senger, D. R., Van de Water, L., Brown, L. F., Nagy, J. A., Yeo, K. T., Yeo, T. K., et al. (1993). Vascular permeability factor (VPF, VEGF) in tumor biology. *Cancer and Metastasis Reviews, 12* (3-4), 303-324.
Senzer, N. N., Soulieres, D., Siu, L., Agarwala, S., Vokes, E., Hidalgo, M., et. al. (2001). Phase 2 evaluation of OSI-774, a potent oral antagonist of the EGFR-RK in patients with advanced squamous cell carcinoma of the head and neck. *Proceedings of the American Society of Clinical Oncology, 20,* Abstract 6.
Seymour, L., & Bezwoda, W. R. (1994). Positive immunostaining for platelet derived growth factor (PDGF) is an adverse prognostic factor in patients with advanced breast cancer. *Breast Cancer Research and Treatment, 32* (2), 229-233.
Shalaby, F., Rossant, J., Yamaguchi, T. P., Gertsenstein, M., Wu, X. F., Breitman, M. L., et al. (1995). Failure of blood-island formation and vasculogenesis in Flk-1-deficient mice. *Nature, 376* (6535), 62-66.
Shawver, L. K., Schwartz, D. P., Mann, E., Chen, H., Tsai, J., Chu, L., et al. (1997). Inhibition of platelet-derived growth factor-mediated signal transduction and tumor growth by N-[4-(trifluoromethyl)-phenyl]5-methylisoxazole-4-carboxamide. *Clinical Cancer Research, 3* (7), 1167-1177.
Shepard, H. M., Lewis, G. D., Sarup, J. C., Fendly, B. M., Maneval, D., Mordenti, J., et al. (1991). Monoclonal antibody therapy of human cancer: taking the HER2 protooncogene to the clinic. *Journal of Clinical Immunology, 11* (3), 117-127.
Sherr, C. J. (1996). Cancer cell cycles. *Science, 274* (5293), 1672-1677.
Sherr, C. J., & Roberts, J. M. (1995). Inhibitors of mammalian G1 cyclin-dependent kinases. *Genes and Development, 9* (10), 1149-1163.
Shibata, T., Kawano, T., Nagayasu, H., Okumura, K., Arisue, M., Hamada, J., et al. (1996). Enhancing effects of epidermal growth factor on human squamous cell carcinoma motility and matrix degradation but not growth. *Tumuor Biol, 17* (3), 168-175.
Shin, D. M., Nemunaitis, J., Zinner, R. G., Donato, N. J., Shin, H .J. C., Myers, J. N., et al. (2001). A phase I clinical and biomarker study of CI-1033, a novel pan-ErbB tyrosine kinase inhibitor in patients with solid tumors. *Proceedings of the American Society of Clinical Oncology, 20,* Abstract 324.
Shing, Y., Folkman, J., Sullivan, R., Butterfield, C., Murray, J., & Klagsbrun, M. (1984). Heparin affinity: purification of a tumor-derived capillary endothelial cell growth factor. *Science, 223* (4642), 1296-1299.
Shoyab, M., Plowman, G. D., McDonald, V. L., Bradley, J. G., & Todaro, G. J. (1989). Structure and function of human amphiregulin: a member of the epidermal growth factor family. *Science, 243* (4894 Pt 1), 1074-1076.
Shull, M. M., Ormsby, I., Kier, A. B., Pawlowski, S., Diebold, R. J., Yin, M., et al. (1992). Targeted disruption of the mouse transforming growth factor-beta 1 gene results in multifocal inflammatory disease. *Nature, 359* (6397), 693-699.
Shusterman, S., Grupp, S. A., Barr, R., Carpentieri, D., Zhao, H., Maris, J. M., et al. (2001). The angiogenesis inhibitor tnp-470 effectively inhibits human neuroblastoma xenograft growth, especially in the setting of subclinical disease. *Clinical Cancer Research, 7* (4), 977-984.
Shweiki, D., Itin, A., Soffer, D., & Keshet, E. (1992). Vascular endothelial growth factor induced by hypoxia may mediate hypoxia-initiated angiogenesis. *Nature, 359* (6398), 843-845.
Siegbahn, A., Hammacher, A., Westermark, B., & Heldin, C. H. (1990). Differential effects of the various isoforms of platelet-derived growth factor on chemotaxis of fibroblasts, monocytes, and granulocytes. *The Journal of Clinical Investigation, 85* (3), 916-920.
Sim, B. K., O'Reilly, M. S., Liang, H., Fortier, A. H., He, W., Madsen, J. W., et al. (1997). A recombinant human angiostatin protein inhibits experimental primary and metastatic cancer. *Cancer Research, 57* (7), 1329-1334.
Singh, Y., Shikata, N., Kiyozuka, Y., Nambu, H., Morimoto, J., Kurebayashi, J., et al. (1997). Inhibition of tumor growth and metastasis by angiogenesis inhibitor TNP-470 on breast cancer cell lines in vitro and in vivo. *Breast Cancer Research and Treatment, 45* (1), 15-27.

Sirotnak, F. M., Zakowsky, M. F., Miller, V. A., Scher, H. I., & Kris, M. G. (2000). Potentiation of cytotoxic agents against human tumors in mice by ZD1839 (Iressa™), an inhibitor of EGFR tyrosine kinase, does not require high levels of expression of EGFR. *Proceedings of the American Association for Cancer Research, 41,* Abstract 3076.
Siu, L. L., Hidalgo, M., Nemunaitis, J., Rizzo, J., Moczygemba, S. G., Eckhardt, S. G., et al. (1999). Dose and schedule-duration escalation of the epidermal growth factor receptor (EGFR) tyrosine kinase (TK) inhibitor CP-358,774: a phase I and pharmacokinetic (PK) study. *Proceedings of the American Society of Clinical Oncology, 18,* Abstract 1498.
Sjöblom, T., Shimizu, A., O'Brien, K. P., Pietras, K., Dal Cin, P., Buchdunger, E., et al. (2001). Growth inhibition of dermatofibrosarcoma protuberans tumors by the platelet-derived growth factor receptor antagonist STI571 through induction of apoptosis. *Cancer Research, 61* (15), 5778-5783.
Slamon, D. J., Clark, G. M., Wong, S. G., Levin, W. J., Ullrich, A., & McGuire, W. L. (1987). Human breast cancer: correlation of relapse and survival with amplification of the HER-2/*neu* oncogene. *Science, 235* (4785), 177-182.
Slamon, D. J., Leyland-Jones, B., Shak, S., Fuchs, H., Paton, V., Bajamonde, A., et al. (2001). Use of chemotherapy plus a monoclonal antibody against HER2 for metastatic breast cancer that overexpresses HER2. *New England Journal of Medicine, 344* (11), 783-792.
Slamon, D. J., Patel, R., Northfelt, R., Pegram, M., Rubin, J., Sebastian, G., et al. (2001). Phase II pilot study of Herceptin combined with taxotere and carboplatin (TCH) in metastatic breast cancer (MBC) patients overexpressing the HER2-neu proto-oncogene a pilot study of the UCLA network. *Proceedings of the American Society of Clinical Oncology, 20,* Abstract 193.
Sledge, G., Miller, K., Novotny, W., Gaudreault, J., Ash, M., & Cobleigh, M. (2000). A Phase II Trial of Single-Agent Rhumab VEGF (Recombinant Humanized Monoclonal Antibody to Vascular Endothelial Cell Growth Factor) in Patients with Relapsed Metastatic Breast Cancer. *Proceedings of the American Society of Clinical Oncology, 19,* Abstract 5C.
Slichenmyer, W. J., Elliott, W. L., & Fry, D. W. (2001). CI-1033, a pan-erbB tyrosine kinase inhibitor. *Seminars in Oncology, 28* (5 Suppl 16), 80-85.
Slichenmyer, W. J., & Fry, D. W. (2001). Anticancer therapy targeting the erbB family of receptor tyrosine kinases. *Seminars in Oncology 28* (5 Suppl 16), 67-79.
Sliwkowski MX, Schaefer G, Akita RW, Lofgren JA, Fitzpatrick VD, Nuijens A, et al. (1994). Coexpression of erbB2 and erbB3 proteins reconstitutes a high affinity receptor for heregulin. *The Journal of Biological Chemistry, 269* (20), 14661-14665.
Smith, G. H., Sharp, R., Kordon, E. C., Jhappan, C., & Merlino, G. (1995). Transforming growth factor-alpha promotes mammary tumorigenesis through selective survival and growth of secretory epithelial cells. *American Journal of Pathology, 147* (4), 1081-1096.
Soriano, P. (1994). Abnormal kidney development and hematological disorders in PDGF beta-receptor mutant mice. *Genes and Development, 8* (16), 1888-1896.
Sporn, M. B., & Roberts A. B. (1985). Autocrine growth factors and cancer. *Nature 313* (6005), 745-747.
Stebbing, J., Benson, C., Eisen, T., Pyle, L., Smalley, K., Bridle, H., et al. (2001). The treatment of advanced renal cell cancer with high-dose oral thalidomide. *British Journal of Cancer, 85* (7), 953-958.
Stefanik, D. F., Rizkalla, L. R., Soi, A., Goldblatt, S. A., & Rizkalla, W. M. (1991). Acidic and basic fibroblast growth factors are present in glioblastoma multiforme. *Cancer Research, 51* (20), 5760-5765.
Takahashi, J. A., Fukumoto, M., Igarashi, K., Oda, Y., Kikuchi, H., & Hatanaka, M. (1992). Correlation of basic fibroblast growth factor expression levels with the degree of malignancy and vascularity in human gliomas. *Journal of Neurosurgery, 76* (5), 792-798.
Takahashi, J. A., Mori, H., Fukumoto, M., Igarashi, K., Jaye, M., Oda, Y., et al. (1990). Gene expression of fibroblast growth factors in human gliomas and meningiomas: demonstration of cellular source of basic fibroblast growth factor mRNA and peptide in tumor tissues. *Proceedings of the National Academy of Sciences USA , 87* (15), 5710-5714.
Takanami, I., Imamura, T., Yamamoto, Y., & Kodaira, S. (1995). Usefulness of platelet-derived growth factor as a prognostic factor in pulmonary adenocarcinoma. *Journal of Surgical Oncology, 58* (1), 40-43.
Talapatra, S., & Thompson, C. B. (2001). Growth factor signaling in cell survival: implications for cancer treatment. *The Journal of Pharmacology and Experimental Therapeutics, 298* (3), 873-878.
Tannheimer, S. L., Rehemtulla, A., & Ethier, S. P. (2000). Characterization of fibroblast growth factor receptor 2 overexpression in the human breast cancer cell line SUM-52PE. *Breast Cancer Research, 2* (4), 311-320.
Thompson, A. M., Murray, D. K., Elliott, W. L., Fry, D. W., Nelson, J. A, Showalter, H. D., et al. (1997). Tyrosine kinase inhibitors. 13. Structure-activity relationships for soluble 7-substituted 4-[(3-bromophenyl)amino]pyrido[4,3-d] pyrimidines designed as inhibitors of the tyrosine kinase activity of the epidermal growth factor receptor. *Journal of Medicinal Chemistry, 40* (24), 3915-3925.
Torrance, C. J., Jackson, P. E., Montgomery, E., Kinzler, K. W., Vogelstein, B., Wissner, A., et al. (2000). Combinatorial chemoprevention of intestinal neoplasia. *Nature Medicine, 6* (9), 1024-1028.

Tosi, P., Zamagni, E., Cellini, C., Ronconi, S., Patriarca, F., Ballerini, F., et al. (2002). Salvage therapy with thalidomide in patients with advanced relapsed/refractory multiple myeloma. *Haematologica, 87* (4), 408-414.
Toyoda, H., Komurasaki, T., Uchida, D., Takayama, Y., Isobe, T., Okuyama, T., et al. (1995). Epiregulin. A novel epidermal growth factor with mitogenic activity for rat primary hepatocytes. *The Journal of Biological Chemistry, 270* (13), 7495-7500.
Tsai, J. C., Goldman, C. K., & Gillespie, G. Y. (1995). Vascular endothelial growth factor in human glioma cell lines: induced secretion by EGF, PDGF-BB, and bFGF. *Journal of Neurosurgery, 82* (5), 864-873.
Tseng, J. E., Glisson, B. S., Khuri, F. R., Shin, D. M., Myers, J. N., El-Naggar, A. K., et al. (2001). Phase II study of the antiangiogenesis agent thalidomide in recurrent or metastatic squamous cell carcinoma of the head and neck. *Cancer, 92* (9), 2364-2373.
Tsurusaki, T., Kanda, S., Sakai, H., Kanetake, H., Saito, Y., Alitalo, K., et al. (1999). Vascular endothelial growth factor-C expression in human prostatic carcinoma and its relationship to lymph node metastasis. *British Journal of Cancer, 80* (1-2), 309-313.
Turkeri, L. N., Erton, M. L., Cevik, I., & Akdas, A. (1998). Impact of the expression of epidermal growth factor, transforming growth factor alpha, and epidermal growth factor receptor on the prognosis of superficial bladder cancer. *Urology, 51* (4), 645-649.
Uegaki, K., Nio, Y., Inoue, Y., Minari, Y., Sato, M., Song, M.-M., et al. (1997). Clinicopathological significance of epidermal growth factor and its receptor in human pancreatic cancer. *Anticancer Research, 17* (5B):3841-3847.
Ueno, N. T., Yu, D., & Hung, M. C. (2001) E1A: tumor suppressor or oncogene? Preclinical and clinical investigations of E1A gene therapy. *Breast Cancer, 8* (4), 285-293.
Ullrich, A., & Schlessinger, J. (1990). Signal transduction by receptors with tyrosine kinase activity. *Cell, 61* (2), 203-212.
Veale, D., Kerr, N., Gibson, G. J., Kelly, P. J., & Harris, A. L. (1993). The relationship of quantitative epidermal growth factor receptor expression in non-small cell lung cancer to long term survival. *British Journal of Cancer, 68* (1), 162-165.
Veikkola, T., & Alitalo, K. (1999). VEGFs, receptors and angiogenesis. *Seminars in Cancer Biology, 9* (3), 211-220.
Verbeek, B. S., Adriaansen-Slot, S. S., Vroom, T. M., Beckers, T., & Rijksen, G. (1998). Overexpression of EGFR and c-erbB2 causes enhanced cell migration in human breast cancer cells and NIH3T3 fibroblasts. *FEBS Letters, 425* (1), 145-150.
Vlahos, C. J., Matter, W. F., Hui, K. Y., & Brown, R. F. (1994). A specific inhibitor of phosphatidylinositol 3-kinase, 2-(4-morpholinyl)-8-phenyl-4H-1-benzopyran-4-one (LY294002). *The Journal of Biological Chemistry, 269* (7), 5241–5248.
Volm, M., Rittgen, W., & Drings, P. (1998). Prognostic value of ERBB-1, VEGF, cyclin A, FOS, JUN, and MYC in patients with squamous cell lung carcinomas. *British Journal of Cancer, 77* (4), 663-669.
Vuky, J., Berg, W., Yu, R., Ginsberg, M., Mazumdar, M., Bacik, J., et al. (2001). Phase II Trial of Thalidomide in Patients with Metastatic Renal Cell Carcinoma (RCC). *Proceedings of the American Society of Clinical Oncology, 20,* Abstract 1056.
Wagner, M., Lopez, M. E., Cahn, M., & Korc, M. (1998). Suppression of fibroblast growth factor receptor signaling inhibits pancreatic cancer growth in vitro and in vivo. *Gastroenterology, 114* (4), 798-807.
Wahl, M., Grant, D., Owen, C., Page, A., Zahachewsky, M., DeMoraes, E., et al. (2001). Acidification Enhances the Effect of Human Recombinant Angiostatin (rhA) on Human Endothelial Cells. *Proceedings of the American Association for Cancer Research, 20,* Abstract 3123.
Wallace, P. K., Romet-Lemonne, J. L., Chokri, M., Kasper, L. H., Fanger, M.W., & Fadul, C. E. (2000). Production of macrophage-activated killer cells for targeting of glioblastoma cells with bispecific antibody to FcgammaRI and the epidermal growth factor receptor. *Cancer Immunology, Immunotherapy, 49* (9), 493-503.
Wang, D., Huang, H. J., Kazlauskas, A., & Cavenee, W. K. (1999). Induction of vascular endothelial growth factor expression in endothelial cells by platelet-derived growth factor through the activation of phosphatidylinositol 3-kinase. *Cancer Research, 59* (7), 1464-1472.
Wang, L., Ma, W., Markovich, R., Lee, W. L., & Wang, P. H. (1998). Insulin-like growth factor I modulates induction of apoptotic signaling in H9C2 cardiac muscle cells. *Endocrinology, 139* (3), 1354-1360.
Wasilenko, W. J., Palad, A. J., Somers, K. D., Blackmore, P. F., Kohn, E. C., Rhim, J. S., et al. (1996). Effects of the calcium influx inhibitor carboxyamido-triazole on the proliferation and invasiveness of human prostate tumor cell lines. *International Journal of Cancer, 68* (2), 259-264.
Watabe, T., Yoshida, K., Shindoh, M., Kaya, M., Fujikawa, K., Sato, H., et al. (1998). The Ets-1 and Ets-2 transcription factors activate the promoters for invasion-associated urokinase and collagenase genes in response to epidermal growth factor. *International Journal of Cancer, 77* (1), 128-137.
Waterfield, M. D. Scrace G. T., Whittle N., Stroobant, P., Johnsson, A., Wasteson, A., et al. (1983). Platelet-derived growth factor is structurally related to the putative transforming protein p28^{sis} of simian sarcoma virus. *Nature, 304* (5921), 35-39.

Weber W. A., Haubner, R., Vabuliene, E., Kuhnast, B., Wester, H. J., & Schwaiger, M. (2001). Tumor angiogenesis targeting using imaging agents. *The Quarterly Journal of Nuclear Medicine, 45* (2), 179-182.

Werner, H., & LeRoith, D. (1996). The role of the insulin-like growth factor system in human cancer. *Advances in Cancer Research, 68,* 183-223.

Werner, H., & Le Roith, D. (2000). New concepts in regulation and function of the insulin-like growth factors: implications for understanding normal growth and neoplasia. *Cellular and Molecular Life Sciences, 57* (6), 932-942.

Westermark, B., Heldin, C. H., & Nister, M. (1995). Platelet-derived growth factor in human glioma. *Glia, 15* (3), 257-263.

Westermark, B., & Sorg, C. (1993) *Biology of platelet-derived growth factor.* Basel: S Karger AG.

Wikstrand, C. J., Hale, L. P., Batra, S. K., Hill, M. L., Humphrey, P. A., Kurpad, S. N., et al. (1995). Monoclonal antibodies against EGFRvIII are tumor specific and react with breast and lung carcinomas and malignant gliomas. *Cancer Research, 55* (14), 3140-3148.

Wikström, P., Damber, J., & Bergh, A. (2001). Role of transforming growth factor-beta1 in prostate cancer. *Microscopy Research and Technique, 52* (4), 411-419.

Woodburn, J., Barker, A., & Wakeling, A. (1996). 6-amino-4(3-methyl-phenylamine)-quinazoline: an EGF receptor tyrosine kinase inhibitor with activity in a range of human tumor xenografts. *Proceedings of the American Association for Cancer Research, 36,* 390-391.

Woodburn, J., Kendrew, J., Fennell, M., et al. (2000). ZD1839 ("Iressa") a selective epidermal growth factor receptor tyrosine kinase inhibitor (EGFR-TKI): inhibition of c-fos mRNA, an intermediate marker of EGFR activation, correlates with tumor growth inhibition. *Proceedings of the American Association for Cancer Research, 41,* Abstract 2552.

Wu X, Rubin M, Fan Z, DeBlasio T, Soos T, Koff A, et al. (1996). Involvement of p27KIP1 in G1 arrest mediated by an anti-epidermal growth factor receptor monoclonal antibody. *Oncogene, 12* (7), 1397-1403.

Yamaguchi, F., Saya, H., Bruner, J. M., & Morrison, R. S. (1994). Differential expression of two fibroblast growth factor-receptor genes is associated with malignant progression in human astrocytomas. *Proceedings of the National Academy of Sciences USA, 91* (2), 484-488.

Yang, R., Thomas, G. R., Bunting, S., Ko, A., Ferrara, N., Keyt, B., et al. (1996). Effects of vascular endothelial growth factor on hemodynamics and cardiac performance. *Journal of Cardiovascular Pharmacology, 27* (6), 838-844.

Yang, X .D., Jia, X. C., Corvalan, J. R., Wang, P., & Davis, C. G. (2001). Development of ABX-EGF, a fully human anti-EGFR receptor monoclonal antibody, for cancer therapy. *Critical Reviews in Oncology/Hematology, 38* (1), 17-23.

Yang, X-D., Jia, X-C., Corvalaln, J.R.F., Wang, P., Jakobovits, A., Davis, C.G., et al. (1999). Potenti anti-tumor activity of ABX-EGF, a fully human monoclonal antibody to the epidermal growth factor receptor. *Proceedings of the American Society of Clinical Oncology, 18,* Abstract 1766.

Yang, X-D., Jia, X-C., Corvalan, J. R., Wang, P., Wu, E., Zhang, L., et al. (2000). Therapeutic potential of ABX-EGF, a fully human anti-EGF receptor monoclonal antibody, for cancer treatment. *Proceedings of the American Society of Clinical Oncology, 19,* Abstract 183.

Yasui, W., Ji, Z. Q., Kuniyasu, H., Ayhan, A., Yokozaki, H., Ito, H., et al. (1992). Expression of transforming growth factor alpha in human tissues: immunohistochemical study and northern blot analysis. *Virchows Archive A: Pathological Anatomy and Histopathology, 421* (6), 513-519.

Yeh, J. R., Mohan, R., & Crews, C. M. (2000). The antiangiogenic agent TNP-470 requires p53 and p21CIP/WAF for endothelial cell growth arrest. *Proceedings of the National Academy of Sciences USA, 97* (23), 12782-12787.

Zhang, K., Sun, J., Liu, N., Wen, D., Chang, D., Thomason, A., et al. (1996). Transformation of NIH 3T3 cells by HER3 or HER4 receptors requires the presence of HER1 or HER2. *The Journal of Biological Chemistry, 271* (7), 3884-3890.

TGF-β SIGNALING ALTERATIONS IN CANCER

YANSONG BIAN, VIRGINIA KAKLAMANI, JENNIFER REICH, AND BORIS PASCHE

1. INTRODUCTION

Transforming growth factor beta (TGF-β) belongs to a large superfamily of structurally related polypeptides that includes bone morphogenic proteins (BMPs), activins and the growth differentiation factors (GDFs) (Massague, 1998). Practically all cells in the body, including epithelial, endothelial, hematopoietic, neuronal, and connective-tissue cells secrete both TGF- β and its cognate receptors. TGF- β regulates biological processes as diverse as cell proliferation, differentiation, embryonic development, angiogenesis, and wound healing. It is a microenvironmental regulatory molecule that mediates cell cycle arrest. The name TGF- β is misleading; it was based on the observation that this factor has the ability to stimulate fibroblast growth in soft agar. However, TGF- β is actually a potent inhibitor of epithelial cell proliferation and hematopoeisis (Pepper, 1997; Fortunel et al., 2000). The actions of TGF- β are complex; unlike classical hormones, members of the TGF- β family produce different effects that depend on the type and state of the cells.

One of the main characteristics of cancer is uncontrolled cell growth. The potential involvement of TGF- β in cancer has been intriguing for cancer biologists from the time its growth inhibitory properties were discovered. It is generally regarded that TGF- β can have both positive and negative effects on tumorigenesis, acting early as a tumor suppressor, but later as a stimulator of tumor invasion. Our current knowledge of the signaling pathway and how this pathway is altered in cancer forms the basis of our understanding of the various and complex biological effects of this cytokine. This evolving knowledge is beginning to provide insights into potential therapeutic interventions to prevent and treat cancer by modulating the TGF- β signaling pathway.

2. TGF- β SIGNAL TRANSDUCTION PATHWAYS

2.1 Ligands

There are three isoforms of TGF-β: TGF- β1, TGF- β2, and TGF- β3. Each isoform is encoded by a distinct gene and expressed in a tissue specific fashion. The amino acid sequences of the three isoforms are 70 to 80% homologous. TGF- β1 is expressed in endothelial, hematopoietic, and connective tissue cells; TGF- β2 in epithelial and neuronal cells and TGF- β3 primarily in mesenchymal cells (Massague, 1998). All three isoforms are highly conserved in mammals, indicating a critical biological function for each isoform. These isoforms have different binding affinities for TGF- β receptors, and the deletion of individual isoforms in mice results in different phenotypes (Massague, 1998). Each TGF-β molecule is synthesized as part of a large precursor molecule containing a propeptide region in addition to TGF-β. After it has been secreted, most TGF-β is stored in the extracellular matrix as a complex of TGF-β, the propeptide, and a protein called latent TGF-β binding protein (LTBP). The attachment of TGF-β to LTBP prevents it from binding to its receptors. There are four different LTBPs, each encoded by a distinct gene and expressed in a tissue-specific fashion (Sinha, Nevett, Shuttleworth, & Kielty, 1998).

The action of TGF-β requires that cells produce and secrete latent TGF-β. Latent TGF-β must be activated to release the mature bioactive TGF-β1 protein, which can bind to TGF-β receptors to elicit a response. Latent TGF-β can be activated by thrombospondin-1 (TSP-I), a glycoprotein secreted by most cells and incorporated into the extracellular matrix (Schultz-Cherry et al., 1995) (Crawford et al., 1998) (Figure 1). The association of the integrin alpha v beta 6 has also been shown to activate latent TGF-β (Munger et al., 1999). Activation of latent TGF-β in cancer constitutes an important but poorly understood step in the regulation of TGF-β signaling.

2.2 Receptors

TGF- β regulates cellular processes by binding to its high-affinity cell-surface receptors. Three major classes of TGF-β receptor proteins have been identified by affinity cross linking of ^{125}I-TGF-β to cell surface proteins (Cheifetz et al.,

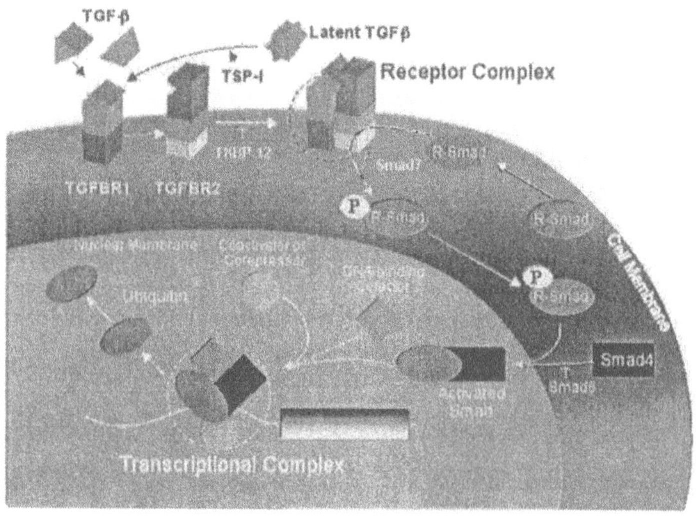

Figure 1: TGF-β signaling pathway

1987) and by cDNA cloning (Lin, Wang, Ng-Eaton, Weinberg, & Lodish, 1992; Franzen et al., 1993; Lopez-Casillas et al., 1991): TGF-β receptors type I-III (abbreviated as TGFβR1, TGFβR2, and TGFβR3, respectively). TGFβR3 is the most abundant receptor type. It functions by first binding TGF-β and transferring the cytokine to its signaling receptors TGFβR1 and TGFβR2. TGFBR3 is not involved in signaling, however, the amount of TGFβR3 that facilitates TGF-β affinity for TGFβR1 and TGFβR2 receptors is an important modifier of TGF-β signaling activity (Brown, Boyer, Runyan, & Barnett, 1999). TGFβR1 and TGFβR2 are serine-threonine protein kinases that contain an extracellular ligand binding domain, a transmembrane domain, and a cytoplasmic serine-threonine kinase domain. Following binding of the ligand to TGFβR1, TGF-β results in the formation of a TGFβR1/TGFβR2 heteromeric complex (Figure 1). Alternatively spliced forms of TGFBR1 and TGFβR2 have been described (Agrotis, Condron, & Bobik, 2000). The alternatively spliced forms of TGFBR1, cloned from vascular smooth muscle cells, are able to transduce TGF-β growth inhibition and gene transcription, but with different potencies. They may account for the multiplicity of effects TGF-β exerts on these cells (Ogasa, Noma, Murata, Kawai, & Nakazawa, 1996). Endoglin is another TGF-β receptor that is abundant on endothelial cells. It contains a transmembrane region and a cytoplasmic tail homologous to TGFβR3. Germline mutations of endoglin are the cause of hereditary hemorrhagic telangiectasia type I (McAllister et al., 1994). Mice lacking endoglin have defective angiogenesis (Li et al., 1999).

2.3 Intracellular signaling through Smads

The SMAD proteins are a family of transcription factors found in vertebrates, insects, and nematodes (Heldin, Miyazono, & Tendijke, 1997). They have demonstrated the ability to propagate signals from the activated receptor complex to the nucleus (Massague, 1998). Intracellular signaling is initiated once TGF-β has induced the formation of a TGFβR1/TGFβR2 heteromeric complex. TGFβR2 phosphorylates TGFβR1 resulting in activation of the TGFβR1 kinase. Activated TGFβR1 specifically recognizes and phosphorylates SMAD2 and SMAD3, a SMAD subgroup known as receptor-activated SMADs (R-SMADs). On their way to the nucleus R-SMADs associate with SMAD4 (Figure 1). SMAD4 is a common partner for the receptor-activated SMADs. It is not required for nuclear accumulation but for the formation of functional transcriptional complexes (Liu, Pouponnot, & Massague, 1997).

3. TGF-β MODULATES CELL CYCLE AND APOPTOSIS

The cell cycle is governed by cyclin-dependent kinases (cdks) that integrate mitogenic and growth inhibitory signals. It has been shown that certain G1 cyclins and cdks may be the targets of the negative signaling pathways induced by TGF-β. TGF-β1 can inhibit the ability of cells to enter S phase when the inhibitory peptide is added to cultures at both early and late points during the prereplicative G1 period (Geng & Weinberg, 1993). In most epithelial, endothelial, and hematopoietic cells, TGF-β mediates G1 cell cycle arrest by inducing or activating cdk inhibitors $p16^{INK4A}$, $p15^{INK4B}$, $p21^{CIP1}$ and/or $p27^{Kip1}$, depending on the cell type (Hannon &

Beach, 1994; Datto et al., 1995). Additional mechanisms contributing to TGF-β mediated growth arrest include the inhibition of the function or production of essential cell-cycle regulators, especially cdk2 and 4 and cyclins A and E. These changes result in decreased phosphorylation of the retinoblastoma gene product pRB, which allows Rb protein to bind to transcription factor E2F and prevent its release. The unreleased E2F is unable to stimulate the expression of genes like *c-myc* and *b-myb* that permit the progression through the cell cycle. TGF-β can also inhibit the expression of c-Myc, CDK4 and CDC25A. High levels of c-Myc render the cells resistant to the growth inhibitory activity of TGF-β, and downregulation of c-Myc is required for the induction of $p15^{INK4B}$, and/or $p21^{CIP1}$. c-Myc may also regulate, at least indirectly, the expression of cyclins E, A, and D1.

In addition to causing cell cycle arrest in some cell types, TGF-β can also induce programmed cell death in others. The SMAD signaling in TGF-β has been shown to induce apoptosis in several cell types. Increased levels of SMAD3 or SMAD4 can induce apoptosis, and dominant negative interference with SMAD3 function protects against apoptosis (Yanagisawa et al., 1998; Dai, Bansal, & Kern, 1999). In addition, SMAD7 can act as both an effector and protector of TGF-β induced cell death, depending on the cell type (Ishisaki et al., 1998; Lallemand et al., 2001).

4. ALTERATION OF TGF-β, ITS RECEPTORS AND SIGNALING PATHWAYS IN CANCER DEVELOPMENT

All epithelial and hematopoietic cell lines are highly sensitive to TGF-β growth inhibitory properties. Hence, in normal cells, TGF-β acts as a tumor suppressor by inhibiting cell growth or promoting cellular differentiation or apoptosis. At some time during the stepwise transition towards malignancy, virtually all cells become, at least partially, resistant to TGF-β growth inhibition. The resistance is believed to be due to inactivating mutations or loss of expression of the genes for one or more known components of the TGF-β signaling pathway. For example, all pancreatic cancers and more than 80% of colon cancers have mutations affecting at least one component of the TGF-β pathway (Villanueva et al., 1998; Grady et al., 1999). Some of these mutations occur in the TGF-β receptors, SMAD4 or SMAD2; others may occur in undetected or yet unknown components of the signaling pathway.

Resistance to the growth inhibitory effect of TGF-β may also result from inactivation of cell cycle mediators involved in TGF-β-induced arrest. For example, inactivation of the RB tumor suppressor gene may prevent or at least limit TGF-β-induced growth inhibition. Loss of TGF-β-induced growth arrest may also result from either the aberrant expression of positive regulators, such as the cyclins and cdks, or the loss of negative regulators, such as the cdk inhibitors. Expression of c-Myc may also be involved in the growth inhibitory response to TGF-β. The downregulation of c-Myc expression by TGF-β has been observed to be lost in epithelial cells as well as in various cancer cell lines, concomitant with the loss of the growth inhibitory response to TGF-β (Chen et al., 2001).

On the other hand, cancer cells in general secrete larger amounts of TGF-β than their normal counterparts. The association of TGF-β with cancer is strongest in the most advanced stages of tumor progression. The increased TGF-β secretion weakens the immune system, exacerbates the malignant phenotype of tumor cells, and contributes to tumor invasion and metastasis.

5. POLYMORPHISMS OF TGF-β1, TGFBR1 AND CARCINOGENESIS

TGF-β1 polymorphisms that may affect the development of osteoporosis, cardiovascular diseases, and lung fibrosis have been recently identified (Yamada et al., 2000; Arkwright et al., 2000; Yokota et al., 2000). This suggests that TGF-β polymorphisms may result in different signaling levels. Recently, genetic polymorphisms of TGF-β1 and TGFBR1 have been associated with altered cancer risk. Evidence of hypomorphic TGF-β signaling association with cancer development arises from both mouse models and clinical epidemiology. Several polymorphisms have been reported within the human TGF-β1 gene. Two are represented by the substitutions of Leucine to Proline (T to C) at the 10th amino acid position and Arginine to Proline (G to C) at the 25th position (Yokota et al., 2000; Yamada et al., 1998). It has been hypothesized that these polymorphisms result in either higher or lower TGF-β signaling levels and are associated with altered cancer susceptibility (Tang et al., 1998). The homozygous *C/C* genotype has been associated with increased serum TGF-β1 levels and a more than 50% decreased incidence of breast cancer when compared with both the *T/T* and the *T/C* genotypes (Ziv, Cauley, Morin, Saiz, & Browner, 2001)(Figure 2). Similarly, a type I TGF-β receptor polymorphism coding for a hypomorphic receptor (*TGFBR1*6A*) has been associated with an increased incidence of human cancers. *TGFBR1*6A* is a polymorphic germline mutation of *TGFBR1* that results in the in-frame deletion of three GCG repeats encoding for alanine (Pasche et al., 1998). TGFBR1*6A mediates TGF-β antiproliferative signals less effectively than TGFBR1 (Chen et al., 1999; Pasche et al., 1999) (Figure 2). Several lines of evidence indicate that *TGFBR1*6A* may act as a tumor susceptibility allele in a variety of cancers including colorectal, ovarian, head and neck and breast cancer (Pasche et al., 1999; Chen, Kang, & Massague, 2001; Knobloch et al., 2001; Chen et al., 2001; Baxter, Choong, Eccles, & Campbell, in press.). The higher than expected *TGFBR1*6A* frequency among tumor samples alludes to the possibility that *TGFBR1*6A* may be somatically acquired mutation in addition to being a common germline polymorphism.

6. MUTATIONS OF TGF-β RECEPTORS

Inactivating mutations in *TGFBR1* have been reported in ovarian cancer, pancreatic and biliary cancer as well as T-cell lymphoma (Chen, Carter, Garrigueantar, & Reiss, 1998; Goggins et al., 1998; Schiemann, Pfeifer, Levi, Kadin, & Lodish, 1999). A *TGFBR1* tumor-specific S387Y mutation has been reported in 40% of metastatic breast cancers though a follow-up study didn't confirm these numbers, suggesting that this is a rare occurrence in breast cancer (Chen et al., 1998; Anbazhagan, Bornman, Johnston, Westra, & Gabrielson, 1999). *TGFBR2* mutations have been found more frequently and in more tumor types than *TGFBR1* mutations. Frameshift mutations of *TGFBR2* encode
truncated proteins that lack the transmembrane and intracellular domains of TGFBR2 resulting in inactivation of downstream signaling (Markowitz et al.,

1995). Mutations of both *TGFBR2* alleles have been observed in 70-90% of colorectal cancers and cancer cell lines with microsatellite instability (MSI), in most gastric tumors and a small proportion of gliomas with MSI, but are less common in MSI positive tumors from the endometrium, pancreatic cancer, liver cancer, and breast cancer (Markowitz et al., 1995; Murata et al., 2000; Myeroff et al., 1995; Parsons et al., 1995; Wang et al., 1995b; Ohue et al., 1996; Renault et al., 1996; Samowitz & Slattery, 1997). *TGFBR1* and *TGFBR2* mutations in the development of carcinomas suggest that both *TGFBR1* and *TGFBR2* may act as tumor supressors.

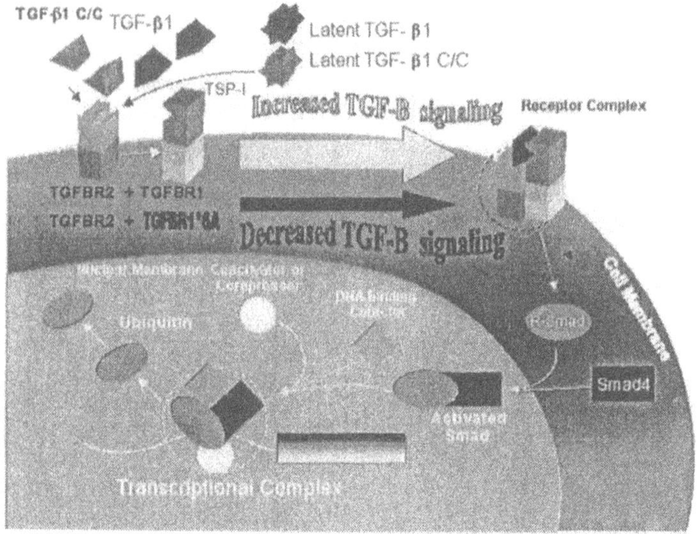

Figure 2: Polymorphisms of the TGF-β signaling pathway associated with modified cancer risk

Mutations in MSI positive colorectal cancer cell lines may partially inactivate TGF-β-induced growth inhibition (Wang et al., 1995a). Whether these mutations represent a consequence of MSI or are truly tumor-specific targets remains to be clarified. A recent report shows that MSI positive colorectal cell lines with homozygous *TGFBR2* mutations still respond to TGF-β growth-inhibition (Ilyas, Efstathiou, Straub, Kim, & Bodmer, 1999). Furthermore, *TGFBR2* mutations in sporadic colorectal polyps are rare suggesting that *TGFBR2* frameshift mutations do not have a pathogenic role in the early stages of colorectal cancer development (Togo et al., 1999; Rashid, Zahurak, Goodman, & Hamilton, 1999). Taken together, the above results cast doubt on the significance of *TGFBR2* mutations observed in colon cancer with MSI. Furthermore, numerous other genes implicated in colon cancer, such as *BAX, IGFRII, hMSH3, hMSH6* and *TCF-4*, are also mutated at the time *TGFBR2* mutations are detected (Duval et al., 1999; Calin et al., 2000). A germline mutation of *TGFBR2* has been observed in Japanese kindred with HNPCC (Lu et al., 1998). However, this finding was not confirmed by a larger analysis of HNPCC patients from Korea (Shin, Park, Park, 2000). The functional significance of this mutation has been further investigated and led to the discovery that the mutant *TGFBR2*, while unable to mediate TGF-β growth inhibition, retains the ability to induce one of the extracellular matrix proteins, plasminogen activator inhibitor type 1, upon TGF-β treatment (Lu, Kawabata, Imamura, Miyazono, & Yuasa, 1999).

Missense and inactive mutations in the kinase domain of TGFBR2 have also been detected in colon cancer without MSI (Park et al., 1994). A *TGFBR2* dominant-negative mutation that is not associated with MSI has been reported in esophageal carcinoma (Tanaka et al., 2000). Although MSI occurs in a third of esophageal carcinomas, *TGFBR2* frameshift mutations have not been reported (Tanaka et al., 2000; Tomita, Miyazato, Tamai, Muto, & Toda, 1999). As in colon cancer, *TGFBR2* frameshift mutations at coding nucleotide repeats are late events in MSI positive gastric cancer and portend a better prognosis (Kim et al., 1999a; Iacopetta, Soong, House, & Hamelin, 1999). In sporadic gastric cancer 10% of tumors harbor *TGFBR2* mutations (Guo et al., 1998). *TGFBR2* mutations have been reported in cervical cancer (Chen et al., 1999). *TGFBR2* mutations are frequent in cell lines but rare in primary lesions, even when microsatellite instability is present (Chu, Lai, Shen, Liu, & Chao, 1999). Human papilloma virus (HPV) has been etiologically linked to cervical cancer. Interestingly, the oncoprotein HPV16 E6 stimulates the TGF-β1 promoter in fibroblasts (Dey, Atcha, & Bagchi, 1997).

Although loss of TGF-β responsiveness provides a distinct advantage for tumor development, most tumors do not have inactivated TGF-β receptors. Transcriptional silencing resulting from loss of expression of TGFBR1 and/or TGFBR2 may be due to hypermethylation of CpG islands within the TGFBR1 and/or TGFBR2 gene promoters. In a number of neoplasms, including gastric cancer cell lines (Park et al., 1994), thyroid tumors (Lazzereschi et al., 1997), intestinal adenomas (Zhang et al., 1997), and small cell lung carcinomas (de Jonge, Garrigue-Antar, Vellucci, & Reiss, 1997), no mutations within the coding region of the gene have been observed among cases showing either reduced expression or failure to express the *TGFBR2* gene at the RNA or protein level. This suggests that defects in the promoter region of the *TGFBR2* gene and/or in the mechanisms regulating the transcription of the *TGFBR2* gene may also play important roles in the aberrant TGFBR2 expression. *TGFBR1* downregulation by means of promoter methylation has also been observed in 13% of primary gastric tumors and in most cell lines (Kang et al., 1999).

7. SMADS AS TUMOR SUPPRESSORS

Functional inactivation of downstream signaling mediators has also been shown to be the basis of the loss of TGF-β responsiveness in various tumors. Inactivation of certain SMADs appears to impart a distinct advantage in tumor progression. Thus, one function of SMADs as downstream effectors of TGF-β signaling is to act as tumor suppressors.

Mutations of *SMAD2* and *SMAD4* genes, but not those of *SMAD3* or the inhibitory *SMAD6* or *SMAD7*, have been detected in several carcinomas (Hata, Shi, & Massague, 1998; Massague & Chen, 2000; Derynck, Akhurst, & Balmain, 2001). The *SMAD2* and *SMAD4* genes were mapped to chromosome 18q21, a region which is frequently mutated or deleted in pancreatic and colon carcinomas (Eppert et al., 1996; Hahn et al., 1996). Inactivation of *SMAD2* and *SMAD4* can be caused by missense mutations, nonsense mutations, small deletions, frameshift mutations, or loss of the entire chromosomal region (Massague et al., 2000; Derynck et al., 2001). Over 90% of pancreatic carcinomas have loss of heterozygosity (LOH) at 18q. Bi-allellic inactivation of *SMAD4* gene at 18q21.1 is seen in about half of pancreatic carcinomas with 18q LOH. In the remaining tumors with 18q LOH, *SMAD4* is not mutated and its expression is unaffected. In these tumors no alterations in the *SMAD2* gene at 18q21.3 have been found. Most *SMAD4* mutations in pancreatic cancer disrupt the molecule's ability to regulate gene transcription (Schutte, 1999). However, different *SMAD4* mutations that do not disrupt activation but induce SMAD4 degradation through the ubiquitin pathway have been described (Xu & Attisano, 2000). Mutations that increase SMAD4 autoinhibition have also been found in pancreatic cancer (Hata, Lo, Wotton, Lagna, & Massague, 1997). Simultaneous homozygous deletions of *TGFBR1* and *SMAD4* have been found in the same pancreatic cells (Goggins et al., 1998). This seemingly redundant inactivation of the TGF-β signaling pathway indicates that different functions of the pathway are targeted during tumor development and progression.

Immunohistochemistry analysis of pancreatic cancer tissues has revealed an increase in SMAD2 that is associated with increased mRNA levels indicating that pancreatic cancer cells have the ability to upregulate SMAD2 expression (Kleeff et al., 1999). Low TGFBR1 levels have been shown to be partly responsible for TGF-β resistance in pancreatic carcinoma cell lines that do not harbor *SMAD4* mutations (Wagner et al., 1998). Despite the well documented high frequency of tumor-specific *SMAD4* mutations in pancreatic cancer, there is no evidence that a germline mutation of *SMAD4* predisposes to this malignancy (Moskaluk et al., 1997).

SMAD4 mutations are not only restricted to pancreatic adenocarcinomas. *SMAD4* mutation screening of pancreatic islet cell tumors showed that 55% of non-functioning endocrine pancreatic carcinomas carried intragenic mutations whereas none were found among insulinomas, gastrinomas and vipomas. This alludes to an important role for *SMAD4* in the tumorigenesis of most non-secreting pancreatic carcinomas (Bartsch et al., 1999).

There is evidence of increased TGF-β signaling in colon cancer when compared with normal tissue as assessed by increased expression of receptor-activated SMAD2 and SMAD3 in a fraction of colorectal cancers. On the contrary, there is no immunostaining for SMAD2, SMAD3 or SMAD5 and only occasional staining for

SMAD1/8 in epithelial mucosa of normal colon (Korchynskyi et al., 1999). Overexpression of the tumor-derived SMAD2.D450E, an unphosphorylable form of SMAD2 found in colorectal and lung cancers, does not abolish TGF-β-mediated growth arrest. However, overexpression of SMAD2.D450E induces cellular invasion, and this effect is enhanced by TGF-β. A similar invasive phenotype is obtained in cells expressing another inactivating mutation in SMAD2, SMAD2.P445H, found in colorectal cancer. This indicates that genetic defects in SMAD2 are sufficient to confer invasion-promoting effects of TGF-β. It also shows that TGF-β acts through SMAD2 to induce cellular invasion by a novel mechanism, activated TGFBR1, which is independent of SMAD2 phosphorylation (Prunier et al., 1999). In summary, these studies suggest a selective upregulation of receptor-activated SMAD proteins in colorectal cancer; its functional consequences remain to be further elucidated.

More than 30% of sporadic colon cancers with distant metastases or distant metastases themselves harbor *SMAD4* mutations while these are not found in colon adenomas. *SMAD4* is one of the true targets of 18q LOH in colon cancer and its inactivation is involved in invasive disease and distant metastasis (Miyaki et al., 1999; Tarafa et al., 2000). Contrary to *TGFBR2* frameshift mutations associated with MSI that portend a good prognosis in colon cancer (Watanabe et al., 2001), *SMAD4* mutations appear to be associated with aggressive disease (Gryfe et al., 2000). This data is the first epidemiological indication that decreased TGF-β signaling at the receptor level downregulates colorectal cancer growth whereas TGF-ß signaling blockade at the SMAD4 level enhances tumor aggressiveness. This is well illustrated by the fact that the tumorigenicity of SW480 colon cancer cell lines in nude mice is suppressed by stable re-expression of SMAD4. Interestingly, in vitro growth of SW480 cells transfected with SMAD4 is not affected when compared to parental cells and resistance towards TGF-β mediated growth-inhibition is retained. Instead, cells exhibit morphological alterations, and adhesion and spreading are accelerated. These phenotypic changes are associated with reduced expression levels of the endogenous urokinase-type plasminogen activator (uPA) and plasminogen-activator-inhibitor-1 (PAI-1) genes, the products of which are implicated in cell adhesion and invasion (Schwarte-Waldhoff et al., 1999). Both *SMAD4* and *APC* appear to play a crucial synergistic role in the progression of colon cancer in mice (Takaku et al., 1998; Haines et al., 2000). These results demonstrate a *SMAD4* tumor suppressive function and suggest a potential role for SMAD4 as a mediator or cell adhesion and invasion that correlates with uPA and PAI-1 expression. Loss of *SMAD4* function by both deletion and silencing as well as inhibition of SMAD2 and SMAD3 function by a hyperactive Ras pathway jointly prevent TGF-β antiproliferative responses in colon cancer cell lines (Calonge & Massague, 1999).

Germline mutations of *SMAD4* account for about one third of juvenile polyposis cases (Howe et al., 1998; Roth et al., 1999; Friedl et al., 1999). In this disease, like in sporadic colorectal cancer, *SMAD4* acts as a tumor suppressor gene as evidenced by *SMAD4* allelic loss in patients' polyps (Woodford-Richens et al., 2000). No mutations have been found in *SMAD1, SMAD2, SMAD3, SMAD5* and *SMAD7* in patients with juvenile polyposis without *SMAD4* mutations (Bevan et al., 1999; Roth et al., 1999). A recent report indicates that alterations of the bone morphogenetic protein (BMP) signaling pathway may also play a key role in controlling epithelial neoplasia (Howe et al., 2001).

SMAD2 and *SMAD4* somatic mutations also occur in hepatic carcinoma. All three of the reported mutations, two in *SMAD4* (Asp332Gly and Cys401Arg) and one in *SMAD2* (Gln407Arg) genes, were A:T to G:C transitions suspected to result from oxidative stress as observed in mitochondrial DNA (Yakicier, Irmak, Romano, Kew, & Ozturk, 1999).

Despite frequent LOH on chromosome 18q, *SMAD4* and *SMAD2* are infrequently mutated in breast (Schutte et al., 1996), ovarian (Zhou et al., 1999), head and neck (Kim et al., 1996; Papadimitrakopoulou et al., 1998) and prostate cancer (Latil et al., 1999).

8. TGF-β EXPRESSION AND CARCINOGENESIS

The different isoforms of TGF-β can exert either positive or negative effects on tumor cells. Exogenous TGF-β has been shown to inhibit the growth of tumor cells in vitro (Ashley, Kong, Bigner, & Hale, 1998) whereas decreased endogenous expression of TGF-β, which leads to a higher incidence of tumor formation, has been observed in a nude mice colon carcinoma model (Wu et al., 1992).

Aberrant expression of TGF-β has been examined in many tumors. Increased TGF-β signaling seems to correlate with a decreased risk of developing breast cancer. Indeed, transgenic mice expressing a constitutively active form of TGF-β1 are resistant to DMBA-induced mammary tumor formation (Pierce, Jr. et al., 1995). The propensity of these mice to develop breast cancer is similarly decreased when crossed with mice that develop mammary tumors at an increased rate because of overexpression of the epithelial mitogen TGF-α (Pierce, Jr. et al., 1995). Conversely, treatment of *Tgfb1* +/- heterozygous mice with tumor induction protocols results in a much higher number of malignant mammary tumors than in *Tgfb1* +/+ mice (Tang et al., 1998). The contribution of TGF-β to the malignant phenotype of breast cancer cells is particularly prominent in cell lines that retain the TGF-β signal transduction system but have lost TGF-β-induced growth inhibition. Such is the case in breast cancer cells with a hyperactive Ras pathway (Oft et al., 1996; Oft, Heider, & Beug, 1998; Yin et al., 1999). A potential molecular mechanism underlying this differential response to TGF-β that favors tumor growth has been attributed to the altered nuclear accumulation of SMADs. Phosphorylation of SMAD2 and SMAD3 by Ras-activated Erk kinases decreases their accumulation in the nucleus reducing TGF-β growth inhibition (Kretzschmar, Doody, Timokhina, & Massague, 1999).

Decreased expression of intracellular TGF-β1 in neoplastic epithelium and increased expression of extracellular TGF-β1 in stroma associated with invasive cervical carcinoma have been reported. This suggests that an early event in the neoplastic transformation of cervical epithelial cells may involve the loss of TGF-β1. Tumor progression may be indirectly promoted by TGF-β1 secreted into or produced by supporting stromal elements. Decreased expression of TGFBR1 is associated with a poor prognosis in patients with bladder transitional cell carcinoma (Tokunaga, Lee, Kim, Wheeler, & Lerner, 1999). Unlike plasma TGF-β1 levels, urinary TGF-β1 and plasma TGF-β2 levels are higher in patients with prostate cancer and may be useful biomarkers of prostate cancer (Perry, Anthony, Case, & Steiner, 1997; Wolff, Fandel, Borchers, & Jakse, 1999).

In contrast to its inhibitory effects, TGF-β can also promote the growth and/or invasiveness of several different tumors. However, the tumor-enhancing effects of

TGF-β are frequently observed when abnormal amounts of TGF-β are secreted by TGF-β sensitive or TGF-β resistant tumor cells. Patients with Epstein-Barr associated nasopharyngeal carcinoma have elevated serum levels of TGF-β1 (Xu et al., 2000) and serum level of TGF-β2 are elevated in patients with metastatic head and neck squamous cell carcinomas (Karcher, Reisser, Daniel, & Herold-Mende, 1999). Patients with lung cancer frequently present with elevated serum levels of TGF-β1. Also, TGF-β1 serum levels correlate with long term outcome in patients with lung carcinoma (Kong, Jirtle, Huang, Clough, & Anscher, 1999). High levels of expression of TGF-β1 in the gastric mucosa of patients with a diagnosis of gastric cancer was recently reported. An interesting finding of the study was that the majority of the patients' first-degree relatives also expressed TGF-β1 in their gastric mucosa. In contrast, only one of 19 individuals without a family history of gastric cancer expressed TGF-β1 in the gastric mucosa. The induction of TGF-β1 expression in first-degree relatives of patients with gastric cancer points to the presence of specific molecular alterations in a subgroup of individuals with an increased risk of developing gastric cancer (Ebert et al., 2000). This agrees with the finding that TGF-β1 expression correlates with the expression of vascular endothelial growth factor and poor prognosis of patients with advanced gastric carcinoma (Saito et al., 1999).

Screening of 96 primary ovarian tumors for expression of TGF-β isoforms showed that TGF-β3 is associated with advanced stages of the disease and reduced survival (Bartlett et al., 1997). Patients with ovarian tumors expressing TGF-β have a worse prognosis (Nakanishi et al., 1997). The biphasic role of TGF-β in skin carcinogenesis is well illustrated in mice with TGF-β1 targeted to keratinocytes. TGF-β1 acts early as a tumor suppressor but later enhances the malignant phenotype. The transgenics are more resistant to chemical induction of benign skin tumors than controls, but the malignant conversion rate is vastly increased (Cui et al., 1996). Melanoma cell lines secrete mostly latent TGF-β but some cell lines secrete high levels of active TGF-β (Bizik, Felnerova, Grofova, & Vaheri, 1996). As compared with healthy controls, patients with melanoma have significantly increased serum levels of TGF-β1 and TGF-β2 but not TGF-β3 (Krasagakis et al., 1998). Analysis of progressing and regressing melanoma lesions shows higher TGF-β1 levels in progressing lesions consistent with increased immunosuppression (Conrad, Ernst, Dummer, Brocker, & Becker, 1999). Expression of TGF-β2 in melanoma correlates with the depth of tumor invasion and metastasis (Reed, McNutt, Prieto, & Albino, 1994; Schmid, Itin, & Rufli, 1995). TGF-β has also been found to enhance adhesion of melanoma cells to the endothelium (Teti et al., 1997). High expression of TGF-β1 and loss of TGF-β receptor expression have been associated with a particularly bad prognosis in patients with prostate cancer (Wikstrom et al., 2000). TGF-β1 has a proliferative effect on the prostate cancer cell line, TSU-PR1, which contains functional TGFBR1 and TGFBR2 receptors and SMADs (Lamm, Sintich, & Lee, 1998; Park et al., 2000). This TGF-β1 proliferative effect is due to oncogenic Ha-Ras-induced activation of the mitogen-activated protein kinase signaling pathway (Park et al., 2000). TGF-β serum levels are elevated in advanced stages of invasive cervical carcinomas (Chopra, Dinh, & Hannigan, 1998). TGF-β1 secretion depends on the tumor histology with adenocarcinomas secreting more TGF-β1 than squamous cell carcinomas (Santin et al., 1997). There is a progressive loss of sensitivity to TGF-β-mediated growth inhibition during cervical carcinoma development (De Geest, Bergman, Turyk, Frank, & Wilbanks, 1994).

9. TGF-β IN METASTATIC CANCER

There is evidence that TGF-β signaling contributes to the metastasis in breast cancer. A soluble form of TGFBR3 that can sequester tumor-secreted TGF-β was expressed in MDA-MB-231 human breast cancer cells, which were then inoculated in athymic nude mice. The tumor incidence and growth rate of TGFBR3 expressing cell lines were lower than those of the control cell lines (Bandyopadhyay et al., 1999). Using the same cell line other investigators have shown that a dominant negative TGFBR2 decreases bone metastasis and a dominant positive TGFBR1 has the opposite effect (Yin et al., 1999). Certain murine renal cancer cells do not express TGFBR2. When transfected with TGFBR2, the tumorigenicity of these cells in vivo is abolished (Engel et al., 1999; Kundu et al., 1998).

Transgenic mice expressing a dominant negative TGFBR2 in the epidermis have an increased sensitivity to chemical carcinogenesis with an earlier appearance and greater number of papillomas than control mice. Increased expression of VEGF, an angiogenesis stimulator, is observed in the transgenic mice. Hence, inactivation of TGFBR2 accelerates skin carcinogenesis at both earlier and later stages, and increases angiogenesis, one of the important mechanisms underlying accelerated tumor growth and metastasis (Go, Li, & Wang, 1999).

10. FUTURE DIRECTIONS AND POTENTIAL THERAPEUTIC TARGETS

Recent findings support aberrant TGF-β expression, its receptors, and other elements of the signaling pathway playing prominent roles in carcinogenesis. Alterations of TGF-ß signaling are emerging as important contributors to both tumor susceptibility as well as tumor progression. Clinical epidemiology as well as a mouse models demonstrate that hypomorphic TGF-ß signaling leads to increased cancer susceptibility. Haploinsufficient *Tgfb1 +/-* mice and *Tgfbr2 +/-* mice are more susceptible to cancer development than their wild type littermates (Tang et al., 1998; Im et al., 2001). Similarly, several case control studies have shown that the hypomorphic *TGFBR1*6A* allele predisposes carriers to a variety of tumors such as breast and colon cancer. (Pasche et al., 1999; Pasche et al., 2001; Baxter et al., 2 A.D.). Conversely, increased TGF-ß signaling is protective against cancer development. Transgenic mice with constitutively active expression of TGF-β1 are less prone to breast cancer development. The clinical correlate of this finding is best exemplified by a recent study showing that a common polymorphism of TGF-ß1, *TGFB1*CC,* which results in higher TGF-ß signaling, is protective against breast cancer (Ziv et al., 2001).

Additional studies are needed to confirm the above results and determine the magnitude of cancer risk modifications due to *TGFBR1*6A* and *TGFB1*CC*. It is likely that a global assessment of TGF-ß signaling may become an important element in cancer risk stratification. Such an approach is appealing because of its feasibility in the era of high throughput screening and the advent of gene expression profiling using DNA arrays. It is conceivable that, in the near future, tumors will be treated based on their acquired and inherited molecular abnormalities, rather than their histology. In this case, germline as well as tumor-specific TGF-β signaling abnormalities should be part of any screening. Indeed, TGF-β is both the most potent naturally occurring inhibitor of cell growth and the most potent naturally occurring suppressor of lymphocyte function.

Endogenous TGF-β can be upregulated in humans by oral intake of substances such as retinoic acid (Comerci et al., 1997). Other agents such as Rapamycin, which blocks FKBP12 binding to TGFBR1, reverses the inhibitory effect of FKBP12 on TGFBR1 phosphorylation thereby resulting in TGFBR1 dowstream signaling, even in the absence of a ligand (Chen, Liu, & Massague, 1997) (Figure 1). In the future, one may consider using such substances in *TGFBR1*6A* carriers to increase basal TGF-β signaling in both primary and secondary prevention of cancers. Likewise, one may envision therapies targeting the molecular abnormalities of the tumor such as restoring SMAD4 function. Several lines of evidence show that the immunosuppressive potential of TGF-β modulates malignant cell growth. This is partly caused by TGF-β-induced interference with the generation of tumor-specific cytotoxic T lymphocytes and by TGF-β-induced promotion of angiogenesis and tumor stroma formation. Until now, significant and long-lasting clinical responses have been difficult to achieve with current cancer immunotherapeutic approaches. One of the possible explanations for this failure is immunosuppression induced by tumor-derived TGF-β (de Visser & Kast, 1999). Specific serine/threonine kinase inhibitors or anti-TGF-β receptor humanized monoclonal antibodies may become useful in clinical settings with an obvious TGF-β overproduction. Indeed, neutralizing TGF-β antibodies increase natural killer cell activity and inhibit human breast cancer cell tumorigenicity in athymic mice (Hurd, Johnson, Forbes, Carty-Dugger, & Arteaga, 1992). This latter approach may prove particularly useful if TGF-β immunosuppressive action turns out to play a predominant role in tumor progression.

In conclusion, TGF-β signaling pathway alterations are implicated in both early and late steps of cancer development. Increased knowledge of this pathway and its ramifications may well offer key therapeutic target in the years to come.

11. ACKNOWLEDGMENTS

This work is supported by grants CA76156-04, CA082516-01A2 and CA89018 from the National Cancer Institute.

Yansong Bian, Virginia Kaklamani, Jennifer Reich, & Boris Pasche
Division of Hematology/Oncology
Department of Medicine
Northwestern University Medical School and
Robert H. Lurie Comprehensive Cancer Center of Northwestern University
Chicago, IL

12. REFERENCES

Agrotis, A., Condron, M., & Bobik, A. (2000). Alternative splicing within the TGF-beta type I receptor gene (ALK-5) generates two major functional isoforms in vascular smooth muscle cells. FEBS Letters, 467, 128-132.

Anbazhagan, R., Bornman, D. M., Johnston, J. C., Westra, W. H., & Gabrielson, E. (1999). The S387Y mutation of the transforming growth factor-beta receptor type I gene is uncommon in metastases of breast cancer and other common types of adenocarcinoma. Cancer Research, 59, 3363-3364.

Arkwright, P. D., Laurie, S., Super, M., Pravica, V., Schwarz, M. J., Webb, A. K., Hutchinson, I. V.. (2000). TGF-beta(1) genotype and accelerated decline in lung function of patients with cystic fibrosis. Thorax, 55, 459-462.

Ashley, D. M., Kong, F. M., Bigner, D. D., & Hale, L. P. (1998). Endogenous expression of transforming growth factor beta-1 inhibits growth and tumorigenicity and enhances fas-mediated apoptosis in a murine high-grade glioma model. Cancer Research, 58, 302-309.

Bandyopadhyay, A., Zhu, Y., Cibull, M. L., Bao, L. W., Chen, C. G., & Sun, L. Z. (1999). A soluble transforming growth factor beta type III receptor suppresses tumorigenicity and metastasis of human breast cancer MDA-MB-231 cells. Cancer Research, 59, 5041-5046.

Bartlett, J. M., Langdon, S. P., Scott, W. N., Love, S. B., Miller, E. P., Katsaros, D., Smyth, J. F., & Miller, W. R. (1997). Transforming growth factor-beta isoform expression in human ovarian tumours. European Journal of Cancer , 33, 2397-2403.

Bartsch, D., Hahn, S. A., Danichevski, K. D., Ramaswamy, A., Bastian, D., Galehdari, H., Barth, P., Schmiegel, W., Simon, B., & Rothmund, M. (1999). Mutations of the DPC4/Smad4 gene in neuroendocrine pancreatic tumors. Oncogene, 18, 2367-2371.

Baxter, S. W., Choong, D. Y. H., Eccles, D. M., & Campbell, I. G. Transforming growth factor-beta receptor-1 polyalanine polymorphism and exon 5 mutation analysis in breast and ovarian cancer. in press. 2-1-0002.

Bevan, S., Woodford-Richens, K., Rozen, P., Eng, C., Young, J., Dunlop, M., Neale, K., Phillips, R., Markie, D., Rodriguez-Bigas, M., Leggett, B., Sheridan, E., Hodgson, S., Iwama, T., Eccles, D., Bodmer, W., Houlston, R., & Tomlinson, I. (1999). Screening SMAD1, SMAD2, SMAD3, and SMAD5 for germline mutations in juvenile polyposis syndrome. Gut, 45, 406-408.

Bizik, J., Felnerova, D., Grofova, M., & Vaheri, A. (1996). Active transforming growth factor-beta in human melanoma cell lines - no evidence for plasmin-related activation of latent tgf- beta. Journal of Cellular Biochemistry, 62, 113-122.

Brown, C. B., Boyer, A. S., Runyan, R. B., & Barnett, J. V. (1999). Requirement of type III TGF-beta receptor for endocardial cell transformation in the heart. Science, 283, 2080-2082.

Calin, G. A., Gafa, R., Tibiletti, M. G., Herlea, V., Becheanu, G., Cavazzini, L., Barbanti-Brodano, G., Nenci, I., Negrini, M., & Lanza, G. (2000). Genetic progression in microsatellite instability high (MSI-H) colon cancers correlates with clinico-pathological parameters: A study of the TGF beta RII, BAX, HMSH3, HMSH6, IGFIIR and BLM genes. International Journal of Cancer, 89, 230-235.

Calonge, M. J. & Massague, J. (1999). Smad4/DPC4 silencing and hyperactive Ras jointly disrupt transforming growth factor-beta antiproliferative responses in colon cancer cells. Journal of Biological Chemistry, 19;274, 33637-33643.

Cardillo, M. R., Petrangeli, E., Perracchio, L., Salvatori, L., Ravenna, L., Di, Silverio, F. (2000). Transforming growth factor-beta expression in prostate neoplasia. Analytical & Quantitative Cytology & Histology, 22, 1-10.

Cheifetz, S., Weatherbee, J. A., Tsang, M. L., Anderson, J. K., Mole, J. E., Lucas, R., & Massague, J. (1987). The transforming growth factor-beta system, a complex pattern of cross-reactive ligands and receptors. Cell, 48, 409-415.

Chen, C. R., Kang, Y., & Massague, J. (2001). Defective repression of c-myc in breast cancer cells: A loss at the core of the transforming growth factor beta growth arrest program. Proceedings of the National Academy of Sciences of the United States of America, 98, 992-999.

Chen, T., de Vries, E. G., Hollema, H., Yegen, H. A., Vellucci, V. F., Strickler, H. D., Hildesheim, A., & Reiss, M. (1999). Structural alterations of transforming growth factor-beta receptor genes in human cervical carcinoma. Int.J Cancer, 82, 43-51.

Chen, T., Triplett, J., Dehner, B., Hurst, B., Colligan, B., Pemberton, J., Graff, J. R., & Carter, J. H. (2001). Transforming growth factor-beta receptor type i gene is frequently mutated in ovarian carcinomas. Cancer Research, 61, 4679-4682.

Chen, T. P., Carter, D., Garrigueantar, L., & Reiss, M. (1998). Transforming growth factor beta type i receptor kinase mutant associated with metastatic breast cancer. Cancer Research, 58, 4805-4810.

Chen, Y. G., Liu, F., & Massague, J. (1997). Mechanism of tgf-beta receptor inhibition by fkbp12. EMBO Journal, 16, 3866-3876.

Chopra, V., Dinh, T. V., & Hannigan, E. V. (1998). Circulating serum levels of cytokines and angiogenic factors in patients with cervical cancer. Cancer Investigation, 16, 152-159.

Chu, T. Y., Lai, J. S., Shen, C. Y., Liu, H. S., & Chao, C. F. (1999). Frequent aberration of the transforming growth factor-beta receptor II gene in cell lines but no apparent mutation in pre-invasive and invasive carcinomas of the uterine cervix. International Journal of Cancer, 80, 506-510.

Comerci, J. T., Runowicz, C. D., Fields, A. L., Romney, S. L., Palan, P. R., Kadish, A. S., & Goldberg, G. L. (1997). Induction of transforming growth factor beta-1 in cervical intraepithelial neoplasia in vivo after treatment with beta- carotene. Clinical Cancer Research, 3, 157-160.

Conrad, C. T., Ernst, N. R., Dummer, W., Brocker, E. B., & Becker, J. C. (1999). Differential expression of transforming growth factor beta 1 and interleukin 10 in progressing and regressing areas of primary melanoma. Journal of Experimental & Clinical Cancer Research, 18, 225-232.

Crawford, S. E., Stellmach, V., Murphyullrich, J. E., Ribeiro, S. F., Lawler, J., Hynes, R. O., Boivin, G. P., & Bouck, N. (1998). Thrombospondin-1 is a major activator of tgf-beta-1 in vivo. Cell, 93, 1159-1170.

Cui, W., Fowlis, D. J., Bryson, S., Duffie, E., Ireland, H., Balmain, A., & Akhurst, R. J. (1996). Tgf-beta-1 inhibits the formation of benign skin tumors, but enhances progression to invasive spindle carcinomas in transgenic mice. Cell, 86, 531-542.

Dai, J. L., Bansal, R. K., & Kern, S. E. (1999). G(1) cell cycle arrest and apoptosis induction by nuclear Smad4/Dpc4: Phenotypes reversed by a tumorigenic mutation. Proceedings of the National Academy of Sciences of the United States of America, 96, 1427-1432.

Datto, M. B., Li, Y., Panus, J. F., Howe, D. J., Xiong, Y., & Wang, X. F. (1995). Transforming growth factor beta induces the cyclin-dependent kinase inhibitor p21 through a p53-independent mechanism. Proceedings of the National Academy of Sciences of the United States of America, 92, 5545-5549.

De Geest, K., Bergman, C. A., Turyk, M. E., Frank, B. S., & Wilbanks, G. D. (1994). Differential response of cervical intraepithelial and cervical carcinoma cell lines to transforming growth factor-beta 1. Gynecologic Oncology, 55,:376-85.

de Jonge, R. R., Garrigue-Antar, L., Vellucci, V. F., & Reiss, M. (1997). Frequent inactivation of the transforming growth factor beta type II receptor in small-cell lung carcinoma cells. Oncol.Res., 9, 89-98.

de Visser, K. E. & Kast, W. M. (1999). Effects of TGF-beta on the immune system: implications for cancer immunotherapy [Review]. Leukemia, 13, 1188-1199.

Dejonge, R. R., Garrigueantar, L., Vellucci, V. F., & Reiss, M. (1997). Frequent inactivation of the transforming growth factor beta type ii receptor in small-cell lung carcinoma cells. Oncology Research, 9, 89-98.

Derynck, R., Akhurst, R. J., & Balmain, A. (2001). TGF-beta signaling in tumor suppression and cancer progression. Nat.Genet., 29, 117-129.

Dey, A., Atcha, I. A., & Bagchi, S. (1997). Hpv16 e6 oncoprotein stimulates the transforming growth factor- beta-1 promoter in fibroblasts through a specific gc-rich sequence. Virology, 228, 190-199.

Duval, A., Gayet, J., Zhou, X. P., Iacopetta, B., Thomas, G., & Hamelin, R. (1999). Frequent frameshift mutations of the TCF-4 gene in colorectal cancers with microsatellite instability. Cancer Research, 59, 4213-4215.

Ebert, M. P. A., Yu, J., Miehlke, S., Fei, G., Lendeckel, U., Ridwelski, K., Stolte, M, Bayerdorffer, E. , Malfertheiner, P. (2000). Expression of transforming growth factor beta-1 in gastric cancer and in the gastric mucose of first-degree relatives of patients with gastric cancer. British Journal of Cancer, 82, 1795-1800.

Eisma, R. J., Spiro, J. D., Vonbiberstein, S. E., Lindquist, R. , & Kreutzer, D. L. (1996). Decreased expression of transforming growth factor beta receptors on head and neck squamous cell carcinoma tumor cells. American Journal of Surgery, 172, 641-645.

Engel, J. D., Kundu, S. D., Yang, T., Yang, S., Goodwin, S., Janulis, L., Cho, J. S., Chang, J., Kim, S. J., & Lee, C. (1999). Transforming growth factor-beta type II receptor confers tumor suppressor activity in murine renal carcinoma (RENCA) cells. urology, 54, 164-170.

Eppert, K., Scherer, S. W., Ozcelik, H., Pirone, R., Hoodless, P., Kim, H., Tsui, L. C., Bapat, B., Gallinger, S., Andrulis, I. L., Thomsen, G. H., Wrana, J. L., & Attisano, L. (1996). Madr2 maps to 18q21 and encodes a tgfbeta-regulated mad-related protein that is functionally mutated in colorectal carcinoma. Cell, 86, 543-552.

Evangelou, A., Jindal, S. K., Brown, T. J., Letarte, M. (2000). Down-regulation of transforming growth factor beta receptors by androgen in ovarian cancer cells. Cancer Research, 60, 929-935.

Fortunel, N., Hatzfeld, J., Kisselev, S., Monier, M. N., Ducos, K., Cardoso, A., Batard, P., Hatzfeld, A. (2000). Release from quiescence of primitive human hematopoietic stem/progenitor cells by blocking their cell-surface TGF-beta type II receptor in a short-term in vitro assay. Stem Cells, 18, 102-111.

Franzen, P., ten Dijke, P., Ichijo, H., Yamashita, H., Schulz, P., Heldin, C. H., & Miyazono, K. (1993). Cloning of a TGF beta type I receptor that forms a heteromeric complex with the TGF beta type II receptor. Cell, 75, 681-692.

Friedl, W., Kruse, R., Uhlhaas, S., Stolte, M., Schartmann, B., Keller, K. M., Jungck, M., Stern, M., Loff, S., Back, W., Propping, P., & Jenne, D. E. (1999). Frequent 4-bp deletion in exon 9 of the SMAD4/MADH4 gene in familial juvenile polyposis patients. Genes, Chromosomes & Cancer, 25, 403-406.

Geng, Y. & Weinberg, R. A. (1993). Transforming growth factor beta effects on expression of G1 cyclins and cyclin-dependent protein kinases. Proc.Natl.Acad.Sci.U.S.A, 90, 10315-10319.

Go, C., Li, P., & Wang, X. J. (1999). Blocking transforming growth factor beta signaling in transgenic epidermis accelerates chemical carcinogenesis: A mechanism associated with increased angiogenesis. Cancer Research, 59, 2861-2868.

Goggins, M., Shekher, M., Turnacioglu, K., Yeo, C. J., Hruban, R. H., & Kern, S. E. (1998). Genetic alterations of the transforming growth factor beta receptor genes in pancreatic and biliary adenocarcinomas. Cancer Research, 58, 5329-5332.

Grady, W. M., Myeroff, L. L., Swinler, S. E., Rajput, A., Thiagalingam, S., Lutterbaugh, J. D., Neumann, A., Brattain, M. G., Chang, J., Kim, S. J., Kinzler, K. W., Vogelstein, B., Willson, J. V., & Markowitz, S. (1999). Mutational inactivation of transforming growth factor beta receptor type II in microsatellite stable colon cancers. Cancer Research, 59, 320-324.

Gryfe, R., Kim, H., Hsieh, E. T. K., Aronson, M. D., Holowaty, E. J., Bull, S. B., Redston, M, Gallinger, S. (2000). Tumor microsatellite instability and clinical outcome in young patients with colorectal cancer. New England Journal of Medicine, 342, 69-77.

Guo, R. J., Wang, Y., Kaneko, E., Wang, D. Y., Arai, H., Hanai, H., Takenoshita, S., Hagiwara, K., Harris, C. C., & Sugimura, H. (1998). Analyses of mutation and loss of heterozygosity of coding sequences of the entire transforming growth factor beta type ii receptor gene in sporadic human gastric cancer. Carcinogenesis, 19, 1539-1544.

Hahn, S. A., Hoque, A. T., Moskaluk, C. A., da Costa, L. T., Schutte, M., Rozenblum, E., Seymour, A. B., Weinstein, C. L., Yeo, C. J., Hruban, R. H., & Kern, S. E. (1996). Homozygous deletion map at 18q21.1 in pancreatic cancer. Cancer Research, 56, 490-494.

Haines, J., Dunford, R., Moody, J., Ellender, M., Cox, R., Silver, A. (2000). Loss of heterozygosity in spontaneous and X-ray-induced intestinal tumors arising in FI hybrid Min mice: Evidence for sequential loss of Apc(+) and Dpc4 in tumor development. Genes, Chromosomes & Cancer, 28, 387-394.

Hannon, G. J. & Beach, D. (1994). P15ink4b is a potential effector of tgf-beta-induced cell cycle arrest [see comments]. Nature, 371, 257-261.

Hata, A., Lo, R. S., Wotton, D., Lagna, G., & Massague, J. (1997). Mutations increasing autoinhibition inactivate tumour suppressors smad2 and smad4. Nature, 388, 82-87.

Hata, A., Shi, Y. G., & Massague, J. (1998). Tgf-beta signaling and cancer - structural and functional consequences of mutations in smads [Review]. Molecular Medicine Today, 4, 257-262.

Heldin, C. H., Miyazono, K., & Tendijke, P. (1997). Tgf-beta signalling from cell membrane to nucleus through smad proteins [Review]. Nature, 390, 465-471.

Hougaard, S., Norgaard, P., Abrahamsen, N., Moses, H. L., Spang-Thomsen, M., & Poulsen, H. S. (1999). Inactivation of the transforming growth factor beta type II receptor in human small cell lung cancer cell lines. British Journal of Cancer, 79, 1005-1011.

Howe, J. R., Bair, J. L., Sayed, M. G., Anderson, M. E., Mitros, F. A., Petersen, G. M., Velculescu, V. E., Traverso, G., & Vogelstein, B. (2001). Germline mutations of the gene encoding bone morphogenetic protein receptor 1A in juvenile polyposis. Nat.Genet., 28, 184-187.

Howe, J. R., Roth, S., Ringold, J. C., Summers, R. W., Jarvinen, H. J., Sistonen, P., Tomlinson, I. M., Houlston, R. S., Bevan, S., Mitros, F. A., Stone, E. M., & Aaltonen, L. A. (1998). Mutations in the smad4/dpc4 gene in juvenile polyposis. Science, 280, 1086-1088.

Hurd, S. D., Johnson, M. D., Forbes, J. T., Carty-Dugger, T. L., & Arteaga, C. L. (1992). NEUTRALIZING TGF BETA ANTIBODIES INCREASE NATURAL KILLER (NK) CELL ACTIVITY AND INHIBIT HUMAN BREAST CANCER CELL TUMORIGENICITY IN ATHYMIC MICE (MEETING ABSTRACT). Proc.Annu.Meet.Am.Assoc.Cancer Res., 33:A481, A481.

Iacopetta, B. J., Soong, R., House, A. K., & Hamelin, R. (1999). Gastric carcinomas with microsatellite instability: Clinical features and mutations to the TGF-beta type II receptor, IGFII receptor, and BAX genes. Journal of Pathology, 187, 428-432.

Ilyas, M., Efstathiou, J. A., Straub, J., Kim, H. C., & Bodmer, W. F. (1999). Transforming growth factor beta stimulation of colorectal cancer cell lines: Type II receptor bypass and changes in adhesion molecule expression. Proceedings of the National Academy of Sciences of the United States of America, 96, 3087-3091.

Im, Y. H., Kim, H. T., Kim, I. Y., Factor, V. M., Hahm, K. B., Anzano, M., Jang, J. J., Flanders, K., Haines, D. C., Thorgeirsson, S. S., Sizeland, A., & Kim, S. J. (2001). Heterozygous Mice for the Transforming Growth Factor-{beta} Type II Receptor Gene Have Increased Susceptibility to Hepatocellular Carcinogenesis. Cancer Research, 61, 6665-6668.

Ishisaki, A., Yamato, K., Nakao, A., Nonaka, K., Ohguchi, M., Tendijke, P., & Nishihara, T. (1998). Smad7 is an activin-inducible inhibitor of activin-induced growth arrest and apoptosis in mouse b cells. Journal of Biological Chemistry, 273, 24293-24296.

Kang, S. H., Bang, Y. J., Im, Y. H., Yang, H. K., Lee, D. A., Lee, H. Y., Lee, H. S., Kim, N. K., & Kim, S. J. (1999). Transcriptional repression of the transforming growth factor-beta type I receptor gene by DNA methylation results in the development of TGF-beta resistance in human gastric cancer. Oncogene, 18, 7280-7286.

Karcher, J., Reisser, C., Daniel, V., & Herold-Mende, C. (1999). Cytokine expression of transforming growth factor-beta 2 and interleukin-10 in squamous cell carcinomas of the head and neck. Comparison of tissue expression and serum levels [German]. HNO, 47, 879-884.

Kim, J. J., Baek, M. J., Kim, L., Kim, N. G., Lee, Y. C., Song, S. Y., Noh, S. H., & Kim, H. (1999a). Accumulated frameshift mutations at coding nucleotide repeats during the progression of gastric carcinoma with microsatellite instability. Laboratory Investigation, 79, 1113-1120.

Kim, S. K., Fan, Y., Papadimitrakopoulou, V., Clayman, G., Hittelman, W. N., Hong, W. K., Lotan, R., & Mao, L. (1996). Dpc4, a candidate tumor suppressor gene, is altered infrequently in head and neck squamous cell carcinoma. Cancer Research, 56, 2519-2521.

Kim, W. S., Park, C., Jung, Y. S., Kim, H. S., Han, J. H., Park, C. H., Kim, K., Kim, J., Shim, Y. M., & Park, K. (1999b). Reduced transforming growth factor-beta type II receptor (TGF-beta RII) expression in adenocarcinoma of the lung. Anticancer Research, 19, 301-306.

Kleeff, J., Friess, H., Simon, P., Susmallian, S., Buchler, P., Zimmermann, A., Buchler, M. W., & Korc, M. (1999). Overexpression of Smad2 and colocalization with TGF-beta(1) in human pancreatic cancer. Digestive Diseases & Sciences, 44, 1793-1802.

Knobloch, T. J., Lynch, M. A., Song, H., Degroff, V. L., Casto, B. C., Adams, E. M., Alam, K. Y., Lang, J. C., Schuller, D. E., & Weghorst, C. M. (2001). Analysis of TGF-beta type I receptor for mutations and polymorphisms in head and neck cancers. Mutat.Res, 479, 131-139.

Kong, F. M., Jirtle, R. L., Huang, D. H., Clough, R. W., & Anscher, M. S. (1999). Plasma transforming growth factor-beta 1 level before radiotherapy correlates with long term outcome of patients with lung carcinoma. Cancer, 86, 1712-1719.

Korchynskyi, O., Landström, M., Stoika, R., Funa, K., Heldin, C. H., ten Dijke, P., & Souchelnytskyi, S. (1999). Expression of Smad proteins in human colorectal cancer. International Journal of Cancer 19;82, 197-202.

Krasagakis, K., Tholke, D., Farthmann, B., Eberle, J., Mansmann, U., & Orfanos, C. E. (1998). Elevated plasma levels of transforming growth factor (Tgf)-Beta-1 and tgf-beta-2 in patients with disseminated malignant melanoma. British Journal of Cancer, 77, 1492-1494.

Kretzschmar, M., Doody, J., Timokhina, I., & Massague, J. (1999). A mechanism of repression of TGF beta/Smad signaling by oncogenic Ras. Genes & Development, 13, 804-816.

Kundu, S. D., Kim, I. Y., Zelner, D., Janulis, L., Goodwin, S., Engel, J. D., & Lee, C. (1998). Absence of expression of transforming growth factor-beta type ii receptor is associated with an aggressive growth pattern in a murine renal carcinoma cell line, renca. Journal of Urology, 160, 1883-1888.

Lallemand, F., Mazars, A., Prunier, C., Bertrand, F., Kornprost, M., Gallea, S., Roman-Roman, S., Cherqui, G., & Atfi, A. (2001). Smad7 inhibits the survival nuclear factor kappaB and potentiates apoptosis in epithelial cells. Oncogene, 20, 879-884.

Lamm, M. G., Sintich, S. M., & Lee, C. (1998). A proliferative effect of transforming growth factor-beta-1 on a human prostate cancer cell line, tsu-pr1. Endocrinology, 139, 787-790.

Lange, D., Persson, U., Wollina, U., ten Dijke, P., Castelli, E., Heldin, C. H., & Funa, K. (1999). Expression of TGF-beta related Smad proteins in human epithelial skin tumors. International Journal of Oncology, 14, 1049-1056.

Latil, A., Pesche, S., Valeri, A., Fournier, G., Cussenot, O., & Lidereau, R. (1999). Expression and mutational analysis of the MADR2/smad2 gene in human prostate cancer. Prostate, 40, 225-231.

Lazzereschi, D., Ranieri, A., Mincione, G., Taccogna, S., Nardi, F., & Colletta, G. (1997). Human malignant thyroid tumors displayed reduced levels of transforming growth factor beta receptor type ii messenger rna and protein. Cancer Research, 57, 2071-2076.

Li, D. Y., Sorensen, L. K., Brooke, B. S., Urness, L. D., Davis, E. C., Taylor, D. G., Boak, B. B., & Wendel, D. P. (1999). Defective angiogenesis in mice lacking endoglin. Science, 284, 1534-1537.

Lin, H. Y., Wang, X. F., Ng-Eaton, E., Weinberg, R. A., & Lodish, H. F. (1992). Expression cloning of the tgf-beta type ii receptor, a functional transmembrane serine/threonine kinase [published erratum appears in cell 1992 sep 18;70(6):following 1068]. Cell, 68, 775-785.

Liu, F., Pouponnot, C., & Massague, J. (1997). Dual role of the smad4/dpc4 tumor suppressor in tgf-beta-inducible transcriptional complexes. Genes & Development, 11, 3157-3167.

Lopez-Casillas, F., Cheifetz, S., Doody, J., Andres, J. L., Lane, W. S., & Massague, J. (1991). Structure and expression of the membrane proteoglycan betaglycan, a component of the TGF-beta receptor system. Cell, 67, 785-795.

Lu, S. L., Kawabata, M., Imamura, T., Akiyama, Y., Nomizu, T., Miyazono, K., & Yuasa, Y. (1998). Hnpcc associated with germline mutation in the tgf-beta type ii receptor gene. Nature Genetics, 19, 17-18.

Lu, S. L., Kawabata, M., Imamura, T., Miyazono, K., & Yuasa, Y. (1999). Two divergent signaling pathways for TGF-beta separated by a mutation of its type II receptor gene. Biochemical & Biophysical Research Communications, 259, 385-390.

Lynch, M. A., Nakashima, R., Song, H. J., Degroff, V. L., Wang, D., Enomoto, T., & Weghorst, C. M. (1998). Mutational analysis of the transforming growth factor beta receptor type ii gene in human ovarian carcinoma. Cancer Research, 58, 4227-4232.

Markowitz, S., Wang, J., Myeroff, L., Parsons, R., Sun, L., Lutterbaugh, J., Fan, R. S., Zborowska, E., Kinzler, K. W., & Vogelstein, B. (1995). Inactivation of the type II TGF-beta receptor in colon cancer cells with microsatellite instability [see comments]. Science, 268, 1336-1338.

Massague, J. (1998). Tgf-beta signal transduction [Review]. Annual Review of Biochemistry, 67, 753-791.

Massague, J. & Chen, Y. G. (2000). Controlling TGF-beta signaling [Review]. Genes & Development, 14, 627-644.

Massague, J., Wotton, D., Receptors, Signal, t., Smad, Tgf, b., & Transcription. (2000). Transcriptional control by the TGF-beta/Smad signaling system [Review]. EMBO Journal, 19, 1745-1754.

McAllister, K. A., Grogg, K. M., Johnson, D. W., Gallione, C. J., Baldwin, M. A., Jackson, C. E., Helmbold, E. A., Markel, D. S., McKinnon, W. C., Murrell, J., & et al (1994). Endoglin, a tgf-beta binding protein of endothelial cells, is the gene for hereditary haemorrhagic telangiectasia type 1. Nature Genetics, 8, 345-351.

Miyaki, M., Iijima, T., Konishi, M., Sakai, K., Ishii, A., Yasuno, M., Hishima, T., Koike, M., Shitara, N., Iwama, T., Utsunomiya, J. , Kuroki, T., & Mori, T. (1999). Higher frequency of Smad4 gene mutation in human colorectal cancer with distant metastasis. Oncogene, %20;18, 3098-3103.

Moskaluk, C. A., Hruban, R. H., Schutte, M., Lietman, A. S., Smyrk, T., Fusaro, L., Fusaro, R., Lynch, J., Yeo, C. J., Jackson, C. E., Lynch, H. T., & Kern, S. E. (1997). Genomic sequencing of dpc4 in the analysis of familial pancreatic carcinoma. Diagnostic Molecular Pathology, 6, 85-90.

Munger, J. S., Huang, X. Z., Kawakatsu, H., Griffiths, M. D., Dalton, S. L., Wu, J. F., Pittet, J. F., Kaminski, N., Garat, C., Matthay, M. A., Rifkin, D. B., & Sheppard, D. (1999). The integrin alpha v beta 6 binds and activates latent TGF beta 1: A mechanism for regulating pulmonary inflammation and fibrosis. Cell, 96, 319-328.

Murata, M., Iwao, K., Miyoshi, Y., Nagasawa, Y., Ohta, T., Shibata, K., Oda, K., Wada, H., Tominaga, S., Matsuda, Y., Ohsawa, M., Nakamura, Y., & Shimano, T. (2000). Molecular and biological analysis of carcinoma of the small intestine: beta-catenin gene mutation by interstitial deletion involving exon 3 and replication error phenotype. American Journal of Gastroenterology, 95, 1576-1580.

Myeroff, L. L., Parsons, R., Kim, S. J., Hedrick, L., Cho, K. R., Orth, K., Mathis, M., Kinzler, K. W., Lutterbaugh, J., Park, K., Bang, Y. J., Lee, H. Y., Park, J. G., Lynch, H. T., Roberts, A. B., Vogelstein, B., & Markowitz, S. D. (1995). A transforming growth factor beta receptor type ii gene mutation common in colon and gastric but rare in endometrial cancers with microsatellite instability. Cancer Research, 55, 5545-5547.

Nakanishi, Y., Kodama, J., Yoshinouchi, M., Tokumo, K., Kamimura, S., Okuda, H., & Kudo, T. (1997). The expression of vascular endothelial growth factor and transforming growth factor-beta associates with angiogenesis in epithelial ovarian cancer. International Journal of Gynecological Pathology, 16, 256-262.

Oft, M., Heider, K. H., & Beug, H. (1998). Tgf-beta signaling is necessary for carcinoma cell invasiveness and metastasis. Current Biology, 8, 1243-1252.

Oft, M., Peli, J., Rudaz, C., Schwarz, H., Beug, H., & Reichmann, E. (1996). Tgf-beta-1 and ha-ras collaborate in modulating the phenotypic plasticity and invasiveness of epithelial tumor cells. Genes & Development, 10, 2462-2477.

Ogasa, H., Noma, T., Murata, H., Kawai, S., & Nakazawa, A. (1996). Cloning of a cdna encoding the human transforming growth factor- beta type ii receptor - heterogeneity of the mrna. Gene, 181, 185-190.

Ohue, M., Tomita, N., Monden, T., Miyoshi, Y., Ohnishi, T., Izawa, H., Kawabata, Y., Sasaki, M., Sekimoto, M., Nishisho, I., Shiozaki, H., & Monden, M. (1996). Mutations of the transforming growth factor beta type II receptor gene and microsatellite instability in gastric cancer. Int.J Cancer, 68, 203-206.

Papadimitrakopoulou, V. A., Oh, Y. , Elnaggar, A., Izzo, J., Clayman, G., & Mao, L. (1998). Presence of multiple incontiguous deleted regions at the long arm of chromosome 18 in head and neck cancer. Clinical Cancer Research, 4, 539-544.

Park, B. J., Park, J. I., Byun, D. S., Park, J. H., Chi, S. G., & sgchi@nms.kyunghee.ac.kr (2000). Mitogenic conversion of transforming growth factor-beta 1 effect by oncogenic Ha-Ras-induced activation of the mitogen-activated protein kinase signaling pathway in human prostate cancer. Cancer Research, 60, 3031-3038.

Park, K., Kim, S. J., Bang, Y. J., Park, J. G., Kim, N. K., Roberts, A. B., & Sporn, M. B. (1994). Genetic changes in the transforming growth factor beta (tgf- beta) type ii receptor gene in human gastric cancer cells: correlation with sensitivity to growth inhibition by tgf-beta. Proceedings of the National Academy of Sciences of the United States of America, 91, 8772-8776.

Parsons, R., Myeroff, L. L., Liu, B., Willson, J. K. V., Markowitz, S. D., Kinzler, K. W., & Vogelstein, B. (1995). Microsatellite instability and mutations of the transforming growth factor beta type ii receptor gene in colorectal cancer. Cancer Research, 55, 5548-5550.

Pasche, B., Bian, Y. S., Reich, J., Rademaker, A., Kolachana, P., & Offit, K. (2001). T{beta}R-I(6A) in colorectal cancer: a new twist? Cancer Research, 61, 8351.

Pasche, B., Kolachana, P., Nafa, K., Satagopan, J., Chen, Y. G., Lo, R. S., Brener, D., Yang, D., Kirstein, L., Oddoux, C., Ostrer, H., Vineis, P., Varesco, L., Jhanwar, S., Luzzatto, L., Massague, J., & Offit, K. (1999). T beta R-I(6A) is a candidate tumor susceptibility allele. Cancer Research, 59, 5678-5682.

Pasche, B., Luo, Y., Rao, P. H., Nimer, S. D., Dmitrovsky, E., Caron, P., Luzzatto, L., Offit, K., Cordoncardo, C., Renault, B., Satagopan, J. M., Murty, V. S., & Massague, J. (1998). Type I transforming growth factor beta receptor maps to 9q22 and exhibits a polymorphism and a rare variant within a polyalanine tract. Cancer Research, 58, 2727-2732.

Pepper, M. S. (1997). Transforming growth factor-beta: vasculogenesis, angiogenesis, and vessel wall integrity. Cytokine Growth Factor Rev., 8, 21-43.

Perry, K. T., Anthony, C. T., Case, T., & Steiner, M. S. (1997). Transforming growth factor beta as a clinical biomarker for prostate cancer. urology, 49, 151-155.

Pierce, D. F., Jr., Gorska, A. E., Chytil, A., Meise, K. S., Page, D. L., Coffey, R. J., Jr., & Moses, H. L. (1995). Mammary tumor suppression by transforming growth factor beta 1 transgene expression. Proceedings of the National Academy of Sciences of the United States of America, 92, 4254-4258.

Prunier, C., Mazars, A., Noe, V., Bruyneel, E., Mareel, M., Gespach, C., & Atfi, A. (1999). Evidence that Smad2 is a tumor suppressor implicated in the control of cellular invasion. Journal of Biological Chemistry, 274, 22919-22922.

Rashid, A., Zahurak, M., Goodman, S. N., & Hamilton, S. R. (1999). Genetic epidemiology of mutated K-ras proto-oncogene, altered suppressor genes, and microsatellite instability in colorectal adenomas. Gut, 44, 826-833.

Reed, J. A., McNutt, N. S., Prieto, V. G., & Albino, A. P. (1994). Expression of transforming growth factor-beta 2 in malignant melanoma correlates with the depth of tumor invasion. implications for tumor progression. American Journal of Pathology, 145, 97-104.

Renault, B., Calistri, D., Buonsanti, G., Nanni, O., Amadori, D., & Ranzani, G. N. (1996). Microsatellite instability and mutations of p53 and tgf-beta rii genes in gastric cancer. Human Genetics, 98, 601-607.

Roth, S., Sistonen, P., Salovaara, R., Hemminki, A., Loukola, A., Johansson, M., Avizienyte, E., Cleary, K. A., Lynch, P., Amos, C. I., Kristo, P., Mecklin, J. P., Kellokumpu, I., Jarvinen, H., & Aaltonen, L. A. (1999). SMAD genes in juvenile polyposis. Genes, Chromosomes & Cancer, 26, 54-61.

Saito, H., Tsujitani, S., Oka, S., Kondo, A., Ikeguchi, M., Maeta, M., & Kaibara, N. (1999). The expression of transforming growth factor-beta 1 is significantly correlated with the expression of vascular endothelial growth factor and poor prognosis of patients with advanced gastric carcinoma. Cancer, 86, 1455-1462.

Samowitz, W. S. & Slattery, M. L. (1997). Transforming growth factor-beta receptor type 2 mutations and microsatellite instability in sporadic colorectal adenomas and carcinomas. American Journal of Pathology, 151, 33-35.

Santin, A. D., Hermonat, P. L., Hiserodt, J. C., Fruehauf, J., Schranz, V., Barclay, D., Pecorelli, S., & Parham, G. P. (1997). Differential transforming growth factor-beta secretion in adenocarcinoma and squamous cell carcinoma of the uterine cervix. Gynecologic Oncology, 64, 477-480.

Schiemann, W. P., Pfeifer, W. M., Levi, E., Kadin, M. E., & Lodish, H. F. (1999). A deletion in the gene for transforming growth factor beta type I receptor abolishes growth regulation by transforming growth factor beta in a cutaneous T-cell lymphoma. Blood, 94, 2854-2861.

Schmid, P., Itin, P., & Rufli, T. (1995). In situ analysis of transforming growth factor-beta-s (tgf-beta-1, tgf-beta-2, tgf-beta-3), and tgf-beta type ii receptor expression in malignant melanoma. Carcinogenesis, 16, 1499-1503.

Schultz-Cherry, S., Chen, H., Mosher, D. F., Misenheimer, T. M., Krutzsch, H. C., Roberts, D. D., & Murphy-Ullrich, J. E. (1995). Regulation of transforming growth factor-beta activation by discrete sequences of thrombospondin 1. Journal of Biological Chemistry, 270, 7304-7310.

Schutte, M. (1999). DPC4/SMAD4 gene alterations in human cancer, and their functional implications. Annals of Oncology, 10, 4-59.

Schutte, M., Hruban, R. H., Hedrick, L., Cho, K. R., Nadasdy, G. M., Weinstein, C. L., Bova, G. S., Isaacs, W. B., Cairns, P., Nawroz, H., Sidransky, D., Casero, R. A., Jr., Meltzer, P. S., Hahn, S. A., & Kern, S. E. (1996). Dpc4 gene in various tumor types. Cancer Research, 56, 2527-2530.

Schwarte-Waldhoff, I., Klein, S., Blass-Kampmann, S., Hintelmann, A., Eilert, C., Dreschers, S. , Kalthoff, H., Hahn, S. A., & Schmiegel, W. (1999). DPC4/SMAD4 mediated tumor suppression of colon carcinoma cells is associated with reduced urokinase expression. Oncogene, 20:18, 3152-3158.

Shin, K. H., Park, Y. J., Park, J. G. (2000). Mutational analysis of the transforming growth factor beta receptor type II gene in hereditary nonpolyposis colorectal cancer and early-onset colorectal cancer patients. Clinical Cancer Research, 6, 536-540.

Sinha, S., Nevett, C., Shuttleworth, C. A., & Kielty, C. M. (1998). Cellular and extracellular biology of the latent transforming growth factor-beta binding proteins [Review]. Matrix Biology, 17, 529-545.

Takaku, K., Oshima, M., Miyoshi, H., Matsui, M., Seldin, M. F., & Taketo, M. M. (1998). Intestinal tumorigenesis in compound mutant mice of both dpc4 (Smad4) And apc genes. Cell, 92, 645-656.

Tanaka, S., Mori, M., Mafune, K., Ohno, S., Sugimachi, K. (2000). A dominant negative mutation of transforming growth factor-beta receptor type II gene in microsatellite stable oesophageal carcinoma. British Journal of Cancer, 82, 1557-1560.

Tang, B., Bottinger, E. P., Jakowlew, S. B., Bagnall, K. M., Mariano, J., Anver, M. R., Letterio, J. J., & Wakefield, L. M. (1998). Transforming growth factor-beta1 is a new form of tumor suppressor with true haploid insufficiency. Nat.Med., 4, 802-807.

Tarafa, G., Villanueva, A., Farre, L., Rodriguez, J., Musulen, E., Reyes, G., Seminago, R., Olmedo, E., Paules, A. B., Peinado, M. A., Bachs, O., Capella, G. (2000). DCC and SMAD4 alterations in human colorectal and pancreatic tumor dissemination. Oncogene, 19, 546-555.

Teti, A., Degiorgi, A., Spinella, M. T., Migliaccio, S., Canipari, R., Muda, A. O., & Faraggiana, T. (1997). Transforming growth factor-beta enhances adhesion of melanoma cells to the endothelium in vitro. International Journal of Cancer, 72, 1013-1020.

Togo, G., Okamoto, M., Shiratori, Y., Yamaji, H., Kato, J., Matsumura, M., Sano, T., Motojima, T., & Omata, M. (1999). Does mutation of transforming growth factor-beta type II receptor gene play an important role in colorectal polyps? Digestive Diseases & Sciences, 44, 1803-1809.

Tokunaga, H., Lee, D. H., Kim, I. Y., Wheeler, T. M., & Lerner, S. P. (1999). Decreased expression of transforming growth factor beta receptor type I is associated with poor prognosis in bladder transitional cell carcinoma patients. Clinical Cancer Research, 5, 2520-2525.

Tomita, S., Miyazato, H., Tamai, O., Muto, Y., & Toda, T. (1999). Analyses of microsatellite instability and the transforming growth factor-beta receptor type II gene mutation in sporadic human gastrointestinal cancer. Cancer Genetics & Cytogenetics, 115, 23-27.

Villanueva, A., Garcia, C., Paules, A. B., Vicente, M., Megias, M., Reyes, G., Devillalonga, P., Agell, N., Lluis, F., Bachs, O., & Capella, G. (1998). Disruption of the antiproliferative tgf-beta signaling pathways in human pancreatic cancer cells. Oncogene, 17, 1969-1978.

Wagner, M., Kleeff, J., Lopez, M. E., Bockman, I., Massaque, J., & Korc, M. (1998). Transfection of the type i tgf-beta receptor restores tgf-beta responsiveness in pancreatic cancer. International Journal of Cancer, 78, 255-260.

Wang, J., Sun, L., Myeroff, L., Wang, X., Gentry, L. E., Yang, J., Liang, J., Zborowska, E., Markowitz, S., Willson, J. K., & . (1995a). Demonstration that mutation of the type II transforming growth factor beta receptor inactivates its tumor suppressor activity in replication error-positive colon carcinoma cells. J Biol.Chem., 270, 22044-22049.

Wang, J., Sun, L. Z., Myeroff, L., Wang, X. F., Gentry, L. E., Yan, J. H., Liang, J. R., Zborowska, E., Markowitz, S., Willson, J. K. V., & Brattain, M. G. (1995b). Demonstration that mutation of the type ii transforming growth factor beta receptor inactivates its tumor suppressor activity in replication error-positive colon carcinoma cells. Journal of Biological Chemistry, 270, 22044-22049.

Watanabe, T., Wu, T. T., Catalano, P. J., Ueki, T., Satriano, R., Haller, D. G., Benson, A. B., III, & Hamilton, S. R. (2001). Molecular predictors of survival after adjuvant chemotherapy for colon cancer. N.Engl.J Med., 344, 1196-1206.

Wikstrom, P., Bergh, A., Damber, J. E., Tgf, b., Regulation of, p. g., Metastasis, Angiogenesis., & Immunosuppression. (2000). Transforming growth factor-beta 1 and prostate cancer [Review]. Scandinavian Journal of Urology & Nephrology, 34, 85-94.

Wolff, J. M., Fandel, T. H., Borchers, H., & Jakse, G. (1999). Serum concentrations of transforming growth factor-beta 1 in patients with benign and malignant prostatic diseases. Anticancer Research, 19, 2657-2659.

Woodford-Richens, K., Williamson, J., Bevan, S., Young, J., Leggett, B., Frayling, I., Thway, Y., Hodgson, S., Kim, J. C., Iwama, T., Novelli, M., Sheer, D., Poulsom, R., Wright, N., Houlston, R., & Tomlinson, I. (2000). Allelic loss at SMAD4 in polyps from juvenile polyposis patients and use of fluorescence in situ hybridization to demonstrate clonal origin of the epithelium. Cancer Research, 60, 2477-2482.

Wu, S. P., Theodorescu, D., Kerbel, R. S., Willson, J. K., Mulder, K. M., Humphrey, L. E., & Brattain, M. G. (1992). Tgf-beta 1 is an autocrine-negative growth regulator of human colon carcinoma fet cells in vivo as revealed by transfection of an antisense expression vector. Journal of Cell Biology, 116, 187-196.

Xu, J. & Attisano, L. (2000). Mutations in the tumor suppressors Smad2 and Smad4 inactivate transforming growth factor beta signaling by targeting Smads to the ubiquitin-proteasome pathway. Proceedings of the National Academy of Sciences of the United States of America, 97, 4820-4825.

Xu, J. W., Ahmad, A., Jones, J. F., Dolcetti, R., Vaccher, E., Prasad, U., & Menezes, J. (2000). Elevated serum transforming growth factor beta 1 levels in Epstein-Barr virus-associated diseases and their correlation with virus-specific immunoglobulin A (IgA) and IgM. Journal of Virology, 74, 2443-2446.

Yakicier, M. C., Irmak, M. B., Romano, A., Kew, M., & Ozturk, M. (1999). Smad2 and Smad4 gene mutations in hepatocellular carcinoma. Oncogene, 18, 4879-4883.

Yamada, S. D., Baldwin, R. L., & Karlan, B. Y. (1999). Ovarian carcinoma cell cultures are resistant to TGF-beta 1-mediated growth inhibition despite expression of functional receptors. Gynecologic Oncology, 75, 72-77.

Yamada, Y., Miyauchi, A., Goto, J., Takagi, Y., Okuizumi, H., Kanematsu, M., Hase, M., Takai, H., Harada, A., & Ikeda, K. (1998). Association of a polymorphism of the transforming growth factor-beta-1 gene with genetic susceptibility to osteoporosis in postmenopausal japanese women. Journal of Bone & Mineral Research, 13, 1569-1576.

Yamada, Y., Okuizumi, H., Miyauchi, A., Takagi, Y., Ikeda, K., & Harada, A. (2000). Association of transforming growth factor beta 1 genotype with spinal osteophytosis in Japanese women. Arthritis & Rheumatism, 43, 452-460.

Yanagisawa, K., Osada, H., Masuda, A., Kondo, M., Saito, T., Yatabe, Y., Takagi, K., & Takahashi, T. (1998). Induction of apoptosis by smad3 and down-regulation of smad3 expression in response to tgf-beta in human normal lung epithelial cells. Oncogene, 17, 1743-1747.

Yin, J. J., Selander, K., Chirgwin, J. M., Dallas, M., Grubbs, B. G., Wieser, R., Massague, J., Mundy, G. R., & Guise, T. A. (1999). TGF-beta signaling blockade inhibits PTHrP secretion by breast cancer cells and bone metastases development. Journal of Clinical Investigation, 103, 197-206.

Yokota, M., Ichihara, S., Lin, T. L., Nakashima, N., Yamada, Y. (2000). Association of a t29 -> C polymorphism of the transforming growth factor-beta 1 gene with genetic susceptibility to myocardial infarction in Japanese. Circulation, 101, 2783-2787.

Zhang, T., Nanney, L. B., Peeler, M. O., Williams, C. S., Lamps, L., Heppner, K. J., Dubois, R. N., & Beauchamp, R. D. (1997). Decreased transforming growth factor beta type ii receptor expression in intestinal adenomas from min/+ mice is associated with increased cyclin d1 and cyclin-dependent kinase 4 expression. Cancer Research, 57, 1638-1643.

Zhou, Y., Kato, H., Shan, D., Minami, R., Kitazawa, S., Matsuda, T., Arima, T., Barrett, J. C., & Wake, N. (1999). Involvement of mutations in the DPC4 promoter in endometrial carcinoma development. Molecular Carcinogenesis, 25, 64-72.

Ziv, E., Cauley, J., Morin, P. A., Saiz, R., & Browner, W. S. (2001). Association between the T29-->C polymorphism in the transforming growth factor beta1 gene and breast cancer among elderly white women: The Study of Osteoporotic Fractures. JAMA, 285, 2859-2863.

NOTCH IN MALIGNANCY

DOUGLAS W. BALL AND STEVEN D. LEACH

1. INTRODUCTION

The Notch signaling pathway plays a remarkable role in biology as a superbly versatile developmental switch. Notch signaling controls numerous cell fate and differentiation decisions in divergent multicellular organisms. Emerging concepts of Notch action in cancer reflect the importance of this pathway in regulating the phenotype of cancer progenitor cells and the capacity of Notch to regulate growth and to act as an oncogene. We will summarize essential features of Notch signaling mechanisms and several well-studied examples of Notch actions in fetal development and post-natal stem cells. The balance of this review will focus on Notch as an oncogene, as a major determinant of the cancer phenotype, and as a potential target for drug therapy.

2. NOTCH SIGNALING PATHWAY-MOLECULAR ASPECTS

2.1 Overview

Elucidating the mechanisms underlying Notch signaling has engaged many laboratories and remains an incomplete story. Essential aspects of Notch signaling, first uncovered in the early to mid 1990's, are unique among signaling systems described in this book. Most notably, Notch proteins are single pass-transmembrane receptors for extracellular ligands, yet they also function as nuclear transcription factors. Physiologic activation of Notch is accomplished through the action of membrane-tethered ligands that trigger a complex sequence of proteolytic events to generate the active intracellular Notch moiety. Truncated forms of Notch such as the Tan1 oncogene are predominantly nuclear and constitutively active (Ellisen,1991). It is convenient to view two phases of Notch signaling: (1) generation of the free Notch intracellular domain (NICD), and (2) nuclear actions of NICD and downstream effectors. Details underlying these processes are described below.

2.2 Generation of the NICD

In mammals, there are four known Notch homologs (see Mumm,2000 for review). The paradigm molecule, Notch1, appears to have the most prominent role in development and neoplasia, to date. The conserved structure of Notch molecules includes a large extracellular domain composed of numerous epidermal growth factor repeats and Lin-Notch repeats, important for ligand binding. Also conserved is the single transmembrane domain, and intracellular domains including two nuclear localization sequences, RAM and ankyrin repeat protein interaction domains, a c-terminal trans-activaton domain and a PEST sequence, involved in Notch degradation. Post-translational processing of the

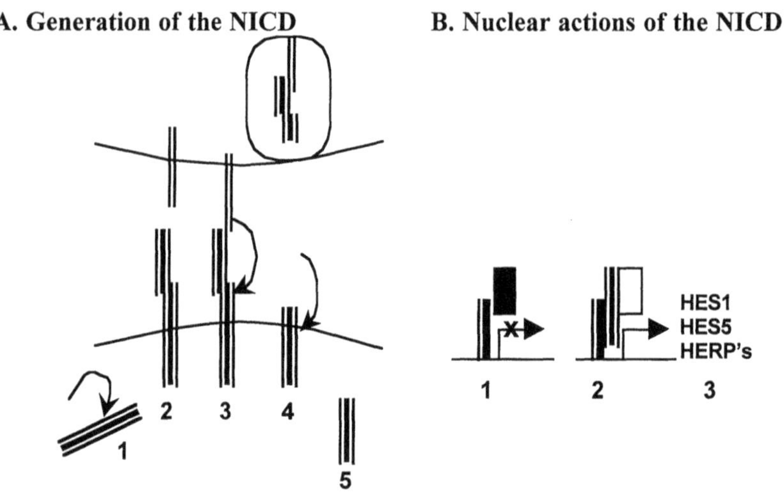

Figure 1. Schematic of Notch signaling pathway. A. 1. The newly synthesized 300 kDa Notch precursor protein is cleaved by furin proteases in the trans-golgi. 2.Notch extracellular and transmembrane fragments linked by a calcium coordinated bond assemble at the membrane. 3. A Notch ligand on an adjoining cell contacts the Notch extracellular domain EGF repeat domain, triggering cleavage of the transmembrane fragment by TACE. 4. The intra-membraneous portion of Notch is cleaved by a complex containing presenilin as the Notch extracellular fragment and ligand are endocytosed in the ligand presenting cell. 5. The NICD is free to migrate to the nucleus. B. Notch as a transcriptional switch. 1. In the absence of Notch, CBF-1 binds a co-repressor complex and silences transcription at target genes. 2. NICD associates with CBF-1 via the ankyrin repeat region, displaces co-repressors and recruits co-activators. 3. Target genes including Hes1, Hes5, Herp1 and Herp2 are activated. Subsequent transcriptional repression by these factors silences multiple target genes. NICD, Notch intracellular domain; TACE, tumor necrosis factor converting enzyme; Hes, Hairy-Enhancer of Split; Herp, Hes- related protein.

Notch protein is critical to its activity. Within the large extracellular region is a recognition site for furin convertases that cleave the 300kDa Notch protein precursor in the trans-Golgi compartment, generating extracellular and transmembrane fragments which undergo linkage at the membrane (Blaumueller,1997) via a calcium-coordinated bond (Rand,2000)(see figure 1). The resulting Notch heterodimer binds to ligands of the DSL (Delta-Serrate- Lag-2) family.

At least eight mammalian Notch ligands have been characterized to date, including Delta1-4, Delta-like 1 and 3, and Jagged1 and 2 (see Table1). These ligands are differentially expressed in a wide variety of tissues. Soluble forms of Notch ligands generally inhibit Notch signaling. Only when an adjoining cell presents the ligand on its surface to a Notch-expressing cell does signaling take place. Figure 1 illustrates the stages of Notch activation by its ligands. Ligand interaction with specific EGF repeat elements within the Notch extracellular domain triggers a series of events including multiple proteolytic steps. Initially, at a site located ~12 amino acids outside of the transmembrane region, enzymes including the TNF-alpha converting enzyme (TACE) cleave the Notch extracellular domain (Brou,2000). The precise mechanism whereby Notch becomes an active substrate for these membrane-associated metalloproteinases is not totally clear. However, dissociation of the extracellular domain or alteration of its configuration appear sufficient to enable the TACE activity (Mumm,2000).

Remarkably, the Notch extracellular domain, when complexed with ligand and cleaved, appears to be "trans-endocytosed" into adjoining ligand-presenting cells (Parks,2000). This ligand-mediated clearance of the Notch extracellular fragment appears essential, since *Drosophila* mutants which are defective in endocytic function exhibit specific Notch loss-of-function phenotypes.

Ligand-mediated cleavage of the Notch extracellular domain, via TACE, exposes the remaining transmembrane Notch molecule to another proteolytic event. The enzymes presenilin 1 and 2 clip Notch within the plasma membrane, a process referred to as regulated intra-membrane proteolysis (see Fortini,2001 for review). Additional presenilin-independent proteins may also contribute to this activation step (Berechid,2002). Recent studies suggest a multiprotein complex involved in this final stage of Notch activation, including both presenilins and nicastrin (Yu,2000).

A number of reports suggest that the activity on Notch of TACE, not presenilin, is the step directly influenced by ligand activation, and that Notch molecules bearing a short extracellular tail can be cleaved constitutively by presenilins (Struhl,2000). Interestingly, presenilins also cleave amyloid precursor proteins. Mutations in PS1 and PS2 account for many cases of hereditary Alzheimer's Disease (Walter,2001). In these instances, accumulation of a cleavage product of amyloid precursor proteins leads to neurotoxicity. Other

Table 1. Conserved elements of Notch signaling in flies, worms, and mammals

	Drosophila	*C. elegans*	*Mammals*
Notch receptors	Notch	lin-12 glp-1	Notch1 Notch2 Notch3 Notch4
DSL ligands	Delta Serrate	lag-2 apx-1	Delta-1 Delta-2 Delta-3 Delta-4 Delta-like 1 (Dll1) Delta-like 3 (Dll3) Jagged-1 (Serrate-1) Jagged-2 (Serrate-2)
Processing enzymes	dfurin Kuzbanian Presenilin	 sup-17 sel-12	Furin Kuzbanian _- secretase/presenilin- 1
CSL proteins	Suppressor of Hairless [Su(H)]	lag-1	CBF-1/RBP-J_
Effectors	Hairy Enhancer of Split [E(spl)] Deltex	lin-22	Hes-1, Hes-5 Hey-1 (HERP2) Hey-2 (HERP1) HeyL Deltex
Co-repressors	Groucho	unc-37	TLE mSin3/N- CoR/HDAC
Modulators	Fringe Numb Nicastrin	 aph-2	lunatic fringe manic fringe radical fringe Numb Numb-like Nicastrin

than a shared involvement of the presenilin enzymes, there is no known role for the Notch pathway in Alzheimer's Disease. Recently-developed inhibitors of presenilin activity (γ-secretase inhibitors) show promise in being able to interrupt ligand-activated Notch signaling (see therapy section below).

2.3 Nuclear actions of the NICD

Following the multi-step cleavage of Notch and liberation of free Notch intracellular domain (NICD) from the inner membrane leaflet, this active c-terminal fragment is transported to the nucleus (Struhl,1998; Schroeter,1998), a process mediated by two nuclear localization sequences. Nuclear localization appears necessary for all known biologic functions of Notch (Jeffries,2000). In the best-characterized model of Notch action, Notch forms a complex with CBF-1, also known as RBPJ-kappa, a DNA binding protein. In the absence of Notch, CBF-1 recruits transcriptional co-repressors including SMRT and CIR, forming a transcriptional repressor complex on specific gene promoters (Zhou,2001). NICD in the nucleus associates with CBF-1 via the ankyrin repeat sequence, and displaces transcriptional co-repressors. In addition, multi-protein complexes including SKIP-1, and other co-activating molecules such as p300, form stabilizing interactions with NICD-CBF-1 (Zhou,2000;Oswald,2001). In this way free, intracellular Notch forms a transcriptional switch, rapidly converting CBF-1 from a transcriptional repressor to an activator.

Knowledge of the range of transcriptional targets of Notch and CBF-1 is currently limited. The best characterized targets to date are four transcription factor genes of the mammalian Hairy-Enhancer of Split family, HES1 (the paradigm factor), HES5, as well as HES-related proteins HERP1 and HERP2. These four proteins function themselves as transcriptional repressors, with heterodimers of HES1 and HERP proteins forming the most potent inhibitory complexes (Iso,2001). These four Notch-sensitive HES family members are a subset of the larger HES family of inhibitory basic Helix Loop Helix (bHLH) transcription factors, which bind to canonical recognition elements termed N-boxes. HES-HERP heterodimers recruit a range of transcriptional repressor proteins to these sites including NCoR, mSin3, and TLE/Groucho-related proteins to silence transcription in N-Box containing promoters (Iso,2001). In addition to the typical interaction of Notch with CBF-1, a variety of CBF-1 independent Notch mechanisms have been identified and partially characterized (Shawber,1996). In one of these recently-described examples, Notch performs its role as a ligand-activated transcriptional switch for the DNA binding protein LEF-1 in a beta catenin-independent manner (Ross,2001). Interestingly, Notch1-LEF-1 heterodimers appear to activate a distinct set of promoters compared to those typically activated by beta catenin-LEF-1 complexes. An additional transcriptional mediator of Notch signaling, apparently independent of CBF-1 and Hes proteins, is the SH3-containing protein, deltex (Yamamoto,2001).

Downstream targets of HES-mediated repression are likely to be very diverse. Although the identity of these targets hasn't been systematically explored in any tissue, numerous studies have implicated bHLH transcription factors as targets of repression. For example, both *in vitro* and in transgenic knockout mice, HES1 appears to inhibit the expression of Mash1/hASH1, the mammalian achaete-scute homolog-1, in the nervous system and developing lung (Ito,2000;Chen,1997; Nakamura,2000). Gut neuroendocrine differentiation, under the control of a series of bHLH factors, is inhibited by Notch acting via HES1 (Jensen,2000). Notch repression of the bHLH proteins E12 and E47 appears essential in the differentiation of T-cells from uncommitted lymphocytic precursors (Ordentlich,1998). Examples of Notch action in a number of classic developmental contexts are discussed in the following section.

3. NOTCH SIGNALING DURING EMBRYONIC DEVELOPMENT

3.1 Overview

During development, tremendous cellular diversity is established among an initially interchangeable population of embryonic cells. Determining how this diversity is generated remains a central issue in developmental biology. One mechanism contributing to this process involves inductive interactions between adjacent cell types. In this regard, Notch-mediated interactions have been shown to play a central role in generating cellular diversity in a wide variety of developing tissues. As noted in Table 1, Notch pathway components are highly conserved among metazoan organisms, reflecting the critical role of this pathway in both vertebrate and invertebrate development.

Classical examples of Notch signaling during development include effects on wing margin formation, leg segmentation, and neurogenesis in *Drosophila*, anchor cell specification during vulvar development in *C. elegans*, somite formation in vertebrates, and regulation of neuroendocrine differentiation in mouse foregut derivatives. As suggested by Bray (Bray,1998), it is useful to group these many influences of Notch into three broad types of developmental events: lateral inhibition, lineage specification, and boundary formation. While these processes all utilize components of the core Notch signaling pathway described above, each process relies on differential modulation of Notch signaling to achieve a distinct developmental outcome. Furthermore, lateral inhibition, lineage specification and boundary formation all may be recapitulated by Notch signaling in cancer.

3.2 Notch-dependent lateral inhibition

Lateral inhibition represents the process by which individual cells within an equivalence group undergo cellular differentiation to achieve a primary cell fate, while similar differentiation is inhibited in adjacent cells. The role of Notch in mediating lateral inhibition was first suggested by Poulson, who observed abnormal hypertrophy of the nervous system at the expense of epidermal structures in flies bearing a mutated Notch allele (Poulson,1937). Because many Notch pathway components were initially identified in mutant fly stocks exhibiting defects in this process, much of the nomenclature involving Notch signaling is derived from descriptions of these mutational phenotypes.

The sensory units of the *Drosophila* peripheral nervous system are externally visible as mechanosensory bristles or chaetae located on the wings, legs, and body of the adult fly (reviewed by Fisher, 1998). The sensory organ is composed of four cell types including a single bipolar neuron and three accessory cells, the trichogen (bristle shaft), the tormogen (bristle socket) and the thecogen (neuronal sheath). Each of these cells is derived from a single sensory organ precursor (SOP) cell which is selected from a field of equivalent epidermal cells, each with the potential to adopt the SOP cell fate. Through a process of lateral inhibition, however, one cell within the equivalence field is singled out to become the SOP, while surrounding cells retain an epidermal cell fate. Changes in the balance of SOP vs. epidermal cells result in changes in the number and concentration of sensory neurons, made externally manifest by associated changes in bristle number.

Several components of the Notch pathway were identified by mutational phenotypes involving this system. Thus the *hairy* mutation is associated with an increased number of bristles, while flies bearing *achaete* or *hairless* mutant alleles exhibit reduced bristle/chaeta number. It is now known that epidermal cells surrounding the SOP are prevented from undergoing neural differentiation through Notch receptor activation initiated by ligands presented on the SOP cell surface. This lateral inhibition of neural differentiation is mediated by transcriptional repression of proneural genes including *achaete, scute* and *atonal.* By virtue of eliminating this lateral inhibitory mechanism and permitting abnormal formation of additional SOP cells, loss-of-function mutations involving the Notch pathway are frequently referred to as neurogenic mutations. Thus "neurogenic" genes such as *Delta, Notch, Suppressor of Hairless, Hairy*, and *Enhancer of Split* generally act to down-regulate expression of proneural genes, resulting in neurogenic phenotypes when mutated. The proneural and neurogenic influences of these genes also appear to regulate development of the mammalian nervous system, in which loss of *atonal*-related genes (e.g. *neurogenin-1, neurogenin-2, neuroD*) results in deficits in neural differentiation (Miyata,1999; Fode,1998; Ma,1998), while mutations in *Notch-1, RBP-J* or *Hes-1* result in phenotypes characterized by excessive and/or premature neurogenesis (de la Pompa,1997; Lutolf,2002; Ishibashi,1995).

Similarly, Notch-mediated lateral inhibition also regulates cellular differentiation during development of the hermaphrodite reproductive organ of *C. elegans*. Two adjacent cells, designated Z1.ppp and Z4.aaa, will ultimately become a terminally differentiated anchor cell, and a ventral uterine precursor cell. Initially, both of these cells carry an equivalent developmental potential, with equal probability that either cell will pursue a given cell fate (Newman,1996). The determination of anchor cell versus ventral uterine cell fate is controlled by Notch signaling, with worms carrying loss-of-function mutations in *lin-12* (a *C. elegans Notch* ortholog) forming two anchor cells, while worms carrying a constitutively active *lin-12* form two ventral uterine precursors. In wild-type worms, subtle differences in Notch pathway activation between Z1.ppp or Z4.aaa dictate which fate will be pursued by which cell, with higher levels of Notch signaling specifying the uterine precursor cell, and lower levels resulting in anchor cell differentiation.

Notch-mediated lateral inhibition thus appears to represent a common component of developmental systems requiring specification of unique cell types within equivalent precursor fields. An important question relates to how apparently identical cells initiate reciprocal changes in Notch activity necessary to exert a lateral inhibitory effect. Recent investigations have suggested that the initiation of biased signaling between similar cell types may be dependent on asymmetric segregation of Numb among adjacent cells. Numb is an intracellular adaptor protein known to inhibit Notch-mediated signals in a cell autonomous manner (Zilian,2001). Inactivation of *numb* results in defective neurogenesis in both the fly and the mouse (Uemura,1989;Zilian,2001), presumably due to unabated Notch signaling. In several developmental systems, evidence suggests that Numb is asymmetrically distributed during precursor cell division, resulting in an inherent bias in Notch signaling potential between otherwise identical daughter cells (Posakony,1994). Once this subtle bias is initiated, a feedback mechanism which includes down-regulation of Delta expression in cells with greater Notch activation results in amplification of these differences, allowing self-reinforcing lateral inhibition to be initiated.

3.3 Notch-dependent lineage specification

In addition to regulating differentiation through lateral inhibition, Notch signaling is frequently employed to further specify cell lineage in a wide variety of developmental contexts. In its simplest form, this process may be viewed as an extension of lateral inhibition among adjacent cell types. In the case of the *Drosophila* SOP, Notch signaling not only regulates selection of the SOP within the proneural cluster, but also regulates subsequent lineage specification during differentiation of the sensory neuron, sensory bristle, bristle shaft and bristle socket. All four of these SOP progeny are formed by two series of asymmetric cell division, with the SOP initially dividing into daughter cells, and these secondary precursors undergoing additional division to form the socket, shaft, sheath and neuron. Inactivation of *Notch* at different points in this process indicates that lineage specification following each of these cell divisions is regulated by Notch, with Notch activation promoting socket cell identity over shaft, and sheath cell identity over the neuronal cell fate. Thus Notch controls differentiation of all four sensory organ cell types by regulating lineage specification during iterative asymmetric cell divisions (Posakony,1994).

In the case of more complex tissues, Notch signaling may also regulate sequential lineage commitment, either by preventing differentiation in a subpopulation of precursor cells or by actively promoting alternate cell fates. The complex roles of Notch in hematopoietic development are reviewed in detail in the section below, "Role of Notch in Stem Cell Biology." Additional systems involving Notch-mediated lineage specification include regulation of neuroendocrine differentiation in mouse endoderm derivatives, including embryonic lung, pancreas, and gut. In each of these tissues, early lineage commitment specifies cells to either an endocrine or non-endocrine lineage. Inactivation of Notch signaling in *Hes1-/-* mice results in precocious and excessive endocrine differentiation at the expense of non-endocrine cell types in lung, pancreas, stomach and intestine (Ito,2000; Jensen,2000). In addition, *Hes1-/-* lung and pancreas have been noted to be hypoplastic compared to wild-type tissues, suggesting that Notch is required not only for differentiation of non-endocrine cell types, but also for reserving a population of undifferentiated cells responsible for normal tissue growth and morphogenesis. In developing pancreas, this population of undifferentiated precursors is depleted not only in *Hes1-/-* mice, but also in *Dll1*, and *RBPJ* knockouts (Apelqvist,1999). In each case, failure to reserve a precursor population characterized by active Notch signaling results in precocious endocrine differentiation and failure to generate non-endocrine cell types. This early endocrine/non-endocrine lineage decision is therefore reminiscent of neural/epidermal lineage specification in *Drosophila*, and underscores the similarity between neural and neuroendocrine differentiation. However, it must be remembered that the differentiating mammalian foregut is vastly more complicated than the Drosophila sensory organ, with multiple lineages arising not by stereotypical asymmetric cell divisions but by the gradual, overlapping emergence of different cell types under the influence of both soluble and cell-contact mediated signals.

Although Notch-mediated lineage specification is well documented in a variety of tissues, the mechanisms by which specific cell types undergo modulation of Notch activity during this process are unknown. Additional work is necessary to determine what tissue-specific or general factors are required to generate different levels of Notch activity among precursor cells in developing mammalian tissues.

3.4 Notch-regulated boundary formation

A third broad category of Notch function during development involves specifying borders and boundaries in developing tissues. This function of Notch appears to underlie the notched wing phenotype associated with haplo-insufficiency in female flies, initially described as a dominant sex-linked allele by Dexter (Dexter,1914). Notch fly stocks are characterized by defects in the wing margin resulting in a notched or scalloped wing contour. More recently, the mechanism underlying this phenotype has been clarified as a defect in dorsal-ventral boundary formation.

The fly wing imaginal disc represents a cluster of undifferentiated epithelial cells derived a reserved pool specified in early embryogenesis (reviewed in [Irvine]). During the larval instars, the imaginal disc cells proliferate, and the disc becomes organized into distinct dorsal and ventral domains through early ventral expression of *wingless*. This initial dorsal/ventral specification divides the wing disc into a dorsal field destined to form the body wall, and a ventral field destined to become wing. Subsequently, the wing field is further divided along the dorsal/ventral axis by regional expression of *apterous* in dorsal cells. With this specification of dorsal and ventral identify, the dorsal/ventral boundary becomes an important organizer and promoter of wing distal outgrowth. Following growth and folding of the wing blade, cells present at this boundary ultimately form the edge of the mature wing, also known as the wing margin, while the dorsal and ventral cells form two opposing cell layers which comprise the wing blade.

Notch signaling plays a critical role in establishing the dorsal/ventral boundary in the developing wing. In contrast to a mechanism of lateral inhibition, this function of Notch involves establishment of a gradually narrowing band of cells which both receive and send Notch signals to and from cells on the opposite side of the boundary. This distinct pattern of Notch activity appears to reflect the activity of *fringe*, a cell-autonomous modulator of Notch activity which is induced in dorsal wing cells by *apterous*. Fringe is a glucosaminyltransferase which transfers GlcNAc to O-fucose residues located within epidermal growth factor-like repeats of Notch (Chen,2001). As a result, Notch is rendered insensitive to activation by Serrate, but shows increased sensitivity to activation by Delta. *Fringe* mutation results in wing margin defects, similar to the wing abnormalities observed in *Notch* fly stocks. Moreover, abnormal juxtaposition of *fringe*+ and *fringe*- cells results in formation and outgrowth of ectopic wing margins at the sight of abnormal *fringe* expression boundaries.

Fringe-modulated Notch activation at the dorsal/ventral boundary results from a combination of compartment-restricted ligand expression and fringe modulation of Notch's ligand sensitivity. While Notch is expressed in both dorsal and ventral cells, *delta* and *serrate* show restricted expression. In the dorsal wing field, *fringe* is expressed with *serrate*, while the ventral field lacks *fringe* and *serrate* but expresses *delta*. As a result, dorsal cells can send effective serrate-mediated signals across the boundary to activate Notch signaling in ventral boundary cells, without activating their *fringe*-expressing dorsal neighbors. Activated Notch induces up-regulated *delta* expression in ventral boundary cells, and these cells can send effective *delta*-mediated signals across the boundary to activate dorsal cells. As a result, Notch is activated in a discrete band of cells on both sides of the dorsal/ventral boundary, with reciprocal signaling resulting in a self-reinforcing positive feedback loop (Irvine,1997). While the precise mechanism by which inactivation of this system results in the notched wing phenotype is unknown, it has been suggested that absence of strong Notch signals in boundary cells alters their survival, proliferative capacity or adhesive properties, leading to cell dropout and margin defects (de Celis,1994).

Three vertebrate orthologs of *fringe* have been described, *manic*, *radical,* and *lunatic Fringe*. In a manner entirely analogous to the role of *fringe* in *Drosophila* wing disc development, *radical fringe* appears to position the apical ectodermal ridge at the dorsal/ventral boundary of the vertebrate limb bud (reviewed in Irvine,1997). In addition to limb patterning, Fringe-modulated Notch signaling is known play a critical role in boundary formation during vertebrate somite formation. Defective somitogenesis is observed in mice bearing knockout mutations in *Notch1, Dll1, RBP-Jκ, presenilin-1, and lunatic fringe* (reviewed in Jiang,1998). During development, vertebrate somites are generated by alternating cohesion and dispersion of cells within the presomitic mesoderm, resulting in a regular pattern of somites and clefts on each side of the midline. Beginning on day E8.0 in the mouse, somites begin to form in a rostral-to-caudal direction at a rate of approximately one somite pair every two hours, until the process is completed on ~E14 with a total of >60 somite pairs. Because of the temporal periodicity with which somites form, it has long been speculated that somite formation might be regulated by patterns of oscillating gene expression in presomitic mesoderm. It now appears that this oscillator involves waves of lunatic Fringe-modulated Notch signaling.

Thus Notch signaling plays critical roles in a diverse array of developmental processes involving lateral inhibition, lineage specification and boundary formation. In the context of the embryo, these influences often involve undifferentiated precursor cells. In light of the growing recognition of multipotent stem cell populations in adult tissues, it is not surprising that Notch also acts as an important regulator of stem cell behavior in the adult.

4. ROLE OF NOTCH IN STEM CELL BIOLOGY

Notch mechanisms in normal stem cells are germane to cancer pathogenesis. Tissue injury frequently leads to the recruitment of multipotent precursor cells, in processes that may be susceptible to neoplastic transformation. By definition, stem cells can undergo asymmetric cell division, generating additional undifferentiated precursors as well as daughters capable of transient amplification and differentiation. In varying contexts, Notch signaling may sustain a progenitor in an uncommitted state or it may switch a cell between two potential differentiation outcomes. As is best illustrated in the role of Notch1 in mammalian hematopoietic differentiation, iterative repeats of Notch activation can guide precursor cells through a complex differentiation cascade, depending on inductive cues from the microenvironment. Notch ligands may be presented either by stromal cells, in the bone marrow, or by adjoining epithelial cells, as in the gut, for example. Advanced differentiation may require silencing of the Notch signal. Conversely, under appropriate conditions, constitutively active forms of Notch may contribute to inhibition of differentiation and alternatively, apoptosis or immortalization of the blocked precursor.

4.1 *Notch signaling in hematopoietic precursors*

The bone marrow is a paradigm for inductive Notch signaling, with a well-characterized requirement for Notch in precursor cell maintenance throughout fetal development and postnatal life. Hematopoietic cells also illustrate the oncogenic potential of constitutively active forms of Notch, which will be discussed in detail in a subsequent section, "Notch as an oncogene." Normal expression of Notch1 occurs throughout the marrow in primitive CD34^{+}lin^{-} hematopoietic stem cells (Milner,1994) Notch1 is also expressed in lymphoid and early erythroid and myeloid progenitor populations, consistent with a role in multiple stages of blood cell differentiation (Milner,1999). Adjoining bone marrow stromal cells express Notch ligands including Delta1 and 4 and Jagged1 (Karanu,2000;Karanu,2001;Li,1998). Notch signaling is also potentially involved in fetal erythropoiesis and granulopoiesis with expression of Jagged1 and Delta1 as early as E12 in the fetal mouse liver (Walker,2001) The essential role of Notch signaling in undifferentiated hematopoietic precursors has been illustrated in both gain-of-function and loss-of-function studies. Numerous gain-of-function studies point to the capacity of Notch1 to maintain and support primitive hematopoietic stem cells. For example, exposure of cultured murine CD34^{+}lin^{-} cells to an active form of Delta1 delays acquisition of differentiation markers, promotes expansion of the multipotent precursor population, and retards apoptosis (Han). Delta4 and Jagged1 have a comparable ability to sustain primitive precursor cells and induce limited growth in culture (Karanu2000;Karanu20001;Li,1998). Transplantation of marrow cultured in the presence of Jagged1 results in enhanced multi-lineage engraftment compared to marrow cultured in the absence of Notch ligand (Karanu,2000).

Compared to ligand-activated Notch signaling, NICD induces a much higher level of Notch activity. Stable expression of NICD in mouse bone marrow cells leads to inhibition of differentiation and precursor cell immortalization with cytokine-dependent growth. Under appropriate signals, NICD-expressing cells can assume early lymphoid or myeloid markers (Varnum-Finney,2000). However, these NICD-expressing precursors are unable to reconstitute the marrow of lethally-irradiated recipient mice, presumably due to a maturation blockade induced by Notch1 in several lineages. Loss-of-function studies to date suggest that there may be subtly different requirements for different Notch homologs in supporting different populations of hematopoietic precursors. Thus, marrow from mice bearing a conditional Notch1 gene deletion is unable to reconstitute T-cells in irradiated recipient animals, but contributes to normal development of other lineages (Radtke,1999).

Beyond the role of Notch signaling in supporting primitive, multipotent hematopoietic precursors, Notch has a well-characterized role in later stages of hematopoietic differentiation. In each of these iterative differentiation steps, Notch ligands presented by bone marrow or thymic stroma function inductively to activate Notch. Notch1 potently restricts myeloid development and favors generation of lymphoid precursors (Robson,2001). In the absence of Notch1, the common lymphoid precursor is shunted to a B-cell identity. Conversely, NICD over-expression or Notch ligand exposure in the thymus promotes a T-cell fate. Highly reminiscent of the Notch loss-of-function phenotype, *Hes1* -/- mice exhibit arrested thymic development at the early $CD4^-CD8^-$ double negative stage (Tomita,1999). Subsequent T-cell developmental choices are also strongly influenced by Notch, including TCR $\alpha\beta/\gamma\delta$ differentiation and CD4/CD8 lineage commitment (reviewed in Milner,1999). Recent studies using conditional knockouts of Notch1 suggest an absolute requirement for Notch1 in specification of early T-cell precursors but not in later T-cell differentiation where additional Notch family members could play a compensatory role (Wolfer,2001).

The downstream targets of Notch signaling relevant to hematopoietic stem cell maintenance have only recently been explored. Up-regulation of the transcription factor GATA-2 appears to be a necessary, but not sufficient, step in the inhibition of myeloid differentiation by Notch1 and Hes1 (Kumano,2001). Well-characterized targets of Notch in the inhibition of B-cell differentiation are the bHLH factors E12 and E47 which promote Ig gene transcription and B-cell differentiation. (Ordentlich,1998) Other critical targets of the Notch pathway in blood development remain to be identified. Manipulation of the Notch pathway in a controlled, conditional fashion is of considerable interest for clinical hematologists as a strategy to amplify and propagate bone marrow stem cell line (Brenner,2000). The consequences of unregulated Notch signaling in leukemogenesis are discussed later.

4.2 Notch signaling in CNS precursors

Although the adult brain had long been considered post-mitotic, there is now unquestioned evidence for the persistence of CNS stem cells far into post-natal life (Gage,2000). CNS stem cells are rare multipotent cells in the nervous system that may divide, with progeny giving rise to neurons, astrocytes and oligodendrocytes. Stem cell populations can be identified in the brain, spinal cord, and retina (Morrison,2001). For example, stem cells isolated from adult rodent hippocampal dentate gyrus can generate new hippocampal neurons and glia, or olfactory neurons depending on the site into which the cells are transplanted (reviewed in Gage,2000). Both Notch1 and Notch3 are expressed and apparently active in this region (Irvin,2001). A second important site of adult CNS stem cells, also expressing Notch genes, is the cortical subventricular zone (Doetsch,1999). A complex set of extrinsic factors appear to influence CNS stem cell differentiation including BMP's, sonic hedgehog, ephrins, FGF's EGF, neurotrophins, thyroid hormone, and other factors (see Morrison,2001 and Anderson,2001 for reviews). In concert with these extracellular cues, cell intrinsic proteins have a profound effect on CNS stem cell differentiation. bHLH transcription factors, such as Mash1 and Neurogenin1, activate the expression of a cascade of genes promoting neurogenesis and actively inhibiting glial differentiation. The Notch pathway, in turn, inhibits proneural bHLH factors, and causes CNS progenitors to adopt a glial fate. Through ligands such as Delta1, expressed in adjoining neurons, Notch may promote glial fate indirectly by down-regulating inhibitors of glial differentiation such as Neurogenin1 (Sun,2001).

Several studies to date suggest that the Notch pathway is involved in maintaining multi-potential CNS stem cells in an undifferentiated state, although the evidence is less clear-cut than for Notch promotion of gliogenesis. For example, the Notch target Hes1 appears to function as a repressor of neuronal commitment in CNS stem cells. Fetal brains from Hes1-/- mice exhibit premature neurogenesis in vivo, Cultured precursor cells from these brains exhibit a reduced ability to divide, survive, and to undergo multi-lineage differentiation (Nakamura,2000). Notch activation by ligand also appears to play a role in maintenance of multi-potential neuroepithelial cells in the fetal retina (Henrique1997). The association between Notch and glial development is provocative in light of unpublished data identifying Notch gene expression in glial-derived tumors such as astrocytoma, oligodendroglioma, and glioblastoma multiforme (Unpublished data from CGAP database). Although a comprehensive understanding of Notch function in CNS stem cell biology is several years away, it appears likely that Notch plays a major role in both maintenance of CNS stem cells as well as in promoting glial differentiation. The role of this pathway, if any, in CNS tumors is unknown.

4.3 Notch signaling in gut epithelial precursors

Although there is strong evidence for an essential role of the Notch pathway in controlling the development of foregut and midgut endoderm, relatively little is known about the contribution of Notch to the control of stem cell function and tissue renewal in the constantly regenerating gut epithelium. It is estimated that a normal adult intestinal colonic crypt contains approximately 4 to 6 stem cells with a larger number of proliferating daughter cells, located at the crypt base in the colon, and several cell diameters up from the crypt base in the small intestine (Booth,1999). There is currently a lack of markers to identify intestinal stem cells and their immediate progeny. Notch1, 2 and 3 and a variety of Notch ligands are expressed in gut epithelium(Jensen,2000). Using Hes1 expression as a marker of Notch signaling, this pathway specifically appears to be active in proliferating intestinal crypt cells, in both fetal and adult mice. In the Hes1-/- strain, the increase in enteroendocrine cells is associated with a decreased number of enterocytes, and a distortion of the normal villous architecture in late gestation. There is also an increase in apoptosis in the crypt regions in these mice (Jensen,2000). The specific identity of the Notch-expressing crypt cells is unclear, as is the contribution of Notch to normal gut renewal, the response to cytotoxic injuries, and the development of tumors in the gut.

5. THE NOTCH PATHWAY IN CANCER

At physiologic levels, normal ligand-activated Notch signaling functions as a discrete switch between two differentiation options. Conventionally, this switch is assumed to be transient, even though downstream events may lead to irreversible changes in cell fate. The Tan1 oncogene, in contrast, is a truncated, predominantly nuclear form of Notch, created as a spontaneous translocation event in T cell neoplasms, that acts in a sustained, cell-autonomous fashion. Subsequent studies have documented other translocation and gene insertion events, altered transcripts, overabundance, and inappropriate expression of Notch genes in a broad range of cancer cell types. Notch has been associated with a variety of pro-neoplastic consequences including cell cycle activation, apoptosis inhibition, and angiogenesis. Paradoxically, certain cancers depending heavily on bHLH factors in order to proliferate may exhibit an anti-mitogenic response to Notch signals. The following section reviews recent studies on the role of Notch in tumorigenesis and in regulating cancer cell phenotypes.

5.1 Notch as an Oncogene

The first definitive indication of a role for Notch in cancer etiology was the discovery in 1991 of Tan1, the product of a t(7;9)(q34;q34.3) chromosomal translocation in a small subset of human pre-T cell acute lymphoblastic leukemia (Ellisen,1991). The translocation juxtaposes DNA encoding the carboxyl-terminal half of Notch1 with the promoter of the T-cell receptor β locus. The resulting fusion gene leads to up-regulated transcription of an mRNA encoding a truncated Notch1 protein that is predominantly nuclear and constitutively active in the absence of ligand. The precise breakpoint occurs in the Notch1 extracellular region, within the proximal EGF repeat domain. Subsequent studies indicate that the Tan1 protein is constitutively cleaved by presenilin without any requirement for ligand-activated TACE. The specific manner in which activated Notch1 contributes to T cell transformation is unclear, although proliferative, anti-apoptotic, and anti-differentiation effects have been cited (see Aster,2001 for review).

An alternative activated form of Notch1 was recently detected in experimental mouse thymomas, resulting from MMTV insertional mutagenesis, together with c-myc overexpression (Hoemann,2000). In this Notch1 mutant, the extracellular and upstream intracellular domains are intact whereas a missense codon results in premature termination near the PEST degradation domain. Preliminary observations suggest that this alternative mutant Notch1 is ligand–dependent, but associated with enhanced protein stability, signaling and tumorigenesis.

The Notch2 gene has also been found to be the target of naturally occurring DNA alterations. In this instance, feline leukemia virus sequences encoding truncated versions of feline Notch2 have been recovered from cat thymic lymphomas. The predicted protein, like Tan1, is truncated, nuclear, and constitutively active (Rohn,1996). Notch3 genomic alterations have recently been reported in cases of non small cell lung cancer and are described below (Dang,2000). Notch4 genomic alterations are seen in a mouse mammary tumor model, the Int-3 insertion site for MMTV. Insertion of MMTV sequences at this locus results in generation of truncated and activated Notch4 proteins, analogous to Tan1 (Gallahan,1997). To date no occurrences of such Notch4 translocations have been documented in human breast cancer, however.

5.2 Transforming Activity of Notch Genes

In cultured mammalian epithelial cells, truncated intracellular forms of Notch 1 and 2 can have transforming activity. Immortalized baby rat kidney (RKE) cells undergo transformation by activated Notch proteins in cooperation with ras to form colonies in semisolid media and form tumors in nude mice (Capobianco,1997). Both nuclear localization and transcriptional activation appear essential for this transforming activity (Jeffries,2000) Similarly, transcriptional activation appears essential for NICD to induce leukemia in marrow cells (Aster,2000). The mechanisms whereby Notch proteins stimulate transforming activity and tumorigenesis are not at all clear, and are likely to be context-dependent. NICD over-expression in a graded fashion can lead to direct up-regulation of cyclin D1 transcription, and consequent increase in CDK2 activity and accelerated entry into S-phase (Ronchini,2001). Although cyclin D1 transcriptional activation by the NICD/CBF-1 heterodimer could be a potent growth promoter, this activity does not appear to be universal in cultured epithelial cells. Thus, in a keratinocyte model system, activated Notch1 has an anti-proliferative affect, mediating up-regulation of p21, inhibition of cyclin-dependent kinases and growth arrest (Rangarajan,2001a). Similarly in small cell lung cancer cells, Notch1 and Notch 2 cause growth arrest through activation of p21 and p27, with no effect on cyclin D1 (Sriuranpong,2001). A second potential mechanism for growth induction by Notch signaling is the potentiation of LEF1 transcriptional activity in a fashion mimicking beta-catenin and the Wnt signaling pathway (Ross,2001) The quantitative impact of Notch on LEF activity and the impact on critical proliferation-related genes is currently unknown, however.

5.3 Notch Regulation of Apoptosis

Several lines of evidence point to potential interactions between Notch signaling and pathways that regulate apoptosis. The emerging picture is that Notch regulation of apoptosis is complex, likely indirect, and context-dependent. Thus Notch can promote apoptosis of B-lymphocyte precursors while promoting survival of the T-cell lineage. Notch1 appears to specifically induce resistance to glucocorticoid-mediated T-cell death. This phenomenon has been reported both in normal maturing $CD4^{+}CD8^{+}$ T cells, as well as in thymic lymphoma cells (Deftos,1998). Instead of modulating glucorticoid signaling in a generic fashion, Notch1 appears to down-regulate a key component of the SWI/SNF chromatin remodeling complex, termed SRG3, which is involved in glucorticoid-mediated T cell apoptosis (Choi,2001). A second example of interaction of Notch with apotosis-related pathways was recently documented in immortalized cervical epithelial cells. Here, activated Notch1 leads to phosphorylation of AKT/Protein kinase B, and resistance to apoptosis upon matrix withdrawal, potentially via the anti-apoptotic actions of NF-kappaB (Rangarajan,2001b). Another interesting connection between Notch and NF-kappaB was described by Bellavia and colleagues (Bellavia,2000). In these studies, an activated form of Notch3, targeted to bone marrow in transgenic mice resulted in apoptosis-resistant T cell populations and T cell leukemia/lymphoma. Increased degradation of IkappaBα via IkappaKinaseα was implicated in this process.

The importance of cellular context in Notch regulation of apoptosis is illustrated in a number of developmental studies. Migrating neural crest precursors which natively express Notch1 can be induced to die in co-culture with Delta-1 expressing cells (Maynard,2000). Conceivably, the reliance of these cells on bHLH factors for differentiation, in analogy to B lymphocytes, could also impact on their reduced survival under strong Notch signaling (Morimura,2000). There is a need for more studies to understand the factors which regulate whether Notch signaling in a given context will be pro-apoptotic or anti-apoptotic. There are limited data to suggest that DNA damage and repair may also promote transduction of Notch signaling. In this instance, the p53-related proteins p73 and p63 (but not p53 itself) can actively induce transcription of the Notch ligands Jagged1 and Jagged2, leading to Hes1 up-regulation in Notch-expressing target cells (Sasaki,2002).

5.4 Notch and Angiogenesis

Vascular endothelial cells express both Notch proteins and ligands. Notch4 expression, for example, appears concentrated in the vasculature (Uyttendaele,2001). Notch4/Notch1 double mutants exhibit severe defects in angiogenic remodeling (Krebs,2000). Notch ligands including Jagged1(Loomes,1991), Delta1 (Beckers,1999) and Delta4 (Mailhos,2001) are frequently expressed in endothelial cells. Jagged1 and Delta1 homozygous mutant embryos die from vascular defects and hemorrhage (Xue,1999) Recently, Delta4 was demonstrated in the early cardiovascular system at sites of arterial growth. Normal adult vessels express very low levels of Delta4, except in areas of vascular proliferation such as the ovarian corpus luteum. Strikingly, Mailhos and colleagues detected high levels of Delta4 mRNA in endothelial cells from every tumor specimen they examined, and in mouse xenograft vessels, but not in surrounding normal tissues. Cultured human vascular endothelial cells produce Delta4 in response to hypoxia, but not in response to VEGF. Thus it appears that Notch signaling is critical to new arterial endothelial cells, perhaps in promoting branching angiogenesis in an inductive fashion. (Mailhos,2001). This function is clearly markedly induced in tumor angiogenesis. Potential interactions between hypoxemia inducible factors and Notch pathway components are a promising topic for study. A remarkable downstream target of Notch signaling in vessels is gridlock, the HES-family member also known as HERP1. The Notch-gridlock pathway functions to regulate the choice of arterial versus venous fate in primitive vessels, apparently by repressing venous fate signaled by the Ephb4 receptor (Zhong,2001). Thus Notch signaling plays a critical role in the development of primitive arteries, and is likely to be critical to tumor angiogenesis as well. Notch-stimulated angiogenesis, in the future, may be a useful therapeutic target in cancer.

5.5 Notch in Hematologic Malignancies

Since the initial discovery of Tan1, a number of groups have sought to characterize the leukemia-inducing properties of Notch proteins in animal model systems and in naturally occurring forms of the disease. It is now clear that over-expression of NICD in rodent bone marrow cells can lead to lymphoid neoplasms (Pear,1996). These neoplasms typically have an immature T-cell phenotype, as circulating leukemia and disseminated T-cell lymphoma. Similarly, activated Notch2 and Notch3 appear to have equivalent leukemia-producing potential (Rohn,1996;Bellavia,2000). Until recently, it was unclear whether persistent ligand-activated Notch signaling would be as potent as NICD in inducing transformation of T-cell precursors. Remarkably, transplantation of Delta4 expressing marrow into lethally- irradiated hosts produces a leukemic phenotype as well. This phenotype is characterized by T-cell lymphoproliferative disease in bone marrow and lymphoid tissues, as well as transplantable monoclonal T-cell leukemia/lymphoma scattered to multiple organs (Yan,2001). As Delta4 is normally highly expressed in the subcapsular cortical region of the thymus, in which immature thymocytes express high levels of Notch1, it's likely that the Notch pathway actively promotes growth and/or retards apoptosis in primitive T-cells (Yan,2001) Thus, rodent model systems indicate that both activated Notch proteins and over-expression of Notch ligands have the potential to initiate primitive T-cell neoplasms. Beyond the rare instances of Tan1-associated T-ALL, there is fairly limited evidence for Notch involvement in naturally-occurring hematologic malignancies in humans. Unpublished data from the Cancer Genome Anatomy Project indicates frequent expression on Notch1 in CLL-derived libraries, as well as in normal marrow and thymus. Although there is evidence for widespread expression of Notch proteins and ligands in AML, the significance of this finding is presently unclear (Tohda,2001)

5.6 Notch in Epithelial Cancers

5.6.1 Cervical Cancer

Although Notch gene alterations have not yet been detected in human cervical cancers, Notch ligands and Notch proteins are known to be expressed in these tumors. In the normal cervix, Notch1, Notch2 Delta-1, Jagged-1 and Jagged-2 are all restricted to the stratum spinosum, a region of proliferating squamous cell precursors (Gray,1999) Such cells are believed to be potential targets for neoplastic transformation. Both *in situ* and invasive cervical adenocarcinoma, and invasive cervical squamous carcinoma appear to express Notch proteins and ligands, frequently at high levels (Gray,1999;Zagouras,1995). Established cervical carcinoma cell lines show a marked increase in growth following over-expression of activated forms of Notch1 (Rangarajan,2001b). A potential pathogenic mechanism for Notch in cervical cancer has recently been identified by Rangarajan and colleagues. Notch1 appears to compliment human papilloma virus E6 and E7 oncogenes, potentially via activation of PI-3kinase and AKT/Protein kinase B. In this setting, Notch signaling appears capable of substituting for activation of the ras pathway.

The combined action of Notch1 and HPV proteins prevented an apoptotic response induced by matrix withdrawal in immortalized cervical epithelial cells. Thus, Notch signaling is a fascinating, though unproven possibility as a cooperating stimulus to virally-induced carcinogenesis of the cervix.

5.6.2 Lung Cancer

In a striking parallel to pancreatic development reviewed earlier in this chapter, Notch signaling also mediates developmental choices between neuroendocrine and non-endocrine epithelial cells in the lung (Ito,2000). An implied assumption in this model is the existence of a common precursor cell population for both endocrine and non-endocrine airway cells. The bHLH transcription factor hASH1/Mash1 is essential for neuroendocrine differentiation in the lung and a hallmark of lung cancers with neuroendocrine features, especially small cell lung cancer (Borges,1997). In contrast, Notch1, Notch3 and Hes1 are expressed in non-endocrine airway cells. A transgenic knockout of *Hes1* is associated with premature and ectopic neuroendocrine differentiation (Ito,2000). Unlike small cell tumors, typical non small cell lung cancer (NSCLC) lacks NE features and hASH1 and exhibits evidence of Notch pathway activation (Chen,1997). Dang and colleagues recently identified Notch3 gene expression in a significant percentage of NSCLC, predominantly adenocarcinomas (Dang,2000). Interestingly, they uncovered a t(15;19) balanced translocation in the tumor DNA of a patient with aggressive NSCLC. The resulting translocation mapped to the 50 kb upstream of the Notch3 gene. In a number of cell lines, chromosome 19 translocation events appeared to correlate with over-expression of wild-type Notch3 transcripts, though the precise association between chromosome 19 events, Notch3 expression and the NSCLC phenotype remains uncertain. Sriuranpong and colleagues explored the consequences of activated Notch1 and Notch2 in small cell lung cancer cells which normally lack significant Notch signaling and utilize hASH1 (Sriuranpong,2001) In these cells, activated Notch1 and Notch2 both induced a growth arrest phenotype, associated with p21 and p27 induction. Notch action in small cell lung cancer led to a rapid loss of hASH1 expression. Surprisingly, hASH1 was silenced both at the level of transcription, and in rapid induction of proteasomal degradation (Sriuanpong,2002). Thus, a competition between bHLH factors and Notch proteins plays an important role in lung development (Ito,2001), reminiscent of previously cited examples in nervous system, lymphocyte, and gut development. The phenotype of lung cancer cells appears to recapitulate this developmental theme, opening the possibility that maneuvers to derail Notch or bHLH signaling may induce arrest or apoptosis of cancers directed in either differentiation pathway. Potential strategies to target Notch signaling are discussed in the concluding section below.

5.6.3 Breast Cancer

Expression of all four of the Notch genes can be detected in mammary glands (Callahan,2001). As described above, the *Notch4* locus is a target for activation by MMTV insertional mutagenesis in mice. The Notch4 intracellular fragment encoded by this mutation confers anchorage-independent growth in soft agar in cultured HC11 mouse mammary epithelial cells (Robbins,1992). In addition, the Notch4 intracellular fragment inhibits the capability of the TAC-2 mammary eptihelial cell line to undergo branching morphogenesis (Uyttendaele,2001). Thus integration of MMTV sequences into exons 21, 22, or 23 of the mouse *Notch4* gene produces a gain-of-function mutation (Gallahan,1997). Based on the role of Notch 4 in mouse model mammary tumors, there has been interest in detecting abnormal Notch activity in human breast tumors as well. Imatani and Callahan detected an abnormal 1.8 Kb Notch4 mRNA species in a subset of human breast cancer cell lines compared to the 6.5 Kb species in normal human tissues. (The shorter 1.8 Kb transcript could be seen in normal testis, possibly in germ cells, and in some colon cancer lines, as well). This variant Notch4 transcript encodes a predicted protein including intracellular portions beginning within the ankyrin repeat region, but lacking the transmembrane and extracellular domains. The truncated form of Notch 4 promotes MCF-10A mammary epithelial cells to grow in soft agar (Imatani,2000). Although this variant Notch4 lacks the RAM interaction domain and part of the ankyrin repeat, it might still be predicted to have constitutive activity. It is currently unclear whether this truncated form of Notch4 would have the full transforming activity of the Notch1 intracellular form seen in the Tan1 oncogene. Further studies are needed to determine the frequency and significance of these naturally-occurring altered Notch gene products in breast cancer and other tumors.

Data from cell lines derived from mouse Notch4/Int-3 tumors further underline the association between Notch signaling and the ras pathway, also noted in cervical cancer. Notch4 -activated mammary tumor cell lines exhibit activation of both ERK1 and 2 and P-I-3 kinase, two arms of the ras pathway (Fitzgerald,2000). It is not known whether independent ras gene mutations occur in these tumors. Thus it is possible that ras pathway activation is a cooperating event that is selected for in Notch-initiated tumorigenesis. Alternatively, activation of the ERK1 and 2 can be seen acutely in response to activated Notch1 and Notch2 in small cell lung cancer, (Sriuranpong,2001) suggesting that direct activation of the ras pathway might also play a role in these Notch-induced tumors.

A novel modulator of Notch signaling activity, SEL1L, has recently been implicated as having a potential role in breast cancer (Orlandi,2002) SEL1L is the human ortholog of the *C. elegans Sel-1* gene, a cytoplasmic protein implicated as a possible repressor of Notch signaling. SEL1L is expressed in normal mammary epithelium, but is variably lost in breast cancers. Reduced or absent SEL1L expression predicted a poor outcome amongst 117 patients with breast cancer, in univariate analysis. Re-introduction of SEL1L into MCF7 cells caused loss of anchorage-independent growth. The importance of SEL1L as a potential tumor suppressor protein in breast cancer and other adenocarcinomas, and the significance of its relationship to Notch in this process remain under investigation.

6. NOTCH AS A TARGET IN CANCER THERAPY

A core strategy of many traditional and investigational cancer therapies, including cytotoxic chemotherapy, radiation, and some hormonal and biologically-based treatments, is the induction of apoptosis in cancer cells. Therapeutic approaches that inhibit Notch action could potentially increase the susceptibility to apoptosis, at least in a subset of Notch-expressing tumor cells (Jang,2000). In addition, Notch-directed therapies could potentially induce tumor necrosis if it can be shown that inhibitors of this pathway block induction of new tumor-associated blood vessels. Predictions of the utility of Notch-directed therapy are based largely on studies in development and Notch gain-of-function experiments in hematologic malignancies, and to a much lesser extent on Notch loss-of-function experiments in any cancer. The critical preclinical experiments to assess the impact of Notch inhibition in model malignancies have not yet been reported. Ideally, candidate inhibitors should have defined activity against wild-type and activated fragments of Notch proteins. Based on limited data on the biochemical similarity of the four human Notch proteins, small molecule inhibitors may not distinguish between Notch1-4. To evaluate the activity and specificity of candidate Notch inhibitors, it will be important to validate intermediate endpoints of Notch function, such as Hes1 and HERP1 expression (Iso,2001). The potential of other signaling pathways, such as ras, to compensate for a loss of Notch signaling has not yet been adequately investigated.

A variety of strategies have been envisioned to inhibit Notch signaling in cancer. Currently, the two best-developed approaches are γ-secretase inhibitors, targeting the final stage in Notch activation, and "decoy" ligand binding antagonists. Other approaches currently under investigation include monoclonal antibodies to Notch1 (Jang,2000;Zlobin,2000), antisense approaches (Garces,1997), and utilization of physiologic Notch modulators, such as the Fringe proteins (Ju,2000;Jang,2000). Effective systemic inhibition of one or more Notch proteins could be predicted to have a number of potential side effects. One likely consequence is transient abnormalities in cellular immunity, based on the essential role of Notch1 in early T-cell commitment and the importance of the Notch family as a whole in T-cell maturation and survival. A profound loss of Notch function would be likely to affect differentiation processes in a number of regenerating tissues, especially the bone marrow, gut and skin. In these settings, depletion of stem cell populations by Notch inhibition could be associated with significant organ toxicity.

6.1 Gamma-secretase inhibitors

As described above, activating intra-membrane cleavage of Notch requires the proteolytic activity of γ-secretase/presenilin-1 (DeStrooper,1999;Fortini,2001). Notably, this enzyme is also responsible for proteolytic production of β-amyloid from amyloid precursor protein (APP), currently felt to represent an initiating event in Alzheimer's disease. Significant interest exists in the development of pharmacologic inhibitors of γ-secretase as therapeutic agents in the treatment and prevention of Alzheimer's Disease. In fact, several of these compounds have completed successful preclinical evaluation and are now being evaluated in phase I clinical trials (Molinoff,2000). With respect to use of these compounds to inhibit cleavage of APP in Alzheimer's patients, associated inhibition of Notch signaling might result in undesired toxicity. However, the ability of available γ-secretase inhibitors to block Notch activation may have desirable effects in the therapy and/or chemoprevention of Notch-associated malignancy.

A variety of pharmacologic γ-secretase inhibitors have been evaluated. One series of inhibitors involves diflouro-ketone peptide analogues designed to mimic the APP peptide domain cleaved by γ-secretase (Wolfe,1999). These compounds have been shown to inhibit γ-secretase-mediated cleavage of both APP and Notch-1, with no apparent effect on either α-secretase or β-secretase activity. Other classes of compounds include non-peptide sulfonamides (Rishton,2000), hydroxyethylene dipeptide transition state analogues (Shearman,2000), and N-arylalanine ester derivatives (Dovey,2001). Although studies suggest that the relative effectiveness of γ-secretase in mediating cleavage of APP versus Notch may be genetically dissociated (Song,1999;Kulic,2000), *in vitro* studies with diflouro-ketone peptide analogues suggest similar IC50's for γ-secretase-mediated cleavage of both APP and Notch. While much of the work characterizing these compounds has been conducted in cell culture systems, two recent reports suggest that γ-secretase inhibition is effective in intact tissues. In mouse embryonic thymus explants, diflouro-ketone peptide analogues dramatically inhibit progression of immature lymphocytes from a CD4-/CD8- population to a double positive CD4+/CD8+ population (Hadland,2001). In addition, γ-secretase inhibition results in accumulation of CD4 single-positive cells at the expense of CD8 single positive cells, consistent with down-regulation of Notch signaling. Similarly, a compound known as DAPT (N-[N-(3,5-difluorophenacetyl)-L-alanyl]-S-phenylglycine t-butyl ester) has been shown to rapidly accumulate in brain following oral administration, and reduce APP cleavage in transgenic mice expressing a pathogenic variant of human APP (Dovey,2001).

6.2 Ligand based approaches to Notch inhibition

The EGF-like repeats in the Notch extracellular ligand-binding domain are a broadly conserved motif in several important proteins. However the apparent specificity of ligand interactions with individual EGF repeats within Notch proteins, and the ability to ablate Notch function with targeted mutations of these repeats has fueled the development of reagents targeting this interaction. Garces, and colleagues reported that a soluble recombinant protein mimicking EGF repeats 11 and 12 of Notch1 could inhibit Notch1 action, presumably by sequestering Notch ligands in a "decoy" fashion. A polyclonal antiserum directed against these repeats led to similar inhibition of Notch action. Significantly, the Notch activity readout in this study was adipocyte differentiation (Garces,1997), rather than a cancer-related outcome. It is difficult evaluate the specificity of these approaches directed at Notch EGF repeats. The use of extracellular decoy molecules to bind and sequester Notch ligands is a potentially attractive approach to Notch-based therapy, however.

7. SUMMARY AND PERSPECTIVES

Impressive progress has been made in understanding Notch molecular mechanisms, Notch activities in development and in stem cell biology. These studies, and data from model malignancies of the blood, and several epithelial tissues such as breast and cervix, suggest that Notch molecules may play an important role in tumor formation and progression. Studies of Notch action in naturally-occurring cancers are lagging however. There is a need for more in-depth analyses of human cancers to detect the hallmarks of active Notch signaling and then determine the benefit (as well as risks) of utilizing the promising tools under development to inhibit or regulate this pathway. Clearly the Notch pathway is a rational and promising target for drug design in the treatment of several forms of human cancer.

Douglas W. Ball
Department of Medicine and the Sidney Kimmel Cancer Center
Johns Hopkins University School of Medicine

Steven D. Leach
Department of Surgery and the Sidney Kimmel Cancer Center
Johns Hopkins University School of Medicine

8. ACKNOWLEDGEMENTS

Supported in part by RO1CA70244 (DWB) and RO1DK61215 (SDL).

9. REFERENCES

Apelqvist, A., Li, H., Sommer, L., Beatus, P., Anderson, D.J., Honjo, T, Hrabe de Angelis, M., Lendahl, U., Edlund, H. (1999) Notch signalling controls pancreatic cell differentiation. Nature, 400:877-881.

Anderson, D.J. (2001) Stem cells and pattern formation in the nervous system: the possible versus the actual. Neuron, 30:19-35.

Aster, J.C., & Pear, W.S. (2001) Notch signaling in leukemia. Curr Opin Hematol, 8:237-244.

Aster, J.C., Xu L., Karnell, F.G., Patriub, V., Pui, J.C., Pear, W.S. (2000) Essential roles for ankyrin repeat and transactivation domains in induction of T-cell leukemia by notch1. Mol Cell Biol, 20:7505-7515.

Beckers, J., Clark, A., Wunsch, K., Hrabe De Angelis, M., Gossler, A. (1999) Expression of the mouse Delta1 gene during organogenesis and fetal development. Mech Dev 84:165-168.

Bellavia, D., Campese, A.F., Alesse, E., et al.(2000) Constitutive activation of NF-kappaB and T-cell leukemia/lymphoma in Notch3 transgenic mice. EMBO J, 19:3337-3348.

Berechid, B.E., Kitzmann, M., Foltz, D.R., Roach, A.H., Seiffert, D., Thompson, L.A., Olson, R.E., Bernstein, A., Donoviel, D.B., Nye, J.S. (2002) Identification and Characterization of Presenilin-Independent Notch Signaling. J Biol Chem, in press.

Blaumueller, C.M., Qi, H., Zagouras, P., Artavanis-Tsakonas, S. (1997) Intracellular cleavage of Notch leads to a heterodimeric receptor on the plasma membrane. Cell, 90:281-291.

Booth, C., O'Shea, J.A., Potten, C.S. (1999) Maintenance of functional stem cells in isolated and cultured adult intestinal epithelium. Exp Cell Res, 249:359-366.

Borges, M., Linnoila, R.I., van de Velde, H.J., Chen, H., Nelkin, B.D., Mabry, M., Baylin, S.B., Ball, D.W. (1997) An achaete-scute homologue essential for neuroendocrine differentiation in the lung. Nature, 386:852-855.

Bray, S. (1998) Notch signalling in Drosophila: three ways to use a pathway. Sem. Cell Devel. Biol., 9:591-597.

Brenner, M. (2000) To be or notch to be. Nature Medicine, 6:1210-1211.

Brou, C., Logeat, F., Gupta, N., Bessia, C., LeBail, O., Doedens, J.R., Cumano, A., Roux, P., Black, R.A., Israel, A. (2000) A novel proteolytic cleavage involved in Notch signaling: the role of the disintegrin-metalloprotease TACE. Mol Cell 5:207-216.

Callahan, R., & Raafat, A. (2001) Notch signaling in mammary gland tumorigenesis. J Mammary Gland Biol Neoplasia, 6:23-36.

Capobianco, A.J., Zagouras, P., Blaumueller, C.M., Artavanis-Tsakonas, S., Bishop, J.M. (1997) Neoplastic transformation by truncated alleles of human NOTCH1/TAN1 and NOTCH2. Mol. Cell. Biol., 17:6265-6273.

Chen, H., Thiagalingam, A., Chopra, H., Borges, M.W., Feder, J.N., Nelkin, B.D., Baylin, S.B., Ball, D.W. (1997) Conservation of the Drosophila lateral inhibition pathway in human lung cancer: a hairy-related protein (HES-1) directly represses achaete-scute homolog-1 expression. Proc Natl Acad Sci U S A, 94:5355-5360.

Chen, J., Moloney, D.J., Stanley, P.(2001) Fringe modulation of Jagged1-induced Notch signaling requires the action of beta 4galactosyltransferase-1. Proc Natl Acad Sci U S A., 98:13716-21.

Choi, Y.I., Jeon, S.H., Jang, J., Han, S., Kim, J.K., Chung, H., Lee, H.W., Chung, H.Y., Park, S.D., Seong, R.H. (2001) Notch1 confers a resistance to glucocorticoid-induced apoptosis on developing thymocytes by down-regulating SRG3 expression. Proc Natl Acad Sci U S A, 98:10267-10272.

Dang, T.P., Gazdar, A.F., Virmani, A.K., Sepetavec, T., Hande, K.R., Minna, J.D., Roberts, J.R., Carbone, D.P. (2000) Chromosome 19 translocation, overexpression of Notch3, and human lung cancer. J Natl Cancer Inst, 92:1355-1357.

De Celis, J.F., Garcia-Bellido, A. (1994) Roles of the Notch gene in Drosophila wing morphogenesis. Mech. Devel., 46:109-122.

De Strooper, B., Annaert, W., Cupers, P., Saftig, P., Craessaerts, K., Mumm, J.S., Schroeter, E.H., Schrijvers, V., Wolfe, M.S., Ray, W.J., Goate, A., Kopan, R. (1999) A presenilin-1-dependent gamma-secretase-like protease mediates release of Notch intracellular domain. Nature, 398:518-522.

Deftos, M.L., He, Y.W., Ojala, E.W., Bevan, M.J. (1998) Correlating notch signaling with thymocyte maturation. Immunity, 9:777-786.

de la Pompa, J.L., Wakeham, A., Correia, K.M., et al. (1997) Development, 124:1139-1148.

Dexter JS. (1914) The analysis of a case of continuous variation in Drosophila by a study of its linkage relations. Am. Naturalist, 48:712-758.

Doetsch, F., Caille, I., Lim, D.A., Garcia-Verdugo, J.M., Alvarez-Buylla, A. (1999) Subventricular zone astrocytes are neural stem cells in the adult mammalian brain. Cell, 97:703-16.

Dovey, H.F., John, V., Anderson, J.P., et al. (2001) Functional gamma-secretase inhibitors reduce beta-amyloid peptide levels in brain. J. Neurochem., 76:173-181.

Ellisen, L.W., Bird, J., West, D.C., et al. (1991) TAN-1, the human homolog of the Drosophila notch gene, is broken by chromosomal translocations in T lymphoblastic neoplasms. Cell 66:649-661.

Fisher, A., & Caudy, M. (1998) The function of hairy-related bHLH repressor proteins in cell fate decisions. Bioessays, 20:298-306.

Fitzgerald, K., Harrington, A., Leder, P. (2000) Ras pathway signals are required for notch-mediated oncogenesis. Oncogene, 19:4191-4198.

Fode, C., Gradwohl, G.,Morin, X., Dierich, A., LeMeur, M., Goridis, C., Guillemot. F. (1998) The bHLH protein NEUROGENIN 2 is a determination factor for epibranchial placode-derived sensory neurons. Neuron, 20: 483-494.

Fortini, M.E. (2001) Notch and presenilin: a proteolytic mechanism emerges. Curr. Opin. Cell Biol., 13:627-634.

Gage, F.H. (2000) Mammalian neural stem cells. Science, 287:1433-1438.

Gallahan, D., & Callahan, R. (1997) The mouse mammary tumor associated gene INT3 is a unique member of the NOTCH gene family (NOTCH4). Oncogene 14:1883-1890.

Garces, C., Ruiz-Hidalgo, M.J., de Mora, J.F., Park, C., Miele, L., Goldstein, J., Bonvini, E., Porras, A., Laborda, J. (1997) Notch-1 controls the expression of fatty acid-activated transcription factors and is required for adipogenesis. J Biol Chem 272:29729-29734.

Gray, G.E., Mann, R.S., Mitsiadis, E, Henrique, D., Carcangiu, M.L., Banks, A., Leiman, J., Ward, D., Ish-Horowitz, D., Artavanis-Tsakonas, S. (1999) Human ligands of the Notch receptor. Am J Pathol, 154:785-794.

Hadland, B.K., Manley, N.R., Su, D., Longmore, G.D., Moore, C.L., Wolfe, M.S., Schroeter, E.H., Kopan, R. (2001) Gamma -secretase inhibitors repress thymocyte development. Proc. Natl. Acad. Sci., 98:7487-7491.

Han, W., Ye, Q., Moore, M.A. (2000) A soluble form of human Delta-like-1 inhibits differentiation of hematopoietic progenitor cells. Blood, 95:1616-1625.

Henrique, D., Hirsinger, E., Adam, J., Le Roux, I., Pourquie, O., Ish-Horowicz, D., Lewis, J. Maintenance of neuroepithelial progenitor cells by Delta-Notch signalling in the embryonic chick retina. (1997) Curr Biol, 7:661-670.

Hoemann, C.D., Beaulieu, N., Girard, L., Rebai, N., Jolicoeur, P. (2000) Two distinct Notch1 mutant alleles are involved in the induction of T-cell leukemia in c-myc transgenic mice. Mol Cell Biol, 20:3831-3842.

Hrabe de Angelis, M., McIntyre, J., Achim, G. (1997) Maintenance of somite borders in mice requires the Delta homologue Dll1. Nature, 386:717-721.

Imatani, A., & Callahan, R. (2000) Identification of a novel NOTCH-4/INT-3 RNA species encoding an activated gene product in certain human tumor cell lines. Oncogene, 19:223-231.

Irvin, D.K., Zurcher, S.D., Nguyen, T., Weinmaster, G., Kornblum, H.I. (2001) Expression patterns of Notch1, Notch2, and Notch3 suggest multiple functional roles for the Notch-DSL signaling system during brain development. J Comp Neurol, 436:167-181.

Irvine, K.D., & Vogt ,T.R. (1997) Dorsal-ventral signaling in limb development. Curr Opin Cell Biol, 9:867-876.

Ishibashi, M., Ang, S.-L., Shiota, K., Nakanishi, S., Kageyama, R., Guillemot, F. (1995)Targeted disruption of mammalian hairy and Enhancer of split homolog-1 (HES-1) leads to up-regulation of neural helix-loop-helix factors, premature neurogenesis, and severe neural tube defects. Genes & Dev, 9:3136-3148.

Iso, T., Sartorelli, V., Poizat, C., Iezzi, S., Wu, H.Y., Chung, G., Kedes, L., Hamamori, Y. (2001) HERP, a novel heterodimer partner of HES/E(spl) in Notch signaling. Mol Cell Biol 21:6080-6089.

Ito, T., Udaka, N., Ikeda, M., Yazawa, T., Kageyama, R., Kitamura, H. (2001) Significance of proneural basic helix-loop-helix transcription factors in neuroendocrine differentiation of fetal lung epithelial cells and lung carcinoma cells. Histol Histopathol, 16:335-343.

Ito, T., Udaka, N., Yazawa, T., et al. (2000) Basic helix-loop-helix transcription factors regulate the neuroendocrine differentiation of fetal mouse pulmonary epithelium. Development,127: 3913-3921.

Jang, M., Zlobin, A., Kast, W.M., Miele, L. (2000) Notch signaling as a target in multimodality cancer therapy. Curr Opin in Mol Therapeutics, 2:55-65.

Jeffries, S., & Capobianco, A.J. (2000) Neoplastic transformation by Notch requires nuclear localization. Mol Cell Biol, 20:3928-3941.

Jensen, J., Pedersen, E.E., Galante, P., et al. (2000) Control of endodermal endocrine development by Hes-1. Nature Genetics, 24: 36-43.

Jiang, Y.J., Smiters, L., Lewis, J. (1998) Vertebrate segmentation: the clock is linked to Notch signaling. Current Biol., 8:R868-R871.

Ju, B.G., Jeong, S., Bae, E., Hyun, S., Carroll, S.B., Yim, J., Kim, J. (2000) Fringe forms a complex with Notch. Nature, 405:191-195.

Karanu, F.N., Murdoch, B., Gallacher, L., Wu, D.M., Koremoto, M., Sakano, S., Bhatia, M. (2000) The notch ligand jagged-1 represents a novel growth factor of human hematopoietic stem cells. J Exp Med, 192:1365-1372.

Karanu, F.N., Murdoch, B., Miyabayashi, T., Ohno, M., Koremoto, M., Gallacher, L., Wu, D., Itoh, A., Sakano, S., Bhatia, M. (2001) Human homologues of Delta-1 and Delta-4 function as mitogenic regulators of primitive human hematopoietic cells. Blood, 97:1960-1967.

Krebs, L.T., Xue, Y., Norton, C.R., et al. (2000) Notch signaling is essential for vascular morphogenesis in mice. Genes Dev 14:1343-1352.

Kulic, L., Walter, J., Multhaup, G., et al. (2000) Separation of presenilin function in amyloid beta-peptide generation and endoproteolysis of Notch. Proc. Natl. Acad. Sci., 97:5913-5918.

Kumano, K., Chiba, S., Shimizu, K., Yamagata, T., Hosoya, N., Saito, T., Takahashi,T., Hamada, Y., Hirai, H. (2001) Notch1 inhibits differentiation of hematopoietic cells by sustaining GATA-2 expression. Blood, 98:3283-3289.

Li, L., Milner, L.A., Deng, Y., Iwata, M., Banta, A, Graf, L., Marcovina, S, Friedman, C., Trask, B.J., Hood, L., Torok-Storb, B. (1998) The human homolog of rat Jagged1 expressed by marrow stroma inhibits differentiation of 32D cells through interaction with Notch1. Immunity, 8:43-55.

Loomes, K.M., Underkoffler, L.A., Morabito, J., Gottlieb, S., Piccoli, D.A., Spinner, N.B., Baldwin, H.S., Oakey, R.J. (1999) The expression of Jagged1 in the developing mammalian heart correlates with cardiovascular disease in Alagille syndrome. Hum Mol Genet, 8:2443-2449.

Lutolf, S., Radtke, F., Aguet, M., Suter, U., Taylor, V. (2002) Notch1 is required for neuronal and glial differentiation in the cerebellum. Development 129:373-385.

Lyman, D.F., & Yedvobnick B. (1995) Drosophila Notch receptor activity suppresses Hairless function during adult external sensory organ development. Genetics, 141:1491-1505.

Ma, Q., Chen, Z., del Barco Barrantes, I., de la Pompa, J.L., Anderson DJ. (1998) Neurogenin 1 is essential for the determination of neuronal precursors for proximal cranial sensory ganglia. Neuron, 20: 469-482.

Mailhos, C., Modlich, U., Lewis, J., Harris, A., Bicknell, R., Ish-Horowicz, D. (2001) Delta4, an endothelial specific notch ligand expressed at sites of physiological and tumor angiogenesis. Differentiation 69:135-144.

Maynard, T.M., Wakamatsu, Y., Weston, J.A. (2000) Cell interactions within nascent neural crest cell populations transiently promote death of neurogenic precursors. Development, 127:4561-4572.

Milner, L.A., & Bigas, A. (1999) Notch as a mediator of cell fate determination in hematopoiesis: evidence and speculation. Blood, 93:2431-2448.
Milner, L.A., Kopan, R., Martin, D.I., Bernstein, I.D. (1994) A human homologue of the Drosophila developmental gene, Notch, is expressed in CD34+ hematopoietic precursors. Blood, 83:2057-2062.
Miyata, T., Maeda, T., Lee, J.E. (1999) NeuroD is required for differentiation of the granule cells in the cerebellum and hippocampus. Genes Devel, 13:1647-1652.
Molinoff, P. B., Felsenstein, K. M., Smith, D. W., Barten, D. M. (2000) A modulation: The next generation of AD therapeutics (World Alzheimer's Congress 2000, Washington, DC, July 9-13, 2000), abstr. no. 615.
Morimura, T, Goitsuka, R., Zhang, Y., Saito, I., Reth, M., Kitamura, D. (2000) Cell cycle arrest and apoptosis induced by Notch1 in B cells. J Biol Chem, 275:36523-36531.
Morrison, S.J. (2001) Neuronal potential and lineage determination by neural stem cells. Curr Opin Cell Biol, 13:666-672.
Mumm, J.S., & Kopan, R. (2000) Notch signaling: from the outside in. Dev Biol, 228:151-165.
Nakamura, Y., Sakakibara, S., Miyata, T., Ogawa, M., Shimazaki,T., Weiss, S., Kageyama, R., Okano, H. (2000) The bHLH gene hes1 as a repressor of the neuronal commitment of CNS stem cells. J Neurosci, 20:283-293.
Newman, A.P., & Sternberg, P.W. (1996) Coordinated morphogenesis of epithelia during development of the Caenorhabditis elegans uterine-vulval connection. Proc. Natl. Acad. Sci USA, 93: 9329-9333.
Ordentlich, P., Lin, A., Shen, C.P., Blaumueller, C., Matsuno, K., Artavanis-Tsakonas, S., Kadesch T. (1998) Notch inhibition of E47 supports the existence of a novel signaling pathway. Mol Cell Biol, 18:2230-2239.
Orlandi, R., Cattaneo, M., Troglio, F., Casalini, P, Ronchini, C., Menard, S., Biunno, I. (2002) SEL1L Expression Decreases Breast Tumor Cell Aggressiveness in Vivo and in Vitro. Cancer Res, 62:567-574.
Oswald, F., Tauber, B., Dobner, T., Bourteele, S., Kostezka, U., Adler, G., Liptay, S., Schmid, R.M. (2001) p300 acts as a transcriptional coactivator for mammalian Notch-1. Mol Cell Biol, 21:7761-7774.
Parks, A.L., Klueg, K.M., Stout, J.R., Muskavitch, MA. (2000) Ligand endocytosis drives receptor dissociation and activation in the Notch pathway. Development, 127:1373-1385.
Pear, W.S., Aster, J.C., Scott, M.L., Hasserjian, R.P., Soffer, B., Sklar, J., Baltimore, D. (1996) Exclusive development of T cell neoplasms in mice transplanted with bone marrow expressing activated Notch alleles. J Exp Med, 183:2283-2291.
Posakony, J.W. (1994) Nature versus nurture: asymmetric cell divisions in Drosophila bristle development. Cell,76: 415-418.
Poulson, D.F. (1937) Chromosomal deficiencies and the embryonic development of Drosophila melanogaster. Proc. Natl. Acad. Sci. USA, 23:133-137.
Radtke, F., Wilson, A., Stark, G., Bauer, M., van Meerwijk, J., MacDonald, H.R., Aguet, M. (1999) Deficient T cell fate specification in mice with an induced inactivation of Notch1. Immunity,10:547-58.
Rand, M.D., Grimm, L.M., Artavanis-Tsakonas, S., Patriub, V., Blacklow, S.C., Sklar, J., Aster, J.C. (2000) Calcium depletion dissociates and activates heterodimeric notch receptors. Mol Cell Biol, 20:1825-1835.
Rangarajan, A., Talora, C., Okuyama, R., et. al. (2001a) Notch signaling is a direct determinant of keratinocyte growth arrest and entry into differentiation. EMBO J, 20:3427-3436.
Rangarajan, A., Syal, R., Selvarajah, S., Chakrabarti, O., Sarin, A., Krishna, S. (2001b) Activated Notch1 signaling cooperates with papillomavirus oncogenes in transformation and generates resistance to apoptosis on matrix withdrawal through PKB/Akt. Virology, 286:23-30.
Rishton, G.M,. Retz, D.M., Tempest, P.A., Novotny, J., Kahn S., Treanor, J.J., Lile, J.D., Citron, M. (2000) Fenchylamine sulfonamide inhibitors of amyloid beta peptide production by the gamma-secretase proteolytic pathway: potential small-molecule therapeutic agents for the treatment of Alzheimer's disease. J Med Chem, 43:2297-2299.
Robbins, J., Blondel, B.J., Gallahan, D., Callahan, R. M. (1992) Mouse mammary tumor gene int-3: a member of the notch gene family transforms mammary epithelial cells. J Virol, 66:2594-2599.
Robson MacDonald, H., Wilson, A., Radtke, F. (2001) Notch1 and T-cell development: insights from conditional knockout mice. Trends Immunol, 22:155-160.
Rohn, J.L., Lauring, A.S., Linenberger, M.L., Overbaugh, J. (1996) Transduction of Notch2 in feline leukemia virus-induced thymic lymphoma. J Virol, 70:8071-80.

Ronchini, C., & Capobianco, A.J. (2001) Induction of cyclin D1 transcription and CDK2 activity by Notch(ic): implication for cell cycle disruption in transformation by Notch(ic). Mol Cell Biol, 21:5925-5934.

Ross D.A., & Kadesch T. (2001) The notch intracellular domain can function as a coactivator for LEF-1. Mol Cell Biol, 21:7537-7544.

Sasaki Y., Ishida S., Morimoto I., Yamashita T., Kojima T., Kihara C., Tanaka, T., Imai, K., Nakamura, Y., Tokino, T. (2002) The p53 family member genes are involved in the Notch signal pathway. J Biol Chem 277:719-724.

Schroeter, E.H., Kisslinger, J.A., Kopan, R. (1998) Notch-1 signalling requires ligand-induced proteolytic release of intracellular domain. Nature, 393:382-386.

Shawber, C., Nofziger, D., Hsieh, J.J., Lindsell, C., Bogler, O., Hayward, D., Weinmaster, G. (1996) Notch signaling inhibits muscle cell differentiation through a CBF1-independent pathway. Development 122:3765-3773.

Shearman, M.S., Beher. D., Clarke, E.E., Lewis, H.D., Harrison. T., Hunt, P., Nadin, A., Smith, A.L., Stevenson, G., Castro, J.L. (2000) L-685,458, an aspartyl protease transition state mimic, is a potent inhibitor of amyloid beta-protein precursor gamma-secretase activity. Biochemistry, 39:8698-8704.

Shou, J., Ross, S., Koeppen, H., de Sauvage, F.J., Gao, W.Q. (2001) Dynamics of notch expression during murine prostate development and tumorigenesis. Cancer Res 61:7291-7297.

Song ,W., Nadeau, P., Yuan, M. (1999) Proteolytic release and nuclear translocation of Notch-1 are induced by presenilin-1 and impaired by pathologic presenilin-1 mutations. Proc. Natl. Acad. Sci. USA, 96:6959-6963.

Sriuranpong, V., Borges, M.W., Ravi, R.K., Arnold, D.R., Nelkin, B.D., Baylin, S.B., Ball, D.W. (2001) Notch signaling induces cell cycle arrest in small cell lung cancer cells. Cancer Res, 61:3200-3205.

Sriuranpong, V., Borges, M.W., Strock, C.L., Nakakura, E.K., Watkins, D.N., Blaumueller, C.M., Nelkin, B.D., and Ball, D.W.(2002) Notch signaling induces rapid degradation of achaete-scute homolog-1. Mol Cell Biol, in press.

Struhl, G., & Adachi, A. (1998) Nuclear access and action of notch in vivo. Cell 93:649-660.

Struhl, G, & Adachi A. (2000) Requirements for presenilin-dependent cleavage of notch and other transmembrane proteins. Mol Cell, 6:625-636.

Sun, Y., Nadal-Vicens, M., Misono, S., Lin, M.Z., Zubiaga, A., Hua, X., Fan, G., Greenberg, M.E. (2001) Neurogenin promotes neurogenesis and inhibits glial differentiation by independent mechanisms. Cell, 104:365-376.

Tohda, S., & Nara, N. (2001) Expression of Notch1 and Jagged1 proteins in acute myeloid leukemia cells. Leuk Lymphoma, 42:467-472.

Tomita, K., Hattori, M., Nakamura, E., Nakanishi, S., Minato, N., Kageyama, R. (1999) The bHLH gene Hes1 is essential for expansion of early T cell precursors. Genes Devel, 13:1203-1210.

Uemura, T., Shepherd, S., Ackerman, L., Jan, L.Y., Jan, Y.N. (1989) numb, a gene required in determination of cell fate during sensory organ formation in *Drosophila* embryos. Cell, 58:349-360.

Uyttendaele, H., Ho, J., Rossant, J., Kitajewski, J. (2001) Vascular patterning defects associated with expression of activated Notch4 in embryonic endothelium. Proc Natl Acad Sci U S A, 98:5643-5648.

Varnum-Finney, B., Xu, L., Brashem-Stein, C., Nourigat, C., Flowers, D., Bakkour, S., Pear, W.S., Bernstein, I.D. (2000) Pluripotent, cytokine-dependent, hematopoietic stem cells are immortalized by constitutive Notch1 signaling. Nat Med, 6:1278-1281.

Walker, L., Carlson, A., Tan-Pertel, H.T., Weinmaster, G., Gasson, J. (2001) The notch receptor and its ligands are selectively expressed during hematopoietic development in the mouse. Stem Cells, 19:543-552.

Walter, J., Kaether, C., Steiner, H., Haass, C. (2001) The cell biology of Alzheimer's disease: uncovering the secrets of secretases. Curr Opin Neurobiol, 11:585-590.

Wolfe, M.S., Xia, W., Moore, C.L., et al. (1999) Peptidomimetic probes and molecular modeling suggest that Alzheimer's gamma-secretase is an intramembrane-cleaving aspartyl protease. Biochemistry,38:4720-4727.

Wolfer, A., Bakker, T., Wilson, A., et al. (2001) Inactivation of Notch 1 in immature thymocytes does not perturb CD4 or CD8T cell development. Nat Immunol,2:235-241.

Xue, Y., Gao, X., Lindsell, C.E., et al. (1999) Embryonic lethality and vascular defects in mice lacking the Notch ligand Jagged1. Hum Mol Genet, 8:723-730.

Yamamoto, N., Yamamoto, S., Inagaki, F., et al. (2001) Role of Deltex-1 as a transcriptional regulator downstream of the Notch receptor. J Biol Chem, 276:45031-45040.

Yan, X.Q., Sarmiento, U., Sun, Y., Huang, G., Guo, J., Juan, T., Van, G., Qi, M.Y., Scully, S., Senaldi, G., Fletcher, F.A. (2001) A novel Notch ligand, Dll4, induces T-cell leukemia/lymphoma when overexpressed in mice by retroviral-mediated gene transfer. Blood, 98:3793-3799.

Yu, G., Nishimura, M., Arawaka, S., et al. (2000) Nicastrin modulates presenilin-mediated notch/glp-1 signal transduction and betaAPP processing. Nature, 407:48-54.
Zagouras, P., Stifani, S., Blaumueller, C.M., Carcangiu, M.L., Artavanis-Tsakonas, S. (1995) Alterations in Notch signaling in neoplastic lesions of the human cervix. Proc Natl Acad Sci U S A, 92:6414-6418.
Zhong, T.P., Childs, S., Leu, J.P., Fishman, M.C. (2001) Gridlock signalling pathway fashions the first embryonic artery. Nature, 414:216-220.
Zhou, S., Fujimuro, M., Hsieh, J.J., Chen, L., Miyamoto, A., Weinmaster, G., Hayward, S.D. (2000) SKIP, a CBF1-associated protein, interacts with the ankyrin repeat domain of NotchIC To facilitate NotchIC function. Mol Cell Biol, 20:2400-2410.
Zhou, S., & Hayward, S.D. (2001) Nuclear localization of CBF1 is regulated by interactions with the SMRT corepressor complex. Mol Cell Biol, 21:6222-6232.
Zilian, O., Saner, C., Hagedorn, L., et al. (2001) Multiple roles of mouse Numb in tuning developmental cell fates. Curr Biol, 11:494-501.
Zlobin, A., Jang, M., Miele, L. (2000) Toward the rational design of cell fate modifiers: Notch signaling as a target for novel biopharmaceuticals. Curr Pharm Biotechnol, 1:83-106.

cAMP SIGNALING IN CANCER GENESIS AND TREATMENT

YOON S. CHO-CHUNG

1. INTRODUCTION

Sutherland's Nobel Prize-winning discovery of cAMP as an intracellular second messenger of hormone action (Sutherland, 1972; Sutherland & Rall, 1957) has led to a rapid generation of literature supporting the role of cAMP in the regulation of cell growth and differentiation for a variety of cell types (Friedman, 1976; Hsie & Puck, 1971; Pastan, Johnson, & Anderson, 1975; Prasad, 1975; Ryan & Heidrick, 1974). Typically, cAMP signaling is activated by the binding of hormone to its receptor. The receptor-hormone complex is then coupled with cellular guanine nucleotide binding protein (G-protein), which interacts with and activates adenlyate cyclase, the enzyme that catalyzes cAMP synthesis (Sutherland, 1972). cAMP then binds to its receptor protein, cAMP-dependent protein kinase (PKA) (Krebs, 1972) and induces reversible phosphorylation of protein substrates that regulate a vast number of cellular processes, including cell growth and differentiation. For more than 25 years, investigators interested in the regulation of cell growth by cAMP have focused on the mechanism of action of the two isoforms of PKA, type I (PKA-I) and type II (PKA-II). However, only during the past decade has experimental evidence revealed distinct functions for PKA-I and PKA-II, providing molecular proof that the intracellular balanced expression between the two isoforms may play a critical role in the control of cell growth and differentiation. It has been established that PKA-I is only transiently overexpressed in normal cells in response to physiological stimuli of cell proliferation, but it is constitutively overexpressed in cancer cells and associated with a worse prognosis in human cancers of different cell types. Conversely, PKA-II is preferentially expressed in normal differentiated tissues (Cho-Chung et al., 1999; Cho-Chung, Pepe, Clair, Budillon, & Nesterova, 1995; Tortora & Ciardiello, 2000).

This review describes how the modulation of each regulatory (R) subunit (RI and RII) of PKA influences the ability of cAMP to regulate growth. The experimental approaches described here include the use of antisense oligonucleotides, gene transfer, transcription factor decoy, 8-Cl-cAMP, and cDNA microarrays. Such approaches not only provide the molecular tools to critically assess cAMP signaling in cancer genesis and progression, but they also contribute to the discovery of target-based drugs for the treatment of cancer.

2. PKA SUBUNITS AND ISOZYME DISTRIBUTION

In the absence of cAMP, mammalian PKA is an inactive tetramer composed of two regulatory subunits (R) and two catalytic subunits (C). Within the holoenzyme, the inhibitory domain of the R subunit inactivates the catalytic activity of the C subunit. When two cAMP molecules bind the R subunit (Corbin et al., 1978), the affinity of the R subunit for the C subunit decreases 10,000–100,000-fold (Døskeland, Maronde, & Gjertsen, 1993), and the tetrametric PKA dissociates into the dimeric R subunit and two monomers of the C subunit (Flockhart & Corbin, 1982; Gettys & Corbin, 1989; Walsh, Perkins, & Krebs, 1968) releasing an active C subunit (Flockhart & Corbin, 1982; Houge, Steinberg, Ogreid, & Doskeland, 1990).

PKA-I and PKA-II are distinguished by their subunits, RI and RII (Beebe & Corbin, 1986). The two isozymes share identical C subunits. Four isoforms of the R subunits (RIα, RIβ, RIIα, and RIIβ) and three isoforms of the C subunit (Cα, Cβ, and Cγ) have been identified (McKnight et al., 1988). However, preferential coexpression of any of the C subunits with RI or RII has not been found (Beebe et al., 1990; Showers & Maurer, 1986). RI and RII differ in molecular weight, isoelectric point, and immunological characteristics. Other differences, such as affinity for cAMP, cAMP analog selectivity, tissue specificity, subcellular localization, and expression in transformation and differentiation, suggest the possibility of differential control by these subunits under various physiological conditions (Beebe & Corbin, 1986; Cho-Chung, Clair, Tortora, Yokozaki, & Pepe, 1991; Cho-Chung et al., 1995; Lohmann & Walter, 1984).

RI and RII contain two tandem cAMP-binding domains at the carboxyl terminus, which is highly conserved. However, these subunits differ significantly in the amino terminus at a proteolytically sensitive hinge region that occupies the catalytic domain of the C subunit (Taylor et al., 1988). In this segment, RII contains an autophosphorylation site, Arg-Arg-X-Ser (Takio, Smith, Krebs, Walsh, & Titani, 1984), which undergoes phosphorylation at the serine residue by the C subunit in the holoenzyme complex (Rosen & Erlichman, 1975). RI, however contains the sequence Arg-Arg-X-Ala (Titani et al., 1984), which does not undergo autophosphorylation but binds with high-affinity to ATP.

2.1 RIα Overexpression and Antisense Inhibition of RIα

Increased expression of RI has been shown to be associated with both chemical and viral carcinogenesis and with oncogene-induced cell transformation. The initiation stage of dimethylbenz (a) anthracene-induced mammary carcinogenesis in rats, (Cho-Chung, Clair, & Shepheard, 1983), the incidence of gastric adenocarcinoma in rats by N-methyl-N'-nitrosguanine, and the trophic action of gastrin on gastric carcinoma production (Yasui & Tahara, 1985) correlate with a sharp increase in RI and PKA-I activity. In another study, only PKA-II is found in normal 3T3 cells, but spontaneously transformed cells and cells transformed with SV40 or with methylcholanthrene express both PKA-I and PKA-II, with an increased level of RI (Gharrett, Malkinson, & Sheppard, 1976; Wehner, Malkinson, Wiser, & Sheppard, 1981). However, these cells exhibit a level of total kinase activity equivalent to that of normal cells. A similar increase in RI and PKA-I expression has been shown in rat 3Y1 cells transformed by human adenovirus type 12, but little or no change occurs in PKA-II following transformation (Ledinko & Chan, 1984). Marked increase in RI expression, with a concomitant decrease in RII expression, has been detected in Ha-MuSV-transformed NIH/3T3 clone 13-3B-4 cells (Clair, Ally, Tagliaferri, Robins, & Cho-Chung, 1987; Tagliaferri, Clair, DeBortoli, & Cho-Chung, 1985), in rat (NRK) kidney cells transformed with TGF or v-Ki-ras oncogene (Tortora et al., 1989), in TGF-induced transformation of mouse mammary epithelial cells (Ciardiello et al., 1990), and in point-mutated c-Ha-ras and c-erbB-2 proto-oncogene–transformed human mammary epithelial cell line MCF-10A HE (Ciardiello et al., 1993).

Overexpression of the RIα subunit has been correlated with multidrug resistance (Yokozaki, Budillon, Clair et al., 1993). In addition, the interaction of the RIα subunit with CoxVb may influence the regulation of cytochrome C oxidase activity, cytochrome C levels, and the release of cytochrome C into the cytoplasm (Yang, Iacono, Tang, & Chin, 1998). RIα also interacts with the ligand-activated epidermal growth factor receptor (EGFR) complex by binding to the SH3 domains of the Grb2 abdaptor protein (Tortora et al., 1997). Thus, overexpression of RIα may cause deregulation of a multitude of cellular functions that regulate cell growth and multidrug resistance. Importantly, expression of the RIα subunit of PKA is increased in various primary human tumors and cell lines, including cancers of the breast (Handschin & Eppenberger, 1979; Miller, Hulme, Cho-Chung, & Elton, 1993; Miller, Watson, Jack, Chetty, & Elton, 1993), ovary (McDaid et al., 1999; Simpson et al., 1996), lung (Young et al., 1995), and colon (Bold, Alpard, Ishizuka, Townsend, & Thompson, 1994; Bradbury, Carter, Miller, Cho-Chung, & Clair, 1994; Gordge, Hulme, Clegg, & Miller, 1996). Furthermore, overexpression of the RIα subunit of PKA correlates with malignancy and poor prognosis in cancer patients (McDaid et al., 1999; Miller, Hulme et al., 1993; Miller, Watson et al., 1993; Simpson et al., 1996). These results suggest that RI may act as a mediator of various mitogenic stimuli and thus represent a potential target for the pharmacological control of cell proliferation.

Nucleic acid therapeutics represent a direct genetic approach to cancer treatment. Such an approach takes advantage of genes known to confer a growth advantage to neoplastic cells and mechanisms that activate these genes (Zamecnik & Stephenson, 1978). Moreover, the ability to block these genes allows the exploration of normal growth regulation in addition to its therapeutic value.

RIα has been overexpressed using vector-mediated infection (Nesterova, Yokozaki, McDuffie, & Cho-Chung, 1996). Overexpression of RIα in cancer cells that have 'inborn' growth-advantageous properties such as hormone-, serum-, and anchorage-independent growth, had no apparent effect on the rate of cell proliferation (Nesterova et al., 1996). However, in non-transformed cells such as FRTL5 rat thyroid cells and immortalized human mammary epithelial cells (MCF-10A), RIα overexpression mimicked the effect of hormone and serum supplement in cell growth in tissue culture, and in cell cycle progression (Tortora, Pepe et al., 1994; Tortora et al., 1993).

If RIα is indeed a mitogenic stimulator, certain mutations in its primary structure should be able to block its mitogenic action. One of the critical structural differences between RI and RII is the presence of an autophosphorylation site in RII (Taylor et al., 1988) at the R·C interaction site. An autophosphorylation site has been introduced into human RIα at alanine 99 via a single nucleotide change, G_T, leading to the replacement of this alanine with serine. The mutant, RIα-P, has been overexpressed in MCF-7 breast cancer cells (G. R. Lee et al., 1999). Overexpression of this mutant inhibits growth and induces apoptosis, and cells overexpressing RIα-P require a higher concentration of cAMP to activate endogenous PKA than do cells overexpressing wild-type RIα or RIIβ (G. R. Lee et al., 1999). RIα-P downregulates PKA-II, unlike wild-type RIα (G. R. Lee et al., 1999). The dominant activity of RIα-P may arise from the ability of RIα-P to trap the endogenous wild-type RIα into inactive dimers, which would block PKA-I activity and thereby inhibit growth.

The possibility that the RI cAMP receptor is a positive regulator of cancer cell growth has been further explored using the antisense strategy. A synthetic RIα antisense oligodeoxynucleotide (ODN) corresponding to the N-terminal seven codons of human RIα (15–30 μM) inhibits growth in breast (MCF-7), colon (LS-174T), and gastric carcinoma (TMK-1), and neuroblastoma (SK-N-SH) cells (Yokozaki, Budillon, Tortora et al., 1993), as well as in HL-60 leukemia cells (Tortora, Yokozaki, Pepe, Clair, & Cho-Chung, 1991), with no sign of cytotoxicity. Furthermore, treatment with an RIα antisense phosphorothioate oligodeoxynucleotide (PS-ODN) brings about a marked reduction in RIα levels with a concomitant increase in RIIβ levels (Yokozaki, Budillon, Tortora et al., 1993). Strikingly, a single-injection of RIα antisense PS-ODN targeted against codons 8–13 of human RIα results in reduction of RIα expression and sustained growth inhibition in LS-174T colon carcinoma in nude mice at up to 14 days of examination (Nesterova & Cho-Chung, 1995). Tumor cells behave like untransformed cells by making less PKA-I (Nesterova & Cho-Chung, 1995).

To address the issue of nonspecific toxicity and side effects associated with antisense PS-ODNs, the polyanionic nature (Agrawal & Zhao, 1998) of the antisense RIα PS-ODN has been minimized, and the immunostimulatory GCGT motif (Krieg et al., 1995) has been blocked in a second generation RNA-DNA RIα antisense (Nesterova & Cho-Chung, 2000). This ODN has improved antisense activity over the PS-ODN (Metelev, Liszlewicz, & Agrawal, 1994; Monia et al., 1993), is more resistant to nucleases, forms more stable duplexes with RNA than the parental PS-ODN (Metelev et al., 1994; Shibahara et al., 1989), and retains the capability to induce RNAse H (Metelev et al., 1994). Thus, in addition to reducing nonspecific effects, the RNA-DNA RIα antisense ODN facilitates the exploration of sequence-specific antisense effects (Nesterova & Cho-Chung, 2000). This modulation ultimately inhibits growth and induces apoptosis in various cancer cell lines and in tumors in nude mice (Alper, Hacker, & Cho-Chung, 1999; Cho et al., In press; Cho-Chung et al., 1997; Cho-Chung et al., 1999; Nesterova & Cho-

Chung, 2000; Nesterova, Noguchi, Park, Lee, & Cho-Chung, 2000; Srivastava, Srivastava, Park, Agrawal, & Cho-Chung, 1998; Srivastava, Srivastava, Seth, Agrawal, & Cho-Chung, 1999; Tortora et al., 2000; Wang et al., 1999).

The target specificity of RIα antisense has been thoroughly addressed. Pulse-chase experiments have revealed that RIα has a relatively short half-life: 17 hr in control cells and 13 hr in antisense-treated cells (i.e., LS-174 colon carcinoma) (Nesterova et al., 2000). The short half-life of RIα, along with its message downregulation, is consistent with the rapid RIα downregulation observed in antisense-treated tumors (Nesterova & Cho-Chung, 1995). In addition, levels of RIIβ protein increase because of a longer half-life (about 5.5 fold) (Nesterova et al., 2000), leading to a decrease in the PKA-I to PKA-II ratio in tumor cells. The half-lives of RIIα and Cα remain unchanged in antisense-treated cells. The RIα antisense-induced stabilization of the RIIβ protein is consistent with results in RIβ and RIIβ knockout mice, in which compensatory stabilization-induced elevation of the RIα protein appears in tissues that normally express the β isoforms of the R subunit (Amieux et al., 1997). These results show a clear correlation between growth inhibition induced by RIα antisense and the target-specific antisense effect, namely, RIα downregulation.

The effects of RIα antisense RNA-DNA ODN on the cAMP-signaling cascade are dependent on the expression of PKA-I and PKA-II in the cell. In LS-174T colon cancer cells and in LNCaP prostate cancer cells, in which both PKA-I and PKA-II are expressed (Nesterova et al., 1996), the antisense-directed loss of RIα results in the expected compensatory stabilization of the RIIβ protein, again because RIIβ's half-life is lengthened (Nesterova et al., 2000). The antisense also triggers an increase in the activity of PDE4 (Nesterova & Cho-Chung, 2000), a cAMP-inducible enzyme (Beavo & Reifsnyder, 1990; Conti, Jin, Monaco, Repaske, & Swinnen, 1991), and nuclear translocation of the PKA Cα subunit (Neary & Cho-Chung, 2001) in the absence of an increase of cellular cAMP. Thus, the loss of RIα activates cAMP signaling by activating PKA-I and bypassing adenylate cyclase. However, in the case of HCT-15 MDR colon carcinoma cells, in which PKA-I is primarily expressed, (Nesterova & Cho-Chung, unpublished data) the antisense directed loss of RIα decreases Cα subunit stability by shortening the half-life of Cα (Nesterova & Cho-Chung, 2000). This leads to reduction in cAMP signaling as evidenced by reduced PDE4 activity (Nesterova & Cho-Chung, 2000). These results are consistent with those observed in S49 lymphoma cells, which express PKA-I only. The RI subunit becomes much more labile in mutant cells lacking a functional C subunit than in wild-type cells, and in cells treated with cAMP analogs than in untreated control cells (Steinberg & Agard, 1981).

These results can be interpreted in the context of cyclic AMP response element (CRE)-directed transcription. PKA activates the transactivation activity of cAMP response element binding protein (CREB) (Montminy & Bilezikjian, 1987) by phosphorylating Ser 133 (Gonzalez, Biggs, Vale, & Montminy, 1989). Phosphorylation at this amino acid is also crucial for growth factor induction of c-*fos* transcription (Ginty, Bonni, & Greenberg, 1994). In transformed cells, the growth factor-mediated phosphorylation of CREB may supersede that mediated by

PKA and therefore stimulate cell growth. However, upon RIα antisense treatment, activated PKA, which is the released Cα subunit, may augment Cα-mediated CREB-phosphorylation, resulting in a switch to the mechanism of CREB phosphorylation from one mediated by growth factors to one mediated by PKA. This switch would inhibit growth factor signals and ultimately inhibit cell growth in LS-174T and LNCaP cancer cells (Nesterova & Cho-Chung, 2000). In HCT-15 MDR cells, the RIα antisense RNA-DNA ODN-directed destabilization of Cα may simply turn off transactivation of CRE, Ap-1, and Sp-1, which are commonly upregulated in HCT-15 MDR cells (Rohlff & Glazer, 1995), and thereby inhibit cell growth (Nesterova & Cho-Chung, 2000). The oral efficacy (Wang et al., 1999) and the growth inhibition exerted by RIα antisense RNA-DNA second generation ODN in cancer cells of a variety of cell types (Alper et al., 1999; Cho et al., In press; Cho-Chung et al., 1997; Cho-Chung et al., 1999; Nesterova & Cho-Chung, 2000; Nesterova et al., 2000; Srivastava, Srivastava et al., 1998; Srivastava et al., 1999; Tortora et al., 2000; Wang et al., 1999) support efforts to test the effects of this antisense ODN on tumors in a clinical setting [GEM 231, an RIα antisense RNA-DNA second generation ODN (Chen et al., 2000)].

2.2 RII Overexpression

The RIIβ cAMP receptor is essential for cAMP-induced growth inhibition and differentiation in cancer cells. An RIIβ antisense ODN blocks the growth inhibition and differentiation induced by cAMP; cells become refractory to the cAMP stimulus and continue to grow in the presence or absence of a cAMP analog (Tortora, Clair, & Cho-Chung, 1990).

The relationship between RIIβ expression and malignancy has been tested using vector-mediated overexpression of RIIβ. Overexpression of RIIβ inhibits growth, with no sign of toxicity, in a variety of cancer cell types, including SK-N-SH neuroblastoma, MCF-7 breast carcinoma, Ki-*ras*-transformed NIH/3T3 clone DT (Cho-Chung, Clair, Tortora, & Yokozaki, 1991; Tortora, Budillon et al., 1994), HL-60 leukemia cells (Tortora, Budillon et al., 1994), and PC12 mutant A-126 cells (Tortora & Cho-Chung, 1990). SK-N-SH, DT, and A-126 cells also display striking changes in morphology. Cells become flat and exhibit an increased ratio of cytoplasm to nucleus (Cho-Chung, Clair, Tortora, & Yokozaki, 1991; Tortora, Budillon et al., 1994; Tortora & Cho-Chung, 1990). This morphology is similar to that induced by exposure of these cells to RIα antisense ODN (Tortora et al., 1991). In SK-N-SH cells, overexpression of RIIβ directly induces growth arrest and reversion of the transformed phenotype; no further treatment with cAMP analogs is required. These results suggest that the RIIβ cAMP receptor may act as a tumor suppressor protein that inhibits growth and promotes differentiation and reverse transformation.

RIIβ shares extensive homology with the cAMP-binding domain of the bacterial catabolite gene activator protein (CAP) (Crombrugghe, Busby, & Buc, 1984). In bacteria, cAMP regulates gene expression by modulating the DNA-binding capability of CAP. The evolutionary conservation between RIIβ and CAP suggests that RIIβ may also bind DNA. Recent studies have demonstrated that RIIβ does bind to the cAMP-responsive element (CRE), through which it activates transcription (Srivastava, Lee et al., 1998). cAMP enhances the ability of RIIβ to bind the CRE, and the mutant RIIβ-P, in which the autophosphorylation site (Ser 114) has been changed to alanine, exhibits reduced ability to bind the CRE and to activate transcription from the CRE (Srivastava, Lee et al., 1998). Although a role for a kinase can not be completely ruled out, these studies nevertheless suggest that RIIβ may mediate the regulation of CRE-directed transcription in eukaryotic cells.

Cells overexpressing RIIβ-P behave as transformed cells (Budillon et al., 1995; Nesterova et al., 1996) and exhibit an increase in a novel, 53-kDa RIIβ protein species that is not detected in parental cells (Nesterova et al., 1996). Decreased RIα levels are also detected in these cells. The RIIα subunit has also been overexpressed in LS-174T human colon carcinoma cells (Nesterova et al., 1996). RIIα protein levels are unaffected, but RIIα mRNA levels increase, indicating a posttranscriptional control mechanism similar to that for RIα. Cells overexpressing RIIβ subunit also exhibit decreased RIα levels, but overexpression of RIα does not affect RIIα expression (Nesterova et al., 1996).

2.3 PKA Isozyme Distribution in Cancer

A correlation between the changing ratio of PKA-I and PKA-II has been shown in ontogenic development and differentiation processes (Cho-Chung, 1990; Lohmann & Walter, 1984). Evidence suggests an interesting correlation regarding the different expression of type I and type II PKA subunits and their mRNAs with neoplastic transformation and tumor growth. The ratio of PKA-I/PKA-II in renal cell carcinomas is about twice that in renal cortex, although the total soluble PKA activity is similar in both tissues (Fossberg, Døskeland, & Ueland, 1978). Surgical specimens of Wilms' tumor exhibit a PKA-I/PKA-II ratio that is twice that found in normal tissue, and the RI/RII ratio in tumors is more than three times that in normal tissue (Nakajima, Imashuku, Wilimas, Champion, & Green, 1984). In a study of pituitary tumors of the rat, RII appears at lower levels in nuclei isolated from tumors than in normal tissue (Piroli, Weisenberg, Grillo, & De Nicola, 1990). In the neoplastically transformed BT5C glioma cell line the ratio of type I/type II PKA is significantly higher than the normal fetal brain cells, but the R and C subunits of protein kinase are expressed to a similar degree in both cell lines (Ekanger et al., 1985). Normal and malignant osteoblasts differ also in their isozyme response to hormones, with a relative predominance of type I activation in malignant cells and of type II in normal cells (Livesey, Kemp, Re, Partridge, & Martin, 1982). In addition, increased expression of PKA-I, compared with PKA-II, has also been correlated with the multidrug resistance (MDR) of cancer cells, (Rohlff & Glazer, 1995; Yokozaki, Budillon, Clair et al., 1993). However, experiments with the retroviral vector-mediated overexpression of R subunits demonstrate that PKA-II formation is highly favored over that of PKA-I. Overexpression of the RII subunit induces a striking shift in PKA isozyme distribution by reducing PKA-I levels and increasing PKA-II levels in LS-174T colon carcinoma cells (Nesterova et al., 1996). PKA-I levels are almost completely eliminated in cells overexpressing RIIβ and RIIβ-P infectants, and different species of PKA-II, which do not appear in parental cells or in cells overexpressing RIIα, are detected in these cells. In contrast, PKA-II levels are unaltered in cells overexpressing RIα, and in cells overexpressing Cα. These data suggest that the R and C subunits are in equilibrium between PKA-I and PKA-II and that PKA-II formation is highly favored.

This preferential formation of PKA-II is not limited to LS-174T cells; such a preference has also been demonstrated in ras-transformed NIH3T3 cells and in AtT20 pituitary cells (McKnight et al., 1988). Most likely, RIIα and Cα associate preferentially in LS-174T cells, and PKA-I is formed only if the C subunit is present in excess over RIIα. Excess free RIα may be degraded; therefore the increase in RIα or PKA-I cannot occur in RIα infectants even though RIα mRNA increases (Nesterova et al., 1996). That the formation of PKA-I over PKA-II increases in cancer cells, in contrast to the favored formation of PKA-II over PKA-I demonstrated by overexpression of the wild-type R subunits, suggests an intrinsic structural alteration in R subunits, possibly at the site of interaction between the R subunit and the C subunit. However, no such mutant of the R subunit has been identified in cancer cells.

The results mentioned above suggest that abnormal expression of R-subunit isoforms of PKA is involved in neoplastic transformation and that suppression of RIα/PKA-I and/or induction of RIIβ/PKA-IIβ can restore growth control in transformed cells. The autophosphorylation mutant RIIβ-P, which has lost the phosphorylation site, fails to mimic the effects of RIIβ (Budillon et al., 1995; Nesterova et al., 1996) and the RIα-P mutant, which has gained the autophosphorylation site, functionally mimics RIIβ (G. R. Lee et al., 1999) suggesting the functional importance of the RIIβ autophosphorylation site in restraining tumor cell growth.

3. OTHER EXPERIMENTAL APPROACHES IN STUDYING cAMP AND PKA

3.1 8-Cl-cAMP

cAMP, at high (millimolar) concentrations, saturates both PKA-I and PKA-II maximally and equally (Beebe & Corbin, 1986). Site-selective cAMP analogs, however, demonstrate selective binding toward either one of two cAMP binding sites, Site A (Site 2) and Site B (Site 1) (Døskeland, 1978; Rannels & Corbin, 1980) in the R subunit, resulting in preferential binding and activation of either PKA isozyme. The use of site-selective cAMP analogs that demonstrate high affinity and selectivity toward protein kinase isozyme makes it possible to correlate the specific effect of PKA isozymes with cAMP-mediated responses in intact cells (Beebe, Holloway, Rannels, & Corbin, 1984). With respect to growth control, site-selective cAMP analogs have been shown to induce growth inhibition and differentiation in a broad spectrum of human cancer cell lines, including carcinomas, sarcomas, and leukemias, without causing cytotoxicity (Katsaros et al., 1987; P.

Tagliaferri et al., 1988; Tortora et al., 1988). Of these, 8-Cl-cAMP, the most potent site-selective cAMP analog, has recently completed several Phase I clinical studies (Tortora et al., 1995). 8-Cl-cAMP, which belongs to the ISD (isozyme site discriminator) class (Cho-Chung, 1990; Øgreid et al., 1985) of site-selective cAMP analogs, activates and downregulates PKA-I, but not PKA-II, by binding to both Site A and B of RI and to Site B of RII (Ally et al., 1988; Cho-Chung, 1990). The mechanism of action of 8-Cl-cAMP has been studied in detail in HL-60 promyelocytic leukemia cells (Rohlff, Clair, & Cho-Chung, 1993). 8-Cl-cAMP downregulates PKA-I by promoting truncation of the 48 kDa RIα subunit to a 34 kDa form. The 34 kDa RIα exists in the PKA-I holoenzyme, suggesting that this molecule is truncated at the C terminus. This mode of truncation of RIα may facilitate rebinding of 8-Cl-cAMP to the reconstituted holoenzyme and subsequent dissociation of the enzyme into its subunits, thus enhancing downregulation of PKA-I without allowing accumulation of the free RIα subunit. The truncation of the 48 kDa form of RIα to the 34 kDa form is a mechanism of action unique to 8-Cl-cAMP; the formation of the 34 kDa protein is not induced in the downregulation of PKA-I by other means, such as treatment with RIα antisense or overexpression of RIIβ. Most likely, treatment with 8-Cl-cAMP activates a protease that breaks the 48 dDa RIα down to 34 kDa.

Several reports in the literature have indicated that the anti-proliferative activity of 8-Cl-cAMP results from its conversion to its hydrolytic metabolites (Lange-Carter, Vuillequez, & Malkinson, 1993; Taylor & Yeoman, 1992; Van Lookeren Campagne, Villalba Diaz, Jastorff, & Kessin, 1991). However, 8-Cl-cAMP hydrolytic activity is largely absent in heat-inactivated fetal calf serum (Van Lookeren Campagne et al., 1991), suggesting that a mechanism other than the hydrolysis of 8-Cl-cAMP promotes the growth inhibitory effect. In fact, HPLC analysis has demonstrated that 8-Cl-5′-AMP and 8-Cl-adenosine are the major metabolites formed after 48 hr in medium containing heat-inactivated fetal calf serum and 8-Cl-cAMP (Rohlff et al., 1993). Each metabolite accounts for only 6 to 7 percent of the total 8-Cl-cAMP present. The remainder is intact 8-Cl-cAMP (Rohlff et al., 1993).

In pre-clinical studies, 8-Cl-cAMP suppresses the expression of c-*myc* and c-*ras* (Cho-Chung et al., 1989), reverses the transformed phenotype (P. Tagliaferri et al., 1988; P Tagliaferri et al., 1988; Tortora, Budillon et al., 1994), and induces apoptotic cell death in human cancer cells (Kim et al., 2000; Tortora, Budillon et al., 1994). Results of a phase I clinical trial suggest that effective plasma levels (determined in pre-clinical studies) of 8-Cl-cAMP can be maintained below the maximum tolerated dose (Tortora et al., 1995). To determine the mechanism of the anti-tumor activity exhibited by 8-Cl-cAMP, two experimental approaches have been employed. One approach has used Bcl-2 overexpression or treatment with ZVAD (a broad-range caspase inhibitor) to specifically block apoptotic cell death without affecting the cell proliferation pathway. At up to 5 days of 8-Cl-cAMP treatment, Bcl-2 is transiently downregulated, and Bad expression continuously increases. Overexpression of Bcl-2 blocks 8-Cl-cAMP-induced apoptosis but has no effect on the accompanying inhibition of cell proliferation (Kim et al., 2000).

Suppression of apoptosis by ZVAD does not abrogate 8-Cl-cAMP-induced inhibition of cell proliferation. The second approach has assessed the effect of 8-Cl-cAMP in cells overexpressing RIIβ. RIIβ overexpressing cells exhibit retarded cell growth and a reverted phenotype (Budillon et al., 1995; Nesterova et al., 1996; Tortora, Budillon et al., 1994) but do not undergo spontaneous apoptosis (Kim et al., 2000). 8-Cl-cAMP exhibits no additive effect on the inhibition of cell proliferation in cells overexpressing RIIβ (Kim et al., 2000).

These results indicate that 8-Cl-cAMP inhibits cancer cell growth through both an antiproliferation and a pro-apoptotic mechanism. Most likely, 8-Cl-cAMP, being a selective activator of PKA-I but not PKA-II (Ally et al., 1988; Cho-Chung, 1990; Cho-Chung et al., 1989; Rohlff et al., 1993) promotes the phosphorylation of Bcl-2, but not Bad, leading to Bcl-2 inactivation and apoptosis. PKA-II phosphorylates Bad in mitochondria leading to the activation of Bcl-2 (Harada et al., 1999). Further studies are required to refine the mechanism of action of 8-Cl-cAMP action in tumor growth inhibition.

3.2 Transcription factor-decoy inhibition of cAMP responsive gene expression and tumor growth

The CRE (cyclic AMP response element)-transcription factor complex is a pleiotropic activator that participates in the induction of a wide variety of cellular and viral genes (Roesler, Vandenbark, & Hanson, 1988).

The synthetic, palindromic, single-stranded CRE oligonucleotide functions as an effective and stable transcription factor decoy to alter gene expression *in vivo* (Park, Nesterova, Agrawal, & Cho-Chung, 1999). Importantly, the CRE-decoy oligonucleotides achieve gene-specific regulation *in vivo* and thereby selectively inhibit cancer cell growth without adversely affecting the growth of normal cells (Park et al., 1999). Several lines of evidence support the specificity of CRE-induced growth inhibition. Treatment with the CRE-decoy oligonucleotide inhibits growth in cancer cells, but not in normal cells, both *in vitro* and *in vivo*. The administration of CRE-decoy oligonucleotides, but not mismatched oligonucleotides, markedly inhibits CRE DNA-protein complex formation, CRE-directed transcription activity, and endogenous cAMP-responsive gene expression in both cancer cells and normal cells. The cellular uptake of decoy oligonucleotides and control oligonucleotides is similar for both cancer cells and normal cells, and the specific growth inhibitory effect of CRE-decoy on cancer cells correlates with the induction of phenotypic change and apoptosis (Alper, Bergmann-Leitner, Abrams, & Cho-Chung, 2001; Park et al., 1999).

Experimental data show that the binding of decoy oligonucleotide at the transcription factor DNA-binding domain is clearly related to the growth-inhibitory effect of the decoy (Park et al., 1999). First, the CRE-decoy produces no growth inhibition in F9 teratocarcinoma cells, which still contain CRE, but it is nonfunctional and thus unresponsive to cAMP (Gonzalez & Montminy, 1989), suggesting that the decoy may inhibit growth, at least in part, through binding to CRE-binding protein (CREB). Second, KCREB, a CREB mutant that contains a mutation of a single amino acid in the DNA-binding domain, does not bind to the native CRE sequence (Walton, Rehfuss, Chrivia, Lochner, & Goodman, 1992), and cancer cells overexpressing KCREB exhibit decreased cell growth and show little or no response to decoy oligonucleotide treatment.

Importantly, the CRE-decoy oligonucleotide brings about a dual blockade (Park et al., 1999); it blocks the CRE-PKA pathway via repression of the PKA genes and the Ap-1-PKC pathway by inhibiting c-*fos* gene expression, which is responsive to CRE (Roesler et al., 1988). This dual blockade may be casually related, at least in part, to the inhibition of cancer cell growth by the CRE-decoy. In addition, the CRE-decoy brings (Park et al., 2001) about a reduction in cyclin D1/Cdk4/retinoblastoma protein signaling by inhibiting cyclin D1 gene expression, which is also CRE-responsive (R. J. Lee et al., 1999).

Initially, only phosphorylation by cAMP-dependent protein kinase was shown to be solely responsible for transactivation increase of CREB, a member of the CREB/ATF family of transcription factors (Montminy & Bilezikjian, 1987). However, it later became apparent that CREB is an *in vivo* substrate for a variety of other kinases including calmodulin kinases II and IV (Sheng, Thompson, & Greenberg, 1991) or RSK2 (Xing, Ginty, & Greenberg, 1996), implying that the CREB/ATF family of transcription factors can activate CRE-transcription in response to cAMP, Ca^{2+}, and growth factors (Ginty et al., 1994; Gonzalez et al., 1989; Sheng et al., 1991; Tan et al., 1996). That the growth factor-stimulated pathways are quiescent in non-cancerous cells could explain, at least in part, the tumor cell-specific growth inhibition demonstrated by the CRE-decoy. Furthermore, CREB interacts with its co-activator CBP (CREB-binding protein) (Chrivia et al., 1993), which is involved in the transcriptional activation of many other genes including p53, Ap-1, and retinoic acid receptors (Arias et al., 1994; Goodman & Smolik, 2000). In fact, CRE-decoy upregulates the wild-type p53 by increasing the half-life of the protein (Lee, Park, Choi, Cho, & Cho-Chung, 2000). CREB, which is directly activated by growth factors, plays an important role in the acquisition of the metastatic phenotype exhibited by human melanoma cells (Xie et al., 1997) and ovarian cancer cells (Alper et al., 2001).

These results together support the ability of the CRE-decoy oligonucleotide to regulate the expression of cAMP-responsive genes underlying tumorigenesis and tumor progression.

3.3 Secreted Protein Kinase A

Various cancer cell types excrete PKA into conditioned medium (Cho, Lee, & Cho-Chung, 2000; Cvijic, Kita, Shih, DiPaola, & Chin, 2000). This extracellular PKA (ECPKA) is present in active, free C subunit form, and its activity is specifically inhibited by the PKA inhibitory protein PKI (Cho, Lee et al., 2000; Cvijic et al., 2000). Compared with serum taken from normal persons, serum taken from cancer patients exhibit marked upregulation of ECPKA expression. Biochemical and immunological characterization have shown that ECPKA is identical to the free Cα subunit of intracellular PKA. The excess PKA-I observed in tumor cells (Cho-

Chung, Clair, Tortora, & Yokozaki, 1991) may reflect the upregulated ECPKA expression in the growth medium of cancer cells and in cancer patients' serum. Importantly, this upregulation is reduced in cancer cells, such as hormone-dependent breast cancer cells, that maintain hormone dependency (a normal cell property); in cancer cells exhibiting a reverted phenotype arising from RIIβ subunit overexpression; and in cells overexpressing a Cα-Ala mutant that lacks myristic acid. The latter result suggests that the N-terminal myristyl group of Cα is required for ECPKA expression (Cho, Park et al., 2000). Thus, regulation of PKA in mammalian cells can occur in the extracellular space, and this phenomenon may add a new dimension in the mode of cAMP/PKA signaling in the regulation of cell growth and differentiation.

3.4 cDNA Microarray Studies

A cDNA microarray (Schena, Shalon, Davis, & Brown, 1995) has been used to investigate sequence-specific antisense effects on global gene expression in cells treated with an RIα antisense ODN and in cells overexpressing the RIα gene (Cho et al., 2001). Expression is altered for approximately 10 percent of the total cDNA elements (2,304) on the array, and these changes in gene expression are comparable in prostate and colon cancer cells, which have vastly different gene expression profiles. Affected genes include genes for transcription factors, protein kinases and phosphatases, cell cycle regulators, proteins involved in DNA synthesis and regulation, G-proteins, and cytoskeleton regulatory proteins. RIα antisense thus directs a cellular regulation that is superimposed on that arising from the Watson-Crick base-pairing mechanism of action.

RIα antisense treatment affects one cluster of genes, or signature, involved in proliferation and another involved in differentiation (Cho et al., 2001). Genes that define the 'proliferation-transformation' signature are highly expressed in untreated control cells and markedly suppressed in cells exposed to antisense treatment. Conversely, genes that define the 'differentiation-reverse transformation' signature are upregulated. Similar proliferation and differentiation signatures are observed in antisense-treated tumors in nude mice, but not in host livers (Cho et al., 2001). These expression signatures, together with other prominent features of the antisense-induced expression profile, appear to reflect the profile of a non-malignant or reverted phenotype (Cho et al., 2001).

4. cAMP-DEPENDENT PROTEIN KINASE IN cAMP SIGNALING

When phytohemagglutinin and Con A are used to stimulate mitosis in lymphocytes, the activation of PKA-I is observed (Byus, Klimpel, Lucas, & Russell, 1977). The addition of DBcAMP activates both PKA isozymes (PKA-I and PKA-II) and thereby inhibits growth (Byus et al., 1977; Klimpel, Byus, Russell, & Lucas, 1979). In mammary tumor cells, the ratio PKA-I to PKA-II activity is two times higher than in normal cells, but the total PKA activity remains constant (Handschin & Eppenberger, 1979). cAMP dissociates PKA-I more easily than PKA-

II (Beebe & Corbin, 1986; Byus et al., 1977; Schwoch, 1978), suggesting that PKA-I may positively regulate cell growth at a decreased level of cAMP. Under these conditions, it is possible that dissociation of PKA-II is hindered and therefore observed only at sufficiently high levels of cAMP. In this scenario, activation of PKA-II may stimulate cell differentiation.

It is likely that PKA activity is integrated with primary, intrinsic regulatory signals and with other second messengers such as calcium and phosphionosides. Furthermore, calcium regulates cAMP metabolism via regulation of adenylate cyclase and phosphodiesterase (Beebe & Corbin, 1986; Boynton & Whitfield, 1983). Crosstalk between the cAMP signaling pathway and the Ras pathway represents another direction in which cAMP exerts its effects on cell growth and cancer. For example, phosphorylation of Raf-1 by PKA may block the Ras pathway (Wu et al., 1993). Thus, Ca^{2+}, phosphoinosides, and the *ras* pathways must be considered in studying the regulation of growth and development.

5. PERSPECTIVE

Signaling via the cAMP pathway may be complex, and biological effects of the pathway in normal cells may depend upon the physiological state of the cells. cAMP and its receptors, cAMP-dependent protein kinase (PKA) function in cell growth and differentiation. Two PKA isozymes, PKA-I and PKA-II, appear in different ratios during ontogenic development, cell differentiation, and transformation. However, the distinct functions of PKA isozymes have been the subjects of debate because these isozymes exhibit an identical catalytic activity in phosphorylating the target protein. Only during the past decade has experimental evidence started to confer distinct functions to PKA-I and PKA-II, showing that their intracellular, balanced expression may play a critical role in the control of cell growth and differentiation.

Although they both have an identical catalytic subunit, PKA isozymes have distinct regulatory subunits (RI for PKA-I and RII for PKA-II). For this reason, pharmacological interventions targeting the R subunits can distinctly modulate these isozymes in the intact cell. Of these pharmacological agents, antisense oligonucleotides (ODN) targeted against the PKA-I subunit of RIα (antisense RIα), from the unmodified ODN to the more sophisticated RNA-DNA second generation ODN, have provided the first direct evidence that the PKA isoforms have opposite roles in cancer cell growth. PKA-I/RIα appears to promote cell growth, and PKA-II/RIIβ inhibits growth and induces differentiation.

In response to the antisense-directed loss of RIα, RIIβ becomes stabilized into the PKA-II holoenzyme complex. This compensatory stabilization of RIIβ may represent an important biochemical mechanism of antisense RIα that ensures the depletion of PKA-I and ultimately inhibits tumor cell growth. PKA-I inhibition is associated with early inhibition in the expression of growth factors and their receptors (such as TGFα, EGFR, and erbB-2), oncogenes (such as *myc* and *ras*), and angiogenic factors (such as VEGF and bFGF). PKA-I inhibition also results in the induction of apoptosis, in differentiation, and, finally, in growth arrest, as demonstrated both *in vitro* and *in vivo* in mouse models (Cho-Chung et al., 1999; Cho-Chung et al., 1995; Tortora & Ciardiello, 2000).

Studies using cDNA microarrays have demonstrated, for the first time, that the novel hybrid RNA-DNA antisense RIα can modulate, in a sequence-specific manner, a wide set of genes related to cell proliferation and transformation. Antisense RIα also modulates the expression of genes involved in growth arrest and differentiation (Cho et al., 2001). The cDNA microarray approach not only has confirmed and extended the findings of 'conventional' biochemical, molecular biology, and translational approaches, but it has also provided opportunities to define the new molecular signatures of cAMP signaling in reverting tumor cells to a normal phenotype.

To date, the mechanistic aspect of the role of PKA-I in cell proliferation and transformation is still under debate. Gene-transfer experiments have shown that PKA-II is the favored form of holoenzyme over PKA-I in the cell. But what causes the increase in PKA-I observed in cancer cells? Does PKA-I simply titrate out the C subunit that otherwise should be available for the growth inhibitory PKA-IIβ, does it phosphorylate selected targets in specific subcellular regions where it may be located, or does the RIα subunit play an independent, growth regulatory function thus far unexplored?

Despite these questions, the important, therapeutically relevant implication is that the downregulation of RIα expression prevents PKA-I formation, favors PKA-II formation, and eventually leads to tumor growth arrest. That the CRE-transcription factor decoy inhibits cancer cell growth, but not normal cell growth, in response to a block in cAMP-responsive gene expression is an intriguing observation. This observation clearly indicates separate and distant cAMP signaling pathways that regulate growth for normal cells versus cancer cells. For example, germline mutations in the RIα subunit of PKA is responsible for a multiple neoplasia syndrome characteristic of Carney Complex (Kirschner et al., 2000). This suggests a role for RIα as a tumor suppressor during the development of normal embryonic cells (Kirschner et al., 2000). On the other hand, the fact that the oncogene RET/ptc2, which is the product of a papillary thyroid carcinoma translocation event, consists of the c-*ret* proto-oncogene fused with the RIα subunit of PKA (Lanzi et al., 1992) suggests a role for RIα as a positive regulator of tumor cell growth.

The diversity and complexity of the cAMP signaling are highly dependent on different stages of normal cellular development and differentiation, and such signaling is disrupted in an abnormal physiology such as cancer. An intervention targeting cAMP-signaling may therefore provide a more selective and effective method of restraining tumor cell growth without affecting normal cell growth.

Yoon S. Cho-Chung, M.D., Ph.D.
Chief, Cellular Biochemistry Section
Basic Research Laboratories, Center for Cancer Research
National Cancer Institute

6. ACKNOWLEDGEMENT

I thank Dr. Frances McFarland of Palladian Partners, Inc. who provided editorial support under contract number NO2-BC-76212/C2700212 with the National Cancer Institute.

7. REFERENCES

Agrawal, S., & Zhao, Q. (1998). Mixed backbone oligonucleotdes: improvement in oligonucleotide-induced toxicity in vivo. *Antisense & Nucleic Acid Drug Dev, 8*, 135-139.

Ally, S., Tortora, G., Clair, T., Grieco, D., Merlo, G., Katsaros, D., Ogreid, D., Døskeland, S. O., Jahnsen, T., & Cho-Chung, Y. S. (1988). Selective modulation of protein kinase isozymes by the site-selective analog 8-chloroadenosine 3',5'-cyclic monophosphate provides a biological means for control of human colon cancer cell growth. *Proc Natl Acad Sci USA, 85*, 6319-6322.

Alper, O., Bergmann-Leitner, E. S., Abrams, S., & Cho-Chung, Y. S. (2001). Apoptosis, growth arrest and suppression of invasiveness by CRE-decoy oligonucleotide in ovarian cancer cells: protein kinase A downregulation and cytoplasmic export of CRE-binding proteins. *Mol Cell Biochem, 218*(1-2), 55-63.

Alper, O., Hacker, N. F., & Cho-Chung, Y. S. (1999). Protein kinase A-Ialpha subunit-directed antisense inhibition of ovarian cancer cell growth: crosstalk with tyrosine kinase signaling pathway. *Oncogene, 18*(35), 4999-5004.

Amieux, P. S., Cummings, D. E., Motamed, K., Brandon, E. P., Wailes, L. A., Le, K., Idzerda, R. L., & McKnight, G. S. (1997). Compensatory regulation of RIalpha protein levels in protein kinase A mutant mice. *J Biol Chem, 272*(7), 3993-3998.

Arias, J., Alberts, A. S., Brindle, P., Claret, F. X., Smeal, T., Karin, M., Feramisco, J., & Montminy, M. (1994). Activation of cAMP and mitogen responsive genes relies on a common nuclear factor. *Nature, 370*(6486), 226-229.

Beavo, J. A., & Reifsnyder, D. H. (1990). Primary sequence of cyclic nucleotide phosphodiesterase isozymes and the design of selective inhibitors. *Trends Pharmacol Sci, 11*(4), 150-155.

Beebe, S. J., & Corbin, J. D. (1986). Cyclic nucleotide-dependent protein kinases, *The Enzymes: Control by Phosphorylation* (Vol. 17, part A, pp. 43-111). New York: Academic.

Beebe, S. J., Holloway, R., Rannels, S. R., & Corbin, J. D. (1984). Two classes of cAMP analogs which are selective for the two different cAMP-binding sites of type II protein kinase demonstrate synergism when added together to intact adipocytes. *J Biol Chem, 259*(6), 3539-3547.

Beebe, S. J., Oyen, O., Sandberg, M., Froysa, A., Hansson, V., & Jahnsen, T. (1990). Molecular cloning of a unique tissue-specific protein kinase Cg from human testis—representing a third isoform for the catalytic subunit of the cAMP-dependent protein kinase. *Mol Endocrinol, 4*, 465-475.

Bold, R. J., Alpard, S., Ishizuka, J., Townsend, C. M., Jr., & Thompson, J. C. (1994). Growth-regulatory effect of gastrin on human colon cancer cell lines is determined by protein kinase a isoform content. *Regul Pept, 53*(1), 61-70.

Boynton, A. L., & Whitfield, J. F. (1983). The role of cyclic AMP in cell proliferation: a critical assessment of the evidence. In P. Greengard & G. A. Robinson (Eds.), *Advances in cyclic nucleotide research* (Vol. 15, pp. 193-294). New York: Raven Press.

Bradbury, A. W., Carter, D. C., Miller, W. R., Cho-Chung, Y. S., & Clair, T. (1994). Protein kinase A (PK-A) regulatory subunit epxression in colorectal cancer and related mucosa. *Br J Cancer, 69*, 738-742.

Budillon, A., Cereseto, A., Kondrashin, A., Nesterova, M., Merlo, G., Clair, T., & Cho-Chung, Y. S. (1995). Point mutation of the autophosphorylation site or in the nuclear location signal causes protein kinase A RIIb regulatory subunit to lose its ability to revert transformed fibroblasts. *Proc Natl Acad Sci USA, 92*(23), 10634-10638.

Byus, C. V., Klimpel, G. R., Lucas, D. O., & Russell, D. H. (1977). Type I and type II cyclic AMP-dependent protein kinase as opposite effectors of lymphocyte mitogenesis. *Nature, 268*, 63-64.

Chen, H. X., Marshall, J. L., Ness, E., Martin, R. R., Dvorchik, B., Rizvi, N., Marquis, I., McKinlay, M., Dahut, W., & Hawkins, M. J. (2000). A safety and pharmacokinetic study of a mixed-backbone oligonucleotide (GEM 231) targeting the type I protein kinase A by 2-hour infusions in patients with refractory solid tumors. *Clin Cancer Res, 6*, 1259-1266.

Cho, Y. S., Kim, M.-K., Cheadle, C., Neary, C., Becker, K. G., & Cho-Chung, Y. S. (2001). Antisense DNAs as multisite genomic modulators identified by DNA microarray. *Proc Natl Acad Sci U S A, 98*, 9819-9823.

Cho, Y. S., Kim, M.-K., Tan, L., Srivastava, R., Agrawal, S., & Cho-Chung, Y. S. (In press). Protein kinase A RIa antisense inhibition of prostate cancer growth: Bcl-2 hyperphosphorylation, Bax Upregulation, and Bad hypophosphorylaton. *Clin Cancer Res.*

Cho, Y. S., Lee, Y. N., & Cho-Chung, Y. S. (2000). Biochemical characterization of extracellular cAMP-dependent protein kinase as a tumor marker. *Biochem Biophys Res Commun, 278*(3), 679-684.

Cho, Y. S., Park, Y. G., Lee, Y. N., Kim, M. K., Bates, S., Tan, L., & Cho-Chung, Y. S. (2000). Extracellular protein kinase A as a cancer biomarker: its expression by tumor cells and reversal by a myristate-lacking Calpha and RIIbeta subunit overexpression. *Proc Natl Acad Sci U S A, 97*(2), 835-840.

Cho-Chung, Y. S. (1990). Role of cyclic AMP receptor proteins in growth, differentiation, and suppression of malignancy: new approaches to therapy. *Cancer Res, 50*, 7093-7100.

Cho-Chung, Y. S., Clair, T., & Shepheard, C. (1983). Anticarcinogenic effect of N6,O2-dibutyryl cyclic adenosine 3':5'-monophosphate on 7,12-dimethylbenz(a)anthracene mammary tumor induction in the rat and its relationship to cyclic adenosine 3':5'-monophosphate metabolism and protein kinase. *Cancer Res, 43*, 2736-2740.

Cho-Chung, Y. S., Clair, T., Tagliaferri, P., Ally, S., Katsaros, D., Tortora, G., Neckers, L., Avery, T. L., Crabtree, G. W., & Robins, R. K. (1989). Site-selective cyclic AMP analogs as new biological tools in growth control, differentiation and proto-oncogene regulation. *Cancer Inv, 7*, 161-177.

Cho-Chung, Y. S., Clair, T., Tortora, G., & Yokozaki, H. (1991). Role of site-selective cAMP analogs in the control and reversal of malignancy. *Pharmac Ther, 50*, 1-33.

Cho-Chung, Y. S., Clair, T., Tortora, G., Yokozaki, H., & Pepe, S. (1991). Suppression of malignancy targeting the intracellular signal transducing proteins of cAMP: the use of site-selective cAMP analogs, antisense strategy, and gene transfer. *Life Sci, 48*, 1123-1132.

Cho-Chung, Y. S., Nesterova, M., Kondrashin, A., Noguchi, K., Srivastava, R. K., & Pepe, S. (1997). Antisense-protein kinase A: a single-gene-based therapeutic approach. *Antisense & Nucleic Acid Drug Dev, 7*, 217-223.

Cho-Chung, Y. S., Nesterova, M., Pepe, S., Lee, G. R., Noguchi, K., Srivastava, R. K., Srivastava, A. R., Alper, O., Park, Y. G., & Lee, Y. N. (1999). Antisense DNA-targeting protein kinase A-RIA subunit: a novel approach to cancer treatment. *Front Biosci, 4*, D898-907.

Cho-Chung, Y. S., Pepe, S., Clair, T., Budillon, A., & Nesterova, M. (1995). cAMP-dependent protein kinase: role in normal and malignant growth. *Crit Rev Oncol Hematol, 21*(1-3), 33-61.

Chrivia, J. C., Kwok, R. P., Lamb, N., Hagiwara, M., Montminy, M. R., & Goodman, R. H. (1993). Phosphorylated CREB binds specifically to the nuclear protein CBP. *Nature, 365*(6449), 855-859.

Ciardiello, F., Pepe, S., Bianco, C., Baldassarre, G., Ruggiero, A., Selvam, M. P., Bianco, A. R., & Tortora, G. (1993). Down-regulation of RIa subunit of cAMP-dependent protein kinase induces growth inhibition of human mammary epithelial cells transformed by c-Ha-ras and c-erbB-2 proto-oncogenes. *Int J Cancer, 53*(3), 438-443.

Ciardiello, F., Tortora, G., Kim, N., Clair, T., Ally, S., Salomon, D. S., & Cho-Chung, Y. S. (1990). 8-Chloro-cAMP inhibits transforming growth factor a transformation of mammary epithelial cells by restoration of the normal mRNA patterns for cAMP-dependent protein kinase regulatory subunit isoforms which show disruption upon transformation. *J Biol Chem, 265*, 1016-1020.

Clair, T., Ally, S., Tagliaferri, P., Robins, R. K., & Cho-Chung, Y. S. (1987). Site-selective cAMP analogs induce nuclear translocation of the RII cAMP receptor protein in Ha-MuSV-transformed NIH/3T3 cells. *FEBS Lett, 224*(2), 377-384.

Conti, M., Jin, S. L., Monaco, L., Repaske, D. R., & Swinnen, J. V. (1991). Hormonal regulation of cyclic nucleotide phosphodiesterases. *Endocr Rev, 12*(3), 218-234.

Corbin, J. D., Sugden, P. H., West, L., Flockhart, D. A., Lincoln, T. M., & McCarthy, D. (1978). Studies on the properties and mode of action of the purified regulatory subunit of bovine heart adenosine 3',5'-monophosphate-dependent protein kinase. *J Biol Chem, 253*(11), 3997-4003.

Crombrugghe, B. D., Busby, S., & Buc, H. (1984). Activation of transcription by the cyclic AMP receptor protein. In R. F. Goodberger & K. R. Yamamoto (Eds.), *Biological regulation and development* (Vol. 3B, pp. 129-167). New York: Plenum Press.

Cvijic, M. E., Kita, T., Shih, W., DiPaola, R. S., & Chin, K. V. (2000). Extracellular catalytic subunit activity of the cAMP-dependent protein kinase in prostate cancer. *Clin Cancer Res, 6*(6), 2309-2317.

Døskeland, S. O. (1978). Evidence that rabbit muscle protein kinase has two kinetically distinct binding sites for adenosine 3',5'-cyclic monophosphate. *Biochem Biophys Res Commun, 83*, 542-549.

Døskeland, S. O., Maronde, E., & Gjertsen, B. T. (1993). The genetic subtypes of cAMP-dependent protein kinase--functionally different or redundant? *Biochim Biophys Acta, 1178*(3), 249-258.

Ekanger, R., Øgreid, D., Evjen, O., Vintermyr, O., Laerum, O. D., & Doskeland, S. O. (1985). Characterization of cyclic adenosine 3':5'-monophosphate-dependent protein kinase isozymes in normal and neoplastic fetal rat brain cells. *Cancer Res, 45*(6), 2578-2583.

Flockhart, D. A., & Corbin, J. D. (1982). Regulatory mechanisms in the control of protein kinases. *CRC Crit Rev Biochem, 12*(2), 133-186.

Fossberg, T. M., Døskeland, S. O., & Ueland, P. M. (1978). Protein kinases in human renal cell carcinoma and renal cortex. A comparison of isozyme distribution and of responsiveness to adenosine 3':5'-cyclic monophosphate. *Arch Biochem Biophys, 189*(2), 272-281.

Friedman, D. L. (1976). Role of cyclic nucleotides in cell growth and differentiation. *Physiol Rev, 56*, 652-708.

Gettys, T., & Corbin, J. D. (1989). The protein kinase family of enzymes. In V. Moudgil (Ed.), *Receptor Phosphorylation* (pp. 40-88). Boca Raton: CRC Press.

Gharrett, A. J., Malkinson, A. M., & Sheppard, J. R. (1976). Cyclic AMP-dependent protein kinases from normal and SV40-transformed 3T3 cells. *Nature, 264*, 673-675.

Ginty, D. D., Bonni, A., & Greenberg, M. E. (1994). Nerve growth factor activates a ras-dependent protein kinase that stimulates c-*fos* transcription via phosphorylation of CREB. *Cell, 77*, 713-725.

Gonzalez, G. A., Biggs, W., III, Vale, W. W., & Montminy, M. R. (1989). A cluster of phosphorylation sites on the cyclic AMP-regulated nucleoar factor CREB predicated by its sequence. *Nature, 337*, 749-752.

Gonzalez, G. A., & Montminy, M. R. (1989). Cyclic AMP stimulates somatostatin gene transcription by phosphorylation of CREB at serine 133. *Cell, 59*, 675-680.

Goodman, R. H., & Smolik, S. (2000). CBP/p300 in cell growth, transformation, and development. *Genes Dev, 14*(13), 1553-1577.

Gordge, P. C., Hulme, M. J., Clegg, R. A., & Miller, W. R. (1996). Elevation of protein kinase A and protein kinase C activities in malignant as compared with normal human breast tissue. *Eur J Cancer, 32A*, 2120-2126.

Handschin, J. S., & Eppenberger, U. (1979). Altered cellular ratio of type I and type II cyclic AMP-dependent protein kinase in human mammary tumors. *FEBS Lett, 106*, 301-304.

Harada, H., Becknell, B., Wilm M, M., M , Huang, L. J., Taylor, S. S., Scott, J. D., & Korsmeyer, S. J. (1999). Phosphorylation and inactivation of BAD by mitochondria-anchored protein kinase A. *Mol Cell, 3*(4), 413-422.

Houge, G., Steinberg, R. A., Ogreid, D., & Doskeland, S. O. (1990). The rate of recombination of the subunits (RI and C) of cAMP-dependent protein kinase depends on whether one or two cAMP molecules are bound per RI monomer. *J Biol Chem, 265*(32), 19507-19516.

Hsie, A. W., & Puck, T. T. (1971). Morphological transformation of Chinese hamster cells by dibutyryl adenosine cyclic 3':5'-monophosphate and testosterone. *Proc Natl Acad Sci USA, 68*, 358-361.

Katsaros, D., Tortora, G., Tagliaferri, P., Clair, T., Ally, S., Neckers, L., Robins, R. K., & Cho-Chung, Y. S. (1987). Site-selective cyclic AMP analogs provide a new approach in the control of cancer cell growth. *FEBS Lett, 223*, 97-103.

Kim, S. N., Kim, S. G., Park, J. H., Lee, M. A., Park, S. D., Cho-Chung, Y. S., & Hong, S. H. (2000). Dual anticancer activity of 8-Cl-cAMP: inhibition of cell proliferation and induction of apoptotic cell death. *Biochem Biophys Res Commun, 273*(2), 404-410.

Kirschner, L. S., Carney, J. A., Pack, S. D., Taymans, S. E., Giatzakis, C., Cho, Y. S., Cho-Chung, Y. S., & Stratakis, C. A. (2000). Mutations of the gene encoding the protein kinase A type I-alpha regulatory subunit in patients with the Carney complex. *Nat Genet, 26*(1), 89-92.

Klimpel, G. R., Byus, C. V., Russell, D. H., & Lucas, D. O. (1979). Cyclic AMP-dependent protein kinase activation and the induction of ornithine decarboxylase during lymphocyte mitogenesis. *J Immunol, 123*(2), 817-824.

Krebs, E. G. (1972). Protein kinases. *Curr Top Cell Regul, 5*, 99-133.

Krieg, A. M., Yi, A. K., Matson, S., Waldschmidt, T. J., Bishop, G. A., Teasdale, R., Koretzky, G. A., & Klinman, D. M. (1995). CpG motifs in bacterial DNA trigger direct B-cell activation. *Nature, 374*(6522), 546-549.

Lange-Carter, C. A., Vuillequez, J. J., & Malkinson, A. M. (1993). 8-Chloroadenosine mediates 8-chloro-cyclic AMP-induced down-regulation of cyclic AMP-dependent protein kinase in normal and neoplastic mouse lung epithelial cells by a cyclic AMP-independent mechanism. *Cancer Res, 53*(2), 393-400.

Lanzi, C., Borrello, M. G., Bongarzone, I., Migliazza, A., Fusco, A., Grieco, M., Santoro, M., Gambetta, R. A., Zunino, F., Della Porta, G., & et al. (1992). Identification of the product of two oncogenic rearranged forms of the RET proto-oncogene in papillary thyroid carcinomas. *Oncogene, 7*(11), 2189-2194.

Ledinko, N., & Chan, I.-J. A. D. (1984). Increase in type I cyclic adenosine 3',5'-monophosphate-dependent protein kinase activity and specific accumulation of type I regulatory subunits in adenovirus type 12-transformed cells. *Cancer Res, 44*, 2622-2627.

Lee, G. R., Kim, S. N., Noguchi, K., Park, S. D., Hong, S. H., & Cho-Chung, Y. S. (1999). Ala99ser mutation in RI alpha regulatory subunit of protein kinase A causes reduced kinase activation by cAMP and arrest of hormone- dependent breast cancer cell growth. *Mol Cell Biochem, 195*(1-2), 77-86.

Lee, R. J., Albanese, C., Stenger, R. J., Watanabe, G., Inghirami, G., Haines, G. K., 3rd, Webster, M., Muller, W. J., Brugge, J. S., Davis, R. J., & Pestell, R. G. (1999). pp60(v-src) induction of cyclin D1 requires collaborative interactions between the extracellular signal-regulated kinase, p38, and Jun kinase pathways. A role for cAMP response element-binding protein and activating transcription factor-2 in pp60(v-src) signaling in breast cancer cells. *J Biol Chem, 274*(11), 7341-7350.

Lee, Y. N., Park, Y. G., Choi, Y. H., Cho, Y. S., & Cho-Chung, Y. S. (2000). CRE-transcription factor decoy oligonucleotide inhibition of MCF-7 breast cancer cells: cross-talk with p53 signaling pathway. *Biochemistry, 39*(16), 4863-4868.

Livesey, S. A., Kemp, B. E., Re, C. A., Partridge, N. C., & Martin, T. J. (1982). Selective hormonal activation of cyclic AMP-dependent protein kinase isoenzymes in normal and malignant osteoblasts. *J Biol Chem, 257*(24), 14983-14987.

Lohmann, S. M., & Walter, U. (1984). Regulation of the cellular and subcellular concentrations and distribution of cyclic nucleotide-dependent protein kinases. In P. Greengard & G. A. Robinson (Eds.), *Advances in cyclic nucleotide and protein phosphorylation research* (Vol. 18, pp. 63-117). New York: Raven Press.

McDaid, H. M., Cairns, M. T., Atkinson, R. I., McAleer, S., Harkin, D. P., Gilmore, P., & Johnston, P. G. (1999). Increased expression of the RIa subunit of the cAMP-dependent protein kinase A is associated with advanced stage of ovarian cancer. *Br. J. Cancer, 79*, 933-939.

McKnight, G. S., Clegg, C. H., Uhler, M. D., Chrivia, J. C., Cadd, G. G., Correll, L. A., & Otten, A. D. (1988). Analysis of the cAMP-dependent protein kinase system using molecular genetic approaches. *Recent Prog Horm Res, 44*, 307-335.

Metelev, V., Liszlewicz, J., & Agrawal, S. (1994). Study of antisense oligonucleotide phosphorothioates containing segments of oligodeoxynucleotides and 2'-O-methyloligoribonucleotides. *Bioorg Medicinal Chem Lett, 4*, 2929-2934.

Miller, W. R., Hulme, M. J., Cho-Chung, Y. S., & Elton, R. A. (1993). Types of cyclic AMP binding proteins in human breast cancers. *Eur J Cancer, 29A*, 989-991.

Miller, W. R., Watson, D. M. A., Jack, W., Chetty, U., & Elton, R. A. (1993). Tumor cyclic AMP binding proteins: An independent prognostic factor for disease recurrence and survival in breast cancer. *Breast Cancer Res Treat, 26*, 89-94.

Monia, B. P., Lesnik, E. A., Gonzalez, C., Lima, W. F., McGee, D., Guinosso, C. J., Kawasaki, A. M., Cook, P. D., & Freier, S. M. (1993). Evaluation of 2'-modified oligonucleotides containing 2'-deoxygaps as antisense inhibitors of gene expression. *J Biol Chem, 268*, 14514-14522.

Montminy, M. R., & Bilezikjian, L. M. (1987). Binding of a nuclear protein to the cyclic-AMP response element of the somatostatin gene. *Nature, 328*(6126), 175-178.

Nakajima, F., Imashuku, S., Wilimas, J., Champion, J. E., & Green, A. A. (1984). Distribution and properties of type I and type II binding proteins in the cyclic adenosine 3':5'-monophosphate-dependent protein kinase system in Wilms' tumor. *Cancer Res, 44*(11), 5182-5187.

Neary, C. L., & Cho-Chung, Y. S. (2001). Nuclear translocation of the catalytic subunit of protein kinase A induced by an antisense oligonucleotide directed against the RIalpha regulatory subunit. *Oncogene, 20*(55), 8019-8024.

Nesterova, M., & Cho-Chung, Y. S. Unpublished.

Nesterova, M., & Cho-Chung, Y. S. (1995). A single-injection protein kinase A-directed antisense treatment to inhibit humor growth. *Nat Med, 1*, 528-633.

Nesterova, M., & Cho-Chung, Y. S. (2000). Oligonucleotide sequence-specific inhibition of gene expression, tumor growth inhibition, and modulation of cAMP signaling by an RNA-DNA hybrid antisense targeted to protein kinase A RIa subunit. *Antisense & Nucleic Acid Drug Development, 10*, 423-433.

Nesterova, M., Noguchi, K., Park, Y. G., Lee, Y. N., & Cho-Chung, Y. S. (2000). Compensatory stabilization of RIIb protein, cell cycle deregulation, and growth arrest in colon and prostate carcinoma cells by antisense-directed down-regulation of protein kinase A RIa protein. *Clinical Cancer Research, 6*, 3434-3441.
Nesterova, M. V., Yokozaki, H., McDuffie, L., & Cho-Chung, Y. S. (1996). Overexpression of RIIb regulatory subunit of protein kinase A in human colon carcinoma cell induces growth arrest and phenotypic changes that are abolished by site-directed mutation of RIIb. *Eur J Cancer, 253*, 486-494.
Øgreid, D., Ekanger, R., Suva, R. H., Muller, J. P., Sturm, P., Corbin, J. D., & Doskeland, S. O. (1985). Activation of protein kinase isozymes by cyclic nucleotide analygs used singly or in combination. *Eur J Biochem, 150*, 219-227.
Park, Y. G., Nesterova, M., Agrawal, S., & Cho-Chung, Y. S. (1999). Dual blockade of cyclic AMP response element- (CRE) and AP-1-directed transcription by CRE-transcription factor decoy oligonucleotide. gene- specific inhibition of tumor growth. *J Biol Chem, 274*(3), 1573-1580.
Park, Y. G., Park, S., Lim, S. O., Lee, M. S., Ryu, C. K., Kim, I., & Cho-Chung, Y. S. (2001). Reduction in cyclin D1/Cdk4/retinoblastoma protein signaling by CRE- decoy oligonucleotide. *Biochem Biophys Res Commun, 281*(5), 1213-1219.
Pastan, I., Johnson, G. S., & Anderson, W. B. (1975). Role of cyclic nucleotides in growth control. *Ann Rev Biochem, 44*, 491 522.
Piroli, G., Weisenberg, L. S., Grillo, C., & De Nicola, A. F. (1990). Subcellular distribution of cyclic adenosine 3',5'-monophosphate- binding protein and estrogen receptors in control pituitaries and estrogen-induced pituitary tumors. *J Natl Cancer Inst, 82*(7), 596-601.
Prasad, K. N. (1975). Differentiation of neuroblastoma cells in culture. *Biol Rev Camb Philos Soc, 50*, 129-165.
Rannels, S. R., & Corbin, J. D. (1980). Two different intrachain cAMP binding sites of cAMP-dependent protein kinases. *J Biol Chem, 255*, 7085-7088.
Roesler, W. J., Vandenbark, G. R., & Hanson, R. W. (1988). Cyclic AMP and the induction of eukaryotic gene transcription. *J Biol Chem, 263*(19), 9063-9066.
Rohlff, C., Clair, T., & Cho-Chung, Y. S. (1993). 8-Cl-cAMP induces truncation and down-regulation of the RIa subunit and up-regulation of the RIIb subunit of cAMP-dependent protein kinase leading to type II holoenzyme-dependent growth inhibition and differentiation of HL-60 leukemia cells. *J Biol Chem, 268*, 5774-5782.
Rohlff, C., & Glazer, R. I. (1995). Regulation of multidrug resistance through the cAMP and EGF signaling pathways. *Cell Signal, 7*, 431-443.
Rosen, O. M., & Erlichman, J. (1975). Reversible autophosphorylation of a cyclic 3':5'-AMP-dependent protein kinase from bovine cardiac muscle. *J Biol Chem, 250*(19), 7788-7794.
Ryan, W. L., & Heidrick, M. L. (1974). Role of cyclic nucleotides in cancer. *Adv Cycl Nucl Res, 4*, 81-116.
Schena, M., Shalon, D., Davis, R. W., & Brown, P. O. (1995). Quantitative monitoring of gene expression patterns with a complementary DNA microarray. *Science, 270*(5235), 467-470.
Schwoch, G. (1978). Differential activation of type-I and type-II adenosine 3':5'-cyclic monophosphate-dependent protein kinases in liver of glucagon-treated rats. *Biochem J, 170*(3), 469-477.
Sheng, M., Thompson, M. A., & Greenberg, M. E. (1991). CREB: a Ca(2+)-regulated transcription factor phosphorylated by calmodulin-dependent kinases. *Science, 252*(5011), 1427-1430.
Shibahara, S., Mukai, S., Morisawa, H., Nakashima, H., Kobayashi, S., & Yamamoto, N. (1989). Inhibition of human immunodeficiency virus (HIV-1) replication by synthetic oligo-RNA derivatives. *Nucleic Acids Res, 17*(1), 239-252.
Showers, M. O., & Maurer, R. A. (1986). A cloned bovine cDNA encodes an alternate form of the catalytic subunit of cAMP-dependent protein kinase. *J Biol Chem, 261*, 16288-16291.
Simpson, B. J. B., Ramage, A. D., Hulme, M. J., Burns, D. J., Katsaros, D., Langdon, S. P., & Miller, W. R. (1996). Cyclic adenosine 3',5'-monophosphate-binding proteins in human ovarian cancer: Correlations with clinicapachological features. *Clin Cancer Res, 2*, 201-206.
Srivastava, R. K., Lee, Y. N., Noguchi, K., Park, Y. G., Ellis, M. J., Jeong, J. S., Kim, S. N., & Cho-Chung, Y. S. (1998). The RIIb regulatory subunit of protein kinase A binds to cAMP response element: an alternative cAMP signaling pathway. *Proc Natl Acad Sci USA, 95*(12), 6687-6692.
Srivastava, R. K., Srivastava, A. R., Park, Y. G., Agrawal, S., & Cho-Chung, Y. S. (1998). Antisense depletion of RIalpha subunit of protein kinase A induces apoptosis and growth arrest in human breast cancer cells. *Breast Cancer Res Treat, 49*(2), 97-107.

Srivastava, R. K., Srivastava, A. R., Seth, P., Agrawal, S., & Cho-Chung, Y. S. (1999). Growth arrest and induction of apoptosis in breast cancer cells by antisense depletion of protein kinase A-RI alpha subunit: p53- independent mechanism of action. *Mol Cell Biochem, 195*(1-2), 25-36.

Steinberg, R. A., & Agard, D. A. (1981). Turnover of regulatory subunit of cyclic AMP-dependent protein kinase in S49 mouse lymphoma cells. Regulation by catalytic subunit and analogs of cyclic AMP. *J Biol Chem, 256*(21), 10731-10734.

Sutherland, E. W. (1972). Studies on the mechanism of hormone action. *Science, 177*(47), 401-408.

Sutherland, E. W., & Rall, T. W. (1957). Properties of an adenine ribonucleotide produced with cellular particles, adenosinetriphosphate, magnesium, and adrenaline or glucagon. *J Am Chem Soc, 79*, 3608.

Tagliaferri, P., Clair, T., DeBortoli, M. E., & Cho-Chung, Y. S. (1985). Two classes of cAMP analogs synergistically inhibit p21 ras protein synthesis and phenotypic transformation of NIH/3T3 cells transfected with Ha-MuSV DNA. *Biochem Biophys Res Commun, 130*, 1193-1200.

Tagliaferri, P., Katsaros, D., Clair, T., Ally, S., Tortora, G., Neckers, L., Rubalcava, B., Parandoosh, Z., Chang, Y. A., Revankar, G. R., & et al. (1988). Synergistic inhibition of growth of breast and colon human cancer cell lines by site-selective cyclic AMP analogues. *Cancer Res, 48*(6), 1642-1650.

Tagliaferri, P., Katsaros, D., Clair, T., Neckers, L., Robins, R. K., & Cho-Chung, Y. S. (1988). Reverse transformation of Harvey murine sarcoma virus-transformed NIH/3T3 cells by site-selective cyclic AMP analogs. *J Biol Chem, 263*, 409-416.

Takio, K., Smith, S. B., Krebs, E. G., Walsh, K. A., & Titani, K. (1984). Amino acid sequence of the regulatory subunit of bovine type II adenosine cyclic 3',5'-phosphate dependent protein kinase. *Biochemistry, 23*(18), 4200-4206.

Tan, Y., Rouse, J., Zhang, A., Cariati, S., Cohen, P., & Comb, M. J. (1996). FGF and stress regulate CREB and ATF-1 via a pathway involving p38 MAP kinase and MAPKAP kinase-2. *Embo J, 15*(17), 4629-4642.

Taylor, C. W., & Yeoman, L. C. (1992). Inhibition of colon tumor cell growth by 8-chloro-cAMP is dependent upon its conversion to 8-chloro-adenosine. *Anticancer Drugs, 3*(5), 485-491.

Taylor, S. S., Bubis, J., Toner-Webb, J., Saraswat, L. D., First, E. A., Buechler, J. A., Knighton, D. R., & Sowadski, J. (1988). cAMP-dependent protein kinase: prototype for a family of enzymes. *FASEB J, 2*, 2677-2685.

Titani, K., Sasagawa, T., Ericsson, L. H., Kumar, S., Smith, S. B., Krebs, E. G., & Walsh, K. A. (1984). Amino acid sequence of the regulatory subunit of bovine type I adenosine cyclic 3',5'-phosphate dependent protein kinase. *Biochemistry, 23*(18), 4193-4199.

Tortora, G., Bianco, R., Damiano, V., Fontanini, G., De Placido, S., Bianco, A. R., & Ciardiello, F. (2000). Oral antisense that targets protein kinase A cooperates with taxol and inhibits tumor growth, angiogenesis, and growth factor production. *Clin Cancer Res, 6*(6), 2506-2512.

Tortora, G., Budillon, A., Yokozaki, H., Clair, T., Pepe, S., Merlo, G., Rohlff, C., & Cho-Chung, Y. S. (1994). Retroviral vector-mediated overexpression of the RIIb subunit of the cAMP-dependent protein kinase induces differentiation in human leukemia cells and reverts the transformed phenotype of mouse fibroblasts. *Cell Growth Differ, 5*(7), 753-759.

Tortora, G., & Cho-Chung, Y. S. (1990). Type II regulatory subunit of protein kinase restores cAMP-dependent transcription in a cAMP-unresponsive cell line. *J Biol Chem, 265*(30), 18067-18070.

Tortora, G., & Ciardiello, F. (2000). Targeting of epidermal growth factor receptor and protein kinase A: molecular basis and therapeutic applications. *Ann Oncol, 11*(7), 777-783.

Tortora, G., Ciardiello, F., Ally, S., Clair, T., Salomon, D. S., & Cho-Chung, Y. S. (1989). Site-selective 8-chloroadenosine 3',5'-cyclic monophosphate inhibits transformation and transforming growth factor alpha production in Ki- ras-transformed rat fibroblasts. *FEBS Lett, 242*(2), 363-367.

Tortora, G., Ciardiello, F., Pepe, S., Tagliaferri, P., Ruggiere, A., Blanco, C., Guarrand, R., Miki, K., & Blanco, R. (1995). Phase I clinical study with 8-chloro-cAMP and evaluation of immunological effects in cancer patients. *Clin Cancer Res, 4*, 377-384.

Tortora, G., Clair, T., & Cho-Chung, Y. S. (1990). An antisense oligodeoxynucleotide targeted against the type RIIb regulatory subunit mRNA of protein kinase inhibits cAMP-induced differentiation in HL-60 leukemia cells without affecting phorbol ester effects. *Proc Natl Acad Sci USA, 87*, 705-708.

Tortora, G., Damiano, V., Bianco, C., Baldassarre, G., Bianco, A. R., Lanfrancone, L., Pelicci, P. G., & Ciardiello, F. (1997). The RIa subunit of protein kinase A (PKA) binds to Grb2 and allows PKA interaction with the activated EGF-receptor. *Oncogene, 14*(8), 923-928.

Tortora, G., Pepe, S., Bianco, C., Baldassarre, G., Budillon, A., Clair, T., Cho-Chung, Y. S., Bianco, A. R., & Ciardiello, F. (1994). The RIa subunit of protein kinase A controls serum dependency and entry into cell cycle of human mammary epithelial cells. *Oncogene, 9*(11), 3233-3240.

Tortora, G., Pepe, S., Cirafici, A. M., Ciardiello, F., Porcellini, A., Clair, T., Colletta, G., Cho-Chung, Y. S., & Bianco, A. R. (1993). Thyroid-stimulating hormone-regulated growth and cell cycle distribution of thyroid cells involve type I isozyme of cyclic AMP- dependent protein kinase. *Cell Growth Differ, 4*(5), 359-365.

Tortora, G., Tagliaferri, P., Clair, T., Colamonici, O., Neckers, L. M., Robins, R. K., & Cho-Chung, Y. S. (1988). Site-selective cAMP analogs at micromolar concentrations induce growth arrest and differentiation of acute promyelocytic, chronic myelocytic, and acute lymphocytic human leukemia cell lines. *Blood, 71*, 230-233.

Tortora, G., Yokozaki, H., Pepe, S., Clair, T., & Cho-Chung, Y. S. (1991). Differentiation of HL-60 leukemia cells by type I regulatory subunit antisense oligodeoxynucleotide of cAMP-dependent protein kinase. *Proc. Natl. Acad. Sci. USA, 88*, 2011-2015.

Van Lookeren Campagne, M. M., Villalba Diaz, F., Jastorff, B., & Kessin, R. H. (1991). 8-Chloroadenosine 3',5'-monophosphate inhibits the growth of Chinese hamster ovary and Molt-4 cells through its adenosine metabolite. *Cancer Res, 51*(6), 1600-1605.

Walsh, D. A., Perkins, J. P., & Krebs, E. G. (1968). An adenosine 3',5'-monophosphate-dependant protein kinase from rabbit skeletal muscle. *J Biol Chem, 243*(13), 3763-3765.

Walton, K. M., Rehfuss, R. P., Chrivia, J. C., Lochner, J. E., & Goodman, R. H. (1992). A dominant repressor of cyclic adenosine 3',5'-monophosphate (cAMP)- regulated enhancer-binding protein activity inhibits the cAMP-mediated induction of the somatostatin promoter in vivo. *Mol Endocrinol, 6*(4), 647-655.

Wang, H., Cai, Q., Zeng, X., Yu, D., Agrawal, S., & Zhang, M. Q. (1999). Antitumor activity and pharmacokenetics of a mixed-backbone antisense oligonucleotide targeted to the RIa subunit of protein kinase A after oral administration. *Proc Natl Acad Sci USA, 96*, 13989-13994.

Wehner, J. M., Malkinson, A. M., Wiser, M. F., & Sheppard, J. R. (1981). Cyclic AMP-dependent protein kinases from Balb 3T3 cells and other 3T3 derived lines. *J Cell Physiol, 108*, 175-184.

Wu, J., Dent, P., Jelinek, T., Wolfman, A., Weber, M. J., & Sturgill, T. W. (1993). Inhibition of the EGF-activated MAP kinase signaling pathway by adenosine 3',5'-monophosphate. *Science, 262*(5136), 1065-1069.

Xie, S., Price, J. E., Luca, M., Jean, D., Ronai, Z., & Bar-Eli, M. (1997). Dominant-negative CREB inhibits tumor growth and metastasis of human melanoma cells. *Oncogene, 15*(17), 2069-2075.

Xing, J., Ginty, D. D., & Greenberg, M. E. (1996). Coupling of the RAS-MAPK pathway to gene activation by RSK2, a growth factor-regulated CREB kinase. *Science, 273*(5277), 959-963.

Yang, W. L., Iacono, L., Tang, W. M., & Chin, K. V. (1998). Novel function of the regulatory subunit of protein kinase A: regulation of cytochrome c oxidase activity and cytochrome c release. *Biochemistry, 37*(40), 14175-14180.

Yasui, W., & Tahara, E. (1985). Effect of gastrin on gastric mucosal cyclic adenosine 3',5'-monophosphate-dependent protein kinase activity in rat stomach carcinogenesis induced by *N*-methyl-*N*-nitro-*N*-nitrosoguanidine. *Cancer Res, 45*, 4763-4767.

Yokozaki, H., Budillon, A., Clair, G. T., Kelley, K., Cowan, K. H., Rohlff, C., Glazer, R. I., & Cho-Chung, Y. S. (1993). 8-chloroadenosine 3',5'-monophosphate as a novel modulator of multidrug resistance. *Int J Oncol, 3*, 423-430.

Yokozaki, H., Budillon, A., Tortora, G., Meissner, S., Beaucage, S. L., Miki, K., & Cho-Chung, Y. S. (1993). An antisense oligodeoxynucleotide that depletes RIa subunit of cyclic AMP-dependent protein kinase induces growth inhibition in human cancer cells. *Cancer Res, 53*, 868-872.

Young, M. R. I., Montpettit, M., Lozano, Y., Djordjevic, A., Devata, S., Matthews, I. P., Yedavalli, S., & Chejfec, G. (1995). Regulation of Lewis lung carcinoma invasion and metastasis by protein kinase A. *Int J Cancer, 61*, 104-109.

Zamecnik, P., & Stephenson, M. (1978). Inhibition of Rous sarcoma virus replication and cell transformation by a specific oligodeoxynucleotide. *Proc Natl Acad Sci USA, 75*(75), 280-284.

PI3K/PTEN/AKT PATHWAY

A critical mediator of oncogenic signaling

JUAN PAEZ AND WILLIAM R. SELLERS

1. INTRODUCTION

Phosphoinositide 3-kinase (PI3K) plays a crucial role in effecting alterations in a broad range of cellular functions in response to extracellular signals. A key downstream effector of PI3K is the serine-threonine kinase Akt which in response to PI3K activation, phosphorylates and regulates the activity of a number of targets including kinases, transcription factors and other regulatory molecules. A causal link between activation of PI3K and the process of cellular transformation was first appreciated in the mid 1980's when the oncogenic activity of Middle T antigen of Polyoma virus was linked to its ability to induce PI3K activity. A major role for PI3K pathway activation in human tumors has been more recently established following both the positional cloning of the *PTEN* tumor suppressor gene, and the discovery that the PTEN protein product was a lipid phosphatase that antagonizes PI3K function and consequently inhibits downstream signaling through Akt.

Subsequently a number of the components of the pathway have been found mutated or deregulated in a wide variety of human cancers highlighting the key role of this pathway in cellular transformation.

A comprehensive review of the PI3K/PTEN/Akt pathway is beyond the scope of this chapter and has been covered elsewhere (Fruman, Meyers, & Cantley, 1998; Katso et al., 2001; Vanhaesebroeck & Waterfield, 1999).

2. THE PATHWAY

2.1. Overview

Phosphoinositides (Ptdlns) are rare lipids. A large family of lipid kinases are capable of phosphorylating these lipids and are sub-classified based upon their structure and preferred substrates. The class I PI3Ks catalyse the conversion of phosphatidylinositol-3,4-bisphosphate (Ptdlns-4,5-P_2) to phosphatidylinositol-3,4,5-trisphosphate (Ptdlns-3,4,5-P_3). Ptdlns-3,4,5-P_3 is absent or undetectable in resting cells but is acutely increased in response to multiple stimuli that activate type I PI3K.

A large number of the plasma membrane receptors, in particular those with tyrosine kinase activity, can activate class I PI3Ks. For instance, binding of insulin-like growth factor-1 (IGF-1) to its cognate receptor IGF1R leads to receptor activation and autophosphorylation on tyrosine residues. This in turn leads, through an adaptor molecule, to the recruitment of PI3K to the membrane. Cytokines and cell attachment to the extracellular matrix also stimulate PI3K activity. Once activated and localized to the membrane, PI3K phosphorylates phosphoinositol lipids on the D3 position of the inositol ring generating Ptdlns-3-phosphates (Ptdlns-3,4-P_2 and

PtdIns-3,4,5-P_3). These specialized lipids serve to recruit pleckstrin homology (PH) domain-containing proteins such as the serine-threonine kinase Akt and PDK1 (phosphoinositide-dependent kinase 1) to the plasma membrane. After recruitment to the membrane, Akt is phophorylated and consequently activated, by PDK. In turn, Akt phosphorylates multiple proteins on serine and threonine residues (see Figure 1 and further below). Through phosphorylation of these targets, Akt carries out its role as a key regulator of a variety of critical cell functions including glucose metabolism, cell proliferation and survival.

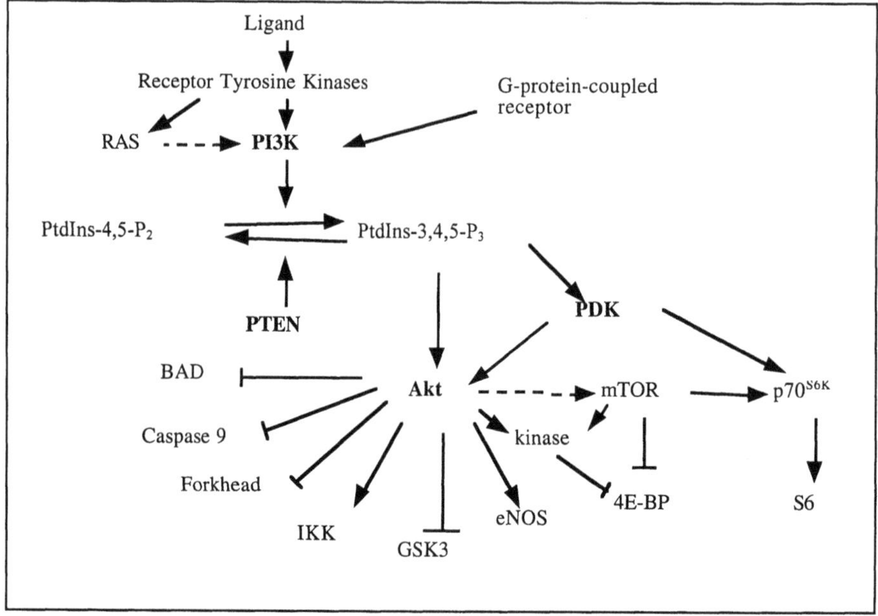

Figure 1. The PI3K/PTEN/Akt pathway. GSK3 (glycogen synthase 3), p70^{S6K} (ribosomal protein S6 kinase), BAD (Bcl-2, Bcl$_{XL}$-antagonist causing cell death), IKK (IκB kinase), eNOS (endothelial nitric oxide synthase), mTOR (mammalian target of rapamycin)4E-BP (eukaryotic translation initiation factor 4E binding protein).

This pathway is highly conserved among different species including *Drosophila melanogaster*, *Caenorhabditis elegans* and mammals. Studies in Drosophila have established the involvement of this pathway in the regulation of cell size and number (Brogiolo et al., 2001; Goberdhan, Paricio, Goodman, Mlodzik, & Wilson, 1999; Huang et al., 1999; Oldham, Bohni, Stocker, Brogiolo, & Hafen, 2000; Verdu, Buratovich, Wilder, & Birnbaum, 1999). Genetic studies in *C. elegans* have linked this pathway to regulation of the dauer formation. The dauer phenotype is a larval state characterised by developmental arrest and reduced metabolic rate triggered by adverse environmental conditions including nutrient deprivation and overcrowding. Genetic dissection of the genes involved in this pathway led to the identification of the *daf* (dauer affected) genes (Lin, Dorman, Rodan, & Kenyon, 1997; Ogg & Ruvkun, 1998), some of which are the homologs of the mammalian components of the insulin-PI3K signaling. Figure 2 depicts the main components of this pathway conserved among different species.

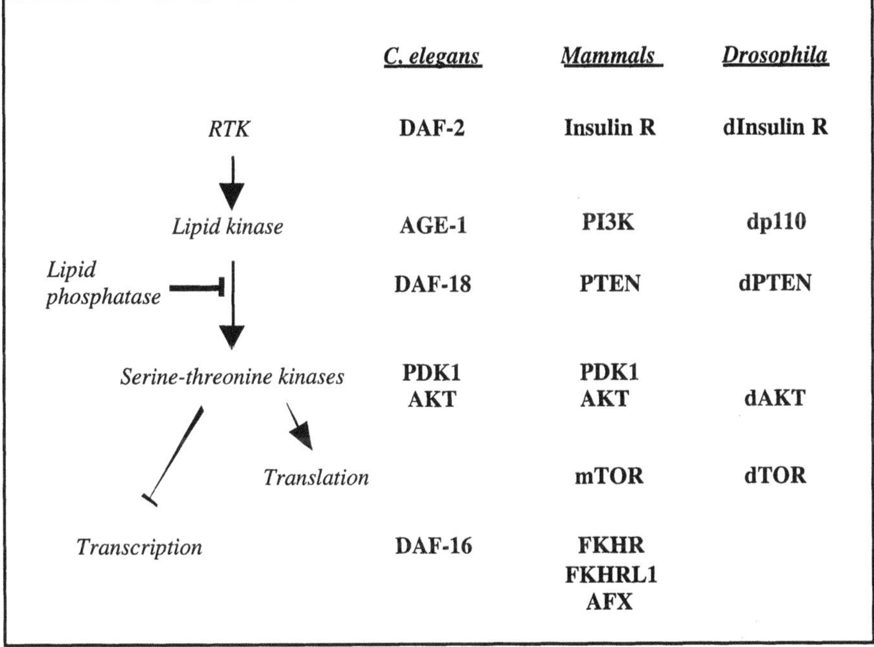

Figure 2. The PI3K/PTEN/Akt pathway in different species.

2.2. Phosphoinositide 3- kinases (PI3K).

PI3K belongs to a large family of PI3K-related kinases or PIKK. Other members of the family include mTOR (mammalian target of rapamycin), ATM (ataxia-telangiectasia mutated), ATR (ATM and RAD3 related), DNA-PK (DNA-dependent protein kinase). All possess the characteristic PI3K-homologous kinase domain and a highly conserved carboxyl-terminal tail (Kuruvilla & Schreiber, 1999). However, only PI3K is known to have an endogenous lipid substrate. Importantly, all members of the PIKK family have been implicated in human cancer both as oncogenes in the case of type I PI3K or as tumor suppressor genes in the case of ATM and ATR.

The PI3K family (see table 1) comprises eight members divided into three classes according to their sequence homology and substrate preference (reviewed in (Fruman et al., 1998; Vanhaesebroeck & Waterfield, 1999). All mammalian cells express representatives of the three groups. The first member of the family was isolated in 1990 (Carpenter et al., 1990).

Class I: four members have been identified and are further subclassified on the basis of their mechanism of activation. Class Ia, including p110α, p110β and p110δ, associate with a p85 regulatory subunit to form a heterodimeric complex.

There are 8 isoforms of p85 encoded by three genes, each containing two SH2 (Src homology) domains that interact with phosphotyrosines on activated RTKs. This results in recruitment of the enzyme to the plasma membrane and activation of the enzymatic activity. For instance, both PDGFR (platelet-derived growth factor receptor) and IR (insulin receptor) have binding sites for p85 and thus strongly activate class Ia PI3K upon binding to their cognate ligands. In addition, activated (GTP-bound) RAS can activate class Ia kinases by direct interaction with the catalytic subunit (Downward, 1998).

Table 1. PI3K family members

Class	Catalitic subunit	Regulatory subunit	Activation	Products
Ia	p110α p110β p110δ	p85	RTK, RAS	PtdIns-3,4,5-P_3 PtdIns-3,4-P_2 PtdIns-3-P
Ib	P110γ	p101	Heterotrimeric G proteins	PtdIns-3,4,5-P_3 PtdIns-3,4-P_2 PtdIns-3-P
II	PI3KC2α PI3KC2β PI3KC2γ		RTK, integrins	PtdIns-3,4,-P_2 PtdIns-3-P
III	VSP34p			PtdIns-3-P

Genetic studies in the mice have highlighted the role of p110α in regulating cell proliferation during embryo development. Indeed, homozygous deletion of the gene encoding p110α (*Pik3ca*) in the mice is embryonic lethal due to a complete lack of proliferation at embryonic day 9.5 (Bi, Okabe, Bernard, Wynshaw-Boris, & Nussbaum, 1999). Interestingly, the p85 regulatory subunit was highly overexpressed in these mice. Thus, a dominant negative effect on the remaining p110β and p110δ cannot be ruled out.

Class Ib has one member, p110γ, which is activated by βγ subunits of the heterotrimeric G proteins, which are released upon activation of seven transmembrane receptors. p110γ is expressed primarily in leukocytes.

Class II comprises three members (PI3KC2α, β and γ) characterised by a carboxyl-terminal phospholipid-binding domain. While no regulatory subunit has been identified, class II enzyme are predominantly membrane bound and activated by membrane receptors including RTKs and integrins.

The Class III kinase VPS34p is responsible for producing the majority of the cellular PtdIns-3-P and is involved in protein trafficking through the lysosome.

2.3. The tumor suppressor PTEN

PTEN (phosphatase and tensin homolog deleted on chromosome 10)/MMAC1 (mutated in multiple advanced cancers)/TEP-1(TGFβ-regulated and epithelial cell-enriched phosphatase) (hereafter referred as to PTEN) is a tumor suppressor gene localized to chromosome 10q23 (Li & Sun, 1997; Li et al., 1997; Steck et al.,

1997). The PTEN protein is both a protein and a lipid phosphatase (reviewed in (Cantley & Neel, 1999; Maehama, Taylor, & Dixon, 2001; Vazquez & Sellers, 2000). The phosphatase domain has homology to protein tyrosine phosphatases, dual-specificity phosphatases, and to tensin and auxilin (Li & Sun, 1997; Li et al., 1997; Steck et al., 1997). The lipid phosphatase activity of PTEN can dephosphorylate the D3 position of PtdIns-3,4-P_2 and PtdIns-3,4,5-P_3, the lipid products of the PI3K lipid kinase activity (Maehama & Dixon, 1998). Thus, PTEN antagonizes signaling through the PI3K pathway. Indeed, cells lacking PTEN function exhibit a two fold increase in PtdIns-3,4,5-P_3 levels (Stambolic et al., 1998; Sun et al., 1999).

PTEN can also dephosphorylate tyrosine-, serine-, and threonine-phosphorylated peptides (Myers & Tonks, 1997). This activity may be related to regulation of cell adhesion and spreading. When overexpressed in cells, PTEN can dephosphorylate focal adhesion kinase (FAK) (Tamura et al., 1999) and the adaptor protein Shc (Gu et al., 1999). In addition, expression of PTEN results in a decrease in cell spreading and motility (Tamura et al., 1998). However, the relevance of the protein phosphatase activity for PTEN tumor suppression is unclear as certain tumor- and germline-derived mutants of PTEN give rise to protein products that retain their protein phosphatase activity(Furnari, Huang, & Cavenee, 1998; Myers et al., 1998; Ramaswamy et al., 1999). These findings suggest that this activity is not sufficient to block tumor development. Indeed, the preponderance of the published data suggests that PTEN's role as a tumor suppressor is mediated largely through its lipid phosphatase activity.

Analysis of PTEN crystal structure shows that in addition to the catalytic domain PTEN has a C2 domain (Lee et al., 1999). The C2 domain binds lipids and thus may serve to position the catalytic domain at the plasma membrane. PTEN also has a C-terminal "tail" that contains a PDZ domain. PDZ domains are protein-protein interaction modules that play a critical role in organizing diverse cell signaling complexes. Phosphorylation of three residues (S380, T382, and T383) within the tail is necessary for maintaining protein stability and also acts inhibiting PTEN function (Adey et al., 2000; Georgescu et al., 2000; Tolkacheva et al., 2001; Vazquez, Ramaswamy, Nakamura, & Sellers, 2000). Phosphorylation of the tail acts as an inhibitory switch. When phosphorylated, PTEN is in a "close", monomeric conformation with low affinity for PDZ-domain containing proteins. Conversely, the unphosphorylated form is in an "open" conformation that allows recruitment to high molecular weight complexes(Vazquez et al., 2001). These complexes comprise PDZ-domain containing proteins, such as MAGI-2, and they are thought to be important for PTEN localization to the plasma membrane (Vazquez et al., 2001; Wu et al., 2000). Once localised to the membrane, PTEN can exert its phospholipid phosphatase activity.

Targeted disruption of *Pten* in the mice leads to embryonic lethality (Di Cristofano, Pesce, Cordon-Cardo, & Pandolfi, 1998; Podsypanina et al., 1999; Stambolic et al., 2000; Sun et al., 1999; Suzuki et al., 1998). Abnormal proliferation but not significant differences in apoptosis are observed in the mutant embryos. Interestingly, $Pten^{+/-}$ mice, as the Cowden's syndrome patients (see further below), are cancer prone and develop a range of neoplasms including tumors of the breast, endometrium prostate, liver, gastrointestinal tract, thyroid and thymus and T-cell lymphomas (Di Cristofano et al., 1998; Podsypanina et al., 1999; Stambolic et al., 2000; Suzuki et al., 1998). The majority of these tumors exhibit loss of the wild type allele, underscoring the importance of loss of PTEN function in tumor formation.

In the fruit fly *Drosophila melanogaster* loss of PTEN function is lethal in the larval stage. Importantly, this lethality can be rescued by a PH domain mutant Akt (Stocker et al., 2002). This Akt mutant has a reduced affinity for PtdIns-3,4,5-P_3 suggesting that PH-domain mediated activation of Akt is the only lethal event triggered by increased levels of PtdIns-3,4,5-P_3 in PTEN-null cells. Thus, *D. melanogaster* Akt appears to be the most critical effector downstream PTEN.

2.4. The serine/threonine protein kinase Akt

The serine-threonine protein kinase Akt (also known as protein kinase B, PKB) mediates many of the downstream effects of PI3K and consequently plays a central role in both normal and pathological signaling by the PI3K pathway.

There are three closely related enzymatic isoforms Akt1 (PKBα), Akt2 (PKBβ) and Akt3 (PKBγ) encoded by three different genes located on chromosomes 14q32, 19q13 and 1q43 respectively. They are similar both in structure and size and are thought to be activated by a common mechanism (Okano, Gaslightwala, Birnbaum, Rustgi, & Nakagawa, 2000). To date, no differences in substrate preference have been established are currently assumed to have identical or similar substrate specificity. The three isoforms are widely expressed though Akt3 tissue distribution seems to be more restricted than 1 and 2, being primarily expressed in brain and testis (Konishi et al., 1995).

The three Akt proteins (henceforth refered to as Akt) contain an N-terminal pleckstrin homology (PH) domain, a central catalytic domain and a C-terminal regulatory region. The PH domains of Akt and related kinases such as BTK (Bruton's tyrosine kinase) can bind specifically to D3-phosphorylated phosphoinositides with high affinity.

Activation of Akt is a multi-step process involving both membrane binding and phosphorylation. Upon PI3K activation and production of PtdIns-3,4,5-P_3 and PtdIns-3,4-P_2, Akt is recruited to the plasma membrane where it binds to the these phosphoinositides through its PH domain (Franke, Kaplan, Cantley, & Toker, 1997). Activation is then thought to involve a conformational change and phosphorylation on two residues. One such phosphorylation site lies within the kinase domain activation loop (Thr 308 in Akt1) and is phosphorylated by another PH-domain containing protein, PDK1 (reviewed in {Alessi, 2001 #2014}. This is thought to be the major activating phosphorylation event. In addition, a second phosphorylation site in the C-terminus (Ser 473 in Akt1) is required for full or maximal activity. The identity of the serine 473 kinase is not firmly established and this phosphorylation event may results from PDK1 itself (Balendran et al., 1999), from integrin-linked kinase (Persad et al., 2001) or from Akt autophosphorylation. A detailed description of the structural features and mechanism of activation can be found elsewhere (Coffer, Jin, & Woodgett, 1998; Datta, Brunet, & Greenberg, 1999; Galetic et al., 1999; Kandel & Hay, 1999).

Growth factor stimulation of PI3K activity leads to Akt activation. Conversely, PI3K inhibition (i.e. using chemical inhibitors such as wortmannin or LY294002) and PTEN mediated dephosphorylation of PtdIns-3,4,5-P_3 and PtdIns-3,4-P_2 results in inhibition of Akt. After activation, Akt can phosphorylate a number of substrates both in the cytoplasm and in the nucleus.

Disruption of the genes for murine *akt1* and *akt2* gives rise to viable mice that show phenotypic differences. *Akt1*$^{-/-}$ mice are smaller and have shorter life span when exposed to genotoxic stress than wild type littermates. In addition, they exhibit increased spontaneous apoptosis in the testis and thymus (Chen et al., 2001) (Cho, Mu et al., 2001). In contrast, Akt2$^{-/-}$ mice show insulin resistance and a diabetes mellitus-like syndrome (Cho, Mu et al., 2001). Whether these differences result from differences in substrate preference or tissue regulation is not clear. In addition, the viability and relatively mild phenotypes of these knockout mice raise the possibility that the three Akt isoforms can, compensate for each other with respect to functions that might compromise organismal viablility. The generation of compound knock-out animals will address this issue.

2.5. *Akt targets*

Akt phosphorylates a variety of substrates involved in the regulation of key cellular functions including cell growth and survival, glucose metabolism and protein translation. These targets include GSK3, IRS-1 (insulin receptor susbtrate-1), PDE-3B (phosphodiesterase-3B), BAD, human caspase 9, Forkhead and NF-κB transcription factors, mTOR, eNOS, Raf protein kinase, BRCA1, and p21$^{Cip1/WAF1}$ (Altiok et al., 1999; Datta et al., 1999; Galetic et al., 1999; Montagnani, Chen, Barr, & Quon, 2001; Zhou et al., 2001; Zimmermann & Moelling, 1999).

One common mechanism through which Akt-mediated phosphorylation results in substrate inhibition is through the regulation of subcellular localization by interaction with 14-3-3 proteins (i.e. BAD, forkhead transcription factors). 14-3-3 proteins are cytoplasmic proteins that bind specifically to phosphoproteins and retain them in the cytoplasm (Yaffe et al., 1997) away from their targets. In particular the Akt consensus phosphorylation site is also a consensus 14-3-3 binding site (Yaffe et al., 2001). For example, BAD phosphorylation by Akt inhibits its proapototic effects. In the unphosphorylated state, BAD is targeted to the mitochondria where it forms a complex with Bcl-2 or Bcl$_{XL}$, inhibiting their anti-apoptotic activity. Conversely, when phosphorylated, BAD associates with 14-3-3 proteins in the cytoplasm.

FKHR, FKHRL1 and AFX transcription factors (henceforth referred to as Forkhead) belong to the winged helix/forkhead transcription factors family characterized by a 100-amino acid, monomeric DNA binding domain (DBD)(reviewed in (Kops & Burgering, 1999; Kops et al., 1999)). These three family members are directly phosphorylated and regulated by Akt. Forkhead transcriptional activity is negatively regulated through Akt-dependent phosphorylation on three conserved residues (Biggs, Meisenhelder, Hunter, Cavenee, & Arden, 1999; Brunet et al., 1999; Kops et al., 1999; Rena, Guo, Cichy, Unterman, & Cohen, 1999). Upon phosphorylation, Forkhead binds to 14-3-3 proteins and remains in the cytoplasm where they are thought to be functionally inactive. Recent data suggests that 14-3-3 acts not merely as a cytoplasmic retention signal, but targets nuclear Forkhead to the nuclear export machinery (Brunet et al., 2002). In cancer cell lines lacking functional PTEN, FKHRL1 and FKHR are constitutively phosphorylated by Akt and are hence constitutively cytoplasmic and unable to activate transcription (Nakamura et al., 2000). Moreover, reconstitution of PTEN to those cells restores nuclear localization of FKHR and restores its ability to activate promoter elements. Mutation of the three Akt phosphorylation sites to alanine renders FKHR independent of Akt activation. Consequently, it remains localized in the nucleus and hence constitutively active. Importantly, this constitutively active form of FKHR (FKHR;A3) is able to replace PTEN function in PTEN-null cells. Specifically, in PTEN-null cells that undergo G1 arrest upon PTEN reconstitution (i.e. 786-0 cells), likewise FKHR;A3 induces a G1 arrest (Medema, Kops, Bos, & Burgering, 2000; Nakamura et al., 2000). On the other hand, in PTEN-null cells that undergo apoptosis upon PTEN reconstitution (i.e. LNCaP cells) FKHR;A3 likewise induces apoptosis. Thus, Forkhead is a critical effector of both cell-cycle progression and apoptosis downstream of PTEN (Nakamura et al., 2000). In addition, other Forkhead family members have also been implicated in the induction of apoptosis both through the upregulation of FasL (Brunet et al., 1999) and through the regulation of the pro-apoptotic Bcl-2 interacting mediator (Bim1) (Dijkers, Medema, Lammers, Koenderman, & Coffer, 2000).

Human Caspase-9, a member of the protease family intimately associated with the initiation of apoptosis, is thought to be phosphorylated and inhibited by Akt.. (Cardone et al., 1998). However, the Akt phosphorylation site is not conserved in the Capase 9 proteins from other mammals making its *in vivo* importance unclear.

In addition to the inhibition of pro-apoptotic factors, Akt can also activate the transcription of anti-apoptotic genes through the activation of the transcription factor NFκB (Kane, Shapiro, Stokoe, & Weiss, 1999; Khwaja, 1999; Ozes et al., 1999; Romashkova & Makarov, 1999). When bound to its inhibitor, termed IκB, NFκB localises to the cytoplasm. Akt associates and activate the IκB kinases (IKKs). Activated IKKs phoshorylate IkB targeting it for degradation by the proteosome. This allows NFκB to translocate to the nucleus and activate transcription of a variety of substrates including anti-apoptotic genes such as the inhibitors of apoptosis (IAP) c-IAP1 and 2.

2.6. FRAP/mTOR

The ribosomal protein S6 kinases (S6Ks) and the mammalian target of rapamycin (mTOR, also known as FRAP) have been linked to the PI3K signalling, though the exact mechanism for this connection remains to be clarified (reviewed in (Gingras, Raught, & Sonenberg, 2001). In response to growth factor stimulation, S6Ks are phosphorylated in multiple sites and, in turn, phosphorylate the ribosomal protein S6 leading to increase translation. The kinases upstream S6K seem to include PDK1 and mTOR among others.

In addition to S6K, mTOR has been reported to phophorylate the eukaryotic translation initiation factor 4E (eIF4E) binding proteins (4E-BPs) positively modulating the initiation of translation. Hypophosphoryated 4E-BPs bind efficiently to eIF-4E forming an inhibited complex. Upon phosphorylation, 4E-BPs dissociates from the complex allowing eIF-4E to incorporate into the translation initiation machinery. A variety of stimuli can activate mTOR kinase activity including mitogens, amino acid availability and ATP levels (Dennis et al., 2001).

In *D. melanogaster*, mutations in the insulin signalling pathway including loss of PTEN act to alter regulation of cell size and cell number. Genetic analysis of this pathway suggests that these effects arise primarily as a consequence of alterations in the function of the TOR homologue in drosophila (Zhang, Stallock, Ng, Reinhard, & Neufeld, 2000). In keeping with these data, in mammalian and avian cells tumors and cancer cell lines harbouring either alterations in PTEN or bearing activated alleles of Akt and PI3K, appear to be exquisitely sensitive to treatment with either rapamycin or the rapamycin analog CCI-779 (Aoki, Blazek, & Vogt, 2001; Neshat et al., 2001; Podsypanina et al., 2001).

2.7 Other PI3K effectors

Other downstream effectors include the small GTPase Rac (Kotani, Hara, Yonezawa, & Kasuga, 1995; Posern, Saffrich, Ansorge, & Feller, 2000) and the serine-threonine kinase ILK (integrin-linked kinases) (Dedhar, Williams, & Hannigan, 1999).

3. PERTURBATIONS IN CANCER

Carcinogenesis is a multi-step process involving genetic and epigenetic alterations that together lead to the acquisition of six common features of the transformed cell. Namely, self-sufficiency in growth signals, insensitivity to growth-inhibitory signals, evasion of apoptosis, limitless replicative potential, sustained angiogenesis, and tissue invasion and metastasis (Hanahan & Weinberg, 2000). In different ways and degrees, the various components of the PI3K/PTEN/Akt pathway have been related to most of those cellular phenotypes.

3.1. PI3K

As mentioned above, most protein tyrosine kinases (both membrane receptors and cytoplasmic) can signal through the PI3K pathway and oncogenic activation of tyrosine kinases observed in multiple human cancers results in deregulated activation of PI3K activity. Other mechanisms of activation include amplification of the gene encoding the catalytic subunit and activating mutations in the regulatory subunit.

Thus, far there is no direct evidence for activating mutations of PI3K catalytic subunit in human cancers, however *PIK3CA*, the gene coding for p110α, is frequently amplified (increased in copy number) in ovarian (Shayesteh et al., 1999) and cervical cancers (Ma et al., 2000). The increased copy number is associated with increased PIK3CA transcription, p110α protein expression and PI3K activity, resulting in increase cell growth and decreased apoptosis. Increased enzymatic activity has been also reported in colorectal tumors (Phillips, St Clair, Munday, Thomas, & Mitchell, 1998).

In addition, somatic mutations in the p85 regulatory subunit leading to constitutively activation of the catalytic subunit have been described in ovarian and colon tumors (Philp et al., 2001).

The avian retroviral oncogene v-p3k, a homolog of p110α, is involved in the induction of hemangiosarcomas in chickens. Here, V-p3k is fused to viral gag proteins resulting in localization to the membrane and, consequently, constitutively enzymatic activation. V-p3k is oncogenic both *in vivo* and *in vitro* (Aoki et al., 2000; Chang et al., 1997). In addition, membrane targeted p110α induces cell cycle entry and in immortalized rodent cells is sufficient for oncogenic transformation (Klippel et al., 1998).

PI3K is also thought to be implicated in the metastatic phenotype. Indeed, several molecules involved in cell migration and cell adhesion can regulate or be regulated by PI3K. For instance, α6β4 integrins can activate PI3K and promote carcinoma invasion (Shaw, Rabinovitz, Wang, Toker, & Mercurio, 1997). This phenotype appears to be independent of Akt activation. Along this lines, recent studies in transgenic mice suggest an Akt-independent mechanism for PI3K-induced metastatic phenotype (Hutchinson, Jin, Cardiff, Woodgett, & Muller, 2001). PI3K can interact and be activated by E-cadherin (Pece, Chiariello, Murga, & Gutkind, 1999), cell surface molecules involved in cell-cell adhesion. PI3K can also activate the small GTPase Rac (Kotani et al., 1995; Posern et al., 2000) and the serine-threonine kinase ILK (integrin-linked kinases) (Dedhar et al., 1999). These downstream effectors seem to be required for PI3K-mediated invasion. However, the specific molecular mechanism by which PI3K signalling mediates or induces a invasive phenotype remains under investigation.

3.2. PTEN

PTEN is one of the genes most commonly mutated in human cancers and LOH at the *PTEN* locus on 10q23 is a frequent event in both primary and metastatic tumors. In addition, germ line mutations of *PTEN* are associated with the hereditary cancer predisposition syndromes known as Cowden's disease and related conditions (Liaw et al., 1997). These findings, together with the studies in animal models, strongly support a critical role of PTEN in tumor suppression.

3.2.1. Germline mutations

Germline mutations in the *PTEN* gene have been reported in two rare autosomal dominant disorders known as Cowden's disease (CD) and Bannayan-Zonana syndrome (BZS). These syndromes are characterized by the development of hamartomas that is lesions characterized by hyperplastic, disorganized and benign tumors. Hamartomas of the outer root sheath of the hair follicle (trichilemmomas) are pathognemonic. In addition, thyroid, breast, skin, and intestinal hamartomas are also found. Loss of the PTEN wild type allele in hamartoma tissue is an early event leading to increased proliferation. In addition, CD patients are prone to develop breast and thyroid cancers (Nelen et al., 1997).

Germline PTEN mutations giving rise to these syndromes comprise frameshift, nonsense, misssense and splice-site mutations typically resulting in the generation of truncated, inactive proteins. Among the missense mutations, a high proportion cluster in the phosphatase domain (Ali, Schriml, & Dean, 1999).

Lhermitte-Duclos disease is a CD associated condition defined by dysplastic gangliocytoma of the cerebellum (Eng et al., 1994). Importantly, it has been recently reported that deletion of PTEN in the mouse brain gives rise to lesions that resemble the histopathology of Lhermitte-Duclos cerebellum (Backman et al., 2001;

Kwon et al., 2001). Neurons lacking PTEN expression exhibit high levels of phosphorylated Akt and show progressive increase in soma size without evidence of abnormal proliferation (Kwon et al., 2001).

3.2.2. Somatic mutations

PTEN is frequently inactivated in sporadic human tumors from various tissues, including endometrium, brain, prostate, and ovary (reviewed in (Ali et al., 1999; Bonneau & Longy, 2000). The most common inactivating events are frameshift and missense mutations and homozygous deletions (Ali et al., 1999).

LOH at chromosome 10q has been reported in 60%-80% of glioblastomas (Bostrom et al., 1998; Rasheed et al., 1997; Steck et al., 1999; Wang et al., 1997). Intragenic mutations in the PTEN gene have been identified in 60% of primary glioblastoma cell lines (Li et al., 1997; Steck et al., 1997) and in approximately 20-40% of glioblastoma multiforme, the most aggressive subtype of astrocytic tumor (Bostrom et al., 1998; Duerr et al., 1998; Li et al., 1997; Liu, James, Frederick, Alderete, & Jenkins, 1997; Rasheed, Wiltshire, Bigner, & Bigner, 1999; Somerville et al., 1998; Steck et al., 1997; Wang et al., 1997). In contrast, in lower grade gliomas (such us anaplastic astrocytomas) although they also harbor chromosome 10q loss mutation of the second PTEN allele is comparatively rare (Bostrom et al., 1998; Duerr et al., 1998). Therefore, PTEN mutation appears to be correlated with higher grade tumors.

In prostate cancer, loss of heterozygosity in the 10q23 interval is found in between 18 and 65% of tumors (reviewed in Ramaswamy S at al., 2000). In addition, *PTEN* promoter methylation and gene silencing has been reported in some prostate cancer xenografts (Whang YE at al., 1998). The PTEN protein is absent in 20% of primary tumor specimens when studied by immunohistochemistry and its absence correlates with advance pathological grade and stage (McMenamin et al., 1999. In addition, as many as 60% of patients with metastatic lesions are found to have a focus of prostate cancer in which PTEN is mutated {Suzuki, 1998 #1457). Thus, *PTEN* loss appears to be a critical step in the development of aggressive and likely lethal forms of prostate cancer.

PTEN mutations occur in 30%-50% of endometrial cancers primarily in the endometrioid sub-type (Ali et al., 1999). Similarly, PTEN is mutated in 24% of ovarian cancers again at higher frequency in the endometrioid type (Obata et al., 1998; Yokomizo et al., 1998). In contrast to other tumor types that sustain PTEN mutations, loss of function PTEN mutations are more common in Grade I or early stage tumors of the ovary. Thus, here PTEN may play a role in the tumor initiation (Levine et al., 1998; Maxwell et al., 1998).

PTEN mutations can be found in 30-40% of malignant melanomas (Guldberg et al., 1997; Tsao, Zhang, Benoit, & Haluska, 1998), correlating with a LOH frequency of 30-50% on chr 10q (Healy et al., 1998; Isshiki, Elder, Guerry, & Linnenbach, 1993). In addition, in specific instances, PTEN mutations were found in metastatic foci, but not in the corresponding primary tumors, again suggesting that PTEN is involved in tumor progression (Guldberg et al., 1997).

3.3. Akt

The first evidence pointing to a role of Akt in tumorigenesis was given by the early studies of the transforming murine virus ATK8 and the finding of *Akt1* and *2* gene amplification in gastric adenocarcinoma (Bellacosa, Testa, Staal, & Tsichlis, 1991; Staal, 1987; Staal & Hartley, 1988). The viral homolog, v-Akt, is a fusion protein containing Gag sequences at its amino terminus (Bellacosa et al., 1991. This fusion creates a myristoylation sequence allowing for a postranslational modification that directs proteins to the plasma membrane {Ahmed, 1993 #1995).

In human cancer, there are several mechanisms that lead to deregulated Akt activity, inappropriate activation of PI3K, *Akt* gene amplification, Akt protein overexpression and loss of PTEN. Given the high frequency of PTEN mutations in human cancer, it is likely that the latter mechanism accounts for the majority of Akt activation events.

Akt1 gene amplification has been found in gastric adenocarcinomas (Staal, 1987). In addition, increased Akt1 kinase activity and its association with a poorer in prostate, ovary and breast carcinomas has been recently described (Sun et al., 2001). In these tumors it is likely that Akt activation resulted from either PTEN loss or PI3K activation rather than direct amplification or activation of Akt (repeat the reference).

Akt2 mutations appear more prevalent or at least, more reproducibly documented in human cancer than Akt 1 or 3. The Akt2 gene is amplified and overexpressed in ovarian carcinomas, both in cell lines and in primary tumors (Cheng et al., 1992); (Bellacosa et al., 1995). Here, amplification was closely associated with an aggressive tumor phenotype. In a recent report, elevated Akt2 kinase activity was found in approximately 40% of primary ovarian cancers (Yuan et al., 2000). Ten percent of pancreatic cancer cells show Akt 2 amplification (Cheng et al., 1996). Moreover, in the same study, expression of an Akt-2 antisense mRNA inhibited tumorigenesis.

Little has been reported on Akt3 thus far. In one study, both Akt3 mRNA levels and enzymatic activity were elevated in breast cancer cell lines and tumors lacking the estrogen receptor as well as in prostate cancer cell lines that are androgen-insensitive. These results indicate that Akt 3 may contribute to the more aggressive phenotype of the hormone-refractory breast and prostate carcinomas (Nakatani et al., 1999).

Myr-Akt is targeted to the plasma membrane and thus constitutively active. Both, preferential location to the membrane and kinase activity are required for oncogenicity by Akt (Aoki, Batista, Bellacosa, Tsichlis, & Vogt, 1998). All three Akts are equally and strongly transforming in chicken embryo fibroblasts (CEFs) and induce the formation of hemangiosarcomas in chicken wing xenograft assays (Mende, Malstrom, Tsichlis, Vogt, & Aoki, 2001). The histology of these tumors is identical to the hemangiosarcomas Myr-p110 PI3K. These data suggest that each Akt family member might mediate transformation downstream of PTEN loss or PI3K activation.

A recent study using transgenic mice overexpressing both an activated mutant of Akt and a PI3K decoupled mutant of polyomavirus middle T antigen shows that Akt can contribute to tumor progression but does not restore the metastatic phenotype observed with the wild type middle T (Hutchinson et al., 2001). These results suggest that PI3K signaling can contribute to the metastatic phenotype via an Akt-independent mechanism as mentioned above.

3.4. Akt targets

Translocations into the genes encoding Forkhead transcription factors have been described. Chromosomal translocations resulting in PAX3-FKHR (Fredericks et al., 1995) and PAX7-FKHR fusion proteins are a common occurrence in alveolar rhabdomyosarcomas (reviewed in (Barr, 2001). The fusion proteins contain PAX3/PAX7 DNA binding domain and FKHR transactivation domain, are expressed at higher levels than the wild type counterparts, and are constitutively nuclear (del Peso, Gonzalez, Hernandez, Barr, & Nunez, 1999). The oncogenic activity of the fusion proteins is thought to be due at least in part to deregulation of PAX3/PAX7 target genes (Barr, 2001).

Similarly, chromosomal translocations involving the MLL gene with AFX (Borkhardt et al., 1997) and FKHRL1 (Hillion, Le Coniat, Jonveaux, Berger, & Bernard, 1997) have been found in acute leukemias. It has been suggested that MLL-FKHRL1 fusion protein may result not only in a MLL gain of function but also in a dominant negative effect on FKHRL1 function (Ayton & Cleary, 2001). Indeed, both loss of growth inhibitory effect of AFX (Medema et al., 2000), and deregulation of FKHRL1 apoptotic target genes (Brunet et al., 1999) can contribute to enhanced survival and tumorigenesis.

The notion that the three Forkhead transcription factors that are substrates of Akt are also targets of translocation in human cancer is intriguing and raises the possibility that the fusion proteins produced from these translocation may serve to interfere with normal Forkhead function.

Other Akt targets involved in cancer include $p70^{S6K}$ which is located at a site of amplification in breast cancer (Barlund et al., 2000) and eIF-4B amplification in head and neck squamous cell carcinomas (Franklin et al., 1999).

4. THERAPEUTIC MANIPULATIONS

The PI3K/PTEN/Akt pathway may be readily amenable to pharmacological manipulations. The recent success in developing relatively selective kinase inhibitors such as Gleevec and Irrissa, and the relatively limited side-effect profile attributed to these agents augers well for future drugs in this class. In this regard, the kinase components of the PI3K pathway are particularly exciting targets for the rational design of small molecules. An open question remains where along the pathway is one most likely to gain therapeutic advantage while minimizing toxicity. Inhibitors against receptor tyrosine kinases are clearly one way by which this pathway can be targeted, but will not be discussed here.

4.1. PI3K

Wortmannin and LY294002 are molecules which disrupt the ATP binding pocket of PI3K and PI3K like enzymes. While wortmannin is an irreversible inhibitor, LY294002 is a competitive inhibitor. Both have been extensively used in cell culture studies and both induce growth inhibition at concentrations that inhibit class Ia PI3Ks. At higher concentrations they induce apoptosis (Yao & Cooper,

1995). For instance, ovarian cancer cells exhibiting activation of the PI3K/Akt pathway undergo apoptosis when treated with either wortmannin or LY294002 (Yuan et al., 2000). Moreover, in ovarian cancers implanted in the murine peritoneum, combinations of LY294002 and paclitaxel are more efficacious than paclitaxel alone (Hu, Hofmann, Lu, Mills, & Jaffe, 2002). Although extensively used in *in vitro* studies neither wortmannin nor LY294002 have been translated to human cancer therapy thus far.

Despite the broad tissue distribution of PI3K isoforms, the evidence of functional specialization within class Ia kinases suggests that isoform-selective inhibitors may have an acceptable therapeutic index. P110β is preferentially involved in insulin signaling whereas p110α is more likely to transmit mitogenic signals. p100γ and δ, more restricted to the lymphocytic compartment and are attractive targets for the development of novel anti-inflammatory drugs (Stein & Waterfield, 2000). While p110α is perhaps the most attractive target, germline deletion in the mouse leads to embryonic lethality. Nonetheless this does not speak to the consequence of inhibition in the adult organism and experiments to temporally delete the catalytic and regulatory subunit genes of PI3K may help to delineate the consequence of PI3K loss to adult animals.

Small molecule inhibitors of PIKKs as potential anticancer drugs is a field of intense research. For example, LY294002-geldanamycin heterodimers have been synthesized with intent of selectively inhibit PI3K and PIKK family members (Chiosis, Rosen, & Sepp-Lorenzino, 2001). In addition, novel pyrrolo-quinoline derivatives exhibiting potent PIKK inhibition have been recently reported (Peng et al., 2002). For a further discussion on PI3K as target for drug development see Stein *et al.* (Stein & Waterfield, 2000).

4.2. PTEN

Overexpression of PTEN in PTEN wild type cells has modest effects on cell signaling, proliferation or viability (Simpson & Parsons, 2001) suggesting that increasing the gene dosage of PTEN in normal cells may be well tolerated. On the other and, restoration of PTEN to PTEN-null cells results in either growth arrest, apoptosis, and inhibition of soft-agar and xenograft growth. Thus restoration of PTEN function to PTEN-null tumors is a possible strategy. Clearly, the rate-limiting step in this approach is the development of effective gene therapy vectors.

4.3. Akt

Akt is an attractive target for the development of novel inhibitors that might prove beneficial in the treatment of cancers in which the PI3K/PTEN/Akt pathway is constitutively activated by any of the aforementioned upstream genetic events (e.g. receptor amplification, PI3KCA amplification, Akt amplification and PTEN deletion). The viability and relatively subtle phenotypes of the Akt1 and 2 knockout mice (Chen et al., 2001; Cho, Thorvaldsen, Chu, Feng, & Birnbaum, 2001) raise the possibility that there may be functional redundancy among these kinase, however, it is clear from these experiments that reduced levels of Akt activity can be tolerated during development and in adult mice. In addition, these data suggest that the Akt-1 and -2 may have evolved functional specifications. Thus, it will be critical to determine whether inhibition or genetic inactivation of specific Akt isoforms reverse the transformed phenotype associated with PTEN loss of PI3K activation. If differences in Akt isoforms are found in such studies then ideally, isoform-specific inhibitors could be generated to exploit such hypothetical differences. The development of Akt3 knockout mouse as well as the disruption of Akt in a pten$^{+/-}$ background will provide further insights into the toxicity of inhibiting Akt activity *in vivo*.

Herbimacyn A and geldanamycin are ansamycin antibiotics that bind to and inhibit the heat-shock protein 90 (Hsp90) function. Hsp90 is a chaperone protein involved in the refolding of proteins during cellular stress and the conformational maturation of certain signaling proteins including Akt, HER2, Raf, EGFR and steroid receptors (Sausville, 2001). Hsp90 inhibition prevents refolding and leads to proteosomal degradation of those signaling molecules including significant reduction of Akt protein levels and a consequent downregulation of signaling through these pathways (Schneider et al., 1996). In addition, Hsp90 binds to and stabilizes the mature HER2 kinase domain. Thus, geldanamycin also stimulates HER2 degradation via disruption of the HER2/Hsp90 association (Xu et al., 2001).

17-allyl-aminogeldanamycin (17-AAG) is a geldanamycin derivative that has anti-tumor activity both in cell lines and xenograft assays. In breast cancer cells, 17-AAG causes RB-dependent G1 arrest and enhances the apoptotic effects of cytotoxic agents such as taxol in breast cancer cell (Munster, Basso, Solit, Norton, & Rosen, 2001). G1 arrest is associated with cyclin D loss and hypophosphorylation of RB.

In breast cancer cells with high levels of HER2, 17-AAG inhibits Akt in a complex manner. In addition to down-regulation of Akt expression, 17-AAG also causes a rapid inhibition of Akt kinase activity prior to proteosomal degradation of HER2 and Akt (Basso, Solit, Munster, & Rosen, 2002). 17-AAG is currently in clinical trials.

4.4. FRAP/mTOR

As mentioned above, the genetic dissection of PI3K signalling in *Drosophila melanogaster* has linked PI3K signalling to the regulation of cell-size and proliferation to the *Drosophila* homologue of mTOR. Furthermore in PTEN-nulls cells there is elevated levels of phosphorylated 4EBP-1, a downstream translation effector of TOR signalling. These data have raised the possibility that rapamycin might have anti-tumor efficacy.

Rapamycin is a natural macrolide isolated from the microorganism Streptomyces hygroscopicus. It binds to the immunophilin FKBP12 and the drug-protein complex in turn binds with high affinity to mTOR. Rapamycin inhibits phosphorylation of mTOR targets p70^{S6K} and 4E-BP resulting in decreased translation resulting in a G1 cell cycle arrest. Though principally a cytostatic drug, rapamacyn can also induce cell death. Rapamycin inhibits immune cell proliferation and thus has been used clinically as an immunosuppressant.

The use of rapamycin has been limited by difficulties in solubility. Newer agents including CCI-779 and 40-O-(2-Hydroxyethyl)-rapamycin are esterified rapamycin derivatives with improved solubility and oral bioavailability. Recent data suggests that tumor lines or murine tumors lacking PTEN are particular sensitive to CCI-779 (Neshat et al., 2001; Podsypanina et al., 2001). Moreover, CEFs that are directly transformed by Akt or PI3K are likewise sensitive to rapamycin when compared to Ras transformed CEFs. These observations suggest that such tumors may depend on continuous TOR activity for either proliferation or survival. Finally, it has been recently reported that immunosuppressive doses of rapamycin can also inhibit tumor growth in mice probably by an anti-angiogenic effect kinked to reduced production of vascular endothelial growth factor (VEGF) (Guba et al., 2002).

In human Phase I trials (dose escalation) treatment with CCI-779 has been associated with decreased platelet counts, diarrhea, vomiting, hypocalcemia and increase triglyceride levels but in general was well tolerated. Phase II trials are under way in glioblastoma multiforme, melanoma, prostate cancer, breast cancer and melanoma. Responses have been seen in a small number of tumors, however phase I trials are not primarily designed to assess efficacy and thus the Phase II data is eagerly awaited.

5. CONCLUSION

In conclusion, direct genetic alterations leading to deregulated PI3K/Akt signalling are common in a significant fraction of human malignancies. The forthcoming decade should witness the development and clinical deployment of a number of novel small molecule inhibitors specifically designed to disrupt the function of members of this pathway. It is hoped and perhaps likely that such inhibitors, either alone or in combination with current therapeutics, will ultimately proof clinically efficacious.

Juan Paez & William R. Sellers
Department of Adult Oncology
Dana-Farber Cancer Institute
Department of Medicine
Brigham and Women's Hospital
Harvard Medical School
Boston, MA 02115

6. REFERENCES

Adey, N. B., Huang, L., Ormonde, P. A., Baumgard, M. L., Pero, R., Byreddy, D. V., Tavtigian, S. V., & Bartel, P. L. (2000). Threonine phosphorylation of the MMAC1/PTEN PDZ binding domain both inhibits and stimulates PDZ binding. *Cancer Res, 60*(1), 35-37.

Ali, I. U., Schriml, L. M., & Dean, M. (1999). Mutational spectra of PTEN/MMAC1 gene: a tumor suppressor with lipid phosphatase activity. *J Natl Cancer Inst, 91*(22), 1922-1932.

Altiok, S., Batt, D., Altiok, N., Papautsky, A., Downward, J., Roberts, T. M., & Avraham, H. (1999). Heregulin induces phosphorylation of BRCA1 through phosphatidylinositol 3-Kinase/AKT in breast cancer cells. *J Biol Chem, 274*(45), 32274-32278.

Aoki, M., Batista, O., Bellacosa, A., Tsichlis, P., & Vogt, P. K. (1998). The akt kinase: molecular determinants of oncogenicity. *Proc Natl Acad Sci U S A, 95*(25), 14950-14955.

Aoki, M., Blazek, E., & Vogt, P. K. (2001). A role of the kinase mTOR in cellular transformation induced by the oncoproteins P3k and Akt. *Proc Natl Acad Sci U S A, 98*(1), 136-141.

Aoki, M., Schetter, C., Himly, M., Batista, O., Chang, H. W., & Vogt, P. K. (2000). The catalytic subunit of phosphoinositide 3-kinase: requirements for oncogenicity. *J Biol Chem, 275*(9), 6267-6275.

Ayton, P. M., & Cleary, M. L. (2001). Molecular mechanisms of leukemogenesis mediated by MLL fusion proteins. *Oncogene, 20*(40), 5695-5707.

Backman, S. A., Stambolic, V., Suzuki, A., Haight, J., Elia, A., Pretorius, J., Tsao, M. S., Shannon, P., Bolon, B., Ivy, G. O., & Mak, T. W. (2001). Deletion of Pten in mouse brain causes seizures, ataxia and defects in soma size resembling Lhermitte-Duclos disease. *Nat Genet, 29*(4), 396-403.

Balendran, A., Casamayor, A., Deak, M., Paterson, A., Gaffney, P., Currie, R., Downes, C. P., & Alessi, D. R. (1999). PDK1 acquires PDK2 activity in the presence of a synthetic peptide derived from the carboxyl terminus of PRK2. *Curr Biol, 9*(8), 393-404.

Barlund, M., Forozan, F., Kononen, J., Bubendorf, L., Chen, Y., Bittner, M. L., Torhorst, J., Haas, P., Bucher, C., Sauter, G., Kallioniemi, O. P., & Kallioniemi, A. (2000). Detecting activation of ribosomal protein S6 kinase by complementary DNA and tissue microarray analysis. *J Natl Cancer Inst, 92*(15), 1252-1259.

Barr, F. G. (2001). Gene fusions involving PAX and FOX family members in alveolar rhabdomyosarcoma. *Oncogene, 20*(40), 5736-5746.

Basso, A. D., Solit, D. B., Munster, P. N., & Rosen, N. (2002). Ansamycin antibiotics inhibit Akt activation and cyclin D expression in breast cancer cells that overexpress HER2. *Oncogene, 21*(8), 1159-1166.

Bellacosa, A., de Feo, D., Godwin, A. K., Bell, D. W., Cheng, J. Q., Altomare, D. A., Wan, M., Dubeau, L., Scambia, G., Masciullo, V., & et al. (1995). Molecular alterations of the AKT2 oncogene in ovarian and breast carcinomas. *Int J Cancer, 64*(4), 280-285.

Bellacosa, A., Testa, J. R., Staal, S. P., & Tsichlis, P. N. (1991). A retroviral oncogene, akt, encoding a serine-threonine kinase containing an SH2-like region. *Science, 254*(5029), 274-277.

Bi, L., Okabe, I., Bernard, D. J., Wynshaw-Boris, A., & Nussbaum, R. L. (1999). Proliferative defect and embryonic lethality in mice homozygous for a deletion in the p110alpha subunit of phosphoinositide 3-kinase. *J Biol Chem, 274*(16), 10963-10968.

Biggs, W. H., 3rd, Meisenhelder, J., Hunter, T., Cavenee, W. K., & Arden, K. C. (1999). Protein kinase B/Akt-mediated phosphorylation promotes nuclear exclusion of the winged helix transcription factor FKHR1. *Proc Natl Acad Sci U S A, 96*(13), 7421-7426.

Bonneau, D., & Longy, M. (2000). Mutations of the human PTEN gene. *Hum Mutat, 16*(2), 109-122.

Borkhardt, A., Repp, R., Haas, O. A., Leis, T., Harbott, J., Kreuder, J., Hammermann, J., Henn, T., & Lampert, F. (1997). Cloning and characterization of AFX, the gene that fuses to MLL in acute leukemias with a t(X;11)(q13;q23). *Oncogene, 14*(2), 195-202.

Bostrom, J., Cobbers, J. M., Wolter, M., Tabatabai, G., Weber, R. G., Lichter, P., Collins, V. P., & Reifenberger, G. (1998). Mutation of the PTEN (MMAC1) tumor suppressor gene in a subset of glioblastomas but not in meningiomas with loss of chromosome arm 10q. *Cancer Res, 58*(1), 29-33.

Brogiolo, W., Stocker, H., Ikeya, T., Rintelen, F., Fernandez, R., & Hafen, E. (2001). An evolutionarily conserved function of the Drosophila insulin receptor and insulin-like peptides in growth control. *Curr Biol, 11*(4), 213-221.

Brunet, A., Bonni, A., Zigmond, M. J., Lin, M. Z., Juo, P., Hu, L. S., Anderson, M. J., Arden, K. C., Blenis, J., & Greenberg, M. E. (1999). Akt promotes cell survival by phosphorylating and inhibiting a Forkhead transcription factor. *Cell, 96*(6), 857-868.

Brunet, A., Kanai, F., Stehn, J., Xu, J., Sarbassova, D., Frangioni, J. V., Dalal, S. N., DeCaprio, J. A., Greenberg, M. E., & Yaffe, M. B. (2002). 14-3-3 transits to the nucleus and participates in dynamic nucleocytoplasmic transport. *J Cell Biol, 156*(5), 817-828.

Cantley, L. C., & Neel, B. G. (1999). New insights into tumor suppression: PTEN suppresses tumor formation by restraining the phosphoinositide 3-kinase/AKT pathway. *Proc Natl Acad Sci U S A, 96*(8), 4240-4245.

Cardone, M. H., Roy, N., Stennicke, H. R., Salvesen, G. S., Franke, T. F., Stanbridge, E., Frisch, S., & Reed, J. C. (1998). Regulation of cell death protease caspase-9 by phosphorylation. *Science, 282*(5392), 1318-1321.

Carpenter, C. L., Duckworth, B. C., Auger, K. R., Cohen, B., Schaffhausen, B. S., & Cantley, L. C. (1990). Purification and characterization of phosphoinositide 3-kinase from rat liver. *J Biol Chem, 265*(32), 19704-19711.

Chang, H. W., Aoki, M., Fruman, D., Auger, K. R., Bellacosa, A., Tsichlis, P. N., Cantley, L. C., Roberts, T. M., & Vogt, P. K. (1997). Transformation of chicken cells by the gene encoding the catalytic subunit of PI 3-kinase. *Science, 276*(5320), 1848-1850.

Chen, W. S., Xu, P. Z., Gottlob, K., Chen, M. L., Sokol, K., Shiyanova, T., Roninson, I., Weng, W., Suzuki, R., Tobe, K., Kadowaki, T., & Hay, N. (2001). Growth retardation and increased apoptosis in mice with homozygous disruption of the Akt1 gene. *Genes Dev, 15*(17), 2203-2208.

Cheng, J. Q., Godwin, A. K., Bellacosa, A., Taguchi, T., Franke, T. F., Hamilton, T. C., Tsichlis, P. N., & Testa, J. R. (1992). AKT2, a putative oncogene encoding a member of a subfamily of protein-serine/threonine kinases, is amplified in human ovarian carcinomas. *Proc Natl Acad Sci U S A, 89*(19), 9267-9271.

Cheng, J. Q., Ruggeri, B., Klein, W. M., Sonoda, G., Altomare, D. A., Watson, D. K., & Testa, J. R. (1996). Amplification of AKT2 in human pancreatic cells and inhibition of AKT2 expression and tumorigenicity by antisense RNA. *Proc Natl Acad Sci U S A, 93*(8), 3636-3641.

Chiosis, G., Rosen, N., & Sepp-Lorenzino, L. (2001). LY294002-geldanamycin heterodimers as selective inhibitors of the PI3K and PI3K-related family. *Bioorg Med Chem Lett, 11*(7), 909-913.

Cho, H., Mu, J., Kim, J. K., Thorvaldsen, J. L., Chu, Q., Crenshaw, E. B., 3rd, Kaestner, K. H., Bartolomei, M. S., Shulman, G. I., & Birnbaum, M. J. (2001). Insulin resistance and a diabetes mellitus-like syndrome in mice lacking the protein kinase Akt2 (PKB beta). *Science, 292*(5522), 1728-1731.

Cho, H., Thorvaldsen, J. L., Chu, Q., Feng, F., & Birnbaum, M. J. (2001). Aktl/PKBalpha is required for normal growth but dispensable for maintenance of glucose homeostasis in mice. *J Biol Chem, 276*(42), 38349-38352.

Coffer, P. J., Jin, J., & Woodgett, J. R. (1998). Protein kinase B (c-Akt): a multifunctional mediator of phosphatidylinositol 3-kinase activation. *Biochem J, 335 (Pt 1)*, 1-13.

Datta, S. R., Brunet, A., & Greenberg, M. E. (1999). Cellular survival: a play in three Akts. *Genes Dev, 13*(22), 2905-2927.

Dedhar, S., Williams, B., & Hannigan, G. (1999). Integrin-linked kinase (ILK): a regulator of integrin and growth-factor signalling. *Trends Cell Biol, 9*(8), 319-323.

del Peso, L., Gonzalez, V. M., Hernandez, R., Barr, F. G., & Nunez, G. (1999). Regulation of the forkhead transcription factor FKHR, but not the PAX3-FKHR fusion protein, by the serine/threonine kinase Akt. *Oncogene, 18*(51), 7328-7333.

Dennis, P. B., Jaeschke, A., Saitoh, M., Fowler, B., Kozma, S. C., & Thomas, G. (2001). Mammalian TOR: a homeostatic ATP sensor. *Science, 294*(5544), 1102-1105.

Di Cristofano, A., Pesce, B., Cordon-Cardo, C., & Pandolfi, P. P. (1998). Pten is essential for embryonic development and tumour suppression. *Nat Genet, 19*(4), 348-355.

Dijkers, P. F., Medema, R. H., Lammers, J. W., Koenderman, L., & Coffer, P. J. (2000). Expression of the pro-apoptotic Bcl-2 family member Bim is regulated by the forkhead transcription factor FKHR-L1. *Curr Biol, 10*(19), 1201-1204.

Downward, J. (1998). Ras signalling and apoptosis. *Curr Opin Genet Dev, 8*(1), 49-54.

Duerr, E. M., Rollbrocker, B., Hayashi, Y., Peters, N., Meyer-Puttlitz, B., Louis, D. N., Schramm, J., Wiestler, O. D., Parsons, R., Eng, C., & von Deimling, A. (1998). PTEN mutations in gliomas and glioneuronal tumors. *Oncogene, 16*(17), 2259-2264.

Eng, C., Murday, V., Seal, S., Mohammed, S., Hodgson, S. V., Chaudary, M. A., Fentiman, I. S., Ponder, B. A., & Eeles, R. A. (1994). Cowden syndrome and Lhermitte-Duclos disease in a family: a single genetic syndrome with pleiotropy? *J Med Genet, 31*(6), 458-461.

Franke, T. F., Kaplan, D. R., Cantley, L. C., & Toker, A. (1997). Direct regulation of the Akt proto-oncogene product by phosphatidylinositol-3,4-bisphosphate. *Science, 275*(5300), 665-668.

Franklin, S., Pho, T., Abreo, F. W., Nassar, R., De Benedetti, A., Stucker, F. J., & Nathan, C. A. (1999). Detection of the proto-oncogene eIF4E in larynx and hypopharynx cancers. *Arch Otolaryngol Head Neck Surg, 125*(2), 177-182.

Fredericks, W. J., Galili, N., Mukhopadhyay, S., Rovera, G., Bennicelli, J., Barr, F. G., & Rauscher, F. J., 3rd. (1995). The PAX3-FKHR fusion protein created by the t(2;13) translocation in alveolar rhabdomyosarcomas is a more potent transcriptional activator than PAX3. *Mol Cell Biol, 15*(3), 1522-1535.

Fruman, D. A., Meyers, R. E., & Cantley, L. C. (1998). Phosphoinositide kinases. *Annu Rev Biochem, 67*, 481-507.

Furnari, F. B., Huang, H. J., & Cavenee, W. K. (1998). The phosphoinositol phosphatase activity of PTEN mediates a serum-sensitive G1 growth arrest in glioma cells. *Cancer Res, 58*(22), 5002-5008.

Galetic, I., Andjelkovic, M., Meier, R., Brodbeck, D., Park, J., & Hemmings, B. A. (1999). Mechanism of protein kinase B activation by insulin/insulin-like growth factor-1 revealed by specific inhibitors of phosphoinositide 3-kinase--significance for diabetes and cancer. *Pharmacol Ther, 82*(2-3), 409-425.

Georgescu, M. M., Kirsch, K. H., Kaloudis, P., Yang, H., Pavletich, N. P., & Hanafusa, H. (2000). Stabilization and productive positioning roles of the C2 domain of PTEN tumor suppressor. *Cancer Res, 60*(24), 7033-7038.

Gingras, A. C., Raught, B., & Sonenberg, N. (2001). Regulation of translation initiation by FRAP/mTOR. *Genes Dev, 15*(7), 807-826.

Goberdhan, D. C., Paricio, N., Goodman, E. C., Mlodzik, M., & Wilson, C. (1999). Drosophila tumor suppressor PTEN controls cell size and number by antagonizing the Chico/PI3-kinase signaling pathway. *Genes Dev, 13*(24), 3244-3258.

Gu, J., Tamura, M., Pankov, R., Danen, E. H., Takino, T., Matsumoto, K., & Yamada, K. M. (1999). Shc and FAK differentially regulate cell motility and directionality modulated by PTEN. *J Cell Biol, 146*(2), 389-403.

Guba, M., von Breitenbuch, P., Steinbauer, M., Koehl, G., Flegel, S., Hornung, M., Bruns, C. J., Zuelke, C., Farkas, S., Anthuber, M., Jauch, K. W., & Geissler, E. K. (2002). Rapamycin inhibits primary and metastatic tumor growth by antiangiogenesis: involvement of vascular endothelial growth factor. *Nat Med, 8*(2), 128-135.

Guldberg, P., thor Straten, P., Birck, A., Ahrenkiel, V., Kirkin, A. F., & Zeuthen, J. (1997). Disruption of the MMAC1/PTEN gene by deletion or mutation is a frequent event in malignant melanoma. *Cancer Res, 57*(17), 3660-3663.

Hanahan, D., & Weinberg, R. A. (2000). The hallmarks of cancer. *Cell, 100*(1), 57-70.

Healy, E., Belgaid, C., Takata, M., Harrison, D., Zhu, N. W., Burd, D. A., Rigby, H. S., Matthews, J. N., & Rees, J. L. (1998). Prognostic significance of allelic losses in primary melanoma. *Oncogene, 16*(17), 2213-2218.

Hillion, J., Le Coniat, M., Jonveaux, P., Berger, R., & Bernard, O. A. (1997). AF6q21, a novel partner of the MLL gene in t(6;11)(q21;q23), defines a forkhead transcriptional factor subfamily. *Blood, 90*(9), 3714-3719.

Hu, L., Hofmann, J., Lu, Y., Mills, G. B., & Jaffe, R. B. (2002). Inhibition of phosphatidylinositol 3'-kinase increases efficacy of paclitaxel in in vitro and in vivo ovarian cancer models. *Cancer Res, 62*(4), 1087-1092.

Huang, H., Potter, C. J., Tao, W., Li, D. M., Brogiolo, W., Hafen, E., Sun, H., & Xu, T. (1999). PTEN affects cell size, cell proliferation and apoptosis during Drosophila eye development. *Development, 126*(23), 5365-5372.

Hutchinson, J., Jin, J., Cardiff, R. D., Woodgett, J. R., & Muller, W. J. (2001). Activation of Akt (protein kinase B) in mammary epithelium provides a critical cell survival signal required for tumor progression. *Mol Cell Biol, 21*(6), 2203-2212.

Isshiki, K., Elder, D. E., Guerry, D., & Linnenbach, A. J. (1993). Chromosome 10 allelic loss in malignant melanoma. *Genes Chromosomes Cancer, 8*(3), 178-184.

Kandel, E. S., & Hay, N. (1999). The regulation and activities of the multifunctional serine/threonine kinase Akt/PKB. *Exp Cell Res, 253*(1), 210-229.

Kane, L. P., Shapiro, V. S., Stokoe, D., & Weiss, A. (1999). Induction of NF-kappaB by the Akt/PKB kinase. *Curr Biol, 9*(11), 601-604.

Katso, R., Okkenhaug, K., Ahmadi, K., White, S., Timms, J., & Waterfield, M. D. (2001). Cellular function of phosphoinositide 3-kinases: implications for development, homeostasis, and cancer. *Annu Rev Cell Dev Biol, 17*, 615-675.

Khwaja, A. (1999). Akt is more than just a Bad kinase. *Nature, 401*(6748), 33-34.

Klippel, A., Escobedo, M. A., Wachowicz, M. S., Apell, G., Brown, T. W., Giedlin, M. A., Kavanaugh, W. M., & Williams, L. T. (1998). Activation of phosphatidylinositol 3-kinase is sufficient for cell cycle entry and promotes cellular changes characteristic of oncogenic transformation. *Mol Cell Biol, 18*(10), 5699-5711.

Konishi, H., Kuroda, S., Tanaka, M., Matsuzaki, H., Ono, Y., Kameyama, K., Haga, T., & Kikkawa, U. (1995). Molecular cloning and characterization of a new member of the RAC protein kinase family: association of the pleckstrin homology domain of three types of RAC protein kinase with protein kinase C subspecies and beta gamma subunits of G proteins. *Biochem Biophys Res Commun, 216*(2), 526-534.

Kops, G. J., & Burgering, B. M. (1999). Forkhead transcription factors: new insights into protein kinase B (c-akt) signaling. *J Mol Med, 77*(9), 656-665.

Kops, G. J., de Ruiter, N. D., De Vries-Smits, A. M., Powell, D. R., Bos, J. L., & Burgering, B. M. (1999). Direct control of the Forkhead transcription factor AFX by protein kinase B. *Nature, 398*(6728), 630-634.

Kotani, K., Hara, K., Yonezawa, K., & Kasuga, M. (1995). Phosphoinositide 3-kinase as an upstream regulator of the small GTP-binding protein Rac in the insulin signaling of membrane ruffling. *Biochem Biophys Res Commun, 208*(3), 985-990.

Kuruvilla, F. G., & Schreiber, S. L. (1999). The PIK-related kinases intercept conventional signaling pathways. *Chem Biol, 6*(5), R129-136.

Kwon, C. H., Zhu, X., Zhang, J., Knoop, L. L., Tharp, R., Smeyne, R. J., Eberhart, C. G., Burger, P. C., & Baker, S. J. (2001). Pten regulates neuronal soma size: a mouse model of Lhermitte-Duclos disease. *Nat Genet, 29*(4), 404-411.

Lee, J. O., Yang, H., Georgescu, M. M., Di Cristofano, A., Maehama, T., Shi, Y., Dixon, J. E., Pandolfi, P., & Pavletich, N. P. (1999). Crystal structure of the PTEN tumor suppressor: implications for its phosphoinositide phosphatase activity and membrane association. *Cell, 99*(3), 323-334.

Levine, R. L., Cargile, C. B., Blazes, M. S., van Rees, B., Kurman, R. J., & Ellenson, L. H. (1998). PTEN mutations and microsatellite instability in complex atypical hyperplasia, a precursor lesion to uterine endometrioid carcinoma. *Cancer Res, 58*(15), 3254-3258.

Li, D. M., & Sun, H. (1997). TEP1, encoded by a candidate tumor suppressor locus, is a novel protein tyrosine phosphatase regulated by transforming growth factor beta. *Cancer Res, 57*(11), 2124-2129.

Li, J., Yen, C., Liaw, D., Podsypanina, K., Bose, S., Wang, S. I., Puc, J., Miliaresis, C., Rodgers, L., McCombie, R., Bigner, S. H., Giovanella, B. C., Ittmann, M., Tycko, B., Hibshoosh, H., Wigler, M. H., & Parsons, R. (1997). PTEN, a putative protein tyrosine phosphatase gene mutated in human brain, breast, and prostate cancer. *Science, 275*(5308), 1943-1947.

Liaw, D., Marsh, D. J., Li, J., Dahia, P. L., Wang, S. I., Zheng, Z., Bose, S., Call, K. M., Tsou, H. C., Peacocke, M., Eng, C., & Parsons, R. (1997). Germline mutations of the PTEN gene in Cowden disease, an inherited breast and thyroid cancer syndrome. *Nat Genet, 16*(1), 64-67.

Lin, K., Dorman, J. B., Rodan, A., & Kenyon, C. (1997). daf-16: An HNF-3/forkhead family member that can function to double the life-span of Caenorhabditis elegans. *Science, 278*(5341), 1319-1322.

Liu, W., James, C. D., Frederick, L., Alderete, B. E., & Jenkins, R. B. (1997). PTEN/MMAC1 mutations and EGFR amplification in glioblastomas. *Cancer Res, 57*(23), 5254-5257.

Ma, Y. Y., Wei, S. J., Lin, Y. C., Lung, J. C., Chang, T. C., Whang-Peng, J., Liu, J. M., Yang, D. M., Yang, W. K., & Shen, C. Y. (2000). PIK3CA as an oncogene in cervical cancer. *Oncogene, 19*(23), 2739-2744.

Maehama, T., & Dixon, J. E. (1998). The tumor suppressor, PTEN/MMAC1, dephosphorylates the lipid second messenger, phosphatidylinositol 3,4,5-trisphosphate. *J Biol Chem, 273*(22), 13375-13378.

Maehama, T., Taylor, G. S., & Dixon, J. E. (2001). PTEN AND MYOTUBULARIN: Novel Phosphoinositide Phosphatases. *Annu Rev Biochem, 70*, 247-279.

Maxwell, G. L., Risinger, J. I., Gumbs, C., Shaw, H., Bentley, R. C., Barrett, J. C., Berchuck, A., & Futreal, P. A. (1998). Mutation of the PTEN tumor suppressor gene in endometrial hyperplasias. *Cancer Res, 58*(12), 2500-2503.

McMenamin, M. E., Soung, P., Perera, S., Kaplan, I., Loda, M., & Sellers, W. R. (1999). Loss of PTEN expression in paraffin-embedded primary prostate cancer correlates with high Gleason score and advanced stage. *Cancer Res, 59*(17), 4291-4296.

Medema, R. H., Kops, G. J., Bos, J. L., & Burgering, B. M. (2000). AFX-like Forkhead transcription factors mediate cell-cycle regulation by Ras and PKB through p27kip1. *Nature, 404*(6779), 782-787.

Mende, I., Malstrom, S., Tsichlis, P. N., Vogt, P. K., & Aoki, M. (2001). Oncogenic transformation induced by membrane-targeted Akt2 and Akt3. *Oncogene, 20*(32), 4419-4423.

Montagnani, M., Chen, H., Barr, V. A., & Quon, M. J. (2001). Insulin-stimulated activation of eNOS is independent of Ca2+ but requires phosphorylation by Akt at Ser(1179). *J Biol Chem, 276*(32), 30392-30398.

Munster, P. N., Basso, A., Solit, D., Norton, L., & Rosen, N. (2001). Modulation of Hsp90 function by ansamycins sensitizes breast cancer cells to chemotherapy-induced apoptosis in an RB- and schedule-dependent manner. See: E. A. Sausville, Combining cytotoxics and 17-allylamino, 17-demethoxygeldanamycin: sequence and tumor biology matters, Clin. Cancer Res., 7: 2155-2158, 2001. *Clin Cancer Res, 7*(8), 2228-2236.

Myers, M. P., Pass, I., Batty, I. H., Van der Kaay, J., Stolarov, J. P., Hemmings, B. A., Wigler, M. H., Downes, C. P., & Tonks, N. K. (1998). The lipid phosphatase activity of PTEN is critical for its tumor supressor function. *Proc Natl Acad Sci U S A, 95*(23), 13513-13518.

Myers, M. P., & Tonks, N. K. (1997). PTEN: sometimes taking it off can be better than putting it on. *Am J Hum Genet, 61*(6), 1234-1238.

Nakamura, N., Ramaswamy, S., Vazquez, F., Signoretti, S., Loda, M., & Sellers, W. R. (2000). Forkhead transcription factors are critical effectors of cell death and cell cycle arrest downstream of PTEN. *Mol Cell Biol, 20*(23), 8969-8982.

Nakatani, K., Thompson, D. A., Barthel, A., Sakaue, H., Liu, W., Weigel, R. J., & Roth, R. A. (1999). Up-regulation of Akt3 in estrogen receptor-deficient breast cancers and androgen-independent prostate cancer lines. *J Biol Chem, 274*(31), 21528-21532.

Nelen, M. R., van Staveren, W. C., Peeters, E. A., Hassel, M. B., Gorlin, R. J., Hamm, H., Lindboe, C. F., Fryns, J. P., Sijmons, R. H., Woods, D. G., Mariman, E. C., Padberg, G. W., & Kremer, H. (1997). Germline mutations in the PTEN/MMAC1 gene in patients with Cowden disease. *Hum Mol Genet, 6*(8), 1383-1387.

Neshat, M. S., Mellinghoff, I. K., Tran, C., Stiles, B., Thomas, G., Petersen, R., Frost, P., Gibbons, J. J., Wu, H., & Sawyers, C. L. (2001). Enhanced sensitivity of PTEN-deficient tumors to inhibition of FRAP/mTOR. *Proc Natl Acad Sci U S A, 98*(18), 10314-10319.

Obata, K., Morland, S. J., Watson, R. H., Hitchcock, A., Chenevix-Trench, G., Thomas, E. J., & Campbell, I. G. (1998). Frequent PTEN/MMAC mutations in endometrioid but not serous or mucinous epithelial ovarian tumors. *Cancer Res, 58*(10), 2095-2097.

Ogg, S., & Ruvkun, G. (1998). The C. elegans PTEN homolog, DAF-18, acts in the insulin receptor-like metabolic signaling pathway. *Mol Cell, 2*(6), 887-893.

Okano, J., Gaslightwala, I., Birnbaum, M. J., Rustgi, A. K., & Nakagawa, H. (2000). Akt/protein kinase B isoforms are differentially regulated by epidermal growth factor stimulation. *J Biol Chem, 275*(40), 30934-30942.

Oldham, S., Bohni, R., Stocker, H., Brogiolo, W., & Hafen, E. (2000). Genetic control of size in Drosophila. *Philos Trans R Soc Lond B Biol Sci, 355*(1399), 945-952.

Ozes, O. N., Mayo, L. D., Gustin, J. A., Pfeffer, S. R., Pfeffer, L. M., & Donner, D. B. (1999). NF-kappaB activation by tumour necrosis factor requires the Akt serine-threonine kinase. *Nature, 401*(6748), 82-85.

Pece, S., Chiariello, M., Murga, C., & Gutkind, J. S. (1999). Activation of the protein kinase Akt/PKB by the formation of E-cadherin-mediated cell-cell junctions. Evidence for the association of phosphatidylinositol 3-kinase with the E-cadherin adhesion complex. *J Biol Chem, 274*(27), 19347-19351.

Peng, H., Kim, D. I., Sarkaria, J. N., Cho, Y. S., Abraham, R. T., & Zalkow, L. H. (2002). Novel pyrrolo-quinoline derivatives as potent inhibitors for PI3-kinase related kinases. *Bioorg Med Chem, 10*(1), 167-174.

Persad, S., Attwell, S., Gray, V., Mawji, N., Deng, J. T., Leung, D., Yan, J., Sanghera, J., Walsh, M. P., & Dedhar, S. (2001). Regulation of protein kinase B/Akt-serine 473 phosphorylation by integrin-linked kinase: critical roles for kinase activity and amino acids arginine 211 and serine 343. *J Biol Chem, 276*(29), 27462-27469.

Phillips, W. A., St Clair, F., Munday, A. D., Thomas, R. J., & Mitchell, C. A. (1998). Increased levels of phosphatidylinositol 3-kinase activity in colorectal tumors. *Cancer, 83*(1), 41-47.

Philp, A. J., Campbell, I. G., Leet, C., Vincan, E., Rockman, S. P., Whitehead, R. H., Thomas, R. J., & Phillips, W. A. (2001). The phosphatidylinositol 3'-kinase p85alpha gene is an oncogene in human ovarian and colon tumors. *Cancer Res, 61*(20), 7426-7429.

Podsypanina, K., Ellenson, L. H., Nemes, A., Gu, J., Tamura, M., Yamada, K. M., Cordon-Cardo, C., Catoretti, G., Fisher, P. E., & Parsons, R. (1999). Mutation of Pten/Mmac1 in mice causes neoplasia in multiple organ systems. *Proc Natl Acad Sci U S A, 96*(4), 1563-1568.

Podsypanina, K., Lee, R. T., Politis, C., Hennessy, I., Crane, A., Puc, J., Neshat, M., Wang, H., Yang, L., Gibbons, J., Frost, P., Dreisbach, V., Blenis, J., Gaciong, Z., Fisher, P., Sawyers, C., Hedrick-Ellenson, L., & Parsons, R. (2001). An inhibitor of mTOR reduces neoplasia and normalizes p70/S6 kinase activity in Pten+/- mice. *Proc Natl Acad Sci U S A, 98*(18), 10320-10325.

Posern, G., Saffrich, R., Ansorge, W., & Feller, S. M. (2000). Rapid lamellipodia formation in nerve growth factor-stimulated PC12 cells is dependent on Rac and PI3K activity. *J Cell Physiol, 183*(3), 416-424.

Ramaswamy, S., Nakamura, N., Vazquez, F., Batt, D. B., Perera, S., Roberts, T. M., & Sellers, W. R. (1999). Regulation of G1 progression by the PTEN tumor suppressor protein is linked to inhibition of the phosphatidylinositol 3-kinase/Akt pathway. *Proc Natl Acad Sci U S A, 96*(5), 2110-2115.

Rasheed, B. K., Stenzel, T. T., McLendon, R. E., Parsons, R., Friedman, A. H., Friedman, H. S., Bigner, D. D., & Bigner, S. H. (1997). PTEN gene mutations are seen in high-grade but not in low-grade gliomas. *Cancer Res, 57*(19), 4187-4190.

Rasheed, B. K., Wiltshire, R. N., Bigner, S. H., & Bigner, D. D. (1999). Molecular pathogenesis of malignant gliomas. *Curr Opin Oncol, 11*(3), 162-167.

Rena, G., Guo, S., Cichy, S. C., Unterman, T. G., & Cohen, P. (1999). Phosphorylation of the transcription factor forkhead family member FKHR by protein kinase B. *J Biol Chem, 274*(24), 17179-17183.

Romashkova, J. A., & Makarov, S. S. (1999). NF-kappaB is a target of AKT in anti-apoptotic PDGF signalling. *Nature, 401*(6748), 86-90.

Sausville, E. A. (2001). Combining cytotoxics and 17-allylamino, 17-demethoxygeldanamycin: sequence and tumor biology matters. Commentary re: P. Munster et al., Modulation of Hsp90 function by ansamycins sensitizes breast cancer cells to chemotherapy-induced apoptosis in an RB- and schedule-dependent manner. Clin. Cancer Res., 7: 2228-2236, 2001. *Clin Cancer Res, 7*(8), 2155-2158.

Schneider, C., Sepp-Lorenzino, L., Nimmesgern, E., Ouerfelli, O., Danishefsky, S., Rosen, N., & Hartl, F. U. (1996). Pharmacologic shifting of a balance between protein refolding and degradation mediated by Hsp90. *Proc Natl Acad Sci U S A, 93*(25), 14536-14541.

Shaw, L. M., Rabinovitz, I., Wang, H. H., Toker, A., & Mercurio, A. M. (1997). Activation of phosphoinositide 3-OH kinase by the alpha6beta4 integrin promotes carcinoma invasion. *Cell, 91*(7), 949-960.

Shayesteh, L., Lu, Y., Kuo, W. L., Baldocchi, R., Godfrey, T., Collins, C., Pinkel, D., Powell, B., Mills, G. B., & Gray, J. W. (1999). PIK3CA is implicated as an oncogene in ovarian cancer. *Nat Genet, 21*(1), 99-102.

Simpson, L., & Parsons, R. (2001). PTEN: life as a tumor suppressor. *Exp Cell Res, 264*(1), 29-41.

Somerville, R. P., Shoshan, Y., Eng, C., Barnett, G., Miller, D., & Cowell, J. K. (1998). Molecular analysis of two putative tumour suppressor genes, PTEN and DMBT, which have been implicated in glioblastoma multiforme disease progression. *Oncogene, 17*(13), 1755-1757.

Staal, S. P. (1987). Molecular cloning of the akt oncogene and its human homologues AKT1 and AKT2: amplification of AKT1 in a primary human gastric adenocarcinoma. *Proc Natl Acad Sci U S A, 84*(14), 5034-5037.

Staal, S. P., & Hartley, J. W. (1988). Thymic lymphoma induction by the AKT8 murine retrovirus. *J Exp Med, 167*(3), 1259-1264.

Stambolic, V., Suzuki, A., de la Pompa, J. L., Brothers, G. M., Mirtsos, C., Sasaki, T., Ruland, J., Penninger, J. M., Siderovski, D. P., & Mak, T. W. (1998). Negative regulation of PKB/Akt-dependent cell survival by the tumor suppressor PTEN. *Cell, 95*(1), 29-39.

Stambolic, V., Tsao, M. S., Macpherson, D., Suzuki, A., Chapman, W. B., & Mak, T. W. (2000). High incidence of breast and endometrial neoplasia resembling human Cowden syndrome in pten+/- mice. *Cancer Res, 60*(13), 3605-3611.

Steck, P. A., Lin, H., Langford, L. A., Jasser, S. A., Koul, D., Yung, W. K., & Pershouse, M. A. (1999). Functional and molecular analyses of 10q deletions in human gliomas. *Genes Chromosomes Cancer, 24*(2), 135-143.

Steck, P. A., Pershouse, M. A., Jasser, S. A., Yung, W. K., Lin, H., Ligon, A. H., Langford, L. A., Baumgard, M. L., Hattier, T., Davis, T., Frye, C., Hu, R., Swedlund, B., Teng, D. H., & Tavtigian, S. V. (1997). Identification of a candidate tumour suppressor gene, MMAC1, at chromosome 10q23.3 that is mutated in multiple advanced cancers. *Nat Genet, 15*(4), 356-362.

Stein, R. C., & Waterfield, M. D. (2000). PI3-kinase inhibition: a target for drug development? *Mol Med Today, 6*(9), 347-357.

Stocker, H., Andjelkovic, M., Oldham, S., Laffargue, M., Wymann, M. P., Hemmings, B. A., & Hafen, E. (2002). Living with Lethal PIP3 Levels: Viability of Flies Lacking PTEN Restored by a PH Domain Mutation in Akt/PKB. *Science.*

Sun, H., Lesche, R., Li, D. M., Liliental, J., Zhang, H., Gao, J., Gavrilova, N., Mueller, B., Liu, X., & Wu, H. (1999). PTEN modulates cell cycle progression and cell survival by regulating phosphatidylinositol 3,4,5,-trisphosphate and Akt/protein kinase B signaling pathway. *Proc Natl Acad Sci U S A, 96*(11), 6199-6204.

Sun, M., Wang, G., Paciga, J. E., Feldman, R. I., Yuan, Z. Q., Ma, X. L., Shelley, S. A., Jove, R., Tsichlis, P. N., Nicosia, S. V., & Cheng, J. Q. (2001). AKT1/PKBalpha kinase is frequently elevated in human cancers and its constitutive activation is required for oncogenic transformation in NIH3T3 cells. *Am J Pathol, 159*(2), 431-437.

Suzuki, A., de la Pompa, J. L., Stambolic, V., Elia, A. J., Sasaki, T., del Barco Barrantes, I., Ho, A., Wakeham, A., Itie, A., Khoo, W., Fukumoto, M., & Mak, T. W. (1998). High cancer susceptibility and embryonic lethality associated with mutation of the PTEN tumor suppressor gene in mice. *Curr Biol, 8*(21), 1169-1178.

Tamura, M., Gu, J., Danen, E. H., Takino, T., Miyamoto, S., & Yamada, K. M. (1999). PTEN interactions with focal adhesion kinase and suppression of the extracellular matrix-dependent phosphatidylinositol 3-kinase/Akt cell survival pathway. *J Biol Chem, 274*(29), 20693-20703.

Tamura, M., Gu, J., Matsumoto, K., Aota, S., Parsons, R., & Yamada, K. M. (1998). Inhibition of cell migration, spreading, and focal adhesions by tumor suppressor PTEN. *Science, 280*(5369), 1614-1617.

Tolkacheva, T., Boddapati, M., Sanfiz, A., Tsuchida, K., Kimmelman, A. C., & Chan, A. M. (2001). Regulation of PTEN binding to MAGI-2 by two putative phosphorylation sites at threonine 382 and 383. *Cancer Res, 61*(13), 4985-4989.

Tsao, H., Zhang, X., Benoit, E., & Haluska, F. G. (1998). Identification of PTEN/MMAC1 alterations in uncultured melanomas and melanoma cell lines. *Oncogene, 16*(26), 3397-3402.

Vanhaesebroeck, B., & Waterfield, M. D. (1999). Signaling by distinct classes of phosphoinositide 3-kinases. *Exp Cell Res, 253*(1), 239-254.

Vazquez, F., Grossman, S. R., Takahashi, Y., Rokas, M. V., Nakamura, N., & Sellers, W. R. (2001). Phosphorylation of the PTEN Tail Acts as an Inhibitory Switch by Preventing Its Recruitment into a Protein Complex. *J Biol Chem, 276*(52), 48627-48630.

Vazquez, F., Ramaswamy, S., Nakamura, N., & Sellers, W. R. (2000). Phosphorylation of the PTEN tail regulates protein stability and function. *Mol Cell Biol, 20*(14), 5010-5018.

Vazquez, F., & Sellers, W. R. (2000). The PTEN tumor suppressor protein: an antagonist of phosphoinositide 3-kinase signaling. *Biochim Biophys Acta, 1470*(1), M21-35.

Verdu, J., Buratovich, M. A., Wilder, E. L., & Birnbaum, M. J. (1999). Cell-autonomous regulation of cell and organ growth in Drosophila by Akt/PKB. *Nat Cell Biol, 1*(8), 500-506.

Wang, S. I., Puc, J., Li, J., Bruce, J. N., Cairns, P., Sidransky, D., & Parsons, R. (1997). Somatic mutations of PTEN in glioblastoma multiforme. *Cancer Res, 57*(19), 4183-4186.

Wu, X., Hepner, K., Castelino-Prabhu, S., Do, D., Kaye, M. B., Yuan, X. J., Wood, J., Ross, C., Sawyers, C. L., & Whang, Y. E. (2000). Evidence for regulation of the PTEN tumor suppressor by a membrane-localized multi-PDZ domain containing scaffold protein MAGI-2. *Proc Natl Acad Sci U S A, 97*(8), 4233-4238.

Xu, W., Mimnaugh, E., Rosser, M. F., Nicchitta, C., Marcu, M., Yarden, Y., & Neckers, L. (2001). Sensitivity of mature Erbb2 to geldanamycin is conferred by its kinase domain and is mediated by the chaperone protein Hsp90. *J Biol Chem, 276*(5), 3702-3708.

Yaffe, M. B., Leparc, G. G., Lai, J., Obata, T., Volinia, S., & Cantley, L. C. (2001). A motif-based profile scanning approach for genome-wide prediction of signaling pathways. *Nat Biotechnol, 19*(4), 348-353.

Yaffe, M. B., Rittinger, K., Volinia, S., Caron, P. R., Aitken, A., Leffers, H., Gamblin, S. J., Smerdon, S. J., & Cantley, L. C. (1997). The structural basis for 14-3-3:phosphopeptide binding specificity. *Cell, 91*(7), 961-971.

Yao, R., & Cooper, G. M. (1995). Requirement for phosphatidylinositol-3 kinase in the prevention of apoptosis by nerve growth factor. *Science, 267*(5206), 2003-2006.

Yokomizo, A., Tindall, D. J., Hartmann, L., Jenkins, R. B., Smith, D. I., & Liu, W. (1998). Mutation analysis of the putative tumor suppressor PTEN/MMAC1 in human ovarian cancer. *Int J Oncol, 13*(1), 101-105.

Yuan, Z. Q., Sun, M., Feldman, R. I., Wang, G., Ma, X., Jiang, C., Coppola, D., Nicosia, S. V., & Cheng, J. Q. (2000). Frequent activation of AKT2 and induction of apoptosis by inhibition of phosphoinositide-3-OH kinase/Akt pathway in human ovarian cancer. *Oncogene, 19*(19), 2324-2330.

Zhang, H., Stallock, J. P., Ng, J. C., Reinhard, C., & Neufeld, T. P. (2000). Regulation of cellular growth by the Drosophila target of rapamycin dTOR. *Genes Dev, 14*(21), 2712-2724.

Zhou, B. P., Liao, Y., Xia, W., Spohn, B., Lee, M. H., & Hung, M. C. (2001). Cytoplasmic localization of p21Cip1/WAF1 by Akt-induced phosphorylation in HER-2/neu-overexpressing cells. *Nat Cell Biol, 3*(3), 245-252.

Zimmermann, S., & Moelling, K. (1999). Phosphorylation and regulation of Raf by Akt (protein kinase B). *Science, 286*(5445), 1741-1744.

WNT SIGNALING IN HUMAN CANCER

PATRICE J. MORIN AND ASHANI T. WEERARATNA

1. INTRODUCTION

From *Drosophila* to humans, the Wnt proteins play crucial roles in cell fate determination and patterning during embryonic development. Defects in this pathway have been shown to cause various embryonic abnormalities in *Drosophila* and animal models and have been implicated in human cancer. In mouse, the deletion of specific Wnts results in the lack of development of specific organs, stressing the importance of Wnts in embryogenesis. Vertebrate wnt genes are expressed in unique but overlapping patterns during gastrulation, and in the adult are expressed in a variety of tissues. It is now recognized that Wnts represent a large family of proteins comprising at least 16 members of various signaling potential and tissue specificity. Several lines of evidence clearly show that inappropriate activation of the Wnt pathway can lead to the development of cancer. First, inappropriate expression of Wnt-1 (initially identified in mouse mammary carcinomas as a target of insertional activation by the mouse mammary tumor virus, MMTV) and other Wnt family members can lead to tumor formation in mice. Second, transfection of many members of the Wnt family (or downstream components) can lead to transformation of C57mg mammary epithelial cells. Third, mutations of many downstream Wnt pathway components have been identified in various human cancers.

In *Drosophila*, Wnt signaling is crucial for both cell morphogenesis and planar cell polarity. There is ample evidence that these dual effects of Wnt are mediated by at least two different downstream pathways (Boutros, Paricio, Strutt, & Mlodzik, 1998; McEwen & Peifer, 2001). Similarly, overexpression of various Wnt in *Xenopus* embryos can lead to either axis duplication or morphogenetic movements, again suggesting the presence of alternative pathways (Kuhl, Sheldahl, Park, Miller, & Moon, 2000). In all systems studied, Wnt signaling can have multiple outcomes corresponding to multiple downstream pathways. Wnt signaling specificity and downstream pathway selection prove to be extremely complex issues, depending not only on the Wnt ligands themselves, but also on their interactions with their receptors and co-receptors. It is currently believed that Wnt proteins can signal through three major pathways: the canonical Wnt pathway (sometimes referred to as the Wnt/β-catenin pathway) and the non-canonical Wnt/Ca^{2+} and Wnt/JNK pathways. Much progress has been made in the past ten years in understanding the downstream effects of Wnt signaling in development and tumorigenesis. In this chapter, we will discuss the molecular pathways by which Wnts mediate their effects, and how these pathways contribute to tumorigenesis.

2. THE WNT PROTEINS AND THE FRIZZLED RECEPTORS: GENERATING THE SIGNAL

2.1. Wnt Proteins

The vertebrate Wnt family of proteins is comprised of at least 16 members located on various chromosomes. Wnt proteins are secreted glycoproteins ranging from about 350 to 400 amino acids in length with an amino-terminal secretory signal peptide. This signal sequence is hydrophobic, and followed by a short domain that is not well conserved. Following this, there is an asparagine-linked oligosaccharide consensus sequence and 22 cysteine-rich regions. The spacing of these cysteine-rich regions is exactly conserved. After translation, Wnts are N-glycosylated, presumably by the porcupine (porc) gene product (Kadowaki, Wilder, Klingensmith, Zachary, & Perrimon, 1996) and this glycosylation appears to be crucial for folding, secretion and biological activity (Smolich, McMahon, McMahon, & Papkoff, 1993). The Wnt proteins have important roles during development, such as in mediating cell-cell interactions during embryogenesis, or regulating morphogenesis and limb development. In normal development, Wnts are expressed both tissue specifically and temporally (Cadigan & Nusse, 1997).

Wnt family members have differing and sometimes antagonistic roles. Indeed, using the C57mg cell model system, Wnt proteins can be divided into three major categories: highly transforming, weakly transforming or non transforming (Jue, Bradley, Rudnicki, Varmus, & Brown, 1992; Wong, Gavin, & McMahon, 1994). Wnts of the group that have high-transforming ability in C57mg cells such as Wnt-1, Wnt-2 and Wnt-3 (referred collectively as Wnt-1-type proteins) signal via the stabilization of β-catenin (Shimizu et al., 1997). In development this pathway is responsible for cell growth as well as cell fate determination (Orsulic & Peifer, 1996; Smalley & Dale, 1999; Sokol, 1999) and is known as the canonical pathway. Wnts with intermediate transforming ability in C57mg such as Wnt-6 and Wnt-7a or low transforming ability such as Wnt-4 Wnt-5a, Wnt-5b, and Wnt-7b are believed to generally signal through non-canonical Wnt pathways, regulating planar cell polarity and convergent extension movements in embryogenesis (Kuhl, Sheldahl, Park et al., 2000; McEwen & Peifer, 2001).

Interestingly, certain intermediate or non-transformers can antagonize the function of Wnt-1 type proteins. For example, during *Xenopus* development the expression of Wnt-5a can cause a failure of Wnt-1 to duplicate the embryonic axis (Torres, 1996). Moreover, in *Drosophila*, Dwnt-4 antagonizes wingless (a Wnt-1-type protein) function in the embryonic ectoderm (Gieseler et al., 1999). In tumorigenesis, C57mg mammary cell transformation by an anti-sense Wnt-5a mimics Wnt-1-mediated transformation (Olson & Gibo, 1998). All these examples are evidence of multiple downstream signals of the Wnt pathways. Further roles for the Wnt proteins were revealed by examining defects in mouse models lacking specific Wnt genes.

2.2. Wnt Knockout animals

Wnt disruption in mice generally results in severe developmental defects. A sampling of the 20 or so Wnt knockout mouse models reported so far confirms this. Wnt-1 knockout mice reveal severe effects on brain development, particularly in the mesencephalon and the metencephalon, implicating Wnt-1 in the induction of these structures (McMahon, 1990; Thomas & Capecchi, 1990). Wnt-2 knockout mice exhibit defects in the vascularisation of the placenta and increased perinatal lethality (Monkley, Delaney, Pennisi, Christiansen, & Wainwright, 1996). Wnt-3 knockouts do not form paraxial mesoderm and develop an excess of neural tubes, demonstrating a fundamental role for Wnt-3 in primary axis formation in the mouse (P. Liu et al., 1999). Wnt-4 knockouts are unable to form kidney tubules, and thus kidneys, demonstrating the importance of Wnt-4 for mesenchyme-epithelial transitions in kidney development (Stark, Vainio, Vassileva, & McMahon, 1994). In addition, Wnt-4 knockout females exibit masculinization associated with the absence of Mullerian duct (Vainio, Heikkila, Kispert, Chin, & McMahon, 1999). Wnt-5a is crucial for outgrowth from the primary body axis as Wnt-5a knockout mice exhibit truncation of the proximal skeleton and absence of distal digits (Yamaguchi, Bradley, McMahon, & Jones, 1999). Wnt-7a ablation in male mice resulted in the inability of these mice to regress the Mullerian duct, the regression of which is necessary in males so that female sex organs do not develop (Parr & McMahon, 1998). In female mice, this knockout results in infertility due to the malformations of the oviduct and uterus, again due to the effects on mesenchymal interactions with the Mullerian ducts. Furthermore these mice also exhibit ventralized limbs (Parr & McMahon, 1995). Similarly, other Wnt knockouts also exhibit various developmental malformations (Parr, Cornish, Cybulsky, & McMahon, 2001; Takada et al., 1994). These numerous knockout experiments unambiguously demonstrate the crucial roles for Wnt proteins in vertebrate development.

2.3. Frizzled Receptors

In order to discuss Wnt signaling, it is important to first describe the receptors for these ligands, the Frizzled proteins. The first Frizzled protein was identified in *Drosophila*, where it was implicated in tissue polarity in the adult cuticle, which is rich in a variety of structures such as bristle sense organs and hair (Vinson & Adler, 1987). Mutations in *frizzled* genes alter the way these structures are oriented in *Drosophila*. These receptors consist of approximately 587 amino acids, the first part of which constitutes a signal peptide. The N terminus of the Frizzled proteins is responsible for mediating Wnt interactions, and is glycosylated. The N-terminus has a conserved, extracellular cysteine-rich domain (CRD), spanning 120 amino acids, which is thought to be responsible for Wnt binding (Bhanot et al., 1996; Cadigan & Nusse, 1997). This is followed by seven transmembrane domains 20 to 25 amino acids each, joined by short, hydrophilic segments. The C-termini, which range in length from 20 amino acids to 200 amino acids, have many regions that could undergo phosphorylation. The overall sequence of the Frizzled receptors bears great homology to a superfamily of proteins known to be G-protein coupled receptors. Only recently however, through the use of bacterial toxins, anti-sense DNA techniques and other molecular strategies, were Frizzled proteins shown to be genuine G-protein-coupled receptors (see below) (Malbon, Wang, & Moon, 2001).

2.4. Frizzled co-receptors

In addition to the Frizzled receptors, a new family of co-receptors has been identified. These co-receptors work together with Frizzled receptors to mediate Wnt signaling. This adds another level of complexity as different receptor and co-receptor combinations can result in the transduction of signals down different pathways. These co-receptors are homologous to low-density lipoprotein receptor (LDLR) and have been named LRP (LDLR related proteins). LRPs have been identified in *Drosophila*, *Xenopus* and mouse (Tamai et al., 2000). LRPs are single transmembrane proteins, that contain epidermal growth factor like repeats and three LDL-receptor type Q repeats in their extracellular region (Pandur & Kuhl, 2001). Intracellularly, these proteins contain a proline-rich region that may bind to SH3-domain-containing proteins. It appears that these co-receptor associate with Frizzled in a Wnt-dependent fashion (Tamai et al., 2000). It is not yet known how exactly these complexes are organized; they may be heterotrimeric complexes of LRP, Frizzled and Wnt, or heterodimeric complexes of just Frizzled and LRP. It may also be that these proteins are important intracellularly, bridging Frizzled and Dsh, or Frizzled and other signaling molecules such as SH-3 domain containing proteins.

The function of these proteins appears to be intricately connected to their Frizzled/Wnt related functions since knocking out these proteins mimics a combination of Wnt knockout phenotypes. For example, LRP6 knockouts exhibit mid and hindbrain defects (Wnt-1), expansion of neural tissue and loss of paraxial mesoderm (Wnt-3a) and ventralization of limbs (Wnt-7a) (Pinson, Brennan, Monkley, Avery, & Skarnes, 2000).

3. THE CANONICAL WNT PATHWAY

3.1. β-catenin stability

Wnt signaling by members of the Wnt family such as Wnt-1 and Wnt-8 results in the regulation of β-catenin stabilization, and it now appears that this pathway is mediated by the binding of Wnt to Frizzled receptors that couple via the G-proteins Gαo and Gαq to the downstream components (Malbon et al., 2001). This is based mostly on evidence obtained with Frizzled-1 but is likely to be a general feature of the canonical pathway (Liu et al., 2001; Liu, Liu, Wang, Moon & Malbon, 1999). In the absence of Wnt signals, cytoplasmic β-catenin is rapidly degraded. In the presence of signal, β-catenin is stabilized and can associate with the T-cell factor (TCF) family of transcription factors to regulate expression of target genes (Figure 1).

The control of β-catenin protein levels is at the heart of signaling through the canonical Wnt pathway. Glycogen synthase kinase-3β (GSK3-β) can phosphorylate β-catenin at specific regulatory sites at its N-terminus. Phosphorylated β-catenin is recognized by the ubiquitin ligase β-TrCP leading to its ubiquitination and eventual destruction by the proteasome complex (Hart et al., 1999; Jiang & Struhl, 1998; Orford, Crockett, Jensen, Weissman, & Byers, 1997; Salomon et al., 1997; Winston et al., 1999). Phosphorylation of β-catenin by GSK3-β occurs in a large complex which contains adenomatous polyposis coli (APC, the gene causing Familial Adenomatous Polyposis), Axin, protein phosphatase 2A and β-TrCP (Behrens et al., 1998; Hart, de los Santos, Albert, Rubinfeld, & Polakis, 1998; Kishida et al., 1998; Seeling et al., 1999). The exact roles of each protein in the complex is still unclear but it appears that APC and Axin provide a scaffold for β-catenin phosphorylation by GSK3-β and subsequent ubiquitination mediated by β-TrCP. It is clear however, that the roles of Axin and APC are more than just providing passive scaffolding and are involved in regulating GSK3-β effects on β-catenin (von Kries et al., 2000). Indeed, Wnt signaling is accompanied by dephosphorylation of Axin leading to the release of β-catenin from the degradation complex (Willert, Shibamoto, & Nusse, 1999). This disengagement of β-catenin from the degradation complex leads to a decrease in its phosphorylation and an increase in its stability.

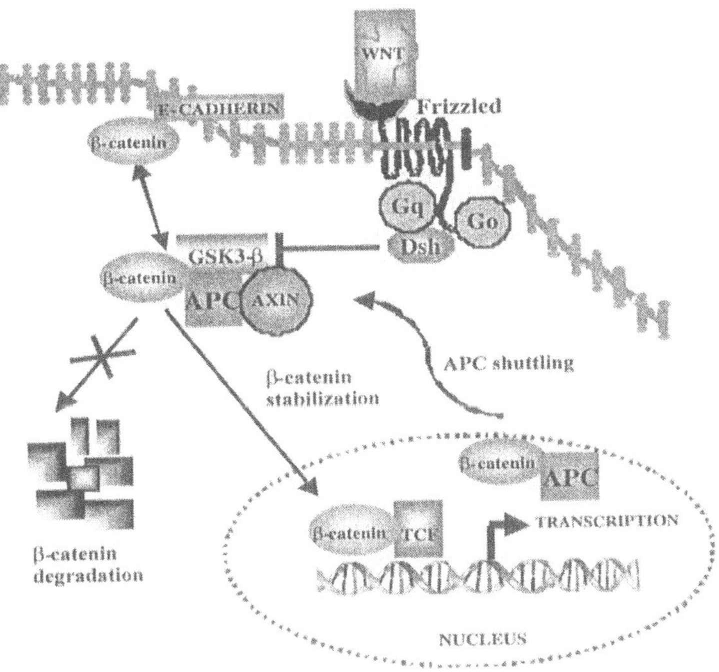

Figure 1. The canonical Wnt pathway

When Wnt binds to the Frizzled receptor, the protein dishevelled (Dsh), a cytoplasmic phosphoprotein that regulates cell proliferation, becomes activated and is recruited to the cell membrane (Axelrod, Miller, Shulman, Moon, & Perrimon, 1998). It is thought that this effect may be mediated by activation of the G-protein subunits Gαo and Gαq (see above). Although the exact mechanism by which Dsh leads to stabilization of β-catenin is unclear, it is known that during Wnt signaling Dsh becomes hyperphosphorylated via multiple kinases such as casein kinase-1 and -2 (Peters, McKay, McKay, & Graff, 1999; Sakanaka, Leong, Xu, Harrison, & Williams, 1999; Willert, Brink, Wodarz, Varmus, & Nusse, 1997). Dsh inhibits GSK3-β phosphorylation of β-catenin, although the enzymatic activity of GSK3-β remains unaffected. Dsh may block Axin either by direct interaction or through change in Axin phosphorylation, perhaps altering it such that GSK3-β cannot access β-catenin or by releasing β-catenin from the complex (Willert et al., 1999). This is consistent with the fact that the N-terminal 200 amino acids of Dsh (including the DIX domain) interact with the N terminus of Axin, but without competing for GSK3-β binding (Behrens et al., 1998; Ikeda et al., 1998; Kishida et al., 1999; Yamamoto et al., 1998; Zeng et al., 1997). Activated Dsh can also inactivate GSK3-β by interacting with GBP/Frat1 which binds to Dsh via its N-terminal PDZ domain and to GSK3-β via its c-terminus (Li et al., 1999). This results in the destruction of the entire Axin complex.

The ultimate result of Wnt signaling via Dsh is the stabilization of β-catenin and its accumulation in the cytoplasm. The free β-catenin in the cytoplasm can then translocate into the nucleus and participate in transcriptional regulation with TCFs, which provide the DNA binding moiety (Clevers & van de Wetering, 1997). It was originally thought that β-catenin may "piggy-back" on TCFs into the nucleus. Recent evidence suggests that β-catenin enters the nucleus through direct interaction with the nuclear pore complex in a manner similar to importin-β (Fagotto, Gluck, & Gumbiner, 1998; Yokoya, Imamoto, Tachibana, & Yoneda, 1999). APC contains two nuclear localization signals and can be found both in the cytoplasm and in the nucleus (Neufeld & White, 1997; Smith et al., 1993; Zhang, White, & Neufeld, 2000). At its N-terminus, APC also contains nuclear export sequences that can interact with the Crm1 nuclear export factor, leading to the hypothesis that APC may be involved in β-catenin shuttling from the nucleus to the degradation machinery in the cytoplasm (Neufeld, Nix et al., 2000; Neufeld, Zhang, Cullen, & White, 2000; Rosin-Arbesfeld, Townsley, & Bienz, 2000).

3.2. TCF/β-catenin transcriptional activity: targets of the pathway

TCF transcription factors (also known as Lef or TCF/Lef) were originally identified as lymphoid specific DNA-binding proteins that recognize a specific sequence-5'CTTTGWW3' (where W= A or T) (Travis, Amsterdam, Belanger, & Grosschedl, 1991; van de Wetering, Oosterwegel, Dooijes, & Clevers, 1991). TCFs bind to DNA via their high mobility group (HMG), which induces a sharp bend in the DNA helix (Giese, Amsterdam, & Grosschedl, 1991; Giese, Cox, & Grosschedl, 1992), but have no transactivation domains in the absence of β-catenin. During Wnt signaling and when interacting with TCFs, β-catenin provides two transcriptional activation domains located in the C and N termini (Hecht, Litterst, Huber, & Kemler, 1999; Hsu, Galceran, & Grosschedl, 1998). In the absence of Wnt signaling, TCFs can actively mediate the repression of Wnt-regulated genes via binding to the co-repressors TLE/groucho (Cavallo et al., 1998; Levanon et al., 1998; Roose & Clevers, 1999; Roose et al., 1998). Groucho, for example, can repress transcription via the recruitment of repressive chromatin through interactions with histone H3 (Cavallo et al., 1998). CBP can antagonize Wnt signaling by directly interacting with TCF, and acetylating a lysine residue in the β-catenin-binding region of dTCF *in vitro*, thus reducing the affinity of TCF for β-catenin (Waltzer & Bienz, 1998). *In vivo*, this may have the practical effect of preventing TCF transcription until the levels of β-catenin have reached a certain level. To add to the complexity, CBP was also found to interact directly with β-catenin to increase transcriptional activity from TCF sites (Hecht, Vleminckx, Stemmler, van Roy, & Kemler, 2000; Miyagishi et al., 2000; Takemaru & Moon, 2000). The rationale for these opposite effects of CBP on Wnt signaling is currently unknown but the role of CBP on signaling may be situation- or promoter-specific. In addition to acetylation, phosphorylation can also affect TCF activity. The MAP kinase related pathway involves a TGF-β activated kinase (TAK1) and NEMO like protein serine kinases which can antagonize β-catenin/TCF signaling by phosphorylating TCF (Ishitani et al., 1999; Rocheleau et al., 1999).

Ultimately, the canonical Wnt pathway regulates the expression of target genes by the TCF/β-catenin transcription factor. Many putative targets of the TCF/β-catenin transcriptional complex have been identified both in development and tumorigenesis (Barker, Morin, & Clevers, 2000; Morin, 1999; Polakis, 1999). In tumorigenesis, c-Myc, cyclin D1 and PPARδ have been identified as targets of the canonical Wnt pathway (He et al., 1998; He, Chan, Vogelstein, & Kinzler, 1999; Shtutman et al., 1999; Tetsu & McCormick, 1999).

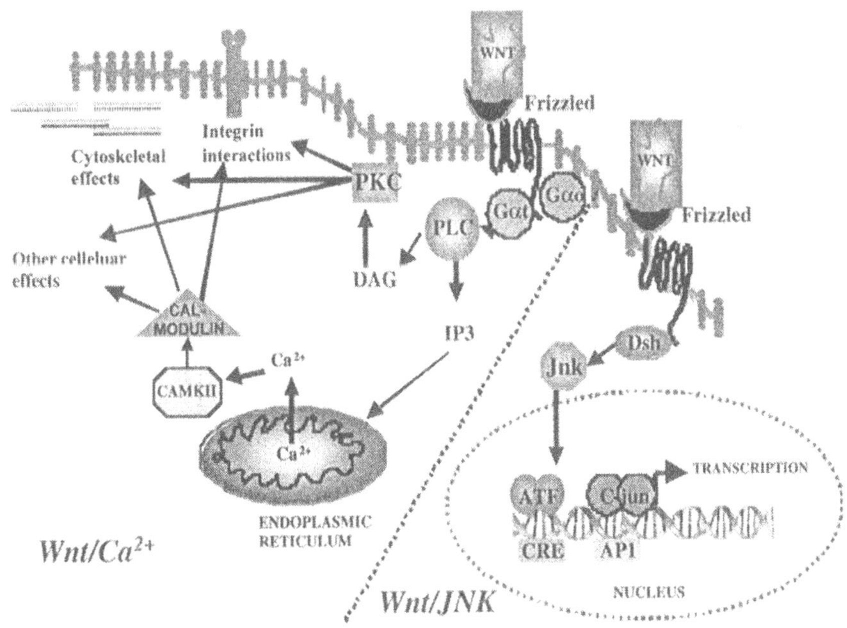

Figure 2. The non-canonical Wnt pathways

These targets have long been known to be important in tumorigenesis and may partially explain the oncogenic effects of Wnt activation. Indeed, transfecting cells with a dominant negative TCF can result in the arrest of colon cancer cells in the G1 phase of the cell cycle, by interfering with the production of cyclin D1 (Tetsu & McCormick, 1999). Other targets of this pathway include the matrix metalloproteinase, matrilysin (Brabletz, Jung, Dag, Hlubek, & Kirchner, 1999) and the transcription factors AP-1, c-jun and fra1 (Mann et al., 1999).

4. WNT/CA^{2+} SIGNALING PATHWAY

The non-canonical Wnt/Ca^{2+} pathway is regulated by the non-transforming members of the Wnt family such as Wnt-5a, Wnt-11 and Wnt-4. These Wnts alter movements and cell adhesion when overexpressed in *Xenopus* embryos (Du, Purcell, Christian, McGrew, & Moon, 1995; Moon et al., 1993). In fact, Wnt-5a was the first member of this family that was suspected to act via a β-catenin-independent pathway, as its overexpression could alter morphogenetic movements and cell adhesion, but could not transform C57mg cells, or cause axis induction in *Xenopus* embryos.

It was observed that the phenotype induced by Wnt-5a expression mimics the phenotype induced by 5HT1c receptor, a serotonin receptor (Ault, Durmowicz, Galione, Harger, & Busa, 1996). Furthermore, the overexpression of 5HT1c activates the release of Ca^{2+} in a G-protein-dependent manner, and it was subsequently demonstrated that Wnt-5a could also cause the release of intracellular Ca^{2+} (Slusarski, Yang-Snyder, Busa, & Moon, 1997). It has now been shown that Wnt-5a can mediate these effects via its interaction with the Frizzled receptor, which results in the activation of heterotrimeric G-proteins (Malbon et al., 2001)(Figure 2). Specifically, Frizzled-2-mediated functions (such as formation of the primitive endoderm in *Xenopus*) was shown to be sensitive to pertussis toxin, and indicated that these functions were controlled by G-protein activation (X. Liu et al., 1999). Using DNA antisense technology it was determined that indeed Frizzled-2 activation utilized heterotrimeric G-protein subunits Gαo and Gαt2. These G-protein subunits then activate phospholipase C, which translocates to the membrane and hydrolyzes membrane phospholipids, causing them to turn over and to initiate phosphatidylinositol signaling (Slusarski, Corces, & Moon, 1997). Inositol 1,4,5-triphosphate (IP_3) interacts with the SERCA-ATPase pump at the membrane of the endoplasmic reticulum, and results in the release of Ca^{2+} from these intracellular stores. Intracellular calcium can increase the expression and activity of calmodulin, and calmodulin kinases such as CAM KII (Kuhl, Sheldahl, Malbon, & Moon, 2000; Kuhl, Sheldahl, Park et al., 2000). Ca^{2+} can also increase the activity of Protein Kinase C (PKC), and this molecule can also be activated directly by diacylgycerol (DAG). Thus, one of the effects of Wnt-5a signaling is an increase in the activity of PKC (Sheldahl, Park, Malbon, & Moon, 1999). PKC activation can lead to a variety of different cellular responses as it is involved in numerous signal transduction pathways.

As mentioned before the complexity of the Wnt signaling pathways can be attributed to the diversity of the responses elicited by different Wnt/Frizzled pairs. For example, work performed in *Xenopus* shows that although Wnt-5a overexpression has been shown to result in the activation of the Ca^{2+} pathway, presumably via its interaction with Frizzled-2, it can also induce the canonical pathway when the Frizzled-5 receptor is overexpressed as well (He et al., 1997). However, the affinity of Wnt-5a for frizzled-5 is much higher than the affinity of Wnt-5a for Frizzled-2, and the induction of the β-catenin mediated pathway in *Xenopus* development by Wnt-5a/Frizzled-5 binding is not complete, perhaps indicating that this particular ligand-receptor pair is signaling via the Ca^{2+} pathway as well. It may be that these interactions are also dependent upon more as yet unidentified co-receptors specific to each pathway or that the pathway selection depends on the stochiometric levels of these receptor-ligand pairs.

4.1. Downstream targets of the Wnt-5a Ca^{2+} pathway

The obvious initial downstream targets after PLC activation and Ca^{2+} release are PKC and calmodulin, which are involved in a variety of signal transduction cascades (Kuhl, Sheldahl, Park et al., 2000). These signal transduction cascades can affect cell motility, morphogenesis, apoptosis, cytoskeletal changes and differentiation. However, other downstream targets of the Wnt/Ca^{2+} pathway have been identified while studying development in various animals. For example, in the development of skeletal muscle, the formation of sub-epithelial cells known as myotomes are the first step towards differentiated skeletal muscle, a process known as myogenic differentiation. It has been shown that this process is mediated by a combination of signaling from the Sonic Hedgehog family of molecules as well as the Wnt family. Two important target genes in this process are Myf 5 and MyoD. Myf5 appears to be activated by Wnt-1, and presumably the Wnt/β-catenin pathway, where MyoD appears to be activated by a Wnt pathway independent of β-catenin, presumably the Wnt/Ca^{2+} pathway (Cossu & Borello, 1999; Tajbakhsh et al., 1998).

Although development provides us with clues as to how molecules signal, human disease also provides an insight into these pathways. For example in rheumatoid arthritis, Wnt-5a has been shown to be an important molecule. Fibroblast-like synoviocytes (FLS, a cell type found in the normal synovium) in patients with rheumatoid arthritis are in an activated state due to their inflammatory environment. However, even when removed from the patient and cultured *in vitro*, they remain in their activated state. It has been found that these cells express high levels of Wnt-5a and Frizzled-5, and this receptor-ligand pair has been shown to be crucial for FLS activation, by upregulating the activation of interleukins such as IL-6 and IL- 15 (Sen, Chamorro, Reifert, Corr, & Carson, 2001).

Because of their importance, Wnt proteins are tightly regulated. One of the most interesting molecules which can activate Wnt/Ca^{2+} pathway is PKC. In a recent study, it was shown that agents which inhibit PKC activity can downregulate Wnt-5a expression, and those which activate PKC can increase Wnt-5a expression, suggesting that Wnt-5a and PKC exist in a positive feedback loop (Jonsson, Smith, & Harris, 1998). It is clear how dysregulation of this loop could lead to disease. In breast cancer, studies have shown that H-ras, can inhibit Wnt-5a expression by over 200-fold (Bui, Tortora, Ciardiello, & Harris, 1997).

5. THE WNT/JNK PATHWAY

Planar cell polarity (PCP) signaling controls the polarity of epithelial cells within a plane orthogonal to their apical-basal axis. *Drosophila* Dsh was initially identified as a member of this pathway before it became also implicated in wingless signaling (canonical Wnt signaling). Although Dsh is common to the canonical and PCP pathways these pathways diverge downstream of Dsh (Figure 2). While the Dix and PDZ domains of Dsh are essential for signaling through the canonical pathway, the DEP domain is required for signaling through the PCP pathway (Axelrod et al., 1998). Genetic analyses in *Drosophila* identified the JNK/MAPK (mitogen-activated protein kinase) cascade as a downstream target of the PCP pathway (Boutros et al., 1998; Paricio, Feiguin, Boutros, Eaton, & Mlodzik, 1999). Although the factors affecting signaling decisions downstream of Dsh are poorly understood, PAR-1, a Dsh associated kinase, may be involved, as it seems to promote the activation of the canonical Wnt pathway while blocking JNK signaling (Sun et al., 2001).

Until recently, it was unclear whether Wnt/JNK signaling was conserved in vertebrates. Recent papers have now showed convincingly that this pathway is important in the regulation convergent extension movements during gastrulation in vertebrate embryos (Moriguchi et al., 1999; Yamanaka et al., 2002). Another variation of this pathway may lead to apoptosis in *Xenopus* embryos but appears to function in a Dsh-independent fashion (Lisovsky, Itoh, & Sokol, 2002).

6. WNT SIGNALING PATHWAYS IN CANCER

Ever since the discovery of Wnt-1 as a site of integration of MMTV in mouse mammary carcinoma (Nusse & Varmus, 1982), the canonical Wnt pathway has been repeatedly implicated in tumorigenesis. Overexpression of various Wnt or Wnt downstream components have been shown to promote transformation of C57mg cells and many mutations in Wnt pathway components have been identified in human cancer. These reports have been mostly restricted to the Canonical Wnt pathway, although there have been some suggestion of involvement non-canonical pathway. For example, Wnt-5a has been found overexpressed in breast cancer and melanoma and may be related to invasion (Bittner et al., 2000; Lejeune, Huguet, Hamby, Poulsom, & Harris, 1995). As mentioned before, activation of the non-canonical pathways can antagonize the effects of the canonical pathway. For a long time this led to the hypothesis that the Wnt/Ca^{2+} pathway might actually suppress tumorigenicity, but this is not necessarily true. Unlike Wnt/β-catenin changes, which occur early in tumorigenesis, Wnt/Ca^{2+} changes tend to occur later, and are thus associated with progression rather than initiation of tumors. To illustrate these points, we will discuss the role of each of these pathways in a few major tumor types.

6.1. Colon cancer

Because of its relatively well-defined progression and molecular mechanisms, colon cancer is particularly useful to illustrate the importance of the Wnt pathway in human cancer. The APC tumor suppressor gene is mutated in familial adenomatous polyposis (FAP) families and in approximately 80% of sporadic colon cancer cases (Kinzler & Vogelstein, 1996). The function of APC was mysterious for several years until it was discovered to associate and down-regulate β-catenin (Munemitsu, Albert, Souza, Rubinfeld, & Polakis, 1995; Rubinfeld et al., 1993; Su, Vogelstein, & Kinzler, 1993). As described above, APC is part of a degradation complex whose function is the degradation of β-catenin, and consequently, leading to the downregulation of the canonical Wnt signal. Strong evidence suggests that downregulation of the Wnt pathway represent the main function of APC. Indeed, β-catenin mutations in the N-terminus of the protein have been identified in tumors with wild-type APC (Morin et al., 1997; Sparks, Morin, Vogelstein, & Kinzler, 1998). These mutations stabilize β-catenin by making it resistant to degradation by the APC complex (Morin, 1999; Polakis, 1999). The fact that β-catenin and APC mutations are mutually exclusive suggests that APC function is the downregualtion of β-catenin. Deregulation of this pathway is believed to be an early event in colon tumorigenesis and alterations of APC or β-catenin account for about 90% of all colon cancer cases (Sparks et al., 1998). Interestingly, mice lacking TCF4, the TCF member implicated downstream of β-catenin in colon cancer (Korinek et al., 1997) are characterized by a lack of intestinal stem cells, suggesting a crucial role of this pathway for stem cell maintenance during development of the gut (Korinek et al., 1998). Inappropriate reactivation of this "stem cell" signaling in adults appears to be highly tumorigenic.

6.2. Melanoma

The canonical Wnt/βcatenin pathway was discovered to be important in melanoma when mutated β-catenin containing a single amino acid substitution at the N terminus was identified as a melanoma-specific antigen (Robbins et al., 1996). The sequence containing the mutation was part of the peptide recognized by a melanoma-specific tumor infiltrating lymphocyte. This constituted the first demonstration that β-catenin could be mutated in human cancer. Subsequently, β-catenin levels were found to be elevated in several melanomas cell lines. These lines were found to contain activating β-catenin mutations or altered APC (Rubinfeld et al., 1997). These results show canonical Wnt signaling is important molecular pathway in melanoma development.

The Wnt/Ca^{2+} pathway may also have some importance in melanoma. In a study that examined the gene expression profiles of melanoma using microarray analysis, Wnt-5a was the gene that best separated highly aggressive melanomas from their less invasive counterparts (Bittner et al., 2000). In highly aggressive melanomas, Wnt-5a was highly overexpressed. When this gene was transfected into less aggressive melanomas, it increased their invasive potential, and also activated PKC (Weeraratna et al., 2002). PKC activation, as well as Ca^{2+} increases have been shown to be important for melanoma invasion and metastasis, and it may be that the overexpression of Wnt-5a in melanoma contributes to these observed increases.

6.3. Prostate cancer

Prostate cancer is one of the few cancers where the activation of the Wnt/β-catenin pathway appears to be a late event. Only a few mutations in β-catenin itself have been found in prostate cancer using single-strand conformation polymorphism (SSCP) (Voeller, Truica, & Gelmann, 1998). Five mutations in the regulatory site of β-catenin were identified in a panel of 104 prostate cancers. However, β-catenin has recently been shown to have specific interactions with the androgen receptor, suggesting that β-catenin may be involved in hormone resistance during prostate cancer progression (Truica, Byers, & Gelmann, 2000; Yang et al., 2002). This interaction is mediated by the binding of the N-terminal and six armadillo repeats to the ligand binding domain of the androgen receptor, and augments the ligand dependent activity of the androgen receptor.
Wnt-5a, which in humans is usually associated with increases in the Ca^{2+} signaling pathway, has been shown to be upregulated in late stage prostate cancer (Iozzo, Eichstetter, & Danielson, 1995). However, the role of this pathway in prostate cancer has not been well studied as of yet.

6.4. Breast Cancer

The Wnt proteins, as mentioned before, were originally identified as a site of integration for MMTV in mouse mammary carcinoma. Nonetheless, the Wnt/β-catenin pathway does not appear to play a large role in human breast cancer, as evidenced by the observation that Wnt-1 expression declines as breast tumor grade increases (Wong et al., 2002) and the fact that β-catenin mutations are rare (Ueda et al., 2001). There is some conflicting evidence as to the role of the Wnt/Ca^{2+} pathway. Initially, Wnt-5a was shown to upregulated in a panel of late-stage breast tumors (Iozzo et al., 1995), but recently a more in depth study suggests that the loss of this protein leases to the risk of relapse and death due to the recurrence of invasive ductal carcinoma (Jonsson, Dejmek, Bendahl, & Andersson, 2002). In MCF-7 cells which have elevated levels of PKC a downstream target of the Wnt/Ca^{2+} pathway, βestradiol can increase Frizzled-10 and Wnt-2 expression, thus implicating them in breast tumorigenesis (Saitoh, Mine, & Katoh, 2002). Interestingly in MCF-7 cells that have abnormally high levels of PKC Wnt-1 expression significantly down-regulated, and β-catenin is less stable, implying perhaps that the Wnt/Ca^{2+} and Wnt/β-catenin act antagonistically in huiman breast cancer.

6.5. Other cancers

In addition to colon, melanoma and prostate mentioned above, activating β-catenin mutations have been identified in a large number of cancers including ovarian, thyroid, medulloblastomas and pilomatricomas (Morin, 1999). In addition, there is growing evidence that non-canonical pathways may prove important in the development of some cancers as well, as evidenced by the identification of Wnt-5a or other "non-canonical" Wnt in human cancers using functional genomic approaches. This demonstrates that, as with many growth factors important in development, dysregulation of the Wnt signaling pathway can contribute to the pathogenesis of a wide variety of human cancer.

7. CONCLUSIONS

Activation of the Wnt pathway can proceed through at least three downstream signaling cascades mediating various cellular effects. We have described several findings that suggest important roles for the Wnt pathway in the development of human cancer. This role is not completely surprising considering the critical importance of this pathway in directing cell proliferation, migration and differentiation during vertebrate embryonic development.

Patrice J. Morin
Laboratory of Cellular and Molecular Biology
National Institute on Aging, NIH
5600 Nathan Shock Drive
Baltimore, MD 21224

Ashani T. Weeraratna
Cancer Genetics Branch
National Human Genome Research Institute, NIH
49 Convent Drive
Bethesda, MD 20892

8. REFERENCES

Ault, K. T., Durmowicz, G., Galione, A., Harger, P. L., & Busa, W. B. (1996). Modulation of Xenopus embryo mesoderm-specific gene expression and dorsoanterior patterning by receptors that activate the phosphatidylinositol cycle signal transduction pathway. *Development, 122*, 2033-2041.

Axelrod, J. D., Miller, J. R., Shulman, J. M., Moon, R. T., & Perrimon, N. (1998). Differential recruitment of Dishevelled provides signaling specificity in the planar cell polarity and Wingless signaling pathways. *Genes Dev, 12*, 2610-2622.

Barker, N., Morin, P. J., & Clevers, H. (2000). The Yin-Yang of TCF/beta-catenin signaling. *Adv Cancer Res, 77*, 1-24.

Behrens, J., Jerchow, B., Wurtele, M., Grimm, J., Asbrand, C., Wirtz, R., Kuhl, M., Wedlich, D., & Birchmeier, W. (1998). Functional interaction of an axin homolog, conductin, with beta-catenin, APC, and GSK3 beta. *Science, 280*, 596-599.

Bhanot, P., Brink, M., Samos, C. H., Hsieh, J.-C., Wang, Y., Macke, J. P., Andrew, D., Nathans, J., & Nusse, R. (1996). A new member of the frizzled family from Drosophila functions as a Wingless receptor. *Nature, 382*, 225-230.

Bittner, M., Meltzer, P., Chen, Y., Jiang, Y., Seftor, E., Hendrix, M., Radmacher, M., Simon, R., Yakhini, Z., Ben-Dor, A., Sampas, N., Dougherty, E., Wang, E., Marincola, F., Gooden, C., Lueders, J., Glatfelter, A., Pollock, P., Carpten, J., Gillanders, E., Leja, D., Dietrich, K., Beaudry, C., Berens, M., Alberts, D., & Sondak, V. (2000). Molecular classification of cutaneous malignant melanoma by gene expression profiling. *Nature, 406*, 536-540.

Boutros, M., Paricio, N., Strutt, D. I., & Mlodzik, M. (1998). Dishevelled activates JNK and discriminates between JNK pathways in planar polarity and wingless signaling. *Cell, 94*, 109-118.

Brabletz, T., Jung, A., Dag, S., Hlubek, F., & Kirchner, T. (1999). beta-catenin regulates the expression of the matrix metalloproteinase-7 in human colorectal cancer. *Am J. Path, 155*, 1033-1038.

Bui, T. D., Tortora, G., Ciardiello, F., & Harris, A. L. (1997). Expression of Wnt5a is downregulated by extracellular matrix and mutated c-Ha-ras in the human mammary epithelial cell line MCF-10A. *Biochem Biophys Res Commun, 239*, 911-917.
Cadigan, K. M., & Nusse, R. (1997). Wnt signaling: a common theme in animal development. *Genes Dev, 11*, 3286-3305.
Cavallo, R. A., Cox, R. T., Moline, M. M., Roose, J., Polevoy, G. A., Clevers, H., Peifer, M., & Bejsovec, A. (1998). Drosophila Tcf and Groucho interact to repress Wingless signalling activity. *Nature, 395*, 604-608.
Clevers, H., & van de Wetering, M. (1997). TCF/LEF factors earn their wings. *Trends Genet, 13*, 485-489.
Cossu, G., & Borello, U. (1999). Wnt signaling and the activation of myogenesis in mammals. *EMBO J, 18*, 6867-6872.
Du, S. J., Purcell, S., Christian, J. L., McGrew, L. L., & Moon, R. T. (1995). Identification of distinct classes and functional domains of Wnts through expression of wild-type and chimeric proteins in Xenopus embryos. *Mol. Cell. Biol., 15*, 2625-2634.
Fagotto, F., Gluck, U., & Gumbiner, B. M. (1998). Nuclear localization signal-independent and importin/karyopherin-independent nuclear import of beta-catenin. *Curr Biol, 8*, 181-190.
Giese, K., Amsterdam, A., & Grosschedl, R. (1991). DNA-binding properties of the HMG domain of the lymphoid-specific transcriptional regulator LEF-1. *Genes Dev, 5*, 2567-2578.
Giese, K., Cox, J., & Grosschedl, R. (1992). The HMG domain of lymphoid enhancer factor 1 bends DNA and facilitates assembly of functional nucleoprotein structures. *Cell, 69*, 185-195.
Gieseler, K., Graba, Y., Mariol, M. C., Wilder, E. L., Martinez-Arias, A., Lemaire, P., & Pradel, J. (1999). Antagonist activity of DWnt-4 and wingless in the Drosophila embryonic ventral ectoderm and in heterologous Xenopus assays. *Mech Dev, 85*, 123-131.
Hart, M., Concordet, J. P., Lassot, I., Albert, I., del los Santos, R., Durand, H., Perret, C., Rubinfeld, B., Margottin, F., Benarous, R., & Polakis, P. (1999). The F-box protein beta-TrCP associates with phosphorylated beta-catenin and regulates its activity in the cell. *Curr Biol, 9*, 207-210.
Hart, M. J., de los Santos, R., Albert, I. N., Rubinfeld, B., & Polakis, P. (1998). Downregulation of beta-catenin by human Axin and its association with the APC tumor suppressor, beta-catenin and GSK3 beta. *Current Biology, 8*, 573-581.
He, T. C., Chan, T. A., Vogelstein, B., & Kinzler, K. W. (1999). PPAR delta is an APC-regulated target of nonsteroidal anti-inflammatory drugs. *Cell, 99*, 335-345.
He, T. C., Sparks, A. B., Rago, C., Hermeking, H., Zawel, L., da Costa, L. T., Morin, P. J., Vogelstein, B., & Kinzler, K. (1998). Identification of c-MYC as a target of the APC pathway. *Science, 281*, 1509-1512.
He, X., St-Jeannet, J.-P., Wang, Nathans, Dawid, & A, V. (1997). A member of the Frizzled protein family mediating axis induction by Wnt-5A. *Science, 275*, 1652.
Hecht, A., Litterst, C. M., Huber, O., & Kemler, R. (1999). Functional characterization of multiple transactivating elements in beta-catenin, some of which interact with the TATA-binding protein in vitro. *J Biol Chem, 274*, 18017-18025.
Hecht, A., Vleminckx, K., Stemmler, M. P., van Roy, F., & Kemler, R. (2000). The p300/CBP acetyltransferases function as transcriptional coactivators of beta-catenin in vertebrates. *EMBO J, 19*, 1839-1850.
Hsu, S. C., Galceran, J., & Grosschedl, R. (1998). Modulation of transcriptional regulation by LEF-1 in response to wnt-1 signaling and association with beta-catenin. *Mol Cell Biol, 18*, 4807-4818.
Ikeda, S., Kishida, S., Yamamoto, H., Murai, H., Koyama, S., & Kikuchi, A. (1998). Axin, a negative regulator of the wnt signaling pathway, forms a complex with GSK-3beta and beta-catenin and promotes GSK-3beta-dependent phosphorylation of beta-catenin. *EMBO J, 17*, 1371-1384.
Iozzo, R. V., Eichstetter, I., & Danielson, K. G. (1995). Aberrant expression of the growth factor Wnt-5A in human malignancy. *Cancer Res, 55*, 3495-3499.
Ishitani, T., Ninomiya-Tsuji, J., Nagai, S., Nishita, M., Meneghini, M., Barker, N., Waterman, M., Bowerman, B., Clevers, H., Shibuya, H., & Matsumoto, K. (1999). The TAK1-NLK-MAPK-related pathway antagonizes signalling between beta- catenin and transcription factor TCF. *Nature, 399*, 798-802.
Jiang, J., & Struhl, G. (1998). Regulation of the Hedgehog and Wingless signalling pathways by the F-box/WD40-repeat protein Slimb. *Nature, 391*, 493-496.
Jonsson, M., Dejmek, J., Bendahl, P. O., & Andersson, T. (2002). Loss of Wnt-5a protein is associated with early relapse in invasive ductal breast carcinomas. *Cancer Res, 62*, 409-416.
Jonsson, M., Smith, K., & Harris, A. L. (1998). Regulation of Wnt5a expression in human mammary cells by protein kinase C activity and the cytoskeleton. *Br J Cancer, 78*, 430-438.

Jue, S. F., Bradley, R. S., Rudnicki, J. A., Varmus, H. E., & Brown, A. M. C. (1992). The mouse Wnt-1 gene can act via a paracrine mechanism in transformation of mammary epithelial cells. *Mol. Cell. Biol., 12*, 321-328.

Kadowaki, T., Wilder, E., Klingensmith, J., Zachary, K., & Perrimon, N. (1996). The segment polarity gene porcupine encodes a putative multitransmembrane protein involved in Wingless processing. *Genes Dev., 10*, 3116-3128.

Kinzler, K. W., & Vogelstein, B. (1996). Lessons from hereditary colorectal cancer. *Cell, 87*, 159-170.

Kishida, S., Yamamoto, H., Hino, S., Ikeda, S., Kishida, M., & Kikuchi, A. (1999). DIX domains of Dvl and Axin are necessary for protein interactions and their ability to regulate beta-catenin stability. *Molec Cell Biol, 19*, 4414-4422.

Kishida, S., Yamamoto, H., Ikeda, S., Kishida, M., Sakamoto, I., Koyama, S., & Kikuchi, A. (1998). Axin, a negative regulator of the Wnt signaling pathway, directly interacts with adenomatous polyposis coli and regulates the stabilization of beta-catenin. *J. Biol. Chem., 273*, 10823-10826.

Korinek, V., Barker, N., Moerer, P., van Donselaar, E., Huls, G., Peters, P. J., & Clevers, H. (1998). Depletion of epithelial stem-cell compartments in the small intestine of mice lacking Tcf-4. *Nat Genet, 19*, 379-383.

Korinek, V., Barker, N., Morin, P. J., van Wichen, D., de Weger, R., Kinzler, K. W., Vogelstein, B., & Clevers, H. (1997). Constitutive transcriptional activation by a beta-catenin-Tcf complex in APC-/- colon carcinoma. *Science, 275*, 1784-1787.

Kuhl, M., Sheldahl, L. C., Malbon, C. C., & Moon, R. T. (2000). Ca(2+)/calmodulin-dependent protein kinase II is stimulated by Wnt and Frizzled homologs and promotes ventral cell fates in Xenopus. *J Biol Chem, 275*, 12701-12711.

Kuhl, M., Sheldahl, L. C., Park, M., Miller, J. R., & Moon, R. T. (2000). The Wnt/Ca2+ pathway: a new vertebrate Wnt signaling pathway takes shape. *Trends Genet, 16*, 279-283.

Lejeune, S., Huguet, E. L., Hamby, A., Poulsom, R., & Harris, A. L. (1995). Wnt5a cloning, expression, and up-regulation in human primary breast cancers. *Clin Cancer Res, 1*, 215-222.

Levanon, D., Goldstein, R. E., Bernstein, Y., Tang, H., Goldenberg, D., Stifani, S., Paroush, Z., & Groner, Y. (1998). Transcriptional repression by AML1 and LEF-1 is mediated by the TLE/Groucho corepressors. *Proc Natl Acad Sci USA, 95*, 11590-11595.

Li, L., Yuan, H. D., Weaver, C. D., Mao, J. H., Farr, G. H., Sussman, D. J., Jonkers, J., Kimelman, D., & Wu, D. Q. (1999). Axin and Frat1 interact with Dvl and GSK, bridging Dvl to GSK in Wnt-mediated regulation of LEF-1. *EMBO J, 18*, 4233-4240.

Lisovsky, M., Itoh, K., & Sokol, S. Y. (2002). Frizzled Receptors Activate a Novel JNK-Dependent Pathway that May Lead to Apoptosis. *Curr Biol, 12*, 53-58.

Liu, P., Wakamiya, M., Shea, M. J., Albrecht, U., Behringer, R. R., & Bradley, A. (1999). Requirement for Wnt3 in vertebrate axis formation. *Nat Genet, 22*(4), 361-365.

Liu, T., DeCostanzo, A. J., Liu, X., Wang, H., Hallagan, S., Moon, R. T., & Malbon, C. C. (2001). G protein signaling from activated rat frizzled-1 to the beta-catenin- Lef-Tcf pathway. *Science, 292*(5522), 1718-1722.

Liu, T., Liu, X. X., Wang, H. Y., Moon, R. T., & Malbon, C. C. (1999). Activation of rat frizzled-1 promotes Wnt signaling and differentiation of mouse F9 teratocarcinoma cells via pathways that require G alpha(q) and G alpha(o) function. *J. Biol Chem., 274*, 33539-33544.

Liu, X., Liu, T., Slusarski, D. C., Yang-Snyder, J., Malbon, C. C., Moon, R. T., & Wang, H. (1999). Activation of a frizzled-2/beta-adrenergic receptor chimera promotes Wnt signaling and differentiation of mouse F9 teratocarcinoma cells via Galphao and Galphat. *Proc Natl Acad Sci USA, 96*, 14383-14388.

Malbon, C. C., Wang, H., & Moon, R. T. (2001). Wnt signaling and heterotrimeric G-proteins: strange bedfellows or a classic romance? *Biochem Biophys Res Commun, 287*(3), 589-593.

Mann, B., Gelos, M., Siedow, A., Hanski, M. L., Gratchev, A., Ilyas, M., Bodmer, W. F., Moyer, M. P., Riecken, E. O., Buhr, H. J., & Hanski, C. (1999). Target genes of beta-catenin-T cell-factor lymphoid-enhancer-factor signaling in human colorectal carcinomas. *Proc. Natl Acad. Sci. USA, 96*, 1603-1608.

McEwen, D. G., & Peifer, M. (2001). Wnt signaling: the naked truth? *Curr Biol, 11*(13), R524-526.

McMahon, B. (1990). The Wnt-1 (int-1) proto-oncogene is required for development of a large region of the mouse brain. *Cell, 62*, 1073.

Miyagishi, M., Fujii, R., Hatta, M., Yoshida, E., Araya, N., Nagafuchi, A., Ishihara, S., Nakajima, T., & Fukamizu, A. (2000). Regulation of Lef-mediated transcription and p53-dependent pathway by associating beta-catenin with CBP/p300. *J Biol Chem, 275*(45), 35170-35175.

Monkley, S. J., Delaney, S. J., Pennisi, D. J., Christiansen, J. H., & Wainwright, B. J. (1996). Targeted disruption of the Wnt2 gene results in placentation defects. *Development, 122*, 3343-3353.

Moon, R. T., Campbell, R. M., Christian, J. L., McGrew, L. L., DeMarais, A. A., Shih, J., & Fraser, S. (1993). Xwnt-5A: a maternal Wnt that affects morphogenetic movements after overexpression in embryos of Xenopus laevis. *Development, 119*, 97-111.

Moriguchi, T., Kawachi, K., Kamakura, S., Masuyama, N., Yamanaka, H., Matsumoto, K., Kikuchi, A., & Nishida, E. (1999). Distinct domains of mouse dishevelled are responsible for the c-Jun N-terminal kinase/stress-activated protein kinase activation and the axis formation in vertebrates. *J Biol Chem, 274*, 30957-30962.

Morin, P. J. (1999). beta-catenin signaling and cancer. *Bioessays, 21*, 1021-1030.

Morin, P. J., Sparks, A. B., Korinek, V., Barker, N., Clevers, H., Vogelstein, B., & Kinzler, K. W. (1997). Activation of beta-catenin-Tcf signaling in colon cancer by mutations in beta-catenin or APC. *Science, 275*, 1787-1790.

Munemitsu, S., Albert, I., Souza, B., Rubinfeld, B., & Polakis, P. (1995). Regulation of intracellular beta-catenin levels by the adenomatous polyposis coli (APC) tumor-suppressor protein. *Proc Natl Acad Sci U S A, 92*, 3046-3050.

Neufeld, K. L., Nix, D. A., Bogerd, H., Kang, Y., Beckerle, M. C., Cullen, B. R., & White, R. L. (2000). Adenomatous polyposis coli protein contains two nuclear export signals and shuttles between the nucleus and cytoplasm. *Proc Natl Acad Sci U S A, 97*(22), 12085-12090.

Neufeld, K. L., & White, R. L. (1997). Nuclear and cytoplasmic localizations of the adenomatous polyposis coli protein. *Proc. Natl. Acad. Sci. USA, 94*, 3034-3039.

Neufeld, K. L., Zhang, F., Cullen, B. R., & White, R. L. (2000). APC-mediated downregulation of beta-catenin activity involves nuclear sequestration and nuclear export. *EMBO Rep, 1*, 519-523.

Nusse, R., & Varmus, H. E. (1982). Many tumors induced by the mouse mammary tumor virus contain a provirus integrated in the same region of the host genome. *Cell, 31*, 99-109.

Olson, D. J., & Gibo, D. M. (1998). Antisense wnt-5a mimics wnt-1-mediated C57MG mammary epithelial cell transformation. *Exp Cell Res, 241*, 134-141.

Orford, K., Crockett, C., Jensen, J. P., Weissman, A. M., & Byers, S. W. (1997). Serine phosphorylation-regulated ubiquitination and degradation of beta-catenin. *J Biol Chem, 272*, 24735-24738.

Orsulic, S., & Peifer, M. (1996). Cell-cell signalling: Wingless lands at last. *Curr Biol, 6*, 1363-1667.

Pandur, P., & Kuhl, M. (2001). An arrow for wingless to take-off. *Bioessays, 23*(3), 207-210.

Paricio, N., Feiguin, F., Boutros, M., Eaton, S., & Mlodzik, M. (1999). The Drosophila STE20-like kinase misshapen is required downstream of the Frizzled receptor in planar polarity signaling. *EMBO J, 18*, 4669-4678.

Parr, B. A., Cornish, V. A., Cybulsky, M. I., & McMahon, A. P. (2001). Wnt7b regulates placental development in mice. *Dev Biol, 237*, 324-332.

Parr, B. A., & McMahon, A. P. (1995). Dorsalizing signal Wnt-7a required for normal polarity of D-V and A-P axes of mouse limb. *Nature, 374*, 350-353.

Parr, B. A., & McMahon, A. P. (1998). Sexually dimorphic development of the mammalian reproductive tract requires Wnt-7a. *Nature, 395*, 707-710.

Peters, J. M., McKay, R. M., McKay, J. P., & Graff, J. M. (1999). Casein kinase I transduces Wnt signals. *Nature, 401*, 345-350.

Pinson, K. I., Brennan, J., Monkley, S., Avery, B. J., & Skarnes, W. C. (2000). An LDL-receptor-related protein mediates Wnt signalling in mice. *Nature, 407*, 535-538.

Polakis, P. (1999). The oncogenic activation of beta-catenin. *Curr Opin Genet & Dev, 9*, 15-21.

Robbins, P. F., El-Gamil, M., Li, Y. F., Kawakami, Y., Loftus, D., Appella, E., & Rosenberg, S. A. (1996). A mutated beta-catenin gene encodes a melanoma-specific antigen recognized by tumor infiltrating lymphocytes. *J. Exp. Med., 183*, 1185-1192.

Rocheleau, C. E., Yasuda, J., Shin, T. H., Lin, R., Sawa, H., Okano, H., Priess, J. R., Davis, R. J., & Mello, C. C. (1999). WRM-1 activates the LIT-1 protein kinase to transduce anterior/posterior polarity signals in C. elegans. *Cell, 97*, 717-726.

Roose, J., & Clevers, H. (1999). TCF transcription factors: molecular switches in carcinogenesis. *Biochim Biophys Acta Rev Cancer, 1424*, M23-M37.

Roose, J., Molenaar, M., Peterson, J., Hurenkamp, J., Brantjes, H., Moerer, P., van de Wetering, M., Destree, O., & Clevers, H. (1998). The Xenopus Wnt effector XTcf-3 interacts with Groucho-related transcriptional repressors. *Nature, 395*, 608-612.

Rosin-Arbesfeld, R., Townsley, F., & Bienz, M. (2000). The APC tumour suppressor has a nuclear export function. *Nature, 406*, 1009-1012.

Rubinfeld, B., Robbins, P., El-Gamil, M., Albert, I., Porfiri, E., & Polakis, P. (1997). Stabilization of b-catenin by genetic defects in melanoma cell lines. *Science, 275*, 1790-1792.
Rubinfeld, B., Souza, B., Albert, I., Muller, O., Chamberlain, S. H., Masiarz, F. R., Munemitsu, S., & Polakis, P. (1993). Association of the APC gene product with beta-catenin. *Science, 262*, 1731-1734.
Saitoh, T., Mine, T., & Katoh, M. (2002). Up-regulation of Frizzled-10 (FZD10) by beta-estradiol in MCF-7 cells and by retinoic acid in NT2 cells. *Int J Oncol, 20*, 117-120.
Sakanaka, C., Leong, P., Xu, L., Harrison, S. D., & Williams, L. T. (1999). Casein kinase I epsilon in the wnt pathway: regulation of beta-catenin function. *Proc Natl Acad Sci U S A, 96*, 12548-12552.
Salomon, D., Sacco, P. A., Roy, S. G., Simcha, I., Johnson, K. R., Wheelock, M. J., & Ben-Ze'ev, A. (1997). Regulation of beta-catenin levels and localization by overexpression of plakoglobin and inhibition of the ubiquitin-proteasome system. *J Cell Biol, 139*, 1325-1335.
Seeling, J. M., Miller, J. R., Gil, R., Moon, R. T., White, R., & Virshup, D. M. (1999). Regulation of beta-catenin signaling by the B56 subunit of protein phosphatase 2A. *Science, 283*, 2089-2091.
Sen, M., Chamorro, M., Reifert, J., Corr, M., & Carson, D. A. (2001). Blockade of Wnt-5A/frizzled 5 signaling inhibits rheumatoid synoviocyte activation. *Arthritis Rheum, 44*, 772-781.
Sheldahl, L. C., Park, M., Malbon, C. C., & Moon, R. T. (1999). Protein kinase C is differentially stimulated by Wnt and Frizzled homologs in a G-protein-dependent manner. *Curr. Biol., 9*, 695-698.
Shimizu, H., Julius, M. A., Giarre, M., Zheng, Z., Brown, A. M., & Kitajewski, J. (1997). Transformation by Wnt family proteins correlates with regulation of beta-catenin. *Cell Growth Differ, 8*, 1349-1358.
Shtutman, M., Zhurinsky, J., Simcha, I., Albanese, C., D'Amico, M., Pestell, R., & Ben-Ze'ev, A. (1999). The cyclin D1 gene is a target of the beta-catenin/LEF-1 pathway. *Proc Natl Acad Sci. USA, 96*, 5522-5527.
Slusarski, D. C., Corces, V. G., & Moon, R. T. (1997). Interaction of Wnt and a Frizzled homologue triggers G-protein-linked phosphatidylinositol signalling. *Nature, 390*(6658), 410-413.
Slusarski, D. C., Yang-Snyder, J., Busa, W. B., & Moon, R. T. (1997). Modulation of embryonic intracellular Ca2+ signaling by Wnt-5a. *Develop. Biol., 182*, 114-120.
Smalley, M. J., & Dale, T. C. (1999). Wnt signalling in mammalian development and cancer. *Cancer Metastasis Rev, 18*, 215-230.
Smith, K. J., Johnson, K. A., Bryan, T. M., Hill, D., Markowitz, S., Willson, J. K., Paraskeva, C., Petersen, G. M., Hamilton, S. R., Vogelstein, B., & Kinzler, K. W. (1993). The APC gene product in normal and tumor cells. *Proc Natl Acad Sci USA, 90*, 2846-2850.
Smolich, B. D., McMahon, J. A., McMahon, A. P., & Papkoff, J. (1993). Wnt family proteins are secreted and associated with the cell surface. *Mol. Cell. Biol., 4*, 1267-1275.
Sokol, S. Y. (1999). Wnt signaling and dorso-ventral axis specification in vertebrates. *Curr Opin Genet. Devel., 9*, 405-410.
Sparks, A. B., Morin, P. J., Vogelstein, B., & Kinzler, K. W. (1998). Mutational Analysis of the APC/beta-Catenin/Tcf Pathway in Colorectal Cancer. *Cancer Research, 58*, 1130-1134.
Stark, K., Vainio, S., Vassileva, G., & McMahon, A. P. (1994). Epithelial transformation of metanephric mesenchyme in the developing kidney regulated by Wnt-4. *Nature, 372*, 679-684.
Su, L. K., Vogelstein, B., & Kinzler, K. W. (1993). Association of the APC tumor suppressor protein with catenins. *Science, 262*, 1734-1737.
Sun, T. Q., Lu, B., Feng, J. J., Reinhard, C., Jan, Y. N., Fantl, W. J., & Williams, L. T. (2001). PAR-1 is a Dishevelled-associated kinase and a positive regulator of Wnt signalling. *Nat Cell Biol, 3*, 628-636.
Tajbakhsh, S., Borello, U., Vivarelli, E., Kelly, R., Papkoff, J., Duprez, D., Buckingham, M., & Cossu, G. (1998). Differential activation of Myf5 and MyoD by different Wnts in explants of mouse paraxial mesoderm and the later activation of myogenesis in the absence of Myf5. *Development, 125*, 4155-4162.
Takada, S., Stark, K. L., Shea, M. J., Vassileva, G., McMahon, J. A., & McMahon, A. P. (1994). Wnt-3a regulates somite and tailbud formation in the mouse embryo. *Genes & Dev., 8*, 174.
Takemaru, K. I., & Moon, R. T. (2000). The transcriptional coactivator CBP interacts with beta-catenin to activate gene expression. *J Cell Biol, 149*, 249-254.
Tamai, K., Semenov, M., Kato, Y., Spokony, R., Liu, C., Katsuyama, Y., Hess, F., Saint-Jeannet, J. P., & He, X. (2000). LDL-receptor-related proteins in Wnt signal transduction. *Nature, 407*, 530-535.
Tetsu, O., & McCormick, F. (1999). Beta-catenin regulates expression of cyclin D1 in colon carcinoma cells. *Nature, 398*, 422-426.

Thomas, K. R., & Capecchi, M. R. (1990). Targeted disruption of the murine int-1 proto-oncogene resulting in severe abnormalities in midbrain and cerebellar development. *Nature, 346*, 847-850.
Torres, Y.-S., Purcell, DeMarais, McGrew, Moon. (1996). Activities of the Wnt-1 class of secreted signaling factors are antagonized by the Wnt-5A class and by a dominant negative cadherin in early Xenopus development. *J. Cell Biol., 133*, 1123.
Travis, A., Amsterdam, A., Belanger, C., & Grosschedl, R. (1991). LEF-1, a gene encoding a lymphoid-specific protein with an HMG domain, regulates T-cell receptor alpha enhancer function [corrected]. *Genes Dev, 5*, 880-894.
Truica, C. I., Byers, S., & Gelmann, E. P. (2000). Beta-catenin affects androgen receptor transcriptional activity and ligand specificity. *Cancer Res, 60*, 4709-4713.
Ueda, M., Gemmill, R. M., West, J., Winn, R., Sugita, M., Tanaka, N., Ueki, M., & Drabkin, H. A. (2001). Mutations of the beta- and gamma-catenin genes are uncommon in human lung, breast, kidney, cervical and ovarian carcinomas. *Br J Cancer, 85*, 64-68.
Vainio, S., Heikkila, M., Kispert, A., Chin, N., & McMahon, A. P. (1999). Female development in mammals is regulated by Wnt-4 signalling. *Nature, 397*, 405-409.
van de Wetering, M., Oosterwegel, M., Dooijes, D., & Clevers, H. (1991). Identification and cloning of TCF-1, a T lymphocyte-specific transcription factor containing a sequence-specific HMG box. *EMBO J., 10*, 123-132.
Vinson, C. R., & Adler, P. N. (1987). Directional non-cell autonomy and the transmission of polarity information by the frizzled gene of Drosophila. *Nature, 329*, 549-551.
Voeller, H. J., Truica, C. I., & Gelmann, E. P. (1998). beta-catenin mutations in human prostate cancer. *Cancer Res, 58*, 2520-2523.
von Kries, J. P., Winbeck, G., Asbrand, C., Schwarz-Romond, T., Sochnikova, N., Dell'Oro, A., Behrens, J., & Birchmeier, W. (2000). Hot spots in beta-catenin for interactions with LEF-1, conductin and APC. *Nat Struct Biol, 7*(9), 800-807.
Waltzer, L., & Bienz, M. (1998). *Drosophila* CBP represses the transcription factor TCF to antagonize Wingless signalling. *Nature, 395*, 521-525.
Weeraratna, A., Jiang, Y., Lueders, J., Hostetter, G., Rosenblatt, K., Duray, P., Bittner, M., & Trent, J. M. (2002). Wnt5a Signaling Directly Affects Cell Motility and Invasion of Metastatic Melanoma. *Cancer Cell, in press.*
Willert, K., Brink, M., Wodarz, A., Varmus, H., & Nusse, R. (1997). Casein kinase 2 associates with and phosphorylates dishevelled. *EMBO J, 16*, 3089-3096.
Willert, K., Shibamoto, S., & Nusse, R. (1999). Wnt-induced dephosphorylation of Axin releases beta-catenin from the Axin complex. *Genes Dev., 13*, 1768-1773.
Winston, J. T., Strack, P., Beer-Romero, P., Chu, C. Y., Elledge, S. J., & Harper, J. W. (1999). The SCF beta-TRCP-ubiquitin ligase complex associates specifically with phosphorylated destruction motifs in I kappa B alpha and beta-catenin and stimulates I kappa B alpha ubiquitination in vitro. *Genes & Dev., 13*, 270-283.
Wong, G. T., Gavin, B. J., & McMahon, A. P. (1994). Differential transformation of mammary epithelial cells by Wnt genes. *Molec. cell. Biol., 14*, 6278-6286.
Wong, S. C., Lo, S. F., Lee, K. C., Yam, J. W., Chan, J. K., & Wendy Hsiao, W. L. (2002). Expression of frizzled-related protein and Wnt-signalling molecules in invasive human breast tumours. *J Pathol, 196*, 145-153.
Yamaguchi, T. P., Bradley, A., McMahon, A. P., & Jones, S. (1999). A Wnt5a pathway underlies outgrowth of multiple structures in the vertebrate embryo. *Development, 126*, 1211-1223.
Yamamoto, H., Kishida, S., Uochi, T., Ikeda, S., Koyama, S., Asashima, M., & Kikuchi, A. (1998). Axil, a member of the Axin family, interacts with both glycogen synthase kinase 3beta and beta-catenin and inhibits axis formation of Xenopus embryos. *Mol Cell Biol, 18*, 2867-2875.
Yamanaka, H., Moriguchi, T., Masuyama, N., Kusakabe, M., Hanafusa, H., Takada, R., Takada, S., & Nishida, E. (2002). JNK functions in the non-canonical Wnt pathway to regulate convergent extension movements in vertebrates. *EMBO Rep, 3*, 69-75.
Yang, F., Li, X., Sharma, M., Sasaki, C. Y., Longo, D. L., Lim, B., & Sun, Z. (2002). Linking beta-catenin to androgen signaling pathway. *J Biol Chem, in press.*
Yokoya, F., Imamoto, N., Tachibana, T., & Yoneda, Y. (1999). beta-catenin can be transported into the nucleus in a Ran-unassisted manner. *Molec Biol Cell, 10*, 1119-1131.
Zeng, L., Fagotto, F., Zhang, T., Hsu, W., Vasicek, T. J., Perry, W. L. r., Lee, J. J., Tilghman, S. M., Gumbiner, B. M., & Costantini, F. (1997). The mouse Fused locus encodes Axin, an inhibitor of the Wnt signaling pathway that regulates embryonic axis formation. *Cell, 90*, 181-192.

Zhang, F., White, R. L., & Neufeld, K. L. (2000). Phosphorylation near nuclear localization signal regulates nuclear import of adenomatous polyposis coli protein. *Proc Natl Acad Sci USA, 97*, 12577-12582.

RAS SIGNALING, DEREGULATION OF GENE EXPRESSION AND ONCOGENESIS

AYLIN S. ÜLKÜ AND CHANNING J. DER

1. INTRODUCTION

The process of carcinogenesis is complex, requiring cells to overcome numerous barriers that limit their responses to stimuli that ensure appropriate function. Decades of cancer research have identified mutations in essential cell checkpoint genes through studies of human disease and animal models. Several lines of evidence have led to the development of a multi-step model of cancer progression in humans (Hanahan and Weinberg, 2000). Driven by dynamic genomic changes, normal cells evolve through a series of premalignant stages to become invasive and mestastatic. Each progressive genetic alteration leads to the deregulation of vital regulatory pathways, which serve as the fundamental defense mechanism of the cell against malignant growth. This model is defined by such genetic changes, resulting in abnormal cell physiology: stimulus-independent proliferation, insensitivity to growth arrest signals, resistance to apoptosis, enhanced angiogenesis, and invasion and metastasis.

The discovery of mutations in two classes of genes has been vital to our understanding of cancer. Mutations in tumor suppressor genes such as p53 and Rb cause loss of function of essential checkpoints that prevent malignant growth. Equally important in tumor progression are mutations in dominant gain of function proto-oncogenes which lead to uncontrolled cell growth and invasion. The most commonly mutated of these oncogenes is *ras*, which is found mutationally activated in 30% of all human cancers (Bos, 1989; Clark and Der, 1993). Addititionally, other oncoproteins (e.g., HER2) or tumor suppressors (e.g., NF1) promote oncogenesis by a Ras-dependent mechanism, thus expanding the importance of aberrant Ras function in cancers where Ras itself is not mutated (Clark and Der, 1995; Cichowski and Jacks, 2001). Therefore, determining the mechanisms by which the Ras oncoprotein facilitates human carcinogenesis will be critical for the development of anti-Ras strategies for cancer treatment.

Our conception of Ras-mediated signaling in cancer has been derived from innumerable animal and cell culture model systems, which in recent years have been recognized as being incomplete and more complicated than once envisioned. First, while a complex array downstream of signaling cascades is now established to be stimulated by Ras, clearly much more remains to be discovered (Shields et al., 2000). Second, it has become apparent that Ras signaling and biology displays striking variation that is influenced by cell-type and species differences as well as genetic context. Third, although deregulation of gene expression is critical for Ras function, the identity of many of the gene targets critical for promoting Ras-mediated oncogenesis remains to be determined. In this review, we summarize our current understanding of these three issues with regards to Ras and oncogenesis.

2. RAS PROTEINS FUNCTION AS MEMBRANE-ASSOCIATED GTPASE SWITCHES

The three human *ras* genes encode four highly homologous 188-189 amino acid (21 kDa) proteins: H-Ras, N-Ras, K-Ras4A and K-Ras4B (due to alternative 4th exon utilization) proteins (Barbacid, 1987). Mutated *ras* genes are associated with 30% of all human cancers, with highest frequencies associated with pancreatic, lung, and colon carcinomas. These mutated *ras* genes encode structurally mutated proteins, most commonly with single amino acid substitutions at residues 12, 13, or 61.

2.1 Ras functions as a GTP/GDP-regulated molecular switch

Ras proteins are GTPases that act as molecular switches, transmitting signals from activated receptors to downstream effectors to mediate cell proliferation, survival and differentiation (Fig. 1). Ras proteins cycle between a GTP-bound (active) and GDP-bound (inactive) state (Bourne et al., 1990). In resting cells, approximately 5% of Ras proteins are GTP-bound. Upon activation by extracellular stimuli, there is a rapid and transient increase (up to 70%) in Ras-GTP levels.

Ras proteins have the intrinsic ability to undergo GDP/GTP cycling. GTPase activity hydrolyzes bound GTP in order to limit proliferative signaling, and nucleotide exchange activity releases GDP to allow GTP binding and activation. However, these intrinsic activities are too low for rapid GDP/GTP cycling, therefore two distinct classes of regulatory proteins accelerate Ras protein cycling (Bourne et al., 1990). First, intrinsic GDP/GTP exchange is enhanced by guanine exchange factors (GEFs) (Fig. 1). Ras GEFs include Sos, RasGRF, and RasGRP. Second, intrinsic GTPase activity is stimulated by GTPase activating proteins (GAPs). These include p120 RasGAP and neurofibromin, the gene product of the NF1 tumor suppressor protein. Mutant Ras proteins are insensitive to GAP-induced GTP hydrolysis, rendering Ras constitutively GTP-bound and active in the absence of extracellular signals (Fig. 1).

2.2 Association with the plasma membrane is critical for Ras function

In addition to GDP/GTP-binding, a second key requirement for Ras function is its association with the inner face of the plasma membrane (Cox and Der, 1997). Ras proteins are synthesized initially as cytosolic, inactive proteins. They then undergo a rapid series of posttranslational modifications that facilitate their association with the inner face of the plasma membrane. These modifications are

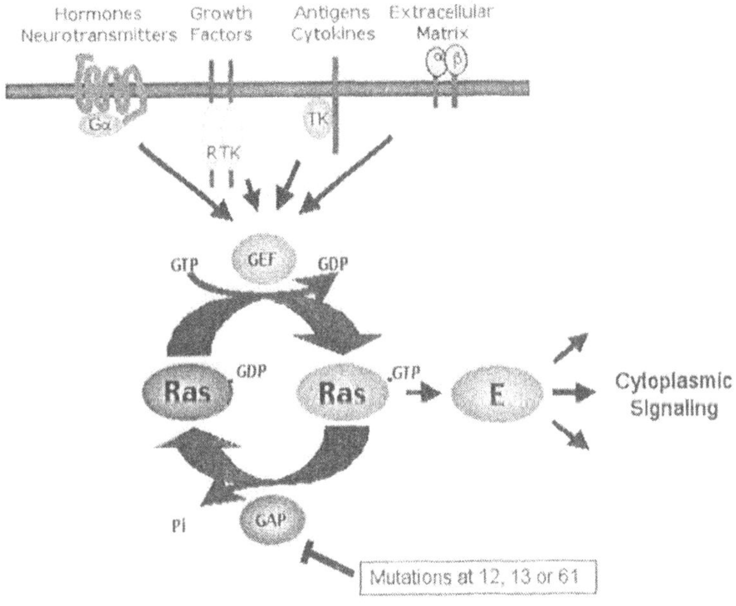

Figure 1. The Ras pathway in cancer

signaled by a carboxyl terminal CAAX tetrapeptide motif found on all Ras proteins, where C = cysteine, A = aliphatic amino acid and X = serine or methionine. First, farnesyltransferase (FTase) catalyzes the addition of a C15 farnesyl isoprenoid to the cysteine residue of the CAAX motif. Second, proteolysis of the AAX residues is mediated by endoprotease activity. Finally, carboxymethylation of the now terminal farnesylated cysteine occurs. H-Ras, N-Ras and K-Ras4A are modified further by carboxyl terminal palmitylation at a cysteine residue(s) positioned upstream of the CAAX motif, whereas the second localization signal for K-Ras4B is provided by a lysine-rich polybasic sequence. The CAAX-mediated modifications, together with these second signals, are necessary and sufficient for plasma membrane localization and Ras function.

The critical requirement for Ras association with the plasma membrane has prompted considerable effort to identify pharmacologic approaches to block the CAAX-mediated modifications to then block Ras function (Oliff, 1999; Cox, 2001). Of these efforts, the development of FTase inhibitors (FTIs) has been the most intensively evaluated and developed. Currently, several FTIs are under evaluation in phase I/II clinical trials. However, a surprising outcome in these efforts has been that, while FTIs have shown impressive anti-tumor activity in preclinical studies, FTIs are believed to inhibit tumor growth by blocking the function of a farnesylated protein(s) either in addition to, or instead of, Ras. Therefore, inhibitors of Ras signaling have been considered as another approach to block Ras function, making a clear delineation of the critical signaling events involved in Ras-mediated oncogenes imperative for the success of these efforts.

2.3 Multiple Ras proteins: redundant or distinct functions?

The different Ras isoforms share significant sequence identity (85%) and biochemical function (common regulators and effectors), and mutated forms of each show comparable transforming activities. This and other evidence initially led to the belief that Ras proteins were functionally identical. However, there are a limited number of observations that suggest some functional differences. For example, mutations in K-*ras* and N-*ras* occur more frequently than H-*ras* in human tumors (Bos, 1989; Clark and Der, 1993). Recently, evidence has arisen that there is differential intracellular trafficking of Ras proteins as well as isoform-specific differences in their association with specific regions of the plasma membrane (Reuther and Der, 2000; Wolfman, 2001). Also, gene knockout studies in mouse models revealed that K-*ras* is necessary for development, whereas H-*ras* and N-*ras* are not (Bar-Sagi, 2001). Finally, whereas H-Ras activity is sensitive to inhibition by FTIs, K-Ras and N-Ras functions are not (Oliff, 1999; Cox, 2001). While these various observations support functional distinctions, clear and significant functional differences important for the mechanism of Ras-mediated oncogenesis remain to be identified.

3. RAS FUNCTIONS AS A SIGNALING NODE

Ras serves as a point of convergence of signaling initiated by diverse extracellular stimuli. This includes stimuli that recognize receptor tyrosine kinases, cytokine receptors, G protein-coupled receptors and integrins. Once activated, Ras interacts with and regulates a complex spectrum of functionally distinct effectors to stimulate a multitude of signaling cascades that regulate cytoplasmic (e.g., actin organization) and nuclear (e.g., gene expression, cell cycle progression) processes important for many normal cellular processes.

3.1 Ras utilizes multiple effectors to mediate diverse cytoplasmic signaling cascades

Normal and oncogenic Ras mediate their biological functions by binding to downstream effectors (Shields et al., 2000). All effectors bind to a core effector loop of Ras proteins (residues 32-40), with additional involvement of residues that change in conformation during GDP/GTP cycling; the switch I (residues 30-38) and switch II (residues 59-76) domains (Marshall, 1996; Campbell et al., 1998). The GTP-bound form displays a significantly greater affinity for effectors. In recent years, the number of Ras effectors and the complexity of downstream pathways that they regulate have grown considerably. We will focus on the contribution of three key Ras effectors to Ras-mediated signaling and transformation.

The first Ras-induced signal transduction cascade to be identified was the Raf>MEK>ERK protein kinase cascade (Marshall, 1996; Campbell et al., 1998).

Activated Ras binds to and promotes the activation of Raf serine/threonine kinases (c-Raf-1, A-Raf and B-Raf). Ras causes activation of Raf, in part, by promoting a translocation of Raf to the plasma membrane, where additional binding and phosphorylation events are necessary for complete Raf activation (Morrison and Cutler, Jr., 1997). Once activated, Raf phosphorylates and activates the MEK1/2 dual specificity kinases that in turn phosphorylate and activate ERK1/2 mitogen-activated protein kinases (MAPKs). Activated ERKs translocate to the nucleus and phosphorylate various transcription factors that include the Ets family member Elk-1.

The second best characterized effector of Ras are phosphatidylinositol 3-kinases (PI3Ks), lipid kinases consisting of a p85 regulatory and a p110 catalytic subunit (Rodriguez-Viciana et al., 1994; Rodriguez-Viciana et al., 1997). PI3K phosphorylates integral membrane phosphotidylinositols (PI) at the 3' position (e.g., phosphatidylinositol 4,5-phosphate; PIP2) to generate various short-lived second messenger products (e.g., phosphatidylinositol 3,4,5-phosphate; PIP3) (Vanhaesebroeck et al., 1997). Membrane-associated PIP3 in turn can regulate the activity of a diverse array of signaling molecules that include the Akt serine/threonine kinase. Akt activation results in complex signaling cascades that lead to the phosphorylation of diverse substrates such as caspases, transcription factors (ATX), and proapoptotic proteins (BAD) that regulate cell survival (Chan et al., 1999). PI3K also mediates antiapoptotic signaling, as well as actin organization, by activating the Rac small GTPase (Bar-Sagi and Hall, 2000). The importance of PI3K in Ras transformation is best characterized in NIH 3T3 mouse fibroblasts. However, PI3K is not required for Ras transformation of other cells, reflecting cell-type differences in Ras effector utilization in transformation (McFall et al., 2001).

The third best understood Ras effectors are Ral GEFs (RalGDS, Rgl, Rlf/Rgl2, etc.) that function as activators of the Ras-related RalA and RalB small GTPases (Feig et al., 1996). RalGEF activation by Ras leads to a GTPase cascade in which activated, GTP-bound Ral binds RalBP1, a putative Rho family GAP. Activated Ral also mediates phosphorylation of the fork head transcription factor AFX, which may provide a link between Ras and the cell cycle (Medema et al., 2000). Whether the effects of RalGEF activation are mediated solely by Ral activation or whether RalGEF has other functions is not clear. RalGEF binding to Ras has been shown to stimulate transcription of transcription factors, proteases and cell cycle components (Reuther and Der, 2000).

Ras proteins bind a large number of other effectors including AF-6, PLCε, PKCζ, Nore1, and RASSF1 (Cullen, 2001; Feig and Buchsbaum, 2002). The roles of these effectors in Ras function are only now being studied. Each different effector pathway contributes distinct aspects of Ras-mediated tumor progression and metastasis. Dissecting these pathways and determining the level of crosstalk has become staggeringly complex but may ultimately increase our understanding of the role of Ras in carcinogenesis and invasion. We will focus on an overview of the contribution of the three main effectors Raf, PI3K and RalGEF to Ras deregulation of proliferation, apoptosis, angiogenesis and invasion/metastasis through gene deregulation.

3.2 Dissecting Ras signal transduction: tools of the trade

In light of the interaction of Ras with multiple effectors, one important issue has been to determine the contribution of each effector in mediating the diverse actions of oncogenic Ras. The ability of activated Raf or MEK alone to cause transformation of NIH 3T3 mouse fibroblasts initially suggested that the Raf>MEK>ERK cascade alone was sufficient for Ras transformation (Marshall, 1996; Campbell et al., 1998). However, it is now clear that Ras causes transformation by utilization of Raf-dependent as well as Raf-independent effector signaling. Another facet that has emerged from these studies is that there can be striking cell-type differences in the contribution of specific effectors to Ras transformation.

One important experimental approach that demonstrated the involvement of Raf-independent effectors in Ras transformation was the identification of effector domain mutants of Ras that showed impaired interaction with a subset of effectors (Rodriguez-Viciana et al., 1997; White et al., 1995; Joneson et al., 1996; Khosravi-Far et al., 1996). These mutants have single mutations at residues E35, E37, and Y40 (Fig. 2). The E35S mutant retains the ability to bind to and activate Raf but is impaired in binding to RalGEF and PI3K. The E37G mutant also lost the ability to activate Raf and PI3K, but retained the ability to activate RalGEF, whereas the Y40C mutant retained the ability to activate PI3K but not Raf or RalGEF. The E37G and Y40C mutants showed impaired ability to bind to and activate Raf, yet they retained the ability to cause tumorigenic transformation of NIH 3T3 cells (Khosravi-Far et al., 1996; Webb et al., 1998). Hence, the transforming activity of 37G or 40C has been attributed to their ability to activate RalGEF or PI3K, respectively. These mutants have been very useful reagents to assess the role of Raf, RalGEF, and PI3K in Ras function.

Constitutively activated effectors have also been useful reagents for assessing the role of each effector in Ras function (Fig. 2). Since Ras promotes effector activation, in part, by promoting their membrane association, the addition of the carboxyl terminal plasma membrane-targeting sequence of Ras onto effectors has been a useful approach to generate constitutively-activated variants of Raf-1, the p110 catalytic subunit of PI3K, and various RalGEFs (Rodriguez-Viciana et al., 1997; Leevers et al., 1994; Stokoe et al., 1994; Wolthuis et al., 1997). The ability of activated PI3K or RalGEF to cooperate with activated Raf and cause synergistic transformation of NIH 3T3 cells has provided evidence for the contribution of each effector to Ras transformation. While activated Raf alone can cause transformation of NIH 3T3 mouse fibroblasts, activated Raf failed to cause transformation of a variety of epithelial cell types, indicating the critical requirement for Raf-independent effectors in transformation of some cell types (Oldham et al., 1996; Gire et al., 1999; Schulze et al., 2001). Constitutively activated substrates of Raf [e.g.,

MEK(ED)], PI3K (e.g., membrane-targeted Akt; Myr-Akt), and RalGEF (e.g., GTPase-deficient mutants of Ral) have also been used for similar analyses (Fig. 2).

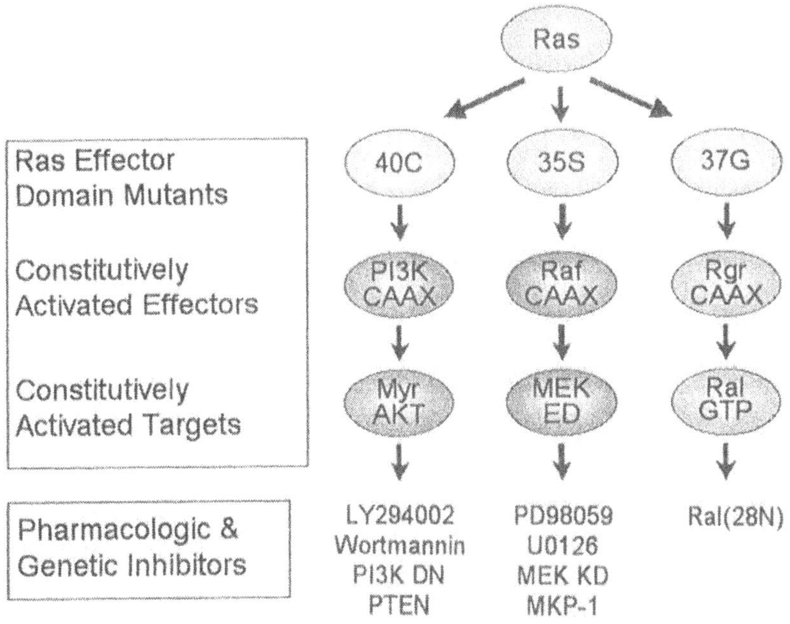

Figure 2. Effectors of Ras function

Pharmacologic or genetic inhibitors of specific effector signaling pathways have also been useful reagents for defining the contribution of specific effectors in Ras transformation (Fig. 2). For example, LY294002 is a specific inhibitor of PI3K, whereas PD98059 and U0126 are specific inhibitors of MEK activation of ERK (Davies et al., 2000). LY294002, but not PD98059, treatment reversed the ability of oncogenic Ras to inhibit suspension-induced apoptosis, or anoikis, in MDCK canine kidney epithelial cells (Khwaja et al., 1997). This demonstrated the critical role of PI3K but not Raf in mediating this important facet of anchorage-independent growth. Finally, kinase-dead mutants of Raf-1, MEK, ERK, Akt, and dominant negative Ral have been useful genetic inhibitors of specific effector signaling pathways (Rodriguez-Viciana et al., 1997; Brtva et al., 1995; Cowley et al., 1994; Khosravi-Far et al., 1995).

3.3 Ras deregulation of gene expression and transformation

As indicated above, signaling initiated by the three main Ras effectors results in the stimulation of a variety of transcription factors (Campbell et al., 1998). Therefore, it is not surprising that Ras transformation has been shown to be dependent on the function of many of these transcription factors. For example, depletion of c-*myc* with specific antisense sequences (Sklar et al., 1991) or expression of dominant negative mutants of Ets (Wasylyk et al., 1998; Langer et al., 1992; Wasylyk et al., 1994), c-Fos (Wick et al., 1992) or c-Jun (Granger-Schnarr et al., 1992) have been shown to block Ras-mediated transformation of NIH 3T3 fibroblasts. Similarly, c-*jun* null mouse embryo fibroblasts were found to be insensitive to Ras-mediated transformation (Johnson et al., 1996). An essential requirement for c-*fos* in Ras-mediated skin tumor formation was shown in c-*fos* knockout mice carrying an H-*ras* transgene (Saez et al., 1995). Finally, inhibition of NF-κB blocked Ras-mediated transformation and resulted in apoptosis of rodent fibroblast cell lines (Finco et al., 1997; Mayo et al., 1997). Taken together, these observations demonstrate the essential role of gene expression changes in Ras-mediated oncogenesis.

At least two broad approaches have been utilized to define the gene targets involved in Ras transformation. First, several techniques to study genome-wide changes in gene expression have been applied to study the transcriptional changes associated with Ras- or Raf-mediated expression or transformation. These techniques include differential display (Liang et al., 1994; McCarthy et al., 1995; Zhang et al., 1998), subtractive suppression hybridization (SSH) (Baba et al., 2000; Zuber et al., 2000), representational difference analysis (RDA) (Shields et al., 2001b; Shields et al., 2001a), and microchip array analyses (Schulze et al., 2001; Habets et al., 2001). These approaches reveal the complexity of gene expression changes associated with Ras transformation. For example, SSH was also employed by Schafer and colleagues to identify genes whose expression was upregulated or downregulated in H-Ras-transformed 208F rat fibroblasts (Zuber et al., 2000). They identified transcriptional stimulation or repression of 244 known genes, 104 ESTs, and 45 novel sequences. Overall, it was estimated that 3 to 8% of all expressed genes were altered in Ras-transformed cells. Interestingly, only a fraction of these gene expression changes were reversed by inhibition of MEK, indicating that Raf>MEK>ERK independent pathways contribute significantly to gene deregulation. This possibility is also supported by RDA analyses that identified gene expression changes caused by activated Ras but not Raf (Shields et al., 2001b; Shields et al., 2001a).

A second approach for defining gene targets of Ras has involved an evaluation of whether the expression of specific genes whose products may contribute to transformation are altered by oncogenic Ras. Included among these are genes encoding proteins that regulate cell proliferation and cell cycle progression, tumor cell invasion and metastasis, and angiogenesis. In the sections below, we summarize some of the findings that have come from these studies. We have not provided a complete summary of this topic. Instead, we have chosen to highlight specific examples of gene targets that may promote oncogenic Ras deregulation of cell proliferation and induction of tumor cell invasion, metastasis, and angiogenesis. These examples also further highlight the role of Raf-independent effectors in Ras oncogenesis as well as cell-type differences in Ras signaling.

4. RAS DEREGULATION OF CELL PROLIFERATION

The significant role of aberrant Ras activation in increased cancer cell growth and proliferation has been well-established. In examining the contribution of Ras to stimulus-independent growth and the inhibition of growth arrest pathways, two themes emerge: deregulation of the cell cycle and induction of growth factor autocrine loops. The first allows Ras-transformed cells to overcome growth arrest imposed by cell cycle checkpoints; the second renders cells self-sufficient by providing a constant stimulus to proliferate. Deregulation of key components of both vital cell regulatory mechanisms can be achieved, in part, by Ras-mediated changes in gene expression.

4.1 Ras regulation of cyclin D1 and cell cycle progression

A number of studies determined that normal Ras is required for mitogen-induced cell cycle progression, while oncogenic Ras promotes growth factor-independent entry into the cell cycle (Marshall, 1999; Pruitt and Der, 2001). Similarly, the mitogen-stimulated regulation of positive (e.g., cyclin D1) and negative (e.g., $p21^{CIP1}$, $p27^{KIP1}$) regulatory components of the cell cycle machinery is well understood (Sherr and Roberts, 1999). Of these, the role of Ras regulation of cyclin D1 expression and function has been the best characterized.

Growth factor stimulation promotes entry into the cell cycle from G_0 to G_1 and facilitates the G_1/S transition partly through D-type cyclin upregulation (Sherr, 1996). Cyclin D1 binds cyclin-dependent kinases (CDKs), enhancing their ability to phosphorylate the Rb tumor suppressor protein that functions as a negative regulator of cell cycle progession. Phosphorylation inactivates Rb, which permits E2F-dependent gene expression necessary for cell proliferation.

Ras mediates upregulation of cyclin D1 by transcriptional activation in a wide variety of cell types (Arber et al., 1996; Filmus et al., 1994; Liu et al., 1995). Transient activation of Ras in rodent fibroblasts and epithelial cells is accompanied by upregulation of cyclin D1 transcription and protein expression (Filmus et al., 1994; Shao et al., 2000; Winston et al., 1996). Serum-stimulated upregulation of cyclin D1 expression is Ras-dependent, and constitutive expression of cyclin D1 overcomes the requirement for Ras activation in NIH 3T3 cell proliferation (Aktas et al., 1997). Finally, Ras transformation of a variety of cell types is associated with sustained upregulation of cyclin D1 protein (Arber et al., 1996; Liu et al., 1995; Shao et al., 2000; Takuwa and Takuwa, 2001; Pruitt et al., 2000).

Oncogenic Ras upregulates cyclin D1 by Raf-dependent and Raf-independent signaling. Although Raf/ERK activation is sufficient to stimulate cyclin D1 gene expression in rodent fibroblasts (Liu et al., 1995; Lavoie et al., 1996; Kerkhoff and Rapp, 1997; Greulich and Erikson, 1998; Cheng et al., 1998; Ladha et al., 1998) additional Ras-mediated pathways may be necessary for cyclin D1 regulation in other cell types (Pruitt et al., 2000; Lavoie et al., 1996). For example, PI3K activation may promote cell cycle entry via post-transcriptional as well as transcriptional regulation of cyclin D1 (Gille and Downward, 1999). Ral GEF-mediated activation of Ral may stimulate the cyclin D1 promoter through activation of NF-κB (Henry et al., 2000). These and other findings suggest that several Ras effector pathways may contribute to distinct aspects of Ras deregulation of the cell cycle in a cell-type specific manner.

4.2 *Ras regulation of TGFα and autocrine growth*

In addition to circumventing growth arrest machinery, Ras-transformed cells become independent of growth factors in order to ensure proliferation. One such mechanism may be oncogenic Ras-induced upregulation of transforming growth factor-α (TGFα) in a variety of cell types (Oldham et al., 1996; Marshall et al., 1985; Ciardiello et al., 1988; Godwin and Lieberman, 1990; Glick et al., 1991; Filmus et al., 1993). TGFα is a member of the epidermal growth factor (EGF) family of mitogens that activate the EGF receptor (EGFR) to promote cell proliferation (Normanno et al., 2001). TGFα-mediated autocrine signaling has been shown to be at least partially responsible for Ras transformation (Filmus et al., 1993; Ciardiello et al., 1990; Gangarosa et al., 1997). Activation of the Raf-MEK-ERK pathway is sufficient for upregulation of TGFα gene expression in some, but not other, cell types (Oldham et al., 1996; Schulze et al., 2001). Although these findings implicate multiple Ras-mediated pathways in the stimulation of the TGFα autocrine loop, the mechanism of TFGα gene upregulation and contribution of TGFα stimulation of EGFR to malignant transformation remain to be determined.

5. RAS TARGETS INVOLVED IN TUMOR CELL ANGIOGENESIS, INVASION AND METASTASIS

In addition to deregulating cell growth and proliferation, oncogenic Ras causes changes in genes that promote malignant transformation. In this section, we highlight several gene targets of Ras whose protein products may contribute to tumor cell angiogenesis (vascular endothelial growth factor; VEGF), invasion and metastasis (matrix metalloproteases; MMPs).

5.1 *Ras, VEGF and tumor cell angiogenesis*

Oncogenic Ras has been observed to be a potent stimulator of vascular endothelial growth factor (VEGF) gene expression (Rak et al., 1995a; Konishi et al., 2000; White et al., 1997). VEGF is one of a number of soluble factors that are mitogens specific for vascular endothelial cells, mediating both normal and pathological angiogenesis. Angiogenesis is required for the growth of microscopic solid tumors beyond 1-2 mm in diameter, providing adequate oxygen and nutrient supplies as well as access to distant sites of metastasis. Tumor cells under hypoxic conditions either commandeer existing vasculature or stimulate endothelial cells to undergo angiogenesis.

The effectors that mediate oncogenic Ras stimulation of VEGF gene expression exhibit significant cell-type differences. For example, the Raf/ERK pathway is sufficient to promote VEGF upregulation in rodent fibroblasts (Grugel et al., 1995; Milanini et al., 1998). Phosphorylation of hypoxia-induced factor-1 (HIF-1) by ERKs may represent one level of integration between Ras-mediated and hypoxia-induced VEGF gene expression. In contrast, in epithelial or other cell types, PI3K is also necessary for Ras-mediated VEGF expression, suggesting that Ras regulation of VEGF may involve several Ras effectors and show cell-type specific differences (Mazure et al., 1997; Rak et al., 2000b).

While upregulation of VEGF may be important for angiogenesis, Ras must regulate the expression of other factors as well to promote tumor angiogenesis. For example, one study found that oncogenic Ras was required for upregulated expression and secretion of VEGF in human colorectal carcinoma cell lines (Okada et al., 1998). Suppression of VEGF expression impaired the tumorigenic growth of these cells, showing the importance of this factor in Ras-induced tumor angiogenesis. However, forced overexpression of VEGF in the absence of mutated Ras was not sufficient to fully restore tumorigenic growth. Similarly, evaluation using a mouse melanoma model showed the importance of continued expression of oncogenic Ras in tumor maintenance (Chin et al., 1999). Expression of Ras was associated with increased tumor vascularization and upregulated expression of VEGF. Loss of Ras expression resulted in apoptosis of endothelial cells lining the tumor vasculature and subsequent tumor cell apoptosis and regression. However, forced VEGF overexpression alone was not sufficient to overcome the need for Ras activity, suggesting that other angiogenic factors in addition to VEGF are regulated by Ras activation. For example, Ras has been shown to downregulate angiogenesis inhibitors such as thrombospondin-1 and tissue inhibitor of matrix metalloproteinase-2 (TIMP-2), adding further complexity to the molecular mechanism for Ras-mediated angiogenesis (Zuber et al., 2000; Laderoute et al., 2000; Tokunaga et al., 2000). Further studies are needed to determine which Ras-mediated pathways are important for VEGF expression in various tumors and to establish the contribution of Ras upregulation of VEGF as well as other factors to angiogenesis.

5.2 Ras and tumor cell invasion/metastasis

Oncogenic Ras can also promote tumor metastasis of a variety of cell types (Thorgeirsson et al., 1985; Vousden et al., 1986; Collard et al., 1987; Treiger and Isaacs, 1988). Metastasis accounts for approximately 90% of cancer mortalities but is the least understood step in the multi-step model of cancer (Woodhouse et al., 1997; Fidler, 1999). The processes that render a benign cancer cell locally invasive as well as metastatic are complex and not yet completely defined. Invading cells must overcome barriers such as basement membranes and interstitial stroma through precisely regulated on-off cycling of adhesion to surrounding matrix and degradation of matrix by proteases.

The contribution of different effector signaling pathways to Ras-induced metastasis has been evaluated. For example, one study utilized Ras effector domain mutants and determined that activation of Raf, but not PI3K or RalGEF, was sufficient for Ras-mediated induction of metastasis of NIH 3T3 mouse fibroblasts (Webb et al., 1998). In contrast, a similar study also used effector domain mutants but found instead a critical role for the RalGEF pathway in promoting metastatic growth in nude mice (Ward et al., 2001). In NIH 3T3 fibroblasts, as well as mouse and human mammary epithelial cells, RalGEF activation promoted aggressive, infiltrating metastases whereas Raf-induced metastases have non-infiltrating borders. While ERK or PI3K activation alone were not sufficient to promote metastasis, it was found that ERK activity was required and cooperated with RalGDS for metastasis. In contrast to these studies, for the *ras* mutation positive HT1080 human fibrosarcoma cell line, PI3K/Akt pathway activation was implicated in mediating increased cell motility and invasion (Kim et al., 2001). Based on these studies, Ras proteins appear to promote invasion through the cooperation or selective activation of several key pathways. However, whether the pathways mediating invasion are cell-type specific or tumor-type specific is still unclear. Furthermore, the mechanisms by which Ras effector activation induce the invasive phenotype and the contribution of gene deregulation to the development of this phenotype remains largely to be determined.

Oncogenic Ras may promote tumor cell invasion and metastasis by causing deregulation of gene expression (Chambers and Tuck, 1993). This includes increased expression or activity of degradative enzymes such as matrix metalloproteinases (MMPs) and cysteine proteinases (cathepsins) as well as decreased expression or activity of their inhibitors (e.g., TIMPs). Of these, MMPs have been relatively well studied as targets for Ras-mediated gene upregulation of invasion-promoting proteins.

MMPs are zinc-dependent endopeptidases that degrade the extracellular matrix (ECM) as well as cleave cell surface molecules to mediate tumor progression, invasion, and angiogenesis. The MMP superfamily is divided into collagenases, stromelysins, gelatinases, transmembrane MMPs, and other MMPs (Coussens and Werb, 1996; Shapiro, 1998; Westermarck and Kahari, 1999; Matrisian, 1999). Most MMPs are secreted as latent precursors that are activated by an initial cleavage of an amino terminal propeptide followed by autocatalytic amino terminal cleavage resulting in full exposure of the catalytic site and protease activity. Four members of specific MMP inhibitors known as tissue inhibitors of MMPs (TIMPs) bind the MMP catalytic domains to inhibit protease activity.

The evidence linking MMP upregulation with invasion and metastasis in a large variety of cancers of different tissue origins is quite extensive. Furthermore, mouse models deficient in specific MMPs exhibit decreased tumor growth, angiogenesis and invasion in response to various carcinogens and tumor-promoting protein expression (Shapiro, 1998; McCawley and Matrisian, 2001). Despite the strong correlation between MMP overexpression and tumor invasion, few mechanistic studies are available that demonstrate the direct role of MMPs in oncogene-stimulated invasion. Furthermore, though most MMPs are induced at the transcriptional level by growth factors, hormones, cell contact to ECM, and oncogenes activation, recent studies have focused on transcription factors and not the cytoplasmic signaling pathways that mediate MMP promoter regulation. This section will focus on the transcriptional upregulation of MMP-2, -3, -7, -9 and –10 by activated Ras and its key effectors.

The best evidence for linking Ras to upregulation of MMPs involves MMP-9/type IV collagenase/gelatinase B (Yanagihara et al., 1995; Ballin et al., 1988; Himelstein et al., 1997; Giambernardi et al., 1998; Bernhard et al., 1990; Baruch et al., 2001; Yang et al., 2001; Gum et al., 1997). Ras-mediated upregulation of MMP-9 enzymatic activity is due primarily to upregulation in gene expression. The MMP-9 promoter contains a variety of Ras-responsive promoter elements, including Ets, AP-1 and NF-κB binding sites (Himelstein et al., 1997; Gum et al., 1996). Although clear cell-type differences in regulation are seen, an important contribution of the Raf/MEK/ERK effector pathway to Ras-mediated MMP-9 upregulation has been determined, but Raf-independent effector function (e.g., PI3K) is also involved (Gum et al., 1997; Gum et al., 1996; Arbiser et al., 1997). Evidence for a functional role for MMP-9 is provided by the observation that forced upregulation of MMP-9 promoted metastasis, whereas suppression of MMP-9 expression in Ras-transformed rodent fibroblasts caused a loss of metastatic growth but not tumorigencity (Bernhard et al., 1994; Hua and Muschel, 1996).

Upregulation of the related MMP-2 (gelatinase A), often together with MMP-9, has also been observed in a variety of cell types transformed by oncogenic Ras (Yanagihara et al., 1995; Baruch et al., 2001; Arbiser et al., 1997; Meade-Tollin et al., 1998; Charvat et al., 1999). Little is known regarding the effector signaling involved in MMP-2 upregulation, and the MMP-2 promoter lacks the Ras-responsive elements seen in the MMP-9 promoter (Westermarck and Kahari, 1999). Evidence for the importance of MMP-2 upregulation in Ras oncogenesis is suggested by the observation that for H-Ras-transformed MCF-10A human mammary epithelial cells, antisense inhibition of MMP-2 gene expression decreased Ras-mediated *in vitro* invasion (Moon et al., 2000). Interestingly, N-Ras transformation of MCF-10A cells preferentially upregulated MMP-9 rather than MMP-2 and did not promote invasion, indicating cell-type differences in MMP-9 involvement in invasion.

MMP-3 (stromelysin-1), a member of the stromelysin subfamily of MMPs, has also been shown to be regulated by Ras in rodent fibroblast cells (Engel et al., 1992; LoSardo et al., 1995). Analyses of differentially-expressed genes identified MMP-3, as well as the related MMP-10 (stromelysin-2), gene as a MEK-dependent upregulated gene in Ras-transformed 208F rat fibroblasts (208F) (Zuber et al., 2000) or as Raf-induced genes in Rat-1 rat fibroblasts (Heinrich et al., 2000). These studies suggest that in fibroblasts, Raf/MEK/ERK pathway activation may be sufficient for MMP-3 and MMP-10 upregulation. Similar to promoter studies performed on the human MMP-9 promoter, MMP-3 promoter analysis revealed Raf/ERK-dependent MMP-9 activation via Ets binding sites and Raf-independent activation via AP-1 binding sites (Kirstein et al., 1996; Jayaraman et al., 1999). The role of activated Ras and its effectors in upregulation of MMP-3 in epithelial cells remains to be clarified.

Perhaps the lease well-studied MMP discussed in this section is MMP-7 (matrilysin). In pancreatic carcinoma cells, MMP-7 transcriptional upregulation is associated with aberrant K-Ras activation (Ohnami et al., 1999; Fukushima et al., 2001). For example, antisense downregulation of *K-ras* expression in a pancreatic cancer cell line was associated with a downregulation of MMP-7 transcript levels. Similarly, K-Ras activation in colon carcinoma cells upregulated MMP-7 transcript in an AP-1 dependent manner (Yamamoto et al., 1995). Although these preliminary studies link Ras activation to MMP-7 upregulation, what effectors may mediate Ras upregulation of MMP-7 has not been identified, nor has the role of MMP-7 in Ras-mediated invasion been determined.

Although many studies illustrate Ras-induced MMP transcriptional upregulation as well as the correlation between Ras-mediated invasion and MMP upregulation, substantial evidence demonstrating MMP upregulation as a mechanism for Ras-mediated invasion is not available. Another complex question that remains unanswered is the vital role that Ras-induced TIMP downregulation may play in the regulation of MMPs by activated Ras. And finally, the interplay between epithelial cells expressing invasion-promoting oncoproteins and their surrounding stroma has only recently come under close scrutiny. Although this review focused on MMP upregulation in tumor cells, recent studies suggest that tumor cells may secrete factors that enhance MMP expression in neighboring stromal tissue. These secreted proteases may then localize to the tumor cell surface or surrounding extracellular environment to promote tumor cell invasion.

6. CONCLUSIONS & PERSPECTIVES

While our understanding of Ras signaling is significant and many of the signaling components and pathways activated by Ras have been delineated, it is also likely that much remains to be determined. The discovery of additional downstream effectors of Ras continues and reveals further diversity and complexity in the cytoplasmic signaling activities of Ras. The recent identification of PLCε as a Ras effector links Ras activity directly to the actions of second messengers, calcium and diacylglycerol, that in turn cause pleotropic cellular responses. Conversely, some effectors of Ras (Norel and RASSF1) may promote apoptosis rather than oncogenesis. How these effectors may contribute to the mechanism of Ras-mediated oncogenesis will be important to establish. One major consequence of these diverse effector signaling events involves changes in gene expression. Some signaling events directly stimulate the activity of specific transcription factors and the number of these factors continues to increase. Other Ras-mediated signaling events, including DNA methylation or histone acetylation, may cause global changes in gene expression. The development and applications of methods, such as microarray analyses and functional proteomics, to evaluate global changes in gene or protein expression will further increase our knowledge of the gene targets of Ras. Hence, this area of Ras research will evolve rapidly in the coming years. The accumulation of information will certainly occur at a pace that greatly exceeds our ability to make sense of these observations. Nevertheless, our utilization of this information will facilitate important advances for understanding the role of Ras in oncogenesis and for the identification of novel therapeutic approaches for cancer diagnosis and treatment.

7. ACKNOWLEDGEMENTS

We thank Misha Rand for manuscript preparation. Our studies are supported by National Institutes of Health (NIH) grants to CJD (CA42978, CA63071, CA67771 and CA69577) and ASU was supported by an NIH training grant (CA71341).

8. REFERENCES

Aktas, H., Cai, H., and Cooper, G.M. (1997). Ras links growth factor signaling to the cell cycle machinery via regulation of cyclin D1 and the Cdk inhibitor $p27^{KIP1}$. Mol.Cell.Biol. *17*, 3850-3857.

Arber, N., Sutter, T., Miyake, M., Kahn, S.M., Venkatraj, V.S., Sobrino, A., Warburton, D., Holt, P.R., and Weinstein, I.B. (1996). Increased expression of cyclin D1 and the Rb tumor suppressor gene in c- K-ras transformed rat enterocytes. Oncogene *12*, 1903-1908.

Arbiser, J.L., Moses, M.A., Fernandez, C.A., Ghiso, N., Cao, Y., Klauber, N., Frank, D., Brownlee, M., Flynn, E., Parangi, S., Byers, H.R., and Folkman, J. (1997). Oncogenic H-ras stimulates tumor angiogenesis by two distinct pathways. Proc.Natl.Acad.Sci.U.S.A. *94*, 861-866.

Baba, I., Shirasawa, S., Iwamoto, R., Okumura, K., Tsunoda, T., Nishioka, M., Fukuyama, K., Yamamoto, K., Mekada, E., and Sasazuki, T. (2000). Involvement of deregulated epiregulin expression in tumorigenesis in vivo through activated Ki-Ras signaling pathway in human colon cancer cells. Cancer Res. *60*, 6886-6889.

Ballin, M., Gomez, D.E., Sinha, C.C., and Thorgeirsson, U.P. (1988). Ras oncogene mediated induction of a 92 kDa metalloproteinase; strong correlation with the malignant phenotype. Biochem.Biophys.Res.Commun. *154*, 832-838.

Bar-Sagi, D. (2001). A Ras by any other name. Mol.Cell Biol. *21*, 1441-1443.

Bar-Sagi, D. and Hall, A. (2000). Ras and Rho GTPases: a family reunion. Cell *103*, 227-238.

Barbacid, M. (1987). *ras* genes. Annu.Rev.Biochem. *56*, 779-827.

Baruch, R.R., Melinscak, H., Lo, J., Liu, Y., Yeung, O., and Hurta, R.A. (2001). Altered matrix metalloproteinase expression associated with oncogene-mediated cellular transformation and metastasis formation. Cell Biol.Int. *25*, 411-420.

Bernhard, E.J., Gruber, S.B., and Muschel, R.J. (1994). Direct evidence linking expression of matrix metalloproteinase 9 (92- kDa gelatinase/collagenase) to the metastatic phenotype in transformed rat embryo cells. Proc.Natl.Acad.Sci.U.S.A. *91*, 4293-4297.

Bernhard, E.J., Muschel, R.J., and Hughes, E.N. (1990). Mr 92,000 gelatinase release correlates with the metastatic phenotype in transformed rat embryo cells. Cancer Res. *50*, 3872-3877.

Bos, J.L. (1989). *ras* oncogenes in human cancer: a review. Cancer Res. *49*, 4682-4689.

Bourne, H.R., Sanders, D.A., and McCormick, F. (1990). The GTPase superfamily: conserved structure and molecular mechanism. Nature *349*, 117-126.

Brtva, T.R., Drugan, J.K., Ghosh, S., Terrell, R.S., Campbell-Burk, S., Bell, R.M., and Der, C.J. (1995). Two distinct Raf domains mediate interaction with Ras. J.Biol.Chem. *270*, 9809-9812.

Campbell, S.L., Khosravi-Far, R., Rossman, K.L., Clark, G.J., and Der, C.J. (1998). Increasing complexity of Ras signaling. Oncogene *17*, 1395-1413.

Chambers, A.F. and Tuck, A.B. (1993). *Ras*-responsive genes and tumor metastasis. Crit.Rev.Oncogenesis *4*, 95-114.

Chan, T.O., Rittenhouse, S.E., and Tsichlis, P.N. (1999). AKT/PKB and other D3 phosphoinositide-regulated kinases: kinase activation by phosphoinositide-dependent phosphorylation. Annu.Rev.Biochem. *68*, 965-1014.

Charvat, S., Le Griel, C., Chignol, M.C., Schmitt, D., and Serres, M. (1999). Ras-transfection up-regulated HaCaT cell migration: inhibition by Marimastat. Clin.Exp.Metastasis *17*, 677-685.

Cheng, M., Sexl, V., Sherr, C.J., and Roussel, M.F. (1998). Assembly of cyclin D-dependent kinase and titration of p27Kip1 regulated by mitogen-activated protein kinase kinase (MEK1). Proc.Natl.Acad.Sci.U.S.A. *95*, 1091-1096.

Chin, L., Tam, A., Pomerantz, J., Wong, M., Holash, J., Bardeesy, N., Shen, Q., O'Hagan, R., Pantginis, J., Zhou, H., Horner, J.W., Cordon-Cardo, C., Yancopoulos, G.D., and DePinho, R.A. (1999). Essential role for oncogenic Ras in tumour maintenance. Nature *400*, 468-472.

Ciardiello, F., Kim, N., Hynes, N., Jaggi, R., Redmond, S., Liscia, D.S., Sanfilippo, B., Merlo, G., Callahan, R., Kidwell, W.R., and . (1988). Induction of transforming growth factor alpha expression in mouse mammary epithelial cells after transformation with a point-mutated c-Ha-ras protooncogene. Mol.Endocrinol. 2, 1202-1216.

Ciardiello, F., McGeady, M.L., Kim, N., Basolo, F., Hynes, N., Langton, B.C., Yokozaki, H., Saeki, T., Elliott, J.W., and Masui, H. (1990). Transforming growth factor-alpha expression is enhanced in

human mammary epithelial cells transformed by an activated c-Ha-ras protooncogene but not by the c-neu protooncogene, and overexpression of the transforming growth factor-alpha complementary DNA leads to transformation. Cell Growth Differ. *1*, 407-420.
Cichowski, K. and Jacks, T. (2001). NF1 tumor suppressor gene function: narrowing the GAP. Cell *104*, 593-604.
Clark, G.J. and Der, C.J. (1993). Oncogenic activation of *Ras* proteins. In GTPases in Biology I. B.F. Dickey and L. Birnbaumer, eds. (Berlin: Springer Verlag), pp. 259-288.
Clark, G.J. and Der, C.J. (1995). Aberrant function of the Ras signal transduction pathway in human breast cancer. Breast Cancer Res.Treat. *35*, 133-144.
Collard, J.G., Schijven, J.F., and Roos, E. (1987). Invasive and metastatic potential induced by ras-transfection into mouse BW5147 T-lymphoma cells. Cancer Res. *47*, 754-759.
Coussens, L.M. and Werb, Z. (1996). Matrix metalloproteinases and the development of cancer. Chem.Biol. *3*, 895-904.
Cowley, S., Paterson, H., Kemp, P., and Marshall, C.J. (1994). Activation of MAP kinase kinase is necessary and sufficient for PC12 differentiation and for transformation of NIH 3T3 cells. Cell *77*, 841-852.
Cox, A.D. (2001). Farnesyltransferase inhibitors: potential role in the treatment of cancer. Drugs *61*, 723-732.
Cox, A.D. and Der, C.J. (1997). Farnesyltransferase inhibitors and cancer treatment: targeting simply Ras? Biochim.Biophys.Acta *1333*, F51-F71
Cullen, P.J. (2001). Ras effectors: Buying shares in Ras plc. Curr.Biol. *11*, R342-R344
Davies, S.P., Reddy, H., Caivano, M., and Cohen, P. (2000). Specificity and mechanism of action of some commonly used protein kinase inhibitors. Biochem.J *351*, 95-105.
Engel, G., Popowicz, P., Marshall, H., Norling, G., Svensson, C., Auer, G., Akusjarvi, G., and Linder, S. (1992). Elevated stromelysin-1 and reduced collagenase-IV expression in invasive rat embryo fibroblasts expressing E1A deletion mutants + T24-H-ras. Int.J.Cancer *51*, 761-766.
Feig, L.A. and Buchsbaum, R.J. (2002). Cell signaling: life or death decisions of ras proteins. Curr.Biol. *12*, R259-R261
Feig, L.A., Urano, T., and Cantor, S. (1996). Evidence for a Ras/Ral signaling cascade. Trends Biochem.Sci. *21*, 438-441.
Fidler, I.J. (1999). Critical determinants of cancer metastasis: rationale for therapy. Cancer Chemother.Pharmacol. *43 Suppl*, S3-10.
Filmus, J., Robles, A.I., Shi, W., Wong, M.J., Colombo, L.L., and Conti, C.J. (1994). Induction of cyclin D1 overexpression by activated ras. Oncogene *9*, 3627-3633.
Filmus, J., Shi, W., and Spencer, T. (1993). Role of transforming growth factor alpha (TGF-α) in the transformation of *ras*-transfected rat intestinal epithelial cells. Oncogene *8*, 1017-1022.
Finco, T.S., Westwick, J.K., Norris, J.L., Beg, A.A., Der, C.J., and Baldwin Jr., A.S. (1997). Oncogenic Ha-Ras-induced signaling activates NF-kB transcriptional activity, which is required for cellular transformation. J.Biol.Chem. *272*, 24113-24116.
Fukushima, H., Yamamoto, H., Itoh, F., Nakamura, H., Min, Y., Horiuchi, S., Iku, S., Sasaki, S., and Imai, K. (2001). Association of matrilysin mRNA expression with K-ras mutations and progression in pancreatic ductal adenocarcinomas. Carcinogenesis *22*, 1049-1052.
Gangarosa, L.M., Sizemore, N., Graves-Deal, R., Oldham, S.M., Der, C.J., and Coffey, R.J. (1997). A Raf-independent epidermal growth factor receptor autocrine loop is necessary for Ras transformation of rat intestinal epithelial cells. J.Biol.Chem. *272*, 18926-18931.
Giambernardi, T.A., Grant, G.M., Taylor, G.P., Hay, R.J., Maher, V.M., McCormick, J.J., and Klebe, R.J. (1998). Overview of matrix metalloproteinase expression in cultured human cells. Matrix Biol. *16*, 483-496.
Gille, H. and Downward, J. (1999). Multiple ras effector pathways contribute to G(1) cell cycle progression. J.Biol.Chem. *274*, 22033-22040.
Gire, V., Marshall, C.J., and Wynford-Thomas, D. (1999). Activation of mitogen-activated protein kinase is necessary but not sufficient for proliferation of human thyroid epithelial cells induced by mutant Ras. Oncogene *18*, 4819-4832.
Glick, A.B., Sporn, M.B., and Yuspa, S.H. (1991). Altered regulation of TGF-beta 1 and TGF-alpha in primary keratinocytes and papillomas expressing v-Ha-ras. Mol.Carcinog. *4*, 210-219.
Godwin, A.K. and Lieberman, M.W. (1990). Early and late responses to induction of rasT24 expression in Rat-1 cells. Oncogene *5*, 1231-1241.
Granger-Schnarr, M., Benusiglio, E., Schnarr, M., and Sassone-Corsi, P. (1992). Transformation and transactivation suppressor activity of the c-Jun leucine zipper fused to a bacterial repressor. Proc.Natl.Acad.Sci.USA *89*, 4236-4239.
Greulich, H. and Erikson, R.L. (1998). An analysis of Mek1 signaling in cell proliferation and transformation. J.Biol.Chem. *273*, 13280-13288.
Grugel, S., Finkenzeller, G., Weindel, K., Barleon, B., and Marmé, D. (1995). Both v-Ha-Ras and v-Raf stimulate expression of the vascular endothelial growth factor in NIH 3T3 cells. J.Biol.Chem. *270*, 25915-25919.
Gum, R., Lengyel, E., Juarez, J., Chen, J.H., Sato, H., Seiki, M., and Boyd, D. (1996). Stimulation of 92-kDa gelatinase B promoter activity by ras is mitogen- activated protein kinase kinase 1-

independent and requires multiple transcription factor binding sites including closely spaced PEA3/ets and AP-1 sequences. J.Biol.Chem. *271*, 10672-10680.
Gum, R., Wang, H., Lengyel, E., Juarez, J., and Boyd, D. (1997). Regulation of 92 kDa type IV collagenase expression by the jun aminoterminal kinase- and the extracellular signal-regulated kinase-dependent signaling cascades. Oncogene *14*, 1481-1493.
Habets, G.G.M., knepper, M., sumortin, J., Choi, Y.J., Sasazuki, T., Shirasawa, S., and Bollag, G. (2001). Chip array screening for Ras-regulated genes. Methods Enzymol. *332*, 245-260.
Hanahan, D. and Weinberg, R.A. (2000). The hallmarks of cancer. Cell *100*, 57-70.
Heinrich, J., Bosse, M., Eickhoff, H., Nietfeld, W., Reinhardt, R., Lehrach, H., and Moelling, K. (2000). Induction of putative tumor-suppressing genes in Rat-1 fibroblasts by oncogenic Raf-1 as evidenced by robot-assisted complex hybridization. J.Mol.Med. *78*, 380-388.
Henry, D.O., Moskalenko, S.A., Kaur, K.J., Fu, M., Pestell, R.G., Camonis, J.H., and White, M.A. (2000). Ral GTPases contribute to regulation of cyclin D1 through activation of NF-kappaB. Mol.Cell Biol *20*, 8084-8092.
Himelstein, B.P., Lee, E.J., Sato, H., Seiki, M., and Muschel, R.J. (1997). Transcriptional activation of the matrix metalloproteinase-9 gene in an H-ras and v-myc transformed rat embryo cell line. Oncogene *14*, 1995-1998.
Hua, J. and Muschel, R.J. (1996). Inhibition of matrix metalloproteinase 9 expression by a ribozyme blocks metastasis in a rat sarcoma model system. Cancer Res. *56*, 5279-5284.
Jayaraman, G., Srinivas, R., Duggan, C., Ferreira, E., Swaminathan, S., Somasundaram, K., Williams, J., Hauser, C., Kurkinen, M., Dhar, R., Weitzman, S., Buttice, G., and Thimmapaya, B. (1999). p300/cAMP-responsive element-binding protein interactions with ets-1 and ets-2 in the transcriptional activation of the human stromelysin promoter. J.Biol.Chem. *274*, 17342-17352.
Johnson, R., Spiegelman, B., Hanahan, D., and Wisdom, R. (1996). Cellular transformation and malignancy induced by ras require c-jun. Mol.Cell.Biol. *16*, 4504-4511.
Joneson, T., White, M.A., Wigler, M.H., and Bar-Sagi, D. (1996). Stimulation of membrane ruffling and MAP kinase activation by distinct effectors of RAS. Science *271*, 810-812.
Kerkhoff, E. and Rapp, U.R. (1997). Induction of cell proliferation in quiescent NIH 3T3 cells by oncogenic c-Raf-1. Mol.Cell.Biol. *17*, 2576-2586.
Khosravi-Far, R., Solski, P.A., Kinch, M.S., Burridge, K., and Der, C.J. (1995). Activation of Rac and Rho, and mitogen activated protein kinases, are required for Ras transformation. Mol.Cell.Biol. *15*, 6443-6453.
Khosravi-Far, R., White, M.A., Westwick, J.K., Solski, P.A., Chrzanowska-Wodnicka, M., Van Aelst, L., Wigler, M.H., and Der, C.J. (1996). Oncogenic Ras activation of Raf/MAP kinase-independent pathways is sufficient to cause tumorigenic transformation. Mol.Cell.Biol. *16*, 3923-3933.
Khwaja, A., Rodriguez-Viciana, P., Wennström, S., Warne, P.H., and Downward, J. (1997). Matrix adhesion and Ras transformation both activate a phosphoinositide 3-OH kinase and protein kinase B/Akt cellular survival pathway. EMBO J. *16*, 2783-2793.
Kim, D., Kim, S., Koh, H., Yoon, S.O., Chung, A.S., Cho, K.S., and Chung, J. (2001). Akt/PKB promotes cancer cell invasion via increased motility and metalloproteinase production. FASEB J. *15*, 1953-1962.
Kirstein, M., Sanz, L., Quinones, S., Moscat, J., Diaz-Meco, M.T., and Saus, J. (1996). Cross-talk between different enhancer elements during mitogenic induction of the human stromelysin-1 gene. J.Biol.Chem. *271*, 18231-18236.
Konishi, T., Huang, C.L., Adachi, M., Taki, T., Inufusa, H., Kodama, K., Kohno, N., and Miyake, M. (2000). The K-ras gene regulates vascular endothelial growth factor gene expression in non-small cell lung cancers. Int.J.Oncol. *16*, 501-511.
Laderoute, K.R., Alarcon, R.M., Brody, M.D., Calaoagan, J.M., Chen, E.Y., Knapp, A.M., Yun, Z., Denko, N.C., and Giaccia, A.J. (2000). Opposing effects of hypoxia on expression of the angiogenic inhibitor thrombospondin 1 and the angiogenic inducer vascular endothelial growth factor. Clin.Cancer Res. *6*, 2941-2950.
Ladha, M.H., Lee, K.Y., Upton, T.M., Reed, M.F., and Ewen, M.E. (1998). Regulation of exit from quiescence by p27 and cyclin D1-CDK4. Mol.Cell Biol. *18*, 6605-6615.
Langer, S.J., Bortner, D.M., Roussel, M.F., Sherr, C.J., and Ostrowski, M.C. (1992). Mitogenic signaling by colony-stimulating factor 1 and *ras* is suppressed by the *ets-2* DNA-binding domain and restored by *myc* overexpression. Mol.Cell.Biol. *12*, 5355-5362.
Lavoie, J.N., L'Allemain, G., Brunet, A., Müller, R., and Pouysségur, J. (1996). Cyclin D1 expression is regulated positively by the p42/p44^{MAPK} and negatively by the p38/HOG ^{MAPK} pathway. J.Biol.Chem. *271*, 20608-20616.
Leevers, S.J., Paterson, H.F., and Marshall, C.J. (1994). Requirement for Ras in Raf activation is overcome by targeting Raf to the plasma membrane. Nature *369*, 411-414.
Liang, P., Averboukh, L., Zhu, W., and Pardee, A.B. (1994). Ras activation of genes: Mob-1 as a model. Proc.Natl.Acad.Sci.U.S.A *91*, 12515-12519.
Liu, J.J., Chao, J.R., Jiang, M.C., Ng, S.Y., Yen, J.J., and Yang-Yen, H.F. (1995). Ras transformation results in an elevated level of cyclin D1 and acceleration of G1 progression in NIH 3T3 cells. Mol.Cell Biol. *15*, 3654-3663.

LoSardo, J.E., Goggin, B.S., Bohoslawec, O., and Neri, A. (1995). Degradation of endothelial cell matrix collagen is correlated with induction of stromelysin by an activated ras oncogene. Clin.Exp.Metastasis *13*, 236-248.

Marshall, C. (1999). How do small GTPase signal transduction pathways regulate cell cycle entry? Curr.Opin.Cell.Biol. *11*, 732-736.

Marshall, C.J. (1996). Ras effectors. Curr.Op.Cell Biol. *8*, 197-204.

Marshall, C.J., Vousden, K., and Ozanne, B. (1985). The involvement of activated ras genes in determining the transformed phenotype. Proc.R.Soc.Lond B Biol.Sci. *226*, 99-106.

Matrisian, L.M. (1999). Cancer biology: extracellular proteinases in malignancy. Curr.Biol. *9*, R776-R778

Mayo, M.W., Wang, C.Y., Cogswell, P.C., Rogers-Graham, K.S., Lowe, S.W., Der, C.J., and Baldwin, A.S.J. (1997). Requirement of NF-kappaB activation to suppress p53-independent apoptosis induced by oncogenic Ras. Science. *278*, 1812-1815.

Mazure, N.M., Chen, E.Y., Laderoute, K.R., and Giaccia, A.J. (1997). Induction of vascular endothelial growth factor by hypoxia is modulated by a phosphatidylinositol 3-kinase/Akt signaling pathway in Ha-ras- transformed cells through a hypoxia inducible factor-1 transcriptional element. Blood *90*, 3322-3331.

McCarthy, S.A., Samuels, M.L., Pritchard, C.A., Abraham, J.A., and McMahon, M. (1995). Rapid induction of heparin-binding epidermal growth factor/diphtheria toxin receptor expression by Raf and Ras oncogenes. Genes Dev. *9*, 1953-1964.

McCawley, L.J. and Matrisian, L.M. (2001). Tumor progression: defining the soil round the tumor seed. Curr.Biol. *11*, R25-R27

McFall, A., Ulku, A., Lambert, Q.T., Kusa, A., Rogers-Graham, K., and Der, C.J. (2001). Oncogenic Ras blocks anoikis by activation of a novel effector pathway independent of phosphatidylinositol 3-kinase. Mol.Cell Biol. *21*, 5488-5499.

Meade-Tollin, L.C., Boukamp, P., Fusenig, N.E., Bowen, C.P., Tsang, T.C., and Bowden, G.T. (1998). Differential expression of matrix metalloproteinases in activated c-ras-Ha-transfected immortalized human keratinocytes. Br.J.Cancer *77*, 724-730.

Medema, R.H., Kops, G.J., Bos, J.L., and Burgering, B.M. (2000). AFX-like Forkhead transcription factors mediate cell-cycle regulation by Ras and PKB through p27kip1. Nature *404*, 782-787.

Milanini, J., Vinals, F., Pouyssegur, J., and Pages, G. (1998). p42/p44 MAP kinase module plays a key role in the transcriptional regulation of the vascular endothelial growth factor gene in fibroblasts. J.Biol.Chem. *273*, 18165-18172.

Moon, A., Kim, M.S., Kim, T.G., Kim, S.H., Kim, H.E., Chen, Y.Q., and Kim, H.R. (2000). H-ras, but not N-ras, induces an invasive phenotype in human breast epithelial cells: a role for MMP-2 in the H-ras-induced invasive phenotype. Int.J.Cancer *85*, 176-181.

Morrison, D.K. and Cutler, R.E., Jr. (1997). The complexity of Raf-1 regulation. Curr.Op.Cell Biol. *9*, 174-179.

Normanno, N., Bianco, C., De Luca, A., and Salomon, D.S. (2001). The role of EGF-related peptides in tumor growth. Front Biosci. *6*, D685-D707

Ohnami, S., Matsumoto, N., Nakano, M., Aoki, K., Nagasaki, K., Sugimura, T., Terada, M., and Yoshida, T. (1999). Identification of genes showing differential expression in antisense K- ras-transduced pancreatic cancer cells with suppressed tumorigenicity. Cancer.Res. *59*, 5565-5571.

Okada, F., Rak, J.W., Croix, B.S., Lieubeau, B., Kaya, M., Roncari, L., Shirasawa, S., Sasazuki, T., and Kerbel, R.S. (1998). Impact of oncogenes in tumor angiogenesis: mutant K-ras up- regulation of vascular endothelial growth factor/vascular permeability factor is necessary, but not sufficient for tumorigenicity of human colorectal carcinoma cells. Proc.Natl.Acad.Sci.U.S.A. *95*, 3609-3614.

Oldham, S.M., Clark, G.J., Gangarosa, L.M., Coffey, R.J., Jr., and Der, C.J. (1996). Activation of the Raf-1/MAP kinase cascade is not sufficient for Ras transformation of RIE-1 epithelial cells. Proc.Natl.Acad.Sci.USA *93*, 6924-6928.

Oliff, A. (1999). Farnesyltransferase inhibitors: targeting the molecular basis of cancer. Biochim.Biophys.Acta *1423*, C19-C30

Pruitt, K. and Der, C.J. (2001). Ras and Rho regulation of the cell cycle and transformation. Cancer Lett. *171*, 1-10.

Pruitt, K., Pestell, R.G., and Der, C.J. (2000). Ras inactivation of the retinoblastoma pathway by distinct mechanisms in NIH 3T3 fibroblast and RIE-1 epithelial cells. J.Biol.Chem. *275*, 40916-40924.

Rak, J., Mitsuhashi, Y., Bayko, L., Filmus, J., Shirasawa, S., Sasazuki, T., and Kerbel, R.S. (1995a). Mutant ras oncogenes upregulate VEGF/VPF expression: implications for induction and inhibition of tumor angiogenesis. Cancer Res. *55*, 4575-4580.

Rak, J., Mitsuhashi, Y., Sheehan, C., Tamir, A., Viloria-Petit, A., Filmus, J., Mansour, S.J., Ahn, N.G., and Kerbel, R.S. (2000b). Oncogenes and tumor angiogenesis: differential modes of vascular endothelial growth factor up-regulation in ras-transformed epithelial cells and fibroblasts. Cancer Res. *60*, 490-498.

Reuther, G.W. and Der, C.J. (2000). The Ras branch of small GTPases: Ras family members don't fall far from the tree. Curr.Opin.Cell Biol. *12*, 157-165.

Rodriguez-Viciana, P., Warne, P.H., Dhand, R., Vanhaesebroeck, B., Gout, I., Fry, M.J., Waterfield, M.D., and Downward, J. (1994). Phosphatidylinositol-3-OH kinase as a direct target of Ras. Nature *370*, 527-532.
Rodriguez-Viciana, P., Warne, P.H., Khwaja, A., Marte, B.M., Pappin, D., Das, P., Waterfield, M.D., Ridley, A., and Downward, J. (1997). Role of phosphoinositide 3-OH kinase in cell transformation and control of the actin cytoskeleton by Ras. Cell *89*, 457-467.
Saez, E., Rutberg, S.E., Mueller, E., Oppenheim, H., Smoluk, J., Yuspa, S.H., and Spiegelman, B.M. (1995). c-fos is required for malignant progression of skin tumors. Cell *82*, 721-732.
Schulze, A., Lehmann, K., Jefferies, H.B., McMahon, M., and Downward, J. (2001). Analysis of the transcriptional program induced by Raf in epithelial cells. Genes Dev. *15*, 981-994.
Shao, J., Sheng, H., DuBois, R.N., and Beauchamp, R.D. (2000). Oncogenic Ras-mediated cell growth arrest and apoptosis is associated with increased ubiquitin-dependent cyclin D1 degradation. J.Biol.Chem.
Shapiro, S.D. (1998). Matrix metalloproteinase degradation of extracellular matrix: biological consequences. Curr.Opin.Cell Biol. *10*, 602-608.
Sherr, C.J. (1996). Cancer cell cycles. Science *274*, 1672-1677.
Sherr, C.J. and Roberts, J.M. (1999). CDK inhibitors: positive and negative regulators of G1-phase progression. Genes Dev. *13*, 1501-1512.
Shields, J.M., Mehta, H., and Der, C.J. (2001a). DNA methylation, and opposing roles of the ERK and p38 mitogen-activated protein kinase cascades, in Ras-mediated downregulation of tropomyosin. Mol.Cell.Biol. *submitted,*
Shields, J.M., Pruitt, K., McFall, A., Shaub, Der, and C.J. (2000). Understanding Ras: "it ain't over 'til it's over". Trends Cell Biol. *10*, 147-153.
Shields, J.M., Rogers-Graham, K., and Der, C.J. (2001b). Loss of transgelin in breast and colon tumors and in RIE-1 cells by Ras deregulation of gene expression through Raf-independent pathways. J Biol Chem *277*, 9790-9799.
Sklar, M.D., Thompson, E., Welsh, M.J., Liebert, M., Harney, J., Grossman, H.B., Smith, M., and Prochownik, E.V. (1991). Depletion of c- *myc* with specific antisense sequences reverses the transformed phenotype in *ras* oncogene-transformed NIH 3T3 cells. Mol.Cell.Biol. *11*, 3699-3710.
Stokoe, D., Macdonald, S.G., Cadwallader, K., Symons, M., and Hancock, J.F. (1994). Activation of Raf as a result of recruitment to the plasma membrane. Science *264*, 1463-1467.
Takuwa, N. and Takuwa, Y. (2001). Regulation of cell cycle molecules by the Ras effector system. Mol.Cell Endocrinol. *177*, 25-33.
Thorgeirsson, U.P., Turpeenniemi-Hujanen, T., Williams, J.E., Westin, E.H., Heilman, C.A., Talmadge, J.E., and Liotta, L.A. (1985). NIH/3T3 cells transfected with human tumor DNA containing activated ras oncogenes express the metastatic phenotype in nude mice. Mol.Cell.Biol. *5*, 259-262.
Tokunaga, T., Tsuchida, T., Kijima, H., Okamoto, K., Oshika, Y., Sawa, N., Ohnishi, Y., Yamazaki, H., Miura, S., Ueyama, Y., and Nakamura, M. (2000). Ribozyme-mediated inactivation of mutant K-ras oncogene in a colon cancer cell line. Br.J.Cancer *83*, 833-839.
Treiger, B. and Isaacs, J. (1988). Expression of a transfected v-Harvey-ras oncogene in a Dunning rat prostate adenocarcinoma and the development of high metastatic ability. J.Urol. *140*, 1580-1586.
Vanhaesebroeck, B., Leevers, S.J., Panayotou, G., and Waterfield, M.D. (1997). Phosphoinositide 3-kinases: a conserved family of signal transducers. Trends.Biochem.Sci. *22*, 267-272.
Vousden, K.H., Eccles, S.A., Purvies, H., and Marshall, C.J. (1986). Enhanced spontaneous metastasis of mouse carcinoma cells transfected with an activated c-Ha-ras-1 gene. Int.J.Cancer *37*, 425-433.
Ward, Y., Wang, W., Woodhouse, E., Linnoila, I., Liotta, L., and Kelly, K. (2001). Signal pathways which promote invasion and metastasis: critical and distinct contributions of extracellular signal-regulated kinase and Ral-specific guanine exchange factor pathways. Mol.Cell Biol. *21* , 5958-5969.
Wasylyk, B., Hagman, J., and Gutierrez-Hartmann, A. (1998). Ets transcription factors: nuclear effectors of the Ras-MAP-kinase signaling pathway. Trends Biochem.Sci. *23*, 213-216.
Wasylyk, C., Maira, S.M., Sobieszczuk, P., and Wasylyk, B. (1994). Reversion of Ras transformed cells by Ets transdominant mutants. Oncogene *9*, 3665-3673.
Webb, C.P., Van Aelst, L., Wigler, M.H., and Woude, G.F. (1998). Signaling pathways in Ras-mediated tumorigenicity and metastasis. Proc.Natl.Acad.Sci.U.S.A. *95*, 8773-8778.
Westermarck, J. and Kahari, V.M. (1999). Regulation of matrix metalloproteinase expression in tumor invasion. FASEB J. *13*, 781-792.
White, F.C., Benehacene, A., Scheele, J.S., and Kamps, M. (1997). VEGF mRNA is stabilized by ras and tyrosine kinase oncogenes, as well as by UV radiation--evidence for divergent stabilization pathways. Growth Factors *14*, 199-212.
White, M.A., Nicolette, C., Minden, A., Polverino, A., Van Aelst, L., Karin, M., and Wigler, M.H. (1995). Multiple Ras functions can contribute to mammalian cell transformation. Cell *80*, 533-541.

Wick, M., Lucibello, F.C., and Müller, R. (1992). Inhibition of Fos- and Ras-induced transformation by mutant Fos proteins with structural alterations in functionally different domains. Oncogene *7*, 859-867.

Winston, J.T., Coats, S.R., Wang, Y.-Z., and Pledger, W.J. (1996). Regulation of the cell cycle machinery by oncogenic *ras*. Oncogene *12*, 127-134.

Wolfman, A. (2001). Ras isoform-specific signaling: location, location, location. Sci.STKE. *2001*, E2

Wolthuis, R.M., de Ruiter, N.D., Cool, R.H., and Bos, J.L. (1997). Stimulation of gene induction and cell growth by the Ras effector Rlf. EMBO J. *16*, 6748-6761.

Woodhouse, E.C., Chuaqui, R.F., and Liotta, L.A. (1997). General mechanisms of metastasis. Cancer *80*, 1529-1537.

Yamamoto, H., Itoh, F., Senota, A., Adachi, Y., Yoshimoto, M., Endoh, T., Hinoda, Y., Yachi, A., and Imai, K. (1995). Expression of matrix metalloproteinase matrilysin (MMP-7) was induced by activated Ki-ras via AP-1 activation in SW1417 colon cancer cells. J.Clin.Lab Anal. *9*, 297-301.

Yanagihara, K., Nii, M., Tsumuraya, M., Numoto, M., Seito, T., and Seyama, T. (1995). A radiation-induced murine ovarian granulosa cell tumor line: introduction of v-ras gene potentiates a high metastatic ability. Jpn.J.Cancer Res. *86*, 347-356.

Yang, J.Q., Zhao, W., Duan, H., Robbins, M.E., Buettner, G.R., Oberley, L.W., and Domann, F.E. (2001). v-Ha-RaS oncogene upregulates the 92-kDa type IV collagenase (MMP-9) gene by increasing cellular superoxide production and activating NF-kappaB. Free Radic.Biol.Med. *31*, 520-529.

Zhang, R., Averboukh, L., Zhu, W., Zhang, H., Jo, H., Dempsey, P.J., Coffey, R.J., Pardee, A.B., and Liang, P. (1998). Identification of rCop-1, a new member of the CCN protein family, as a negative regulator for cell transformation. Mol.Cell Biol. *18*, 6131-6141.

Zuber, J., Tchernitsa, O.I., Hinzmann, B., Schmitz, A.C., Grips, M., Hellriegel, M., Sers, C., Rosenthal, A., and Schafer, R. (2000). A genome-wide survey of RAS transformation targets. Nat.Genet. *24*, 144-152.

ROLE OF THE RB TUMOR SUPPRESSOR IN CANCER

LILI YAMASAKI

1. INTRODUCTION

The retinoblastoma tumor suppressor, referred to as pRB, is the prototypic member of a small group of proteins known to inhibit neoplasia in humans, and the inactivation of which facilitates tumorigenesis. In fact, the *RB* gene encoding pRB is mutated in approximately half of all human tumors. Furthermore, genes encoding upstream regulators of pRB are mutated or overexpressed in the remaining half of all human tumors. These observations strongly suggest that there is a pRB tumor suppressor pathway that must be inactivated for neoplastic progression. In fact, this pathway is a delicately balanced network of oncogenes and tumor suppressors that oppose each other's function in normal cells. Deregulation of these components due to loss-of-function mutations in tumor suppressors or gain-of-function mutations in oncogenes facilitate cellular transformation and tumorigenesis. This chapter will review the basic components of the pathways, recent insights on how pRB actually controls cell growth through transcription and the new mutant mouse models which have been engineered to analyze the function of the pRB tumor suppressor pathway *in vivo.*

2. DISCOVERY OF THE pRB TUMOR SUPPRESSOR

2.1 *Retinoblastomas and the "Two-Hit Hypothesis"*

Retinoblastomas are rare pediatric tumors affecting 1/20,000 live births, affecting children up until six or seven years of age. These tumors are usually detected by four years of age, and are fatal unless treated by removal of the eye, followed by radiation and chemotherapy. They arise from the embryonic retinal layer, which later gives rise to the photoreceptor rod and cone cells, and display a differentiated morphology referred to as Flexner-Wintersteiner rosettes (Cotran R.S. et al. 1994). Retinoblastomas are known to occur in two separate populations of patients, sporadic cases with no family history of this disease and inherited cases exhibiting definite familial predisposition (40% of all cases). The frequencies of tumor incidence between these two populations differed dramatically, familial carriers having a greatly increased risk of developing retinoblastoma. Furthermore, retinoblastomas in the sporadic cases are unilateral and unifocal, while in the inherited cases, retinoblastomas were bilateral and multifocal. In inherited cases, susceptibility to retinoblastoma is transmitted as an autosomal dominant trait.

The identification of chromosomal abnormalities involving loss of Chr 13q14 in a subset of sporadic (25%) as well as inherited (5%) cases of retinoblastomas, strongly suggested that the inactivation of a putative tumor suppressor gene at Chr 13q14 was the answer. Alfred Knudson in 1971 predicted that the different frequencies of tumor development could be explained by the existence of a putative *RB* tumor suppressor gene, which required two mutations or "two hits" to inactivate in the sporadic cases and only one mutation or "one hit" in the inherited cases (Knudson 1971). He correctly surmised that the familial cases already inherited a germline mutation which inactivated one allele of this proposed *RB* tumor suppressor gene, so only one additional mutation would be necessary to inactivate the remaining functional allele. This notion was supported by studies in which tumor DNA from a subset of inherited retinoblastomas showed abnormalities involving loss of both Chr13q14 chromosomal subregions, while normal cells from these same patients displayed loss of only one Chr13q14 subregion (Francke and Kung 1976; Knudson et al. 1976). Thus, although tumor susceptibility was inherited dominantly, tumor development was recessive, since both copies of *RB* required inactivation for retinoblastoma to occur.

2.2 *Identification of the RB Tumor Suppressor Gene*

The isolation of the retinoblastoma tumor suppressor gene, termed *RB*, involved classical human genetics, positional cloning, DNA tumor virology and cellular and molecular biology. The identification of DNA markers mapping within this Chr13q14 subregion allowed investigators to search for candidate genes mutated in retinoblastomas. Using these markers, loss-of-heterozygosity (LOH) could be seen in tumors from inherited cases, consistent with the concept that inactivation of a tumor suppressor was responsible for the increased incidence in familial cases of retinoblastomas. A physical map of genomic clones representing Chr 13q14 was established, and the smallest deletion lying within this genomic region in retinoblastomas helped the search for candidate genes encoded by this locus. Using a genomic probe derived from this physical map of Chr13q14 (Dryja et al. 1986; Dryja et al. 1984), the *RB* gene with its 27 exons spanning ~200 kB, was identified (Dunn et al. 1988; Friend et al. 1986; Fung et al. 1987; Lee et al. 1987). Numerous retinoblastomas failed to express the *RB* mRNA due to large deletions of coding exons, while other retinoblastomas without any obvious chromosomal abnormality at Chr13q14 were shown to carry fine mutations that mapped within the coding exons of *RB*, presumably inactivating the function of this novel protein, referred to as pRB. Most *RB* mutations identified-to-date are high penetrance mutations, since individuals carrying these mutations in their germline develop retinoblastomas with high frequency. There are however, *RB* mutations known as "low penetrance" alleles, in which the mutations map either in the coding region or in the *RB* promoter, and families carrying these low penetrance mutations in their germline develop retinoblastomas much less frequently.

2.3 *Clinical Human Tumor Spectrum of RB Mutations*

Children which have developed inherited retinoblastoma are at increased risk for developing osteosarcomas later in adolescence. Mutation of the remaining normal *RB* allele or loss-of-heterozygosity at the *RB* locus has occurred in these tumors, demonstrating that pRB normally functions to suppress neoplasia in bone as well as retina. Using DNA probes encoding the *RB* gene, researchers surveyed numerous classes of human adult tumors to determine if mutations in *RB* were involved in other forms of sporadic neoplasia. Subsequently carcinomas of the bladder (33%), breast (10%) and prostate were shown to carry *RB* mutations with high frequency. In addition, nearly all small cell lung carcinomas (SCLC) carry *RB* mutations. Taken together, the large number of tumor types in which the *RB* locus was mutated strongly suggested the retinoblastoma tumor suppressor, pRB, played a central role in inhibiting neoplasia in a variety tissues far beyond the developing retina (Bookstein et al. 1990; Friend et al. 1986; Hansen et al. 1985; Harbour et al. 1988; Horowitz et al. 1990; Lee et al. 1988; T'Ang et al. 1988; Takahashi et al. 1991).

2.4 *pRB Growth Suppression and Phosphorylation*

Once the sequence of the *RB* gene had been determined, little if anything could be predicted about the function of pRB, and even less was known about how this 105 kilodalton protein (Figure 1) suppressed neoplasia. Our understanding of the pRB tumor suppressor pathway was facilitated greatly by ongoing studies about cyclin/Cdk-complexes and control of cell cycle progression via phosphorylation. Passage from the G1-phase of the cell cycle into S-phase, or the G1/S-transition marks an important time in the cell cycle, beyond which much energy must be expended and numerous cellular products must be synthesized to begin DNA replication. Just prior to the G1/S-transition, there is a "restriction point" (Pardee 1974), which marks the "commitment" of cells to replicate their genome, one of the critical decision points during the cell cycle. Prior to the restriction point, cells in G1-phase are sensitive to the presence or absence of growth factors or inhibitory factors, which indicate whether or not the environment is conducive to cell division. After the restriction point, cells become insensitive to the presence or absence of growth factors, and is instead committed to enter S-phase.

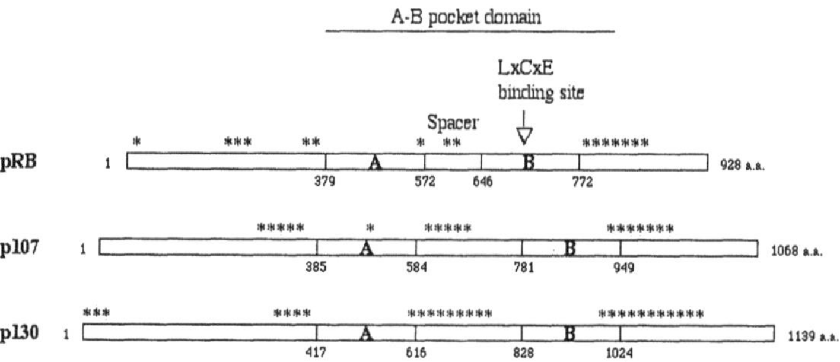

Figure 1. pRB Family Members. Linear structures of the pRB family members are shown with 'A' and 'B' conserved pocket regions indicated. Also potential S/T-P phosphorylation sites are indicated by asterisks. For actual phosphorylated residue numbers, see Ashizawa et al., 2001.

Initial studies on pRB showed that it is a nuclear phosphoprotein, the phosphorylation of which fluctuates through the cell cycle (Buchkovich et al. 1989; Chen et al. 1989; DeCaprio et al. 1989; Mihara et al. 1989). Cells in G0 or G1 have low but detectable levels of pRB phosphorylation on serine and threonine residues, while cells in S phase have high levels of pRB phosphorylation on these amino acids. The accumulation of phosphorylated residues on pRB continues throughout the cell cycle, and is reversed in mitosis by the action of a type 1 protein phosphatase PP1α2 (Durfee et al. 1993; Rubin et al. 2001). Passage through the restriction point involves the sequential action of cyclin D - Cdk4/6 complexes in mid-G1 and cyclin E-Cdk2 complexes, which phosphorylate pRB, thereby altering its conformation and growth suppressive capabilities (Dowdy et al. 1993; Ewen et al. 1993; Harbour et al. 1999; Hatakeyama et al. 1994; Hinds et al. 1992; Kato et al. 1993; Zarkowska and Mittnacht 1997). Overexpression of pRB is able to suppress the growth of tumor cell lines (Bookstein et al. 1990; Huang et al. 1988; Sumegi et al. 1990) by blocking cell cycle progression in G1, and most tumor-derived mutants of pRB are incapable of suppressing growth, which is now thought to involve the induction of a more differentiated state. In early G1, hypophosphorylated pRB is able to suppress growth, and after the G1/S-transition, hyperphosphorylated pRB is much less capable of suppressing growth. There are 16 potential Cdk-phosphorylation sites on pRB, and multiple phosphorylation site mutants of pRB bearing 8 or more alanine substitutions in potential Cdk-sites are more capable of inducing G1-phase arrest (Ashizawa et al. 2001; Hamel et al. 1992). To a large part, the ability of pRB to suppress growth resides in its capacity to bind transcription factors repressing the activity of some (e.g., E2F/DP) and stimulating the activity of others (e.g., C/EBP). The release of a subset of these cellular proteins from pRB occurs upon its phosphorylation at the G1/S transition.

2.5 Interaction with DNA Tumor Viral Oncoproteins

A major breakthrough came in 1988, when researchers discovered that pRB is targeted and inactivated by DNA tumor viral oncoproteins. Upon viral infection, DNA tumor viruses recruit the cellular machinery for DNA replication to replicate its own viral DNA as episomes by forcing infected cells to enter S-phase. This is accomplished by the action of viral early region oncoproteins that commandeers the host cell cycle and replication machinery. Abortive viral infections can lead to cellular transformation when viral DNA integrates into host DNA and the action of early region oncoprotein products is uncoupled from viral replication.

The adenoviral early region E1A protein binds specifically to pRB, and non-transforming mutants of E1A or tumor-derived mutants of pRB failed to show this interaction (Whyte et al. 1988). The large T antigen of SV40 and the E7 protein of human papilloma virus (HPV) also bind pRB specifically, using oncoprotein domains required for cellular transformation (DeCaprio et al. 1988; Dyson et al. 1989; Munger et al. 1989). SV40-T specifically binds only the hypophosphorylated form of pRB (Ludlow et al. 1989). The regions of these divergent viral oncoproteins required for pRB binding contain a sequence motif, LxCxE (where L = leucine, C=cysteine, E = glutamic acid and x=any amino acid), and mutation of these key viral residues interferes with binding to pRB. The interaction of these 3 oncoproteins from distinct virus families with pRB strongly suggested that pRB normally restrained cell transformation and oncoprotein binding inactivates the tumor suppressor function of pRB, leading to deregulation of the host cell cycle.

In addition to inactivating the pRB tumor suppressor, these 3 viruses have oncoproteins which act on other cellular proteins to transform cells (i.e., p53 and p300). Specifically, the adenoviral E1B (55K) protein, SV40-T and the E6 oncoprotein of HPV inactivate the p53 tumor suppressor by different mechanisms, promoting cellular transformation. Importantly, it is the coordinated inactivation of both the pRB and p53 tumor suppressor pathways, which facilitates cellular transformation, since the inactivation of pRB without the inactivation of p53 would signal ectopic proliferation leading to apoptotic cell death. This point will be re-visited towards the end of this review.

2.6 *pRB Homologues and the Pocket Domain*

Understanding growth regulation via the pRB tumor suppressor pathway is complicated by the existence of numerous homologues at each level of the pathway. Besides pRB, there are 2 pRB family members that were isolated by low stringency hybridization, p107 and p130 (Ewen et al. 1991; Li et al. 1993; Mayol et al. 1993; Zhu et al. 1993). Sequence comparisons between these 3 pRB family members have shown that all 3 proteins share conserved domains referred to as the A-B "pocket" and C-terminal domains (Figure 1) (Livingston et al. 1993). However, p107 and p130 share even a greater degree of homology with each other, within conserved regions in the N-terminus and spacer region bridging the A and B pocket domains, indicating that the genes encoding p107 and p130 have more recently diverged from each other than either gene from RB. This higher degree of homology correlates with mutant mouse data showing that p130 and p107 share overlapping function in vivo (see Section 5). Inactivation of pRB function in high penetrance tumor-derived *RB* mutations occurs by the deletion of exons or substitution of residues within the A and B conserved domains of the pocket region.

This A-B pocket is a large conformational structure rich in alpha-helices into which numerous proteins are known to bind, including DNA tumor viral oncoproteins. The crystal structure of a fragment of pRB (including the A-spacer-B pocket and C-terminus) bound to an LxCxE containing peptide from the HPV-E7 oncoprotein has been solved (Lee et al. 1998). This study has shown that the actual contact sites of pRB with the LxCxE motif of HPV-E7 lie in the B domain and are surrounded by a patch of lysine residues. The importance of the A domain is to dictate the conformation of the B-domain, and therefore tumor-derived mutations lying in A or B destroy pRB structure and function. Mutation of the lysines in this LxCxE binding region of pRB decreases the intramolecular binding of the phosphorylated C-terminus of pRB (Harbour et al. 1999) and blocks the association of pRB with viral oncoproteins without changing the interaction of pRB with other cellular proteins (Brown and Gallie 2002; Dick et al. 2000). Similarly, the crystal structure of the A-B domains of pRB bound to the N-terminus of SV40-T has been solved (Kim et al. 2001) and shows that all contacts with SV40-T lie within the B-domain of the pocket.

In contrast to the frequent mutation of the *RB* gene in human tumors, the gene encoding p107 has been reported mutated in a single B-cell lymphoma (Ichimura et al. 2000). Two separate studies have reported that the gene encoding p130 has been found mutated in isolated lung tumors (Claudio et al. 2000; Helin et al. 1997). Overexpression of p107 and p130 suppresses the growth of Saos-2 cells as discussed previously for pRB; however, there are clear differences between how these pRB family members suppress growth. In contrast to pRB, p107 and p130 use their N-terminal domains and their spacer regions, which each contains a cyclin-binding motif also found in cyclin-dependent kinase inhibitors of the CIP/KIP family, to suppress growth through the sequestration of cyclins (Zhu et al. 1995). p130 complexes are most abundant in G0 arrested cells and are thought to be important in maintaining the quiescent state. p107 complexes are most abundant in S-phase; yet the S-phase accumulation of p107 complexes that are thought to function as growth suppressors, is still not understood.

3. UPSTREAM REGULATORS OF pRB

Although the function of the retinoblastoma tumor suppressor will be discussed below, it will be helpful here to discuss the tumor spectrum seen with mutations in genes encoding upstream regulators of pRB. Inactivation of pRB is accomplished every cell cycle by the concerted action of a group of cyclin-dependent kinases or Cdks, which temporally regulate the ability of pRB to restrain the cell cycle. The activation and specificity of these Cdks are controlled positively by the association of a cyclin subunit, and controlled negatively by the association of an inhibitor or a cyclin-dependent kinase inhibitor, referred to as a CKI. The concerted action of these Cdks in the G1-phase of the cell cycle results in the hyperphosphorylation of pRB, which changes its ability to restrain cell cycle progression by altering its capacity to interact directly with cellular targets of pRB (Figure 2).

Specifically in early G1, cyclin D1-3 associate and activate Cdk4 or Cdk6 kinases, while in mid G1, cyclin E1 or E2 associate and activate Cdk2. All of these Cdk complexes display kinase activity directed towards pRB. Controlling these G1 Cdk-complexes in G1 are two families of CKIs, the CIP/KIP family and the INK4 family of inhibitors. Regulation of these proteins and their dysregulation in human tumors is discussed below.

3.1 G1 Cyclins and Cdk Complexes

Cyclin D1, D2 and D3 share 60% amino acid sequence identity, and all three D-type cyclins can activate Cdk4 or Cdk6 kinases, which specifically phosphorylates the C-terminus of pRB. Overexpression of cyclin D1 result in the hyperphosphorylation of pRB, and shortens the G1-phase of the cell cycle presumably by inactivating pRB's control of G1. In fact, the gene encoding cyclin D1, known as *CCND1/BCL1/PRAD1* is an oncogene and gain-of-function mutations (translocations or amplifications) of the cyclin D1 locus resulting in overexpression have been found in lymphomas, parathyroid adenomas and breast carcinomas (reviewed in (Peters 1994)). Cyclin D2 overexpression occurs in some ovarian and testicular germ cell tumors (Sicinski et al. 1996). Amplification of the gene encoding Cdk4 has been found in glioblastomas, anaplastic astrocytomas and in sarcomas (Khatib et al. 1993; Schmidt et al. 1994). In a subset of these tumors, the neighboring *GLI* and *HDM2* genes are also amplified. Overexpression of Cdk6 has been detected in T-lymphoblastic lymphomas and splenic marginal zone B-cell lymphomas (Chilosi et al. 1998; Corcoran et al. 1999). Additionally gene mutations which make the Cdk4 subunit insensitive to the p16INK4A have been isolated in familial and sporadic melanomas (Wolfel et al. 1995; Zuo et al. 1996).

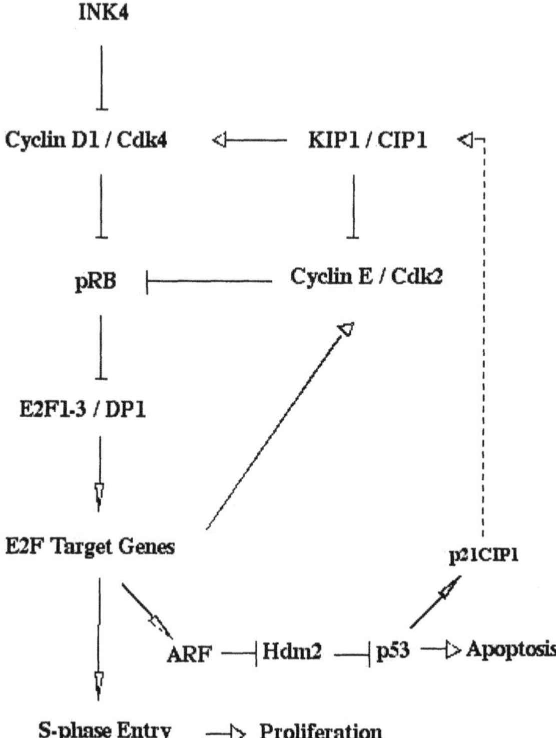

Figure 2. pRB Tumor Suppressor Pathway

Thus, overactivation of the cyclin D1/Cdk4-6 kinases clearly facilitates tumor progression, presumably because increased cyclin D1/Cdk4-6 kinase activity inactivates the tumor suppressor activity of pRB.

Cyclin E1 and E2 share 47% sequence identity and both activate the Cdk2 kinase, which specifically phosphorylates pRB. Overexpression of cyclin E1 hyperphosphorylates pRB, and shortens the G1-phase of the cell cycle presumably by inactivating pRB's control of G1, similarly to cyclin D1. Overexpression of cyclin E1 has been found in a wide range of human carcinomas, including breast carcinomas (Keyomarsi et al. 1994; Nielsen et al. 1996), a portion of which also overexpress cyclin E2 (Geng et al. 2001). Additionally, cyclin E2 is overexpressed in non-SCLC and SCLC (Gudas et al. 1999), many of which also overexpress cyclin E1. Cyclin E1 is normally degraded by ubiquitin-mediated proteolysis (Moberg et al. 2001; Schwab and Tyers 2001; Strohmaier et al. 2001), and stabilization of E1 results in the activation of cyclin E1/Cdk2 complexes and pRB hyperphosphorylation.

3.2 The CIP/KIP and the INK4 Families of CKIs

Upstream of cyclin D/Cdk4 or Cdk6 complexes lie the CKI proteins that help interpret the growth signals in the environment, which engage or disengage the pRB tumor suppressor pathway. There are two classes of cyclin-dependent kinase inhibitors (CKIs) that function in G1 to regulate the phosphorylation state of pRB. Those are the CIP/KIP family of CKIs (i.e., p27KIP1, p21CIP1 and p57KIP2), and the INK4 family of CKIs (p16INK4A, p15INK4B, p18INK4C and p19INK4D). The CIP/KIP family members act as inhibitors of cyclin/Cdk2 or Cdc2 complexes, yet also as assembly factors for the cyclin D/Cdk4 or Cdk6 complexes (Cheng et al. 1999; LaBaer et al. 1997). In contrast, the INK4 family members are small ankyrin-repeat containing proteins that inhibit Cdk4 or Cdk6 kinases exclusively, and do not require cyclin D association with the kinase subunit for inhibition.

The signals controlling the CIP/KIP and the INK4 families of CKIs are quite different. The p21CIP1 inhibitor is a transcriptional target of p53, and thus, levels of p21CIP1 increase following DNA damage, which block cyclin/Cdk2 complexes, causing a G1- and/or a G2-arrest (el-Deiry et al. 1993; Gu et al. 1993; Noda et al. 1994; Xiong et al. 1993). Inactivating mutations in the *CIP1* gene have not been detected in human tumors. The p27KIP1 inhibitor responds to cellular environmental signals such as the presence or absence of growth factors, cell anchorage and contact inhibition (Polyak et al. 1994). Loss of even one allele of the *KIP1* gene have rarely been detected in human tumors. However, levels of p27KIP1 are controlled during the cell cycle post-translationally by its Cdk-mediated phosphorylation and ubiquitin-mediated degradation via the Skp2-ubiquitin ligase subunit (Carrano et al. 1999; Pagano et al. 1995), which subsequently allows the activation of cyclin E/Cdk2 complexes and thus, hyperphosphorylation of pRB. Increased ubiquitin-mediated degradation of p27KIP1 occurs in many human tumors, and p27 levels act as an independent poor prognostic marker of survival (Loda et al.

1997). Genomic imprinting at chromosome 11p15.5 controls the expression of the *KIP2* locus, as well as other genes (*H19, IGF2* and *KCNQ10T1*), and aberrations at this complex genetic locus are associated with Beckwith-Wiedemann syndrome, which includes overgrowth, congenital malformations, and predisposition to childhood tumors (Hatada et al. 1996; Matsuoka et al. 1996).

In contrast, the signals controlling the INK4 family of inhibitors are quite distinct. Levels of p16INK4A increase with cell passage number and the onset of cellular senescence or premature senescence induced by the expression of activated *Ras* (Palmero et al. 1997; Serrano et al. 1997). Transcription of the *INK4A* gene is increased by the action of Ets transcription factors, and decreased by Id1(Ohtani et al. 2001). The p15INK4B inhibitor accumulates following TGFβ-treatment (Hannon and Beach 1994; Reynisdottir et al. 1995), and is mediated transcriptionally via a Myc / Miz transcription factor complex (Seoane et al. 2001; Staller et al. 2001). Levels of p18INK4C and p19INK4D display tissue-specific patterns of expression during development, when p16INK4A and p15INK4B are not detectable (Zindy et al. 1997).

3.3 Clinical Tumor Spectrum of Chr 9p21 Mutations

Genes encoding *INK4A* (also known as *MTS1*) and *INK4B* (MTS2), are closely linked at chromosomal position 9p21, one of the most commonly mutated loci found in human tumors, particularly familial melanomas and pancreatic carcinomas (reviewed in (Ruas and Peters 1998)). Large deletions at this complex genetic locus frequently delete both the *INK4A* and *INK4B* genes, and finer deletions and point mutations have been mapped within the *INK4A* coding sequence itself, establishing that p16INK4A is indeed a human tumor suppressor (Kamb et al. 1994). Inactivating mutations in p16INK4A result in overactive cyclin D/Cdk4 or Cdk6 kinase complexes, which in turn hyperphosphorylate and inactivate pRB. Interestingly, human tumors appear to sustain either mutations in the *RB* gene or mutations in the *INK4A* gene (Peters 1994; Sherr 1996). For instance, nearly all human SCLCs carry *RB* mutations, while almost all human non-SCLCs contain *INK4A* mutations (Harbour et al. 1988). The mutual exclusivity of this mutational pattern strongly suggests that the *INK4A* and *RB* genes form a genetic pathway for tumor suppression.

However, the 9p21 locus encodes another gene, *ARF*, in which the second and third exons overlap with those of the *INK4A* gene, encoding a novel p14ARF protein (p19ARF in mice) in an alternative reading frame (reviewed in (Sherr 2000)). The *INK4A* gene has a unique exon 1α, while the *ARF* gene has a unique exon 1β, and each gene has its own promoter driving its expression. The p14ARF protein is a intimate regulator of the p53 tumor suppressor pathway. p14ARF is a nucleolar protein, which inactivates the Hdm2 oncogene (known as Mdm2 in mice). Since Hdm2 is a ring-finger-containing ubiquitin ligase specific for p53, p14ARF concommitantly stabilizes p53 when it inactivates Hdm2. This intricate network of p14ARF is disrupted when large deletions or finer mutations occur at 9p21, inactivating both the *INK4A* and *ARF* genes. Furthermore, *ARF* is a target gene of E2F1 (Bates et al. 1998; DeGregori et al. 1997) and links pRB-mediated repression with p53-mediated apoptosis. Thus, the complex *INK4A/ARF* locus at 9p21 simultaneously regulates the pRB and p53 tumor suppressor pathways at numerous levels. Both *INK4A* and *ARF* encode tumor suppressor genes, an important point which has been extensively tested using mutant mouse models (reviewed in (Sherr 2001); and see section 5).

4. DOWNSTREAM EFFECTORS OF RB

4.1 pRB Interactors

Currently there are 110 published interactors of pRB, many for which the binding has been shown to occur in vitro and in vivo (reviewed in (Morris and Dyson 2001)). The collection of pRB interactors includes kinases, transcription factors, structural proteins and other proteins. This impressive array of interactions along with the identity of the interactors of pRB suggest that pRB integrates a wide variety of signalling pathways within cells. In the absence of a demonstrated interaction *in vivo* for many of these potential pRB interactors, it is also possible that pRB binds non-specifically or with low affinity to many proteins. To a large part, the ability of pRB to suppress growth resides in its capacity to bind transcription factors repressing the activity of some {e.g., E2F/DP (reviewed in (Dyson 1998)), Elf-1 (Wang et al. 1993) , c-ski (Tokitou et al. 1999) and Id2 (Lasorella et al. 2000)} and stimulating the activity of others {e.g., MyoD (Gu et al. 1993), C/EBP (Chen et al. 1996) (Chen PL, 1996b), and NF-IL6 (Chen et al. 1996)}. This review focuses on what is known about the best characterized set of pRB interactors, the cell cycle regulated family of E2F/DP transcription factors. Repression of the E2F/DP family can account for much of the ability of pRB to suppress growth and thereby neoplasia. Importantly, it is very likely that pRB simultaneously promotes cellular differentiation as it suppresses growth, and a number of the pRB interactions that stimulate transcription also promote differentiation. Low penetrance mutant alleles of *RB* encode proteins fail to bind E2F, but still promote differentiation, underscoring the importance of integrating growth and differentiation signalling (Sellers et al. 1998).

4.2 The E2F/DP Transcription Factor Family

4.2.1 E2F Activity

The best characterized set of pRB-interactors is the cell cycle regulated E2F/DP transcription factor family. E2F activity was defined as the E1A-inducible cellular protein(s) needed to activate the adenoviral E2 promoter (Kovesdi et al. 1986; Yee et al. 1987). Downregulation of a similar activity (DRTF) was described upon differentiation of embryonal carcinoma cells(La Thangue and Rigby 1987). The consensus E2F DNA binding site, 5'-TTT(C/G)(G/C)CGC-3', is often found in overlapping and/or tandem repeats in TATA-less promoters within close proximity to Sp1 binding sites. The presence of pRB or the loss of the E2F site can lead either to an increase or decrease in target gene expression, suggesting that E2F sites act as positive and negative regulatory elements in promoters(Weintraub et al. 1992). It is clear that pRB bound to an E2F/DP complex acts as a repressor, while the free E2F/DP heterodimer activates transcription. Cyclin/Cdk-mediated phosphorylation of pRB or viral oncoprotein association with pRB releases E2F activity, which then activates target gene expression.

4.2.2 E2F and DP Family Members

The E2F/DP transcription factor family is composed of six known E2F family members and 2 DP subunits (reviewed in (Dyson 1998; Trimarchi and Lees 2002)). High affinity DNA binding requires heterodimerization of an E2F family member with a DP family member. The E2F and DP domains required for DNA binding and heterodimerization lie in the middle of each protein and show minimal homology (see figure), suggesting that these proteins are distantly related to one another (Girling et al. 1993). The crystal structure of E2F4/DP2 DNA binding domains reveal that both proteins contain a winged-helix DNA-binding motif responsible for E2F site recognition (Zheng et al. 1999).

An 18 amino acid epitope which is required and sufficient for interaction with pRB family members maps to the extreme C-terminal residues and overlaps the transactivation domain in five out of six E2F family members (see figure). Thus, binding of pRB family members minimally can block E2F-mediated transactivation through the basal transcription factor machinery due to steric hindrance. Three distinct subclasses of E2Fs exist. The first includes E2F1-3, which bind with high specificity to pRB, and each of these contain unique N-terminal domains and nuclear localization signals (NLS). The second subclass includes E2F4 and 5, which bind preferentially to p107 and p130, lack an N-terminal extension and an NLS. E2F4, the most abundant form of E2F in most cell types and tissues, can also be found in complexes with pRB. Although E2F6 (the third subclass) does not bind any pRB family member, it forms only a repressive E2F complex in conjunction with the polycomb complex. In contrast to the specificity of the E2F family members, DP1 and DP2 bind all 6 E2F members without restriction, and thus can be found in complexes with all 3 pRB family members. DP1 is expressed abundantly in most tissues, while DP2 is found in alternatively spliced forms only in a subset of tissues.

4.2.3 E2F Target Genes

E2F binding sites lie in the promoters of numerous genes including those required for initiating and executing DNA replication (e.g., *ORC1*, *MCM*, *DHFR*, *RNR*,

TK, *TS* and *POL*α), cell cycle progression (e.g., genes encoding cyclin A, cyclin E, Cdc2, E2F1-3, *RB*, p107), and apoptosis (e.g., *MYC*, *ARF*, *APAF*). Mutation of the E2F site in different cell cycle-regulated promoters changes the timing, amplitude and direction of transcriptional expression ((Lam and Watson 1993; Slansky et al. 1993) for examples). Since levels of E2F1-3 are limiting during G1 and E2F sites lie in the promoters for E2F1-3, release of E2F/DP from pRB at the G1/S-transition triggers an amplification of E2F1-3 transcription (Hsiao et al. 1994; Johnson et al. 1994; Sears et al. 1997). Actually, E2F3 exists in two forms (E2F3a and E2F3b) driven by two separate promoters, only one of which is growth-regulated, leading to the accumulation of E2F3a at the G1/S-transition (Adams et al. 2000; Leone et al. 1998). The sharp accumulation of E2F1-3 at the G1/S-transition stimulates the transcription of gene products involved in firing origins of replication and replicating DNA, leading to S-phase entry. From numerous recent screens to identify E2F target genes, it appears that besides controlling replication, cell cycle progression, and apoptosis, E2Fs also control the expression of genes involved in DNA repair and chromosome dynamics, G2/M checkpoints and mitotic regulation, development and differentiation (Ishida et al. 2001; Kalma et al. 2001 Mar 15; Ma et al. 2002; Muller et al. 2001; Weinmann et al. 2002; Wells et al. 2002).

4.2.4 Induction of Proliferation and Apoptosis

Overexpression of E2F1-3 stimulates S-phase entry, and subsequent cellular proliferation (Johnson et al. 1993; Muller et al. 1997; Verona et al. 1997). In fact, overexpression of E2F1 or DP1 in conjunction with activated *Ras* leads to cellular transformation, and tumor formation when injected into nude mice. Thus, E2F1 and DP1 are oncogenes and their deregulation can contribute to neoplastic progression. However, under conditions of low serum, overexpression of E2F1-3 leads to apoptosis, particularly in the case of E2F1 likely due to its greater potential for transactivation. This E2F1-induced cell death can be either p53-mediated (Wu and Levine 1994) (Kowalik et al. 1995; Qin et al. 1995; Shan and Lee 1994) or p53-independent (Hsieh et al. 1997; Nip et al. 1997; Phillips et al. 1997). Induction of p53-mediated apoptosis involves the accumulation of p53 via induction of p14ARF (p19ARF in mice) by E2F1(Bates et al. 1998; DeGregori et al. 1997). The ability of E2F1 to induce both proliferation and apoptosis may be linked to the paucity of E2F1 mutations in human tumors.

Since the levels of E2F1, in particular, control a molecular switch between cellular proliferation and death, controlling the level of E2F1 is important and several mechanisms exist to decrease free E2F1 activity. First, phosphorylation of the E2F1/DP1 heterodimer by cyclin A/Cdk2 induces a loss of DNA-binding activity (Dynlacht et al. 1994; Krek et al. 1994; Xu et al. 1994) and is involved in an S-phase checkpoint (Krek et al. 1995). Second, E2F1 is regulated by ubiquitin-mediated degradation, and binding to pRB protects the E2F1/DP1 heterodimer from degradation (Hateboer et al. 1996; Hofmann et al. 1996). Degradation is reported to result from an E2F1 N-terminal interaction with the Skp2 ubiquitin ligase subunit

(Marti et al. 1999). Interestingly, phosphorylation of serine 31 in the N-terminus of E2F1 by the ATM kinase following DNA damage stabilizes E2F1 against ubiquitin-mediated degradation (Lin et al. 2001). Furthermore, E2F1 and E2F2 have also been shown to interact with Nbs1, a component of the Mre11/Rad50 complex which act with ATM to invoke an S-phase checkpoint important for DNA repair (Maser et al. 2001). However the E2F1/Nbs1 interaction mapped to an E2F1 domain downstream of the N-terminus.

4.3 Histone Deacetylases and Chromatin Remodeling Complexes

What is becoming increasingly clear as more detailed analyses of the pRB interactions become available, is that pRB co-exists in higher order complexes with more than one class of the interactors at once. For instance, pRB associates with the E2F1/DP1 transcription factor, and simultaneously interacts with histone deacetylases (HDACs) as demonstrated by several groups (Brehm et al. 1998; Luo et al. 1998; Magnaghi-Jaulin et al. 1998). In some cases bridging proteins (e.g., RBP1) are also present (Lai et al. 2001; Lai et al. 1999). Clearly, the pRB family represses E2F/DP-mediated gene expression through a number of mechanisms, steric hindrance of E2F interaction with the basal transcription factor machinery (TFIID and TAF), and recruitment of HDACs to promoters, using its E2F association to position the complex. The recruitment of HDACs to pRB is thought to involve the pocket domain of pRB interacting with the LxCxE binding motif on HDAC or an intermediary protein (RBP1 or RbAp48) which binds pRB through its LxCxE motif and also binds to HDACs. HDACs repress gene expression through deacetylation of histones within nucleosomes, causing tighter folding of the chromatin, and thereby inhibiting gene expression. Additionally it is possible that HDACs act on the pRB and E2F components of this repression complex, since both E2F1 and pRB have been shown to be acetylated (Brown and Gallie 2002; Chan et al. 2001; Martinez-Balbas et al. 2000; Marzio et al. 2000).

Beyond HDAC interaction, there is increasing evidence that pRB controls cell growth through interaction with BRG-1/hbrm (Dunaief et al. 1994; Strobeck et al. 2000; Trouche et al. 1997; Zhang et al. 2000) in SWI/SNF complexes and Sin3a chromatin-remodeling complexes (Tokitou et al. 1999), involving RbAp46 and RbAp48 (Nicolas et al. 2000; Qian and Lee 1995). Additionally, pRB also controls gene expression through interaction with the SUV39H1 histone methyltransferase, which help silence transcription (Nielsen et al. 2001; Vandel et al. 2001). Simultaneous binding of transcription factors and these chromatin-remodeling complexes allows pRB to select its target promoters for growth suppression and promotion of differentiation. In this way pRB can regulate global levels of transcription by changing the ultrastructural state of the genome.

5. MOUSE MODELS INVOLVING THE pRB TUMOR SUPPRESSOR PATHWAY

Insight into the pRB tumor suppressor pathway has been gained from the construction and evaluation of knockout mice with mutations in genes encoding pRB and E2F family members, cyclins, Cdk4, CKIs, and p19ARF. Additionally, transgenic mice overexpressing wildtype products and knock-in mice expressing mutant protein products have been characterized which shed light on the tumor suppressor function of this network. What is clear is that the pRB tumor suppressor pathway is a tightly interwoven set of controls that balance positively acting proto-oncogenes with negatively acting tumor suppressors (Table 1).

5.1 Mouse Models with pRB Family Members

Inactivation of the *Rb* gene in mice leads to mid-gestational embryonic lethality between E13.5 and E15.5, with neuronal and erythropoietic defects (Clarke et al. 1992; Jacks et al. 1992; Lee et al. 1992). Apoptosis and ectopic proliferation visible in the *Rb*-deficient CNS and nucleated erythrocytes in the fetal liver strongly suggest that pRB normally controls differentiation and/or cell cycle exit in these tissues. Partial rescue of the *Rb*-deficient embryos to late gestation with an *Rb*-transgene has uncovered additional role for *Rb* in skeletal muscle differentiation (Zacksenhaus et al. 1996). The mid-gestational lethality of the *Rb*-deficient embryos demonstrates that the pRB tumor suppressor pathway is not critical or essential for the execution of all cell cycles or in all tissues during development. Double knockout chimaeras with high contribution (>90%) of *Rb* deficient cells in all tissues survive to late gestation, suggesting that only a small population of wildtype cells are required within the embryo to overcome the midgestation lethality (Maandag et al. 1994; Williams et al. 1994).

Importantly, the role of pRB as a tumor suppressor is strongly supported by phenotype of the *Rb+/-* mice, which develop neuroendocrine tumors: pituitary adenocarcinomas (100% penetrant arising from the intermediate lobe), thyroid C-cell adenomas and pheochromacytomas (Harrison et al. 1995; Hu et al. 1994; Jacks et al. 1992; Nikitin et al. 1999; Williams et al. 1994). As in human tumors involving mutations of the *RB* gene, loss-of-heterozygosity at the mouse *Rb* locus has occurred, demonstrating the importance of pRB in the suppression of these neuroendocrine tumors. Therefore, the high penetrance of the *Rb+/-* tumor phenotype makes the *Rb+/-* mice an excellent model for studying the importance of the pRB tumor suppressor pathway, despite the fact that these mice do not develop retinoblastomas. Double knockout chimaeras made with *Rb*-deficient ES cells develop pituitary tumors with 100% penetrance with faster onset, demonstrating that loss of the wildtype *Rb* allele is rate-limiting for tumorigenesis(Maandag et al. 1994; Williams et al. 1994). Recently, chimaeras made with *Rb*-mutant ES cells expressing only the extreme N-terminus of pRB fail to develop pituitary tumors,

TABLE 1. SUMMARY OF MUTANT MOUSE PHENOTYPES

Genotype	*Viability*	*Description of Phenotype*
Rb-/-	no	lethality (E13.5-E15.5), CNS and liver apoptosis
p107-/-	yes	tumor-free survival
p130-/-	yes	tumor-free strain-specific survival
E2f1-/-	yes	tissue atrophy and tumor predisposition
E2f2-/-	yes	abnormal hematopoietic differentiation
E2f3-/-	partial	decreased MEF proliferation, heart failure,
E2f4-/-	yes	abnormal hematopoietic differentiation
E2f5-/-	yes	juvenile death with hydroencephaly
D1-/-	yes	retinal and mammary hypoplasia
D2-/-	yes	gonadal hypoplasia and infertility
Cdk4-/-	yes	insulin-deficient diabetes
Cdk4(R24C)	yes	increased tumor predisposition
Cip1-/-	yes	decreased DNA damage response of MEFs
Kip1-/-	yes	gigantism, pituitary adenomas
Kip2-/-	no	midline closure defects at E17.5
Ink4a-/-/Arf-/-	yes	tumor prone, immortalized MEFs
Arf-/-	yes	tumor prone, immortalized MEFs
Ink4a-/-	yes	tumor prone, non-immortalized MEFs
Ink4b-/-	yes	epithelial cell hyperplasia
Ink4c-/-	yes	gigantism, pituitary adenomas
Ink4d-/-	yes	testicular atrophy
Rb+/-	yes	pituitary and thyroid tumors by 12 months
Rb+/-;E2f1-/-	yes	lessened *Rb+/-* tumors, longer survival
Rb+/-;Cip1-/-	yes	worsened *Rb+/-* tumors, shortened survival
Rb+/-;Kip1-/-	yes	worsened *Rb+/-* tumors, shortened survival
Ink4c-/-;Kip1-/-	yes	highly prone to neuroendocrine tumors
Ink4c-/-;Cip1-/-	yes	prone to wide tumor spectrum
Ink4b-/-;Ink4c-/-	yes	little difference from single mutants

strongly suggesting that tumor suppression can involve both the N-terminus and pocket domains of pRB (Yang et al. 2002).

Inactivation of pRB family members p107 or p130 does not lead to increased tumorigenesis, but rather to tumor-free survival (Cobrinik et al. 1996; Lee et al. 1996). However, on a Balb/c background, p107-deficient mice exhibit growth retardation and myeloid proliferation, and p130-deficient mice die in utero, defects which are clearly not observed on a C57BL/6 background (LeCouter et al. 1998; LeCouter et al. 1998). Compound inactivation of p107 and p130 on a C57BL/6 background leads to perinatal death with limb defects, suggesting that the loss of function from inactivation of either p107 or p130 alone is compensated by the remaining member. Inactivation of p107 in an *Rb+/-* background leads to retinal hyperplasia (Lee et al. 1996) and chimaeras made with embryonic stem cells deficient for both pRB and p107, actually develop retinoblastomas and numerous other tumors arise with high frequency (Robanus-Maandag et al. 1998). Mouse embryonic fibroblasts (MEFs) that are deleted for *Rb* as well as p107 and/or p130 are immortalized and are unable to arrest in G1 in response to DNA damage despite increases in p53 and p21CIP1 (Dannenberg et al. 2000; Peeper et al. 2001; Sage et al. 2000).

Overexpression of pRB in transgenic mice leads to dwarfism, demonstrating the role of pRB in numerous tissues for overall body growth (Bignon et al. 1993). Transgenic expression of a multisite phosphorylation mutant of pRB ("super-repressor") in mammary glands limits ductal expansion and promotes differentiation (Jiang and Zacksenhaus 2002). However, some of these transgenic females developed mammary adenocarcinomas, suggesting that increased survival of the ductal epithelium facilitated the accumulation of additional cancer pre-disposing mutations.

5.2 Mouse Models with E2F Family Members

Inactivation of *E2F* family members in mice results in a range of diverse phenotypes. *E2f1*-deficient mice display tissue-specific atrophy (e.g., testes, thyroid) and tumor predisposition (e.g., lymphoma, lung adenocarcinoma, uterine sarcoma) (Field et al. 1996; Yamasaki et al. 1996). Inactivation of *E2f2* results in viable adults, which when crossed to *E2f1*-deficient mice are highly tumor prone (Zhu et al. 2001). Loss of *E2f3* in mice results in strain-dependent embryonic lethality and congestive heart failure in those surviving *E2f3*-deficient adults without obvious tumor predisposition (Cloud et al. 2002; Humbert et al. 2000). Combination of the *E2f3*-deficiency with *E2f1*-deficiency accentuates the phenotype of either single mutant (Cloud et al. 2002). MEFs that are triply deficient for *E2f1-3* are unable to proliferate demonstrating the importance of those E2Fs with high affinity to pRB for cell cycle progression (Wu et al. 2001). Loss of *E2f4* in mice leads to neonatal death with abnormal hematopoiesis and intestinal defects(Humbert et al. 2000; Rempel et al. 2000), while loss of *E2f5* in mice leads to juvenile hydrocephaly due to a defect in cerebral spinal fluid by the choroid plexus (Lindeman et al. 1998). The simultaneous inactivation of *E2f4* and *E2f5* in mice results in late embryonic lethality, and MEFs deficient for *E2f4* and *E2f5* fail to arrest with p16INK4A (Gaubatz et al. 2000). Clearly, individual E2F family members have restricted and unique roles *in vivo*, and loss of any single member still allows at least a portion of each mutant population to survive until birth.

Genetic interaction between pRB and E2Fs has been demonstrated using the *Rb*-mutant mice, emphasizing that loss of pRB function deregulates E2F activity *in vivo*. Loss of *E2f1* or *E2f3* lessens the defects in the nervous system and fetal liver seen in the *Rb*-deficient embryos (Tsai et al. 1998; Ziebold et al. 2001). Furthermore, loss of *E2f1* reduces the penetrance of the pituitary and thyroid tumorigenesis observed in *Rb+/-* mice, demonstrating that E2F1 can function as a tissue-specific oncogene (Yamasaki et al. 1998).

Establishing lines of transgenic mice that overexpress E2F1 has been difficult to accomplish, presumably due to the induction of p53-dependent and/or -independent apoptosis in critical tissues. Lines that have been successfully generated are discussed below. Transgenic mice expressing E2F1 under the general control of the HMG-CoA reductase promoter develop testicular atrophy that is p53-independent (Holmberg et al. 1998). Transgenic mice in which E2F1 expression is driven by the keratin K5 promoter mainly in the epidermis display hyperproliferation and p53-dependent apoptosis, and in a p53-deficient background, K5-E2F1 transgenics develop skin papillomas (Pierce et al. 1998). However, p19ARF-deficiency does not decrease the extent of apoptosis in the K5-E2F1 transgenic epidermis (Russell et al. 2002).

5.3 Mouse Models with Cyclins D and E

The role of G1 cyclins D1-3 and E1-2 in activating Cdk4/6 and Cdk2 complexes respectively, which subsequently phosphorylate pRB suggested that these G1 cyclins would be absolutely required during development. However, inactivation of cyclin D1 in mice leads to viable mice which exhibit neurological disorders and defects in the development of the retina and mammary gland (Fantl et al. 1995; Sicinski et al. 1995). Cyclin D2-deficient mice are viable, but display male and female gonadal hypoplasia (Sicinski et al. 1996). Transgenic mice expressing cyclin D1 under the control of the mouse mammary tumor virus results in mammary hyperplasia and adenocarcinomas (Wang et al. 1994) and transgenic mice expressing cyclin D1 under the control of the parathyroid hormone promoter develop hyperparathyroidism (Imanishi et al. 2001). These studies demonstrate the role of cyclins D1 and D2 in promoting cellular proliferation, presumably through its ability to activate Cdk4 or Cdk6 complexes, which specifically phosphorylate sites on pRB, leading to its inactivation. However, knock-in of the cyclin E1 gene into the cyclin D1 locus rescues the hypoproliferative retinal and mammary gland defects of the cyclin D1-deficient mice (Geng et al. 1999), raising the possibility that the actual sites phosphorylated by cyclin D1/Cdk4 or Cdk6 are not critical.

Cyclins E1 and E2 are expressed similarly during development, and are both deregulated by loss of pRB (Geng et al. 2001). Loss-of-function models do not yet exist for cyclins E1 or E2. Transgenic mice expressing cyclin E1 in thymocytes develop lymphoid hyperplasia, which progresses to lymphoma if animals are treated with MNU (Karsunky et al. 1999). Similarly expression of cyclin E1 under the control of β-lactoglobulin in lactating mice drives mammary gland hyperplasia and the development of mammary carcinomas (Bortner and Rosenberg 1997). In summary, the oncogenic potential of different D- and E-type cyclins *in vivo* is consistent with their known abilities to inactivate the tumor suppressive function of pRB.

5.4 Mouse Models with Cdk4

Cdk4-deficient mice are viable, yet are smaller and have proliferative defects in testicular Leydig cells, ovarian luteal cells and pancreatic β-cells, the latter of which leads to insulin-deficient diabetes (Moons et al. 2002; Rane et al. 1999; Tsutsui et al. 1999). MEFs lacking Cdk4 show delays in cell cycle entry and increased p27KIP1 activity. Mice bearing a mutant form of Cdk4, Cdk4(Arg24Cys), which is insensitive to *INK4* inhibitors, develop a wide spectrum of tumors, and are highly tumor-prone when treated with various chemical carcinogens (Rane et al. 2002; Sotillo et al. 2001). Additionally, MEFs from these animals are immortal, and transformed by activated *Ras* expression. These studies strongly suggest that Cdk4 is required to regulate proliferation via pRB family members in a wide variety of tissues, and overactivity of Cdk4 facilitates tumorigenesis.

5.5 Mouse Models with CKIs

Not all CKIs are expressed in all cell types throughout development and adult life, which may help interpret the complex phenotypes of the CKI mutant mice, which have been generated for both the *CIP/KIP* and *INK4* families of CKIs. Inactivation of *Kip1*, encoding p27, leads to viable mice which display gigantism in most organs due to increased cellularity, and pituitary adenomas (Fero et al. 1996; Kiyokawa et al. 1996; Nakayama et al. 1996). At least in mice, *Kip1* is haploinsufficient for tumor development, since both *Kip1*-deficient and *Kip1+/-* mice are tumor-prone after irradiation or carcinogen treatment(Fero et al. 1998). Mice lacking *Cip1*, encoding p21, are viable and tumor-free, yet MEFs from these mice show defects in their ability to arrest in G1 following DNA damage (Brugarolas et al. 1995; Deng et al. 1995). Inactivation of *Kip2,* encoding p57, leads to strain-specific neonatal death with placental and midline closure defects (Zhang et al. 1997). Simultaneous inactivation of *Cip1* and *Kip1* in MEFs results in a failure to assemble cyclin D/Cdk complexes, demonstrating that the CIP/KIP family members act as assembly factors for cyclin D/Cdk4 or Cdk6 complexes, as well as inhibitors of cyclin/Cdk2 complexes (Cheng et al. 1999). Surprisingly however, these doubly deleted *Cip1*- and *Kip1*-deficient MEFs showed no obvious cell cycle defects. Combination of either p27KIP1 or p21CIP1 deficiency in *Rb+/-* mice leads to earlier onset of pituitary tumorigenesis, suggesting that the *Rb* tumor suppressor pathway and a CIP/KIP suppressor pathway cooperate in the intermediate lobe to suppress neoplastic progression (Brugarolas et al. 1998; Park et al. 1999).

Inactivation of the INK4 family of inhibitors has demonstrated that rather than being essential for viability, INK4 inhibitors are more important for restraining proliferation in the adult. As in the complex human multiple tumor suppressor loci at 9p21, mice have the syntenic region on chromosome 4 containing the gene encoding p15INK4B and the overlapping genes encoding p16INK4A and p19ARF. Inactivation of the common exon 2 of the p16INK4A/p19ARF locus resulted in highly tumor-prone mice, spontaneously immortalized MEFs and escape from activated *Ras* induced senescence (Serrano et al. 1996). However, inactivation of exon 1β, which is specific for p19ARF, leads to these exact same phenotypes (Kamijo et al. 1997). Inactivation of exon 1α, which is specific for p16INK4A or truncation of p16INK4A, while not affecting expression of p19ARF leads to MEFs which display only a low level of immortalization and activated *Ras*-induced senescence, suggesting that these cellular phenotypes in the original exon 2-deficient mice resulted from the loss of p19ARF function (Krimpenfort et al. 2001; Sharpless et al. 2001). However, the loss of exon 1α or truncation mutant of p16INK4A still leads to mice which are predisposed to spontaneous as well as carcinogen-induced tumor-predisposition, albeit at lower frequency than that originally reported. Taken together, these studies demonstrate that p16INK4A and p19ARF both function as tumor suppressors and their concomitant loss compromises tumor surveillance by separable pathways involving pRB and p53 tumor suppressors (Sherr 2001). Since mice triply-deficient for p19ARF, p53 and mdm2 develop a larger number of tumors than p53-deficient mice or mice doubly deficient in p53 and mdm2, *ARF* must also have functions p53-independent routes for tumor suppression (Weber et al. 2000). Likewise, inactivation of *Arf* alone does not rescue the p53-mediated apoptosis in *Rb*-deficient embryos, suggesting that ARF-independent pathways to induce p53 exist in the developing CNS (Tsai et al. 2002).

Inactivation studies involving the remaining INK4 family members demonstrate the importance of these inhibitors for proper maintenance of specific tissues *in vivo*. Inactivation of *Ink4b*, encoding p15, leads to hyperproliferation in various epithelial tissues (Latres et al. 2000). Loss of *Ink4c*, encoding p18, results in gigantism and organomegaly, while also predisposing animals to pituitary adenomas (Franklin et al. 1998; Latres et al. 2000). Simultaneous loss of *Ink4b* and *Ink4c* had little additional effect. Combining the loss of *Ink4c* with that of *Kip1* results in highly neuroendocrine tumor-prone mice; while inactivation of *Ink4c* and *Cip1* results in less severe and distinct tumor predispositions (Franklin et al. 1998; Franklin et al. 2000). Loss of *Ink4d*, encoding p19, leads to viable mice with testicular atrophy, although embryonic lethality has been reported (Zindy et al. 2000)(Pei, X.-H. and Xiong Y. CSH Cell Cycle 2002 Abstract#154). Loss of *Ink4d* and *INK4C* result in male infertility (Zindy et al. 2001). With regards to tumor suppression, these studies suggest that loss of two INK4 family members is tolerated much better than loss of a single INK4 member and a single CIP/KIP family member.

6. SUMMARY

Apart from their coordinated inactivation by DNA tumor viral oncoproteins, the pRB and p53 tumor suppressor pathways were not known to be connected ten years ago. Within the last decade, our appreciation of how these pathways are interconnected has grown substantially. The checks and balances that exist between pRB and p53 involve the regulation of the G1/S transition and its checkpoints, and much of this is under the control of the E2F transcription factor family. Following DNA damage, the p53-dependent induction of p21CIP1 regulates cyclin E/Cdk2 and cyclin A/Cdk2 complexes both of which phosphorylate pRB, leading to E2F-mediated activation. Similarly, E2F1-dependent induction of p19ARF antagonizes the ability of mdm2 to degrade p53, leading to p53 stabilization and potentially p53-mediated apoptosis or cell cycle arrest. From the existing mouse models discussed above, we also know that proliferation, cell death and differentiation of distinct tissues are also intimately linked through entrance and exit from the cell cycle, and thus through pRB and p53 pathways. Virtually all human tumors deregulate either the pRB or p53 pathway, and often times both pathways simultaneously, which is critical for crippling cellular defense against neoplasia. The next decade of cancer research will likely see these two tumor suppressor pathways only merge even more.

7. ACKNOWLEDGEMENTS

LY is supported by grants from NIH-NCI, Pew Scholars Program in the Biomedical Sciences, March of Dimes and Human Frontiers Science Program. She is grateful for the support and patience of Michele and Isabella Pagano.

8. REFERENCES

Adams, M. R., Sears, R., Nuckolls, F., Leone, G., and Nevins, J. R. 2000. Complex transcriptional regulatory mechanisms control expression of the E2F3 locus. *Mol Cell Biol* **20:**, 3633-9.

Ashizawa, S., Nishizawa, H., Yamada, M., Higashi, H., Kondo, T., Ozawa, H., Kakita, A., and Hatakeyama, M. Biol Chem 2001 Apr 6. Collective inhibition of pRB family proteins by phosphorylation in cells with p16INK4a loss or cyclin E overexpression. *J Biol Chem* **276:**, 11362-70.

Bates, S., Phillips, A. C., Clark, P. A., Stott, F., Peters, G., Ludwig, R. L., and Vousden, K. H. 1998. p14ARF links the tumour suppressors RB and p53. *Nature* **395:**, 124-5.

Bignon, Y. J., Chen, Y., Chang, C. Y., Riley, D. J., Windle, J. J., Mellon, P. L., and Lee, W. H. 1993. Expression of a retinoblastoma transgene results in dwarf mice. *Genes Dev* **7:**, 1654-62.

Bookstein, R., Rio, P., Madreperla, S. A., Hong, F., Allred, C., Grizzle, W. E., and Lee, W. H. 1990. Promoter deletion and loss of retinoblastoma gene expression in human prostate carcinoma. *Proc Natl Acad Sci U S A* **87:**, 7762-6.

Bookstein, R., Shew, J. Y., Chen, P. L., Scully, P., and Lee, W. H. 1990. Suppression of tumorigenicity of human prostate carcinoma cells by replacing a mutated RB gene. *Science* **247:**, 712-5.
Bortner, D. M., and Rosenberg, M. P. 1997. Induction of mammary gland hyperplasia and carcinomas in transgenic mice expressing human cyclin E. *Mol Cell Biol* **17:**, 453-9.
Brehm, A., Miska, E. A., McCance, D. J., Reid, J. L., Bannister, A. J., and Kouzarides, T. 1998. Retinoblastoma protein recruits histone deacetylase to repress transcription. *Nature* **391:**, 597-601.
Brown, V. D., and Gallie, B. L. 2002. The B-Domain Lysine Patch of pRB Is Required for Binding to Large T Antigen and Release of E2F by Phosphorylation. *Mol. Cell. Biol.* **22:**, 1390-401.
Brugarolas, J., Bronson, R. T., and Jacks, T. 1998. p21 is a critical CDK2 regulator essential for proliferation control in Rb-deficient cells. *J Cell Biol* **141:**, 503-14.
Brugarolas, J., Chandrasekaran, C., Gordon, J. I., Beach, D., Jacks, T., and Hannon, G. J. 1995. Radiation-induced cell cycle arrest compromised by p21 deficiency. *Nature* **377:**, 552-7.
Buchkovich, K., Duffy, L. A., and Harlow, E. 1989. The retinoblastoma protein is phosphorylated during specific phases of the cell cycle. *Cell* **58:**, 1097-105.
Carrano, A. C., Eytan, E., Hershko, A., and Pagano, M. 1999. SKP2 is required for ubiquitin-mediated degradation of the CDK inhibitor p27. *Nat Cell Biol* **1:**, 193-9.
Chan, H. M., Krstic-Demonacos, M., Smith, L., Demonacos, C., and La Thangue, N. B. 2001. Acetylation control of the retinoblastoma tumour-suppressor protein. *Nat Cell Biol* **3:**, 667-74.
Chen, P. L., Riley, D. J., Chen, Y., and Lee, W. H. 1996. Retinoblastoma protein positively regulates terminal adipocyte differentiation through direct interaction with C/EBPs. *Genes Dev* **10:**, 2794-804.
Chen, P. L., Riley, D. J., Chen-Kiang, S., and Lee, W. H. 1996. Retinoblastoma protein directly interacts with and activates the transcription factor NF-IL6. *Proc Natl Acad Sci U S A* **93:**, 465-9.
Chen, P. L., Scully, P., Shew, J. Y., Wang, J. Y., and Lee, W. H. 1989. Phosphorylation of the retinoblastoma gene product is modulated during the cell cycle and cellular differentiation. *Cell* **58:**, 1193-8.
Cheng, M., Olivier, P., Diehl, J. A., Fero, M., Roussel, M. F., Roberts, J. M., and Sherr, C. J. 1999. The p21(Cip1) and p27(Kip1) CDK 'inhibitors' are essential activators of cyclin D-dependent kinases in murine fibroblasts. *Embo J* **18:**, 1571-83.
Chilosi, M., Doglioni, C., Yan, Z., Lestani, M., Menestrina, F., Sorio, C., Benedetti, A., Vinante, F., Pizzolo, G., and Inghirami, G. 1998. Differential expression of cyclin-dependent kinase 6 in cortical thymocytes and T-cell lymphoblastic lymphoma/leukemia. *Am J Pathol* **152:**, 209-17.
Clarke, A. R., Maandag, E. R., van Roon, M., van der Lugt, N. M., van der Valk, M., Hooper, M. L., Berns, A., and te Riele, H. 1992. Requirement for a functional Rb-1 gene in murine development. *Nature* **359:**, 328-30.
Claudio, P. P., Howard, C. M., Pacilio, C., Cinti, C., Romano, G., Minimo, C., Maraldi, N. M., Minna, J. D., Gelbert, L., Leoncini, L., Tosi, G. M., Hicheli, P., Caputi, M., Giordano, G. G., and Giordano, A. 2000. Mutations in the retinoblastoma-related gene RB2/p130 in lung tumors and suppression of tumor growth in vivo by retrovirus-mediated gene transfer. *Cancer Res* **60:**, 372-82.
Cloud, J. E., Rogers, C., Reza, T. L., Ziebold, U., Stone, J. R., Picard, M. H., Caron, A. M., Bronson, R. T., and Lees, J. A. 2002. Mutant Mouse Models Reveal the Relative Roles of E2F1 and E2F3 In Vivo. *Mol Cell Biol* **22:**, 2663-2672.
Cobrinik, D., Lee, M. H., Hannon, G., Mulligan, G., Bronson, R. T., Dyson, N., Harlow, E., Beach, D., Weinberg, R. A., and Jacks, T. 1996. Shared role of the pRB-related p130 and p107 proteins in limb development. *Genes Dev* **10:**, 1633-44.
Corcoran, M. M., Mould, S. J., Orchard, J. A., Ibbotson, R. E., Chapman, R. M., Boright, A. P., Platt, C., Tsui, L. C., Scherer, S. W., and Oscier, D. G. 1999. Dysregulation of cyclin dependent kinase 6 expression in splenic marginal zone lymphoma through chromosome 7q translocations. *Oncogene* **18:**, 6271-7.
Cotran R.S., Kumar, V., and Robbins, S. L. (1994). Pathologic Basis of Disease, 5th. Edition, F. J. Schoen, ed. (Philadelphia: W. B. Saunders Company).
Dannenberg, J. H., van Rossum, A., Schuijff, L., and te Riele, H. 2000. Ablation of the retinoblastoma gene family deregulates G(1) control causing immortalization and increased cell turnover under growth-restricting conditions. *Genes Dev* **14:**, 3051-64.
DeCaprio, J. A., Ludlow, J. W., Figge, J., Shew, J. Y., Huang, C. M., Lee, W. H., Marsilio, E., Paucha, E., and Livingston, D. M. 1988. SV40 large tumor antigen forms a specific complex with the product of the retinoblastoma susceptibility gene. *Cell* **54:**, 275-83.

DeCaprio, J. A., Ludlow, J. W., Lynch, D., Furukawa, Y., Griffin, J., Piwnica-Worms, H., Huang, C. M., and Livingston, D. M. 1989. The product of the retinoblastoma susceptibility gene has properties of a cell cycle regulatory element. *Cell* **58:**, 1085-95.

DeGregori, J., Leone, G., Miron, A., Jakoi, L., and Nevins, J. R. 1997. Distinct roles for E2F proteins in cell growth control and apoptosis. *Proc Natl Acad Sci U S A* **94:**, 7245-50.

Deng, C., Zhang, P., Harper, J. W., Elledge, S. J., and Leder, P. 1995. Mice lacking p21CIP1/WAF1 undergo normal development, but are defective in G1 checkpoint control. *Cell* **82:**, 675-84.

Dick, F. A., Sailhamer, E., and Dyson, N. J. 2000. Mutagenesis of the pRB pocket reveals that cell cycle arrest functions are separable from binding to viral oncoproteins. *Mol Cell Biol* **20:**, 3715-27.

Dowdy, S. F., Hinds, P. W., Louie, K., Reed, S. I., Arnold, A., and Weinberg, R. A. 1993. Physical interaction of the retinoblastoma protein with human D cyclins. *Cell* **73:**, 499-511.

Dryja, T. P., Rapaport, J. M., Joyce, J. M., and Petersen, R. A. 1986. Molecular detection of deletions involving band q14 of chromosome 13 in retinoblastomas. *Proc Natl Acad Sci U S A* **83:**, 7391-4.

Dryja, T. P., Rapaport, J. M., Weichselbaum, R., and Bruns, G. A. 1984. Chromosome 13 restriction fragment length polymorphisms. *Hum Genet* **65:**, 320-4.

Dunaief, J. L., Strober, B. E., Guha, S., Khavari, P. A., Alin, K., Luban, J., Begemann, M., Crabtree, G. R., and Goff, S. P. 1994. The retinoblastoma protein and BRG1 form a complex and cooperate to induce cell cycle arrest. *Cell* **79:**, 119-30.

Dunn, J. M., Phillips, R. A., Becker, A. J., and Gallie, B. L. 1988. Identification of germline and somatic mutations affecting the retinoblastoma gene. *Science* **241:**, 1797-800.

Durfee, T., Becherer, K., Chen, P. L., Yeh, S. H., Yang, Y., Kilburn, A. E., Lee, W. H., and Elledge, S. J. 1993. The retinoblastoma protein associates with the protein phosphatase type 1 catalytic subunit. *Genes Dev* **7:**, 555-69.

Dynlacht, B. D., Flores, O., Lees, J. A., and Harlow, E. 1994. Differential regulation of E2F transactivation by cyclin/cdk2 complexes. *Genes Dev* **8:**, 1772-86.

Dyson, N. 1998. The regulation of E2F by pRB-family proteins. *Genes Dev* **12:**, 2245-62.

Dyson, N., Howley, P. M., Munger, K., and Harlow, E. 1989. The human papilloma virus-16 E7 oncoprotein is able to bind to the retinoblastoma gene product. *Science* **243:**, 934-7.

el-Deiry, W. S., Tokino, T., Velculescu, V. E., Levy, D. B., Parsons, R., Trent, J. M., Lin, D., Mercer, W. E., Kinzler, K. W., and Vogelstein, B. 1993. WAF1, a potential mediator of p53 tumor suppression. *Cell* **75:**, 817-25.

Ewen, M. E., Sluss, H. K., Sherr, C. J., Matsushime, H., Kato, J., and Livingston, D. M. 1993. Functional interactions of the retinoblastoma protein with mammalian D-type cyclins. *Cell* **73:**, 487-97.

Ewen, M. E., Xing, Y. G., Lawrence, J. B., and Livingston, D. M. 1991. Molecular cloning, chromosomal mapping, and expression of the cDNA for p107, a retinoblastoma gene product-related protein. *Cell* **66:**, 1155-64.

Fantl, V., Stamp, G., Andrews, A., Rosewell, I., and Dickson, C. 1995. Mice lacking cyclin D1 are small and show defects in eye and mammary gland development. *Genes Dev* **9:**, 2364-72.

Fero, M. L., Randel, E., Gurley, K. E., Roberts, J. M., and Kemp, C. J. 1998. The murine gene p27Kip1 is haplo-insufficient for tumour suppression. *Nature* **396:**, 177-80.

Fero, M. L., Rivkin, M., Tasch, M., Porter, P., Carow, C. E., Firpo, E., Polyak, K., Tsai, L. H., Broudy, V., Perlmutter, R. M., Kaushansky, K., and Roberts, J. M. 1996. A syndrome of multiorgan hyperplasia with features of gigantism, tumorigenesis, and female sterility in p27(Kip1)-deficient mice. *Cell* **85:**, 733-44.

Field, S. J., Tsai, F. Y., Kuo, F., Zubiaga, A. M., Kaelin, W. G., Livingston, D. M., Orkin, S. H., and Greenberg, M. E. 1996. E2F-1 functions in mice to promote apoptosis and suppress proliferation. *Cell* **85:**, 549-61.

Francke, U., and Kung, F. 1976. Sporadic bilateral retinoblastoma and 13q- chromosomal deletion. *Med Pediatr Oncol* **2:**, 379-85.

Franklin, D. S., Godfrey, V. L., Lee, H., Kovalev, G. I., Schoonhoven, R., Chen-Kiang, S., Su, L., and Xiong, Y. 1998. CDK inhibitors p18(INK4c) and p27(Kip1) mediate two separate pathways to collaboratively suppress pituitary tumorigenesis. *Genes Dev* **12:**, 2899-911.

Franklin, D. S., Godfrey, V. L., O'Brien, D. A., Deng, C., and Xiong, Y. 2000. Functional collaboration between different cyclin-dependent kinase inhibitors suppresses tumor growth with distinct tissue specificity. *Mol Cell Biol* **20:**, 6147-58.

Friend, S. H., Bernards, R., Rogelj, S., Weinberg, R. A., Rapaport, J. M., Albert, D. M., and Dryja, T. P. 1986. A human DNA segment with properties of the gene that predisposes to retinoblastoma and osteosarcoma. *Nature* **323:**, 643-6.

Fung, Y. K., Murphree, A. L., T'Ang, A., Qian, J., Hinrichs, S. H., and Benedict, W. F. 1987. Structural evidence for the authenticity of the human retinoblastoma gene. *Science* **236:**, 1657-61.

Gaubatz, S., Lindeman, G. J., Ishida, S., Jakoi, L., Nevins, J. R., Livingston, D. M., and Rempel, R. E. 2000. E2F4 and E2F5 play an essential role in pocket protein-mediated G1 control. *Mol Cell* **6:**, 729-35.

Geng, Y., Whoriskey, W., Park, M. Y., Bronson, R. T., Medema, R. H., Li, T., Weinberg, R. A., and Sicinski, P. 1999. Rescue of cyclin D1 deficiency by knockin cyclin E. *Cell* **97:**, 767-77.

Geng, Y., Yu, Q., Whoriskey, W., Dick, F., Tsai, K. Y., Ford, H. L., Biswas, D. K., Pardee, A. B., Amati, B., Jacks, T., Richardson, A., Dyson, N., and Sicinski, P. 2001. Expression of cyclins E1 and E2 during mouse development and in neoplasia. *Proc Natl Acad Sci U S A* **98:**, 13138-43.

Girling, R., Partridge, J. F., Bandara, L. R., Burden, N., Totty, N. F., Hsuan, J. J., and La Thangue, N. B. 1993. A new component of the transcription factor DRTF1/E2F. *Nature* **362:**, 83-7.

Gu, W., Schneider, J. W., Condorelli, G., Kaushal, S., Mahdavi, V., and Nadal-Ginard, B. 1993. Interaction of myogenic factors and the retinoblastoma protein mediates muscle cell commitment and differentiation. *Cell* **72:**, 309-24.

Gu, Y., Turck, C. W., and Morgan, D. O. 1993. Inhibition of CDK2 activity in vivo by an associated 20K regulatory subunit. *Nature* **366:**, 707-10.

Gudas, J. M., Payton, M., Thukral, S., Chen, E., Bass, M., Robinson, M. O., and Coats, S. 1999. Cyclin E2, a novel G1 cyclin that binds Cdk2 and is aberrantly expressed in human cancers. *Mol Cell Biol* **19:**, 612-22.

Hamel, P. A., Gill, R. M., Phillips, R. A., and Gallie, B. L. 1992. Transcriptional repression of the E2-containing promoters EIIaE, c-myc, and RB1 by the product of the RB1 gene. *Mol Cell Biol* **12:**, 3431-8.

Hannon, G. J., and Beach, D. 1994. p15INK4B is a potential effector of TGF-beta-induced cell cycle arrest. *Nature* **371:**, 257-61.

Hansen, M. F., Koufos, A., Gallie, B. L., Phillips, R. A., Fodstad, O., Brogger, A., Gedde-Dahl, T., and Cavenee, W. K. 1985. Osteosarcoma and retinoblastoma: a shared chromosomal mechanism revealing recessive predisposition. *Proc Natl Acad Sci U S A* **82:**, 6216-20.

Harbour, J. W., Lai, S. L., Whang-Peng, J., Gazdar, A. F., Minna, J. D., and Kaye, F. J. 1988. Abnormalities in structure and expression of the human retinoblastoma gene in SCLC. *Science* **241:**, 353-7.

Harbour, J. W., Luo, R. X., Dei Santi, A., Postigo, A. A., and Dean, D. C. 1999. Cdk phosphorylation triggers sequential intramolecular interactions that progressively block Rb functions as cells move through G1. *Cell* **98:**, 859-69.

Harrison, D. J., Hooper, M. L., Armstrong, J. F., and Clarke, A. R. 1995. Effects of heterozygosity for the Rb-1t19neo allele in the mouse. *Oncogene* **10:**, 1615-20.

Hatada, I., Ohashi, H., Fukushima, Y., Kaneko, Y., Inoue, M., Komoto, Y., Okada, A., Ohishi, S., Nabetani, A., Morisaki, H., Nakayama, M., Niikawa, N., and Mukai, T. 1996. An imprinted gene p57KIP2 is mutated in Beckwith-Wiedemann syndrome. *Nat Genet* **14:**, 171-3.

Hatakeyama, M., Brill, J. A., Fink, G. R., and Weinberg, R. A. 1994. Collaboration of G1 cyclins in the functional inactivation of the retinoblastoma protein. *Genes Dev* **8:**, 1759-71.

Hateboer, G., Kerkhoven, R. M., Shvarts, A., Bernards, R., and Beijersbergen, R. L. 1996. Degradation of E2F by the ubiquitin-proteasome pathway: regulation by retinoblastoma family proteins and adenovirus transforming proteins. *Genes Dev* **10:**, 2960-70.

Helin, K., Holm, K., Niebuhr, A., Eiberg, H., Tommerup, N., Hougaard, S., Poulsen, H. S., Spang-Thomsen, M., and Norgaard, P. 1997. Loss of the retinoblastoma protein-related p130 protein in small cell lung carcinoma. *Proc Natl Acad Sci U S A* **94:**, 6933-8.

Hinds, P. W., Mittnacht, S., Dulic, V., Arnold, A., Reed, S. I., and Weinberg, R. A. 1992. Regulation of retinoblastoma protein functions by ectopic expression of human cyclins. *Cell* **70:**, 993-1006.

Hofmann, F., Martelli, F., Livingston, D. M., and Wang, Z. 1996. The retinoblastoma gene product protects E2F-1 from degradation by the ubiquitin-proteasome pathway. *Genes Dev* **10:**, 2949-59.

Holmberg, C., Helin, K., Sehested, M., and Karlstrom, O. 1998. E2F-1-induced p53-independent apoptosis in transgenic mice. *Oncogene* **17:**, 143-55.

Horowitz, J. M., Park, S. H., Bogenmann, E., Cheng, J. C., Yandell, D. W., Kaye, F. J., Minna, J. D., Dryja, T. P., and Weinberg, R. A. 1990. Frequent inactivation of the retinoblastoma anti-oncogene is restricted to a subset of human tumor cells. *Proc Natl Acad Sci U S A* **87:**, 2775-9.

Hsiao, K. M., McMahon, S. L., and Farnham, P. J. 1994. Multiple DNA elements are required for the growth regulation of the mouse E2F1 promoter. *Genes Dev* **8:**, 1526-37.

Hsieh, J. K., Fredersdorf, S., Kouzarides, T., Martin, K., and Lu, X. 1997. E2F1-induced apoptosis requires DNA binding but not transactivation and is inhibited by the retinoblastoma protein through direct interaction. *Genes Dev* **11:**, 1840-52.

Hu, N., Gutsmann, A., Herbert, D. C., Bradley, A., Lee, W. H., and Lee, E. Y. 1994. Heterozygous Rb-1 delta 20/+mice are predisposed to tumors of the pituitary gland with a nearly complete penetrance. *Oncogene* **9:**, 1021-7.

Huang, H. J., Yee, J. K., Shew, J. Y., Chen, P. L., Bookstein, R., Friedmann, T., Lee, E. Y., and Lee, W. H. 1988. Suppression of the neoplastic phenotype by replacement of the RB gene in human cancer cells. *Science* **242:**, 1563-6.

Humbert, P. O., Rogers, C., Ganiatsas, S., Landsberg, R. L., Trimarchi, J. M., Dandapani, S., Brugnara, C., Erdman, S., Schrenzel, M., Bronson, R. T., and Lees, J. A. 2000. E2F4 is essential for normal erythrocyte maturation and neonatal viability. *Mol Cell* **6:**, 281-91.

Humbert, P. O., Verona, R., Trimarchi, J. M., Rogers, C., Dandapani, S., and Lees, J. A. 2000. E2f3 is critical for normal cellular proliferation. *Genes Dev* **14:**, 690-703.

Ichimur, K., Hanafusa, H., Takimoto H., Ohgama, Y., Akagi, T., and Shimizu, K. 2000 Structure of the human retinoblastoma-related p107 gene and its intragenic deletion in a B-cell lymphma cell line. *Gene* 251:37-43.

Imanishi, Y., Hosokawa, Y., Yoshimoto, K., Schipani, E., Mallya, S., Papanikolaou, A., Kifor, O., Tokura, T., Sablosky, M., Ledgard, F., Gronowicz, G., Wang, T. C., Schmidt, E. V., Hall, C., Brown, E. M., Bronson, R., and Arnold, A. 2001. Primary hyperparathyroidism caused by parathyroid-targeted overexpression of cyclin D1 in transgenic mice. *J Clin Invest* **107:**, 1093-102.

Ishida, S., Huang, E., Zuzan, H., Spang, R., Leone, G., West, M., and Nevins, J. R. 2001. Role for E2F in control of both DNA replication and mitotic functions as revealed from DNA microarray analysis. *Mol Cell Biol* **21:**, 4684-99.

Jacks, T., Fazeli, A., Schmitt, E. M., Bronson, R. T., Goodell, M. A., and Weinberg, R. A. 1992. Effects of an Rb mutation in the mouse. *Nature* **359:**, 295-300.

Jiang, Z., and Zacksenhaus, E. 2002. Activation of retinoblastoma protein in mammary gland leads to ductal growth suppression, precocious differentiation, and adenocarcinoma. *J Cell Biol* **156:**, 185-98.

Johnson, D. G., Ohtani, K., and Nevins, J. R. 1994. Autoregulatory control of E2F1 expression in response to positive and negative regulators of cell cycle progression. *Genes Dev* **8:**, 1514-25.

Johnson, D. G., Schwarz, J. K., Cress, W. D., and Nevins, J. R. 1993. Expression of transcription factor E2F1 induces quiescent cells to enter S phase. *Nature* **365:**, 349-52.

Kalma, Y., Marash, L., Lamed, Y., and Ginsberg, D. 2001 Mar 15. Expression analysis using DNA microarrays demonstrates that E2F-1 up-regulates expression of DNA replication genes including replication protein A2. *Oncogene* **20:**, 1379-87.

Kamb, A., Gruis, N. A., Weaver-Feldhaus, J., Liu, Q., Harshman, K., Tavtigian, S. V., Stockert, E., Day, R. S. r., Johnson, B. E., and Skolnick, M. H. 1994. A cell cycle regulator potentially involved in genesis of many tumor types. *Science* **264:**, 436-40.

Kamijo, T., Zindy, F., Roussel, M. F., Quelle, D. E., Downing, J. R., Ashmun, R. A., Grosveld, G., and Sherr, C. J. 1997. Tumor suppression at the mouse INK4a locus mediated by the alternative reading frame product p19ARF. *Cell* **91:**, 649-59.

Karsunky, H., Geisen, C., Schmidt, T., Haas, K., Zevnik, B., Gau, E., and Moroy, T. 1999. Oncogenic potential of cyclin E in T-cell lymphomagenesis in transgenic mice: evidence for cooperation between cyclin E and Ras but not Myc. *Oncogene* **18:**, 7816-24.

Kato, J., Matsushime, H., Hiebert, S. W., Ewen, M. E., and Sherr, C. J. 1993. Direct binding of cyclin D to the retinoblastoma gene product (pRb) and pRb phosphorylation by the cyclin D-dependent kinase CDK4. *Genes Dev* **7:**, 331-42.

Keyomarsi, K., O'Leary, N., Molnar, G., Lees, E., Fingert, H. J., and Pardee, A. B. 1994. Cyclin E, a potential prognostic marker for breast cancer. *Cancer Res* **54:**, 380-5.

Khatib, Z. A., Matsushime, H., Valentine, M., Shapiro, D. N., Sherr, C. J., and Look, A. T. 1993. Coamplification of the CDK4 gene with MDM2 and GLI in human sarcomas. *Cancer Res* **53:**, 5535-41.

Kim, H. Y., Ahn, B. Y., and Cho, Y. 2001. Structural basis for the inactivation of retinoblastoma tumor suppressor by SV40 large T antigen. *Embo J* **20:**, 295-304.

Kiyokawa, H., Kineman, R. D., Manova-Todorova, K. O., Soares, V. C., Hoffman, E. S., Ono, M., Khanam, D., Hayday, A. C., Frohman, L. A., and Koff, A. 1996. Enhanced growth of mice lacking the cyclin-dependent kinase inhibitor function of p27(Kip1). *Cell* **85:**, 721-32.

Knudson, A. G., Jr. 1971. Mutation and cancer: statistical study of retinoblastoma. *Proc Natl Acad Sci U S A* **68:**, 820-3.

Knudson, A. G., Jr., Meadows, A. T., Nichols, W. W., and Hill, R. 1976. Chromosomal deletion and retinoblastoma. *N Engl J Med* **295:**, 1120-3.

Kovesdi, I., Reichel, R., and Nevins, J. R. 1986. Identification of a cellular transcription factor involved in E1A trans-activation. *Cell* **45:**, 219-28.

Kowalik, T. F., DeGregori, J., Schwarz, J. K., and Nevins, J. R. 1995. E2F1 overexpression in quiescent fibroblasts leads to induction of cellular DNA synthesis and apoptosis. *J Virol* **69:**, 2491-500.

Krek, W., Ewen, M. E., Shirodkar, S., Arany, Z., Kaelin, W. G., Jr., and Livingston, D. M. 1994. Negative regulation of the growth-promoting transcription factor E2F-1 by a stably bound cyclin A-dependent protein kinase. *Cell* **78:**, 161-72.

Krek, W., Xu, G., and Livingston, D. M. 1995. Cyclin A-kinase regulation of E2F-1 DNA binding function underlies suppression of an S phase checkpoint. *Cell* **83:**, 1149-58.

Krimpenfort, P., Quon, K. C., Mooi, W. J., Loonstra, A., and Berns, A. 2001. Loss of p16Ink4a confers susceptibility to metastatic melanoma in mice. *Nature* **413:**, 83-6.

La Thangue, N. B., and Rigby, P. W. 1987. An adenovirus E1A-like transcription factor is regulated during the differentiation of murine embryonal carcinoma stem cells. *Cell* **49:**, 507-13.

LaBaer, J., Garrett, M. D., Stevenson, L. F., Slingerland, J. M., Sandhu, C., Chou, H. S., Fattaey, A., and Harlow, E. 1997. New functional activities for the p21 family of CDK inhibitors. *Genes Dev* **11:**, 847-62.

Lai, A., Kennedy, B. K., Barbie, D. A., Bertos, N. R., Yang, X. J., Theberge, M. C., Tsai, S. C., Seto, E., Zhang, Y., Kuzmichev, A., Lane, W. S., Reinberg, D., Harlow, E., and Branton, P. E. 2001. RBP1 recruits the mSIN3-histone deacetylase complex to the pocket of retinoblastoma tumor suppressor family proteins found in limited discrete regions of the nucleus at growth arrest. *Mol Cell Biol* **21:**, 2918-32.

Lai, A., Lee, J. M., Yang, W. M., DeCaprio, J. A., Kaelin, W. G., Jr., Seto, E., and Branton, P. E. 1999. RBP1 recruits both histone deacetylase-dependent and -independent repression activities to retinoblastoma family proteins. *Mol Cell Biol* **19:**, 6632-41.

Lam, E. W., and Watson, R. J. 1993. An E2F-binding site mediates cell-cycle regulated repression of mouse B-myb transcription. *Embo J* **12:**, 2705-13.

Lasorella, A., Noseda, M., Beyna, M., Yokota, Y., and Iavarone, A. 2000. Id2 is a retinoblastoma protein target and mediates signalling by Myc oncoproteins. *Nature* **407:**, 592-8.

Latres, E., Malumbres, M., Sotillo, R., Martin, J., Ortega, S., Martin-Caballero, J., Flores, J. M., Cordon-Cardo, C., and Barbacid, M. 2000. Limited overlapping roles of P15(INK4b) and P18(INK4c) cell cycle inhibitors in proliferation and tumorigenesis. *Embo J* **19:**, 3496-506.

LeCouter, J. E., Kablar, B., Hardy, W. R., Ying, C., Megeney, L. A., May, L. L., and Rudnicki, M. A. 1998. Strain-dependent myeloid hyperplasia, growth deficiency, and accelerated cell cycle in mice lacking the Rb-related p107 gene. *Mol Cell Biol* **18:**, 7455-65.

LeCouter, J. E., Kablar, B., Whyte, P. F., Ying, C., and Rudnicki, M. A. 1998. Strain-dependent embryonic lethality in mice lacking the retinoblastoma-related p130 gene. *Development* **125:**, 4669-79.

Lee, E. Y., Chang, C. Y., Hu, N., Wang, Y. C., Lai, C. C., Herrup, K., Lee, W. H., and Bradley, A. 1992. Mice deficient for Rb are nonviable and show defects in neurogenesis and haematopoiesis. *Nature* **359:**, 288-94.

Lee, E. Y., To, H., Shew, J. Y., Bookstein, R., Scully, P., and Lee, W. H. 1988. Inactivation of the retinoblastoma susceptibility gene in human breast cancers. *Science* **241:**, 218-21.

Lee, J. O., Russo, A. A., and Pavletich, N. P. 1998. Structure of the retinoblastoma tumour-suppressor pocket domain bound to a peptide from HPV E7. *Nature* **391:**, 859-65.

Lee, M. H., Williams, B. O., Mulligan, G., Mukai, S., Bronson, R. T., Dyson, N., Harlow, E., and Jacks, T. 1996. Targeted disruption of p107: functional overlap between p107 and Rb. *Genes Dev* **10:**, 1621-32.

Lee, W. H., Bookstein, R., Hong, F., Young, L. J., Shew, J. Y., and Lee, E. Y. 1987. Human retinoblastoma susceptibility gene: cloning, identification, and sequence. *Science* **235:**, 1394-9.

Leone, G., DeGregori, J., Yan, Z., Jakoi, L., Ishida, S., Williams, R. S., and Nevins, J. R. 1998. E2F3 activity is regulated during the cell cycle and is required for the induction of S phase. *Genes Dev* **12:**, 2120-30.

Li, Y., Graham, C., Lacy, S., Duncan, A. M., and Whyte, P. 1993. The adenovirus E1A-associated 130-kD protein is encoded by a member of the retinoblastoma gene family and physically interacts with cyclins A and E. *Genes Dev* **7:**, 2366-77.

Lin, W. C., Lin, F. T., and Nevins, J. R. 2001. Selective induction of E2F1 in response to DNA damage, mediated by ATM-dependent phosphorylation. *Genes Dev* **15:**, 1833-44.
Lindeman, G. J., Dagnino, L., Gaubatz, S., Xu, Y., Bronson, R. T., Warren, H. B., and Livingston, D. M. 1998. A specific, nonproliferative role for E2F-5 in choroid plexus function revealed by gene targeting. *Genes Dev* **12:**, 1092-8.
Livingston, D. M., Kaelin, W., Chittenden, T., and Qin, X. 1993. Structural and functional contributions to the G1 blocking action of the retinoblastoma protein. (the 1992 Gordon Hamilton Fairley Memorial Lecture). *Br J Cancer* **68:**, 264-8.
Loda, M., Cukor, B., Tam, S. W., Lavin, P., Fiorentino, M., Draetta, G. F., Jessup, J. M., and Pagano, M. 1997. Increased proteasome-dependent degradation of the cyclin-dependent kinase inhibitor p27 in aggressive colorectal carcinomas. *Nat Med* **3:**, 231-4.
Ludlow, J. W., DeCaprio, J. A., Huang, C. M., Lee, W. H., Paucha, E., and Livingston, D. M. 1989. SV40 large T antigen binds preferentially to an underphosphorylated member of the retinoblastoma susceptibility gene product family. *Cell* **56:**, 57-65.
Luo, R. X., Postigo, A. A., and Dean, D. C. 1998. Rb interacts with histone deacetylase to repress transcription. *Cell* **92:**, 463-73.
Ma, Y., Croxton, R., Moorer, R. L., Jr., and Cress, W. D. 2002. Identification of novel E2F1-regulated genes by microarray. *Arch Biochem Biophys* **399:**, 212-24.
Maandag, E. C., van der Valk, M., Vlaar, M., Feltkamp, C., O'Brien, J., van Roon, M., van der Lugt, N., Berns, A., and te Riele, H. 1994. Developmental rescue of an embryonic-lethal mutation in the retinoblastoma gene in chimeric mice. *Embo J* **13:**, 4260-8.
Magnaghi-Jaulin, L., Groisman, R., Naguibneva, I., Robin, P., Lorain, S., Le Villain, J. P., Troalen, F., Trouche, D., and Harel-Bellan, A. 1998. Retinoblastoma protein represses transcription by recruiting a histone deacetylase. *Nature* **391:**, 601-5.
Marti, A., Wirbelauer, C., Scheffner, M., and Krek, W. 1999. Interaction between ubiquitin-protein ligase SCFSKP2 and E2F-1 underlies the regulation of E2F-1 degradation. *Nat Cell Biol* **1:**, 14-9.
Martinez-Balbas, M. A., Bauer, U. M., Nielsen, S. J., Brehm, A., and Kouzarides, T. 2000. Regulation of E2F1 activity by acetylation. *Embo J.* **19:**, 662-71.
Marzio, G., Wagener, C., Gutierrez, M. I., Cartwright, P., Helin, K., and Giacca, M. 2000. E2F family members are differentially regulated by reversible acetylation. *J Biol Chem* **275:**, 10887-92.
Maser, R. S., Mirzoeva, O. K., Wells, J., Olivares, H., Williams, B. R., Zinkel, R. A., Farnham, P. J., and Petrini, J. H. 2001. Mre11 complex and DNA replication: linkage to E2F and sites of DNA synthesis. *Mol Cell Biol* **21:**, 6006-16.
Matsuoka, S., Thompson, J. S., Edwards, M. C., Bartletta, J. M., Grundy, P., Kalikin, L. M., Harper, J. W., Elledge, S. J., and Feinberg, A. P. 1996. Imprinting of the gene encoding a human cyclin-dependent kinase inhibitor, p57KIP2, on chromosome 11p15. *Proc Natl Acad Sci U S A* **93:**, 3026-30.
Mayol, X., Grana, X., Baldi, A., Sang, N., Hu, Q., and Giordano, A. 1993. Cloning of a new member of the retinoblastoma gene family (pRb2) which binds to the E1A transforming domain. *Oncogene* **8:**, 2561-6.
Mihara, K., Cao, X. R., Yen, A., Chandler, S., Driscoll, B., Murphree, A. L., T'Ang, A., and Fung, Y. K. 1989. Cell cycle-dependent regulation of phosphorylation of the human retinoblastoma gene product. *Science* **246:**, 1300-3.
Moberg, K. H., Bell, D. W., Wahrer, D. C., Haber, D. A., and Hariharan, I. K. 2001. Archipelago regulates Cyclin E levels in Drosophila and is mutated in human cancer cell lines. *Nature* **413:**, 311-6.
Moons, D. S., Jirawatnotai, S., Tsutsui, T., Franks, R., Parlow, A. F., Hales, D. B., Gibori, G., Fazleabas, A. T., and Kiyokawa, H. 2002. Intact follicular maturation and defective luteal function in mice deficient for cyclin- dependent kinase-4. *Endocrinology* **143:**, 647-54.
Morris, E. J., and Dyson, N. J. 2001. Retinoblastoma protein partners. *Adv Cancer Res* **82:**, 1-54.
Muller, H., Bracken, A. P., Vernell, R., Moroni, M. C., Christians, F., Grassilli, E., Prosperini, E., Vigo, E., Oliner, J. D., and Helin, K. 2001. E2Fs regulate the expression of genes involved in differentiation, development, proliferation, and apoptosis. *Genes Dev* **15:**, 267-85.
Muller, H., Moroni, M. C., Vigo, E., Petersen, B. O., Bartek, J., and Helin, K. 1997. Induction of S-phase entry by E2F transcription factors depends on their nuclear localization. *Mol Cell Biol* **17:**, 5508-20.
Munger, K., Werness, B. A., Dyson, N., Phelps, W. C., Harlow, E., and Howley, P. M. 1989. Complex formation of human papillomavirus E7 proteins with the retinoblastoma tumor suppressor gene product. *Embo J* **8:**, 4099-105.

Nakayama, K., Ishida, N., Shirane, M., Inomata, A., Inoue, T., Shishido, N., Horii, I., Loh, D. Y., and Nakayama, K. 1996. Mice lacking p27(Kip1) display increased body size, multiple organ hyperplasia, retinal dysplasia, and pituitary tumors. *Cell* **85:**, 707-20.

Nicolas, E., Morales, V., Magnaghi-Jaulin, L., Harel-Bellan, A., Richard-Foy, H., and Trouche, D. 2000. RbAp48 belongs to the histone deacetylase complex that associates with the retinoblastoma protein. *J Biol Chem* **275:**, 9797-804.

Nielsen, N. H., Arnerlov, C., Emdin, S. O., and Landberg, G. 1996. Cyclin E overexpression, a negative prognostic factor in breast cancer with strong correlation to oestrogen receptor status. *Br J Cancer* **74:**, 874-80.

Nielsen, S. J., Schneider, R., Bauer, U. M., Bannister, A. J., Morrison, A., O'Carroll, D., Firestein, R., Cleary, M., Jenuwein, T., Herrera, R. E., and Kouzarides, T. 2001. Rb targets histone H3 methylation and HP1 to promoters. *Nature* **412:**, 561-5.

Nikitin, A. Y., Juarez-Perez, M. I., Li, S., Huang, L., and Lee, W. H. 1999. RB-mediated suppression of spontaneous multiple neuroendocrine neoplasia and lung metastases in Rb+/- mice. *Proc Natl Acad Sci U S A* **96:**, 3916-21.

Nip, J., Strom, D. K., Fee, B. E., Zambetti, G., Cleveland, J. L., and Hiebert, S. W. 1997. E2F-1 cooperates with topoisomerase II inhibition and DNA damage to selectively augment p53-independent apoptosis. *Mol Cell Biol* **17:**, 1049-56.

Noda, A., Ning, Y., Venable, S. F., Pereira-Smith, O. M., and Smith, J. R. 1994. Cloning of senescent cell-derived inhibitors of DNA synthesis using an expression screen. *Exp Cell Res* **211:**, 90-8.

Ohtani, N., Zebedee, Z., Huot, T. J., Stinson, J. A., Sugimoto, M., Ohashi, Y., Sharrocks, A. D., Peters, G., and Hara, E. 2001. Opposing effects of Ets and Id proteins on p16INK4a expression during cellular senescence. *Nature* **409:**, 1067-70.

Pagano, M., Tam, S. W., Theodoras, A. M., Beer-Romero, P., Del Sal, G., Chau, V., Yew, P. R., Draetta, G. F., and Rolfe, M. 1995. Role of the ubiquitin-proteasome pathway in regulating abundance of the cyclin-dependent kinase inhibitor p27. *Science* **269:**, 682-5.

Palmero, I., McConnell, B., Parry, D., Brookes, S., Hara, E., Bates, S., Jat, P., and Peters, G. 1997. Accumulation of p16INK4a in mouse fibroblasts as a function of replicative senescence and not of retinoblastoma gene status. *Oncogene* **15:**, 495-503.

Pardee, A. B. 1974. A restriction point for control of normal animal cell proliferation. *Proc Natl Acad Sci U S A* **71:**, 1286-90.

Park, M. S., Rosai, J., Nguyen, H. T., Capodieci, P., Cordon-Cardo, C., and Koff, A. 1999. p27 and Rb are on overlapping pathways suppressing tumorigenesis in mice. *Proc Natl Acad Sci U S A* **96:**, 6382-7.

Peeper, D. S., Dannenberg, J. H., Douma, S., te Riele, H., and Bernards, R. 2001. Escape from premature senescence is not sufficient for oncogenic transformation by Ras. *Nat Cell Biol* **3:**, 198-203.

Peters, G. 1994. The D-type cyclins and their role in tumorigenesis. *J Cell Sci Suppl* **18:**, 89-96.

Phillips, A. C., Bates, S., Ryan, K. M., Helin, K., and Vousden, K. H. 1997. Induction of DNA synthesis and apoptosis are separable functions of E2F-1. *Genes Dev* **11:**, 1853-63.

Pierce, A. M., Gimenez-Conti, I. B., Schneider-Broussard, R., Martinez, L. A., Conti, C. J., and Johnson, D. G. 1998. Increased E2F1 activity induces skin tumors in mice heterozygous and nullizygous for p53. *Proc Natl Acad Sci U S A* **95:**, 8858-63.

Polyak, K., Lee, M. H., Erdjument-Bromage, H., Koff, A., Roberts, J. M., Tempst, P., and Massague, J. 1994. Cloning of p27Kip1, a cyclin-dependent kinase inhibitor and a potential mediator of extracellular antimitogenic signals. *Cell* **78:**, 59-66.

Qian, Y. W., and Lee, E. Y. 1995. Dual retinoblastoma-binding proteins with properties related to a negative regulator of ras in yeast. *J Biol Chem* **270:**, 25507-13.

Qin, X. Q., Livingston, D. M., Ewen, M., Sellers, W. R., Arany, Z., and Kaelin, W. G., Jr. 1995. The transcription factor E2F-1 is a downstream target of RB action. *Mol Cell Biol* **15:**, 742-55.

Rane, S. G., Cosenza, S. C., Mettus, R. V., and Reddy, E. P. 2002. Germ line transmission of the Cdk4(R24C) mutation facilitates tumorigenesis and escape from cellular senescence. *Mol Cell Biol* **22:**, 644-56.

Rane, S. G., Dubus, P., Mettus, R. V., Galbreath, E. J., Boden, G., Reddy, E. P., and Barbacid, M. 1999. Loss of Cdk4 expression causes insulin-deficient diabetes and Cdk4 activation results in beta-islet cell hyperplasia. *Nat Genet* **22:**, 44-52.

Rempel, R. E., Saenz-Robles, M. T., Storms, R., Morham, S., Ishida, S., Engel, A., Jakoi, L., Melhem, M. F., Pipas, J. M., Smith, C., and Nevins, J. R. 2000. Loss of E2F4 activity leads to abnormal development of multiple cellular lineages. *Mol Cell* **6:**, 293-306.

Reynisdottir, I., Polyak, K., Iavarone, A., and Massague, J. 1995. Kip/Cip and Ink4 Cdk inhibitors cooperate to induce cell cycle arrest in response to TGF-beta. *Genes Dev* **9:**, 1831-45.

Robanus-Maandag, E., Dekker, M., van der Valk, M., Carrozza, M. L., Jeanny, J. C., Dannenberg, J. H., Berns, A., and te Riele, H. 1998. p107 is a suppressor of retinoblastoma development in pRb-deficient mice. *Genes Dev* **12:**, 1599-609.

Ruas, M., and Peters, G. 1998. The p16INK4a/CDKN2A tumor suppressor and its relatives. *Biochim Biophys Acta* **1378:**, F115-77.

Rubin, E., Mittnacht, S., Villa-Moruzzi, E., and Ludlow, J. W. 2001. Site-specific and temporally-regulated retinoblastoma protein dephosphorylation by protein phosphatase type 1. *Oncogene* **20:**, 3776-85.

Russell, J. L., Powers, J. T., Rounbehler, R. J., Rogers, P. M., Conti, C. J., and Johnson, D. G. 2002. ARF Differentially Modulates Apoptosis Induced by E2F1 and Myc. *Mol. Cell. Biol.* **22:**, 1360-8.

Sage, J., Mulligan, G. J., Attardi, L. D., Miller, A., Chen, S., Williams, B., Theodorou, E., and Jacks, T. 2000. Targeted disruption of the three Rb-related genes leads to loss of G(1) control and immortalization. *Genes Dev* **14:**, 3037-50.

Schmidt, E. E., Ichimura, K., Reifenberger, G., and Collins, V. P. 1994. CDKN2 (p16/MTS1) gene deletion or CDK4 amplification occurs in the majority of glioblastomas. *Cancer Res* **54:**, 6321-4.

Schwab, M., and Tyers, M. 2001. Cell cycle. Archipelago of destruction. *Nature* **413:**, 268-9.

Sears, R., Ohtani, K., and Nevins, J. R. 1997. Identification of positively and negatively acting elements regulating expression of the E2F2 gene in response to cell growth signals. *Mol Cell Biol* **17:**, 5227-35.

Sellers, W. R., Novitch, B. G., Miyake, S., Heith, A., Otterson, G. A., Kaye, F. J., Lassar, A. B., and Kaelin, W. G., Jr. 1998. Stable binding to E2F is not required for the retinoblastoma protein to activate transcription, promote differentiation, and suppress tumor cell growth. *Genes Dev* **12:**, 95-106.

Seoane, J., Pouponnot, C., Staller, P., Schader, M., Eilers, M., and Massague, J. 2001. TGFbeta influences Myc, Miz-1 and Smad to control the CDK inhibitor p15INK4b. *Nat Cell Biol* **3:**, 400-8.

Serrano, M., Lee, H., Chin, L., Cordon-Cardo, C., Beach, D., and DePinho, R. A. 1996. Role of the INK4a locus in tumor suppression and cell mortality. *Cell* **85:**, 27-37.

Serrano, M., Lin, A. W., McCurrach, M. E., Beach, D., and Lowe, S. W. 1997. Oncogenic ras provokes premature cell senescence associated with accumulation of p53 and p16INK4a. *Cell* **88:**, 593-602.

Shan, B., and Lee, W. H. 1994. Deregulated expression of E2F-1 induces S-phase entry and leads to apoptosis. *Mol Cell Biol* **14:**, 8166-73.

Sharpless, N. E., Bardeesy, N., Lee, K. H., Carrasco, D., Castrillon, D. H., Aguirre, A. J., Wu, E. A., Horner, J. W., and DePinho, R. A. 2001. Loss of p16Ink4a with retention of p19Arf predisposes mice to tumorigenesis. *Nature* **413:**, 86-91.

Sherr, C. J. 1996. Cancer cell cycles. *Science* **274:**, 1672-7.

Sherr, C. J. 2001. Parsing Ink4a/Arf: "pure" p16-null mice. *Cell* **106:**, 531-4.

Sherr, C. J. 2000. The Pezcoller lecture: cancer cell cycles revisited. *Cancer Res.* **60:**, 3689-95.

Sicinski, P., Donaher, J. L., Geng, Y., Parker, S. B., Gardner, H., Park, M. Y., Robker, R. L., Richards, J. S., McGinnis, L. K., Biggers, J. D., Eppig, J. J., Bronson, R. T., Elledge, S. J., and Weinberg, R. A. 1996. Cyclin D2 is an FSH-responsive gene involved in gonadal cell proliferation and oncogenesis. *Nature* **384:**, 470-4.

Sicinski, P., Donaher, J. L., Parker, S. B., Li, T., Fazeli, A., Gardner, H., Haslam, S. Z., Bronson, R. T., Elledge, S. J., and Weinberg, R. A. 1995. Cyclin D1 provides a link between development and oncogenesis in the retina and breast. *Cell* **82:**, 621-30.

Slansky, J. E., Li, Y., Kaelin, W. G., and Farnham, P. J. 1993. A protein synthesis-dependent increase in E2F1 mRNA correlates with growth regulation of the dihydrofolate reductase promoter. *Mol Cell Biol* **13:**, 1610-8.

Sotillo, R., Dubus, P., Martin, J., de la Cueva, E., Ortega, S., Malumbres, M., and Barbacid, M. 2001. Wide spectrum of tumors in knock-in mice carrying a Cdk4 protein insensitive to INK4 inhibitors. *Embo J.* **20:**, 6637-47.

Staller, P., Peukert, K., Kiermaier, A., Seoane, J., Lukas, J., Karsunky, H., Moroy, T., Bartek, J., Massague, J., Hanel, F., and Eilers, M. Cell Biol 2001 Apr. Repression of p15INK4b expression by Myc through association with Miz-1. *Nat* **3:**, 392-9.

Strobeck, M. W., Knudsen, K. E., Fribourg, A. F., DeCristofaro, M. F., Weissman, B. E., Imbalzano, A. N., and Knudsen, E. S. 2000. BRG-1 is required for RB-mediated cell cycle arrest. *Proc Natl Acad Sci U S A* **97:**, 7748-53.

Strohmaier, H., Spruck, C. H., Kaiser, P., Won, K. A., Sangfelt, O., and Reed, S. I. 2001. Human F-box protein hCdc4 targets cyclin E for proteolysis and is mutated in a breast cancer cell line. *Nature* **413:**, 316-22.
Sumegi, J., Uzvolgyi, E., and Klein, G. 1990. Expression of the RB gene under the control of MuLV-LTR suppresses tumorigenicity of WERI-Rb-27 retinoblastoma cells in immunodefective mice. *Cell Growth Differ* **1:**, 247-50.
T'Ang, A., Varley, J. M., Chakraborty, S., Murphree, A. L., and Fung, Y. K. 1988. Structural rearrangement of the retinoblastoma gene in human breast carcinoma. *Science* **242:**, 263-6.
Takahashi, R., Hashimoto, T., Xu, H. J., Hu, S. X., Matsui, T., Miki, T., Bigo-Marshall, H., Aaronson, S. A., and Benedict, W. F. 1991. The retinoblastoma gene functions as a growth and tumor suppressor in human bladder carcinoma cells. *Proc Natl Acad Sci U S A* **88:**, 5257-61.
Tokitou, F., Nomura, T., Khan, M. M., Kaul, S. C., Wadhwa, R., Yasukawa, T., Kohno, I., and Ishii, S. 1999. Viral ski inhibits retinoblastoma protein (Rb)-mediated transcriptional repression in a dominant negative fashion. *J Biol Chem* **274:**, 4485-8.
Trimarchi, J. M., and Lees, J. A. 2002. Sibling rivalry in the E2F family. *Nat. Rev. Mol. Cell. Biol.* **3:**, 11-20.
Trouche, D., Le Chalony, C., Muchardt, C., Yaniv, M., and Kouzarides, T. 1997. RB and hbrm cooperate to repress the activation functions of E2F1. *Proc Natl Acad Sci U S A* **94:**, 11268-73.
Tsai, K. Y., Hu, Y., Macleod, K. F., Crowley, D., Yamasaki, L., and Jacks, T. 1998. Mutation of E2f-1 suppresses apoptosis and inappropriate S phase entry and extends survival of Rb-deficient mouse embryos. *Mol Cell* **2:**, 293-304.
Tsai, K. Y., MacPherson, D., Rubinson, D. A., Crowley, D., and Jacks, T. 2002. ARF is not required for apoptosis in Rb mutant mouse embryos. *Curr Biol.* **12:**, 159-63.
Tsutsui, T., Hesabi, B., Moons, D. S., Pandolfi, P. P., Hansel, K. S., Koff, A., and Kiyokawa, H. 1999. Targeted disruption of CDK4 delays cell cycle entry with enhanced p27(Kip1) activity. *Mol Cell Biol* **19:**, 7011-9.
Vandel, L., Nicolas, E., Vaute, O., Ferreira, R., Ait-Si-Ali, S., and Trouche, D. 2001. Transcriptional repression by the retinoblastoma protein through the recruitment of a histone methyltransferase. *Mol Cell Biol* **21:**, 6484-94.
Verona, R., Moberg, K., Estes, S., Starz, M., Vernon, J. P., and Lees, J. A. 1997. E2F activity is regulated by cell cycle-dependent changes in subcellular localization. *Mol Cell Biol* **17:**, 7268-82.
Wang, C. Y., Petryniak, B., Thompson, C. B., Kaelin, W. G., and Leiden, J. M. 1993. Regulation of the Ets-related transcription factor Elf-1 by binding to the retinoblastoma protein. *Science* **260:**, 1330-5.
Wang, T. C., Cardiff, R. D., Zukerberg, L., Lees, E., Arnold, A., and Schmidt, E. V. 1994. Mammary hyperplasia and carcinoma in MMTV-cyclin D1 transgenic mice. *Nature* **369:**, 669-71.
Weber, J. D., Jeffers, J. R., Rehg, J. E., Randle, D. H., Lozano, G., Roussel, M. F., Sherr, C. J., and Zambetti, G. P. 2000. p53-independent functions of the p19(ARF) tumor suppressor. *Genes Dev* **14:**, 2358-65.
Weinmann, A. S., Yan, P. S., Oberley, M. J., Huang, T. H., and Farnham, P. J. 2002. Isolating human transcription factor targets by coupling chromatin immunoprecipitation and CpG island microarray analysis. *Genes Dev* **16:**, 235-44.
Weintraub, S. J., Prater, C. A., and Dean, D. C. 1992. Retinoblastoma protein switches the E2F site from positive to negative element. *Nature* **358:**, 259-61.
Wells, J., Graveel, C. R., Bartley, S. M., Madore, S. J., and Farnham, P. J. 2002. The identification of E2F1-specific target genes. *Proc Natl Acad Sci U S A* **99:**, 3890-5.

Whyte, P., Buchkovich, K. J., Horowitz, J. M., Friend, S. H., Raybuck, M., Weinberg, R. A., and Harlow, E. 1988. Association between an oncogene and an anti-oncogene: the adenovirus E1A proteins bind to the retinoblastoma gene product. *Nature* **334:**, 124-9.
Williams, B. O., Remington, L., Albert, D. M., Mukai, S., Bronson, R. T., and Jacks, T. 1994. Cooperative tumorigenic effects of germline mutations in Rb and p53. *Nat Genet* **7:**, 480-4.
Williams, B. O., Schmitt, E. M., Remington, L., Bronson, R. T., Albert, D. M., Weinberg, R. A., and Jacks, T. 1994. Extensive contribution of Rb-deficient cells to adult chimeric mice with limited histopathological consequences. *Embo J* **13:**, 4251-9.
Wolfel, T., Hauer, M., Schneider, J., Serrano, M., Wolfel, C., Klehmann-Hieb, E., De Plaen, E., Hankeln, T., Meyer zum Buschenfelde, K. H., and Beach, D. 1995. A p16INK4a-insensitive CDK4 mutant targeted by cytolytic T lymphocytes in a human melanoma. *Science* **269:**, 1281-4.
Wu, L., Timmers, C., Maiti, B., Saavedra, H. I., Sang, L., Chong, G. T., Nuckolls, F., Giangrande, P., Wright, F. A., Field, S. J., Greenberg, M. E., Orkin, S., Nevins, J. R., Robinson, M. L., and Leone,

G. 2001. The E2F1-3 transcription factors are essential for cellular proliferation. *Nature* **414:**, 457-62.
Wu, X., and Levine, A. J. 1994. p53 and E2F-1 cooperate to mediate apoptosis. *Proc Natl Acad Sci U S A* **91:**, 3602-6.
Xiong, Y., Hannon, G. J., Zhang, H., Casso, D., Kobayashi, R., and Beach, D. 1993. p21 is a universal inhibitor of cyclin kinases. *Nature* **366:**, 701-4.
Xu, M., Sheppard, K. A., Peng, C. Y., Yee, A. S., and Piwnica-Worms, H. 1994. Cyclin A/CDK2 binds directly to E2F-1 and inhibits the DNA-binding activity of E2F-1/DP-1 by phosphorylation. *Mol Cell Biol* **14:**, 8420-31.
Yamasaki, L., Bronson, R., Williams, B. O., Dyson, N. J., Harlow, E., and Jacks, T. 1998. Loss of E2F-1 reduces tumorigenesis and extends the lifespan of Rb1(+/-)mice. *Nat Genet* **18:**, 360-4.
Yamasaki, L., Jacks, T., Bronson, R., Goillot, E., Harlow, E., and Dyson, N. J. 1996. Tumor induction and tissue atrophy in mice lacking E2F-1. *Cell* **85:**, 537-48.
Yang, H., Williams, B. O., Hinds, P. W., Shih, T. S., Jacks, T., Bronson, R. T., and Livingston, D. M. 2002. Tumor suppression by a severely truncated species of retinoblastoma protein. *Mol Cell Biol* **22:**, 3103-10.
Yee, A. S., Reichel, R., Kovesdi, I., and Nevins, J. R. 1987. Promoter interaction of the E1A-inducible factor E2F and its potential role in the formation of a multi-component complex. *Embo J* **6:**, 2061-8.
Zacksenhaus, E., Jiang, Z., Chung, D., Marth, J. D., Phillips, R. A., and Gallie, B. L. 1996. pRb controls proliferation, differentiation, and death of skeletal muscle cells and other lineages during embryogenesis. *Genes Dev* **10:**, 3051-64.
Zarkowska, T., and Mittnacht, S. 1997. Differential phosphorylation of the retinoblastoma protein by G1/S cyclin-dependent kinases. *J Biol Chem* **272:**, 12738-46.
Zhang, H. S., Gavin, M., Dahiya, A., Postigo, A. A., Ma, D., Luo, R. X., Harbour, J. W., and Dean, D. C. 2000. Exit from G1 and S phase of the cell cycle is regulated by repressor complexes containing HDAC-Rb-hSWI/SNF and Rb-hSWI/SNF. *Cell* **101:**, 79-89.
Zhang, P., Liegeois, N. J., Wong, C., Finegold, M., Hou, H., Thompson, J. C., Silverman, A., Harper, J. W., DePinho, R. A., and Elledge, S. J. 1997. Altered cell differentiation and proliferation in mice lacking p57KIP2 indicates a role in Beckwith-Wiedemann syndrome. *Nature* **387:**, 151-8.
Zheng, N., Fraenkel, E., Pabo, C. O., and Pavletich, N. P. 1999. Structural basis of DNA recognition by the heterodimeric cell cycle transcription factor E2F-DP. *Genes Dev* **13:**, 666-74.
Zhu, J. W., Field, S. J., Gore, L., Thompson, M., Yang, H., Fujiwara, Y., Cardiff, R. D., Greenberg, M., Orkin, S. H., and DeGregori, J. 2001. E2F1 and E2F2 determine thresholds for antigen-induced T-cell proliferation and suppress tumorigenesis. *Mol Cell Biol* **21:**, 8547-64.
Zhu, L., Enders, G., Lees, J. A., Beijersbergen, R. L., Bernards, R., and Harlow, E. 1995. The pRB-related protein p107 contains two growth suppression domains: independent interactions with E2F and cyclin/cdk complexes. *Embo J* **14:**, 1904-13.
Zhu, L., van den Heuvel, S., Helin, K., Fattaey, A., Ewen, M., Livingston, D., Dyson, N., and Harlow, E. 1993. Inhibition of cell proliferation by p107, a relative of the retinoblastoma protein. *Genes Dev* **7:**, 1111-25.
Ziebold, U., Reza, T., Caron, A., and Lees, J. A. 2001. E2F3 contributes both to the inappropriate proliferation and to the apoptosis arising in Rb mutant embryos. *Genes Dev.* **15:**, 386-91.
Zindy, F., den Besten, W., Chen, B., Rehg, J. E., Latres, E., Barbacid, M., Pollard, J. W., Sherr, C. J., Cohen, P. E., and Roussel, M. F. 2001. Control of spermatogenesis in mice by the cyclin D-dependent kinase inhibitors p18(Ink4c) and p19(Ink4d). *Mol Cell Biol* **21:**, 3244-55.
Zindy, F., Soares, H., Herzog, K. H., Morgan, J., Sherr, C. J., and Roussel, M. F. 1997. Expression of INK4 inhibitors of cyclin D-dependent kinases during mouse brain development. *Cell Growth Differ* **8:**, 1139-50.
Zindy, F., van Deursen, J., Grosveld, G., Sherr, C. J., and Roussel, M. F. 2000. INK4d-deficient mice are fertile despite testicular atrophy. *Mol Cell Biol* **20:**, 372-8.
Zuo, L., Weger, J., Yang, Q., Goldstein, A. M., Tucker, M. A., Walker, G. J., Hayward, N., and Dracopoli, N. C. 1996. Germline mutations in the p16INK4a binding domain of CDK4 in familial melanoma. *Nat Genet* **12:**, 97-9.

THE Rel/NF-κB/IκB SIGNAL TRANSDUCTION PATHWAY AND CANCER

THOMAS D. GILMORE

1. INTRODUCTION

Most cancers are the result of the coordinate misregulation of a variety of cellular and organismal processes, including growth control (oncogenes and tumor supressor genes), survival (anti-apoptosis), angiogenesis, and immune recognition. Similarly, signal transduction pathways invariably regulate an array of cellular processes, often by affecting the activity of individual transcription factors that control the expression of specific sets of genes. As such, it is not surprising that mutations that result in the misregulation of signaling proteins, especially transcription factors, are frequently involved in oncogenesis. This chapter will focus on a family of eukaryotic transcription factors, the Rel/NF-κB family, which has been implicated in the development of many human cancers, and more recently, has been a target for molecular intervention for a variety of malignancies.

1.1 Rel/NF-κB Proteins and Structures

The Rel/NF-κB family of transcription factors includes several proteins, which are highly conserved structurally and functionally from insects to humans (reviewed in Gilmore, 1999a). The evolutionarily conserved function of Rel/NF-κB factors in insects and mammals appears to be to control the expression of genes involved in the innate immune response (reviewed in Ghosh & May, 1999; Silverman & Maniatis, 2001). In mammals, activation of innate immunity by, for example, bacterial infection results in the rapid synthesis of anti-microbial molecules and cytokines (e.g., interleukins, tumor necrosis factor [TNF]). However, in vertebrates, Rel/NF-κB transcription factors also regulate many other sets of genes, including ones encoding molecules of acquired immunity (e.g., the immunoglobulin κ light chain), adhesion molecules, and proteins involved in the control of cell growth and programmed cell death (apoptosis).

The vertebrate Rel family includes c-Rel, RelA (p65), RelB, p50/p100, p52/p100, and the retroviral oncoprotein v-Rel (Figure 1). (In this review, genes/proteins in all capital letters [e.g., *REL*/REL] refer to human versions, while lowercase [e.g., c-*rel*/c-Rel] is used for other species or general nomenclature.) Cellular Rel/NF-κB proteins can form homodimers or heterodimers, which bind to DNA sites (called κB sites) with high affinity. In many cells, the most common dimer of this family is a p50-RelA heterodimer, which is specifically referred to as NF-κB.

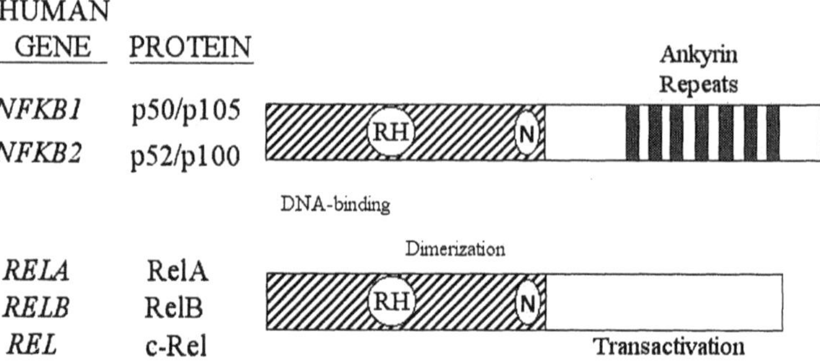

Figure 1. Vertebrate Rel/NF-κB proteins. Shown are the generalized structures of cellular Rel/NF-κB proteins. All Rel/NF-κB proteins contain an N-terminal Rel homology (RH) domain (hatched) that contains sequences important for DNA binding (towards the N-terminal half of the RH domain), the formation of dimers (towards the C-terminal half of the RH domain), and nuclear localization (N; at the extreme C terminus of the RH domain). One class of Rel/NF-κB protein contains C-terminal domains with ankyrin repeats (shaded), which block DNA binding by the full-length protein; the shorter version of these proteins lack the C-terminal sequences and can bind DNA. Members of the second class of Rel/NF-κB protein have C-terminal transactivation domains. To the left, the names of the human genes encoding the indicated Rel/NF-κB proteins are listed.

Cellular Rel/NF-κB proteins are related through a conserved N-terminal domain, called the Rel Homology (RH) domain, which contains sequences essential for DNA binding, dimerization, and nuclear localization (Figure 1). Rel/NF-κB proteins can be subdivided into two classes based on sequences C-terminal to the RH domain. Members of one class (p50/p105 and p52/p100) can exist in two forms: short forms (p50 and p52) that bind DNA and long forms (p105 and p100, respectively) that act as inhibitors of DNA binding (see Section 1.2, below). Members of the second class (c-Rel, RelA, RelB) have C-terminal sequences that contain transcriptional activation domains. Thus, dimers such as p50-p50 (which lack transactivation domains) often repress transcription, whereas dimers that include RelA, c-Rel, or RelB usually activate transcription.

The X-ray crystal structures of several Rel/NF-κB dimers (p50-p50, p50-RelA, RelA-RelA, c-Rel-c-Rel) bound to DNA have been solved (reviewed in Chen & Ghosh, 1999). These structures show that the dimer is essentially wrapped around the target DNA and makes multiple contacts both with specific bases within the major groove and nonspecifically with the phosphate backbone. These multiple specific and nonspecific DNA contacts account for the high affinity with which Rel/NF-κB dimers bind to DNA. The κB sites that are bound by different Rel/NF-κB dimers can vary considerably, and some dimers prefer 9 bp sites whereas others prefer 10 bp ones (Huang et al., 2001a).

1.2. Activation of the Rel/NF-κB Signaling Pathway

Rel/NF-κB complexes are regulated by direct interaction with a second family of proteins called IκB proteins, which generally act as inhibitors of Rel/NF-κB complexes. IκB proteins include IκBα, IκBβ, IκBε, IκBγ, Bcl-3, and the p105 and p100 proteins (reviewed in Karin, 1999). All IκB proteins contain 7 to 8 ankyrin repeats, which are essential for interaction with Rel/NF-κB complexes. The interaction of an IκB protein with a Rel/NF-κB complex generally has two consequences: 1) the IκB blocks DNA binding, and 2) IκB causes the complex to be localized primarily in the cytoplasm.

Many extracellular signals and intracellular stresses can activate Rel/NF-κB complexes (reviewed in Pahl, 1999). These signals include cytokines, growth factors, viral infection, and irradiation, among others. Pathways leading to activation of Rel/NF-κB complexes by these diverse signals usually converge at the point of activation of an IκB kinase (IKK) that phosphorylates IκB and targets IκB for degradation. This sequence of events enables NF-κB to enter the nucleus, bind to DNA, and regulate gene transcription.

There are (at least) two distinct, but related, pathways for induction of nuclear Rel/NF-κB activity (see Figure 2). In one case, there are complexes that contain two Rel/NF-κB subunits (such as p50-RelA) bound to a self-contained IκB protein (such as IκBα); in these complexes, the full IκB protein is degraded. In the second case, a dimer such as p100-RelA undergoes partial proteolysis, in which only the C-terminal sequences of p100 are degraded to yield an active p52-RelA dimer.

The regulation of NF-κB by IκBα is now known in some detail (Figure 2) (reviewed in Silverman & Maniatis, 2001). In most cells, the p50-RelA NF-κB dimer is in an inactive form in the cytoplasm where it is complexed with IκBα. The X-ray crystal structure of the NF-κB-IκBα complex reveals that IκBα blocks the ability of NF-κB to bind DNA by directly covering residues involved in this activity (Huxford et al., 1998; Jacobs & Harrison, 1998). Although it was originally thought that IκBα also covered the nuclear localization sequence of NF-κB to keep it in the cytoplasm, it is now more generally believed that the NF-κB-IκBα complex is continually cycling between the nucleus and the cytoplasm. The NF-κB-IκBα complex is primarily cytoplasmic due to a strong nuclear export

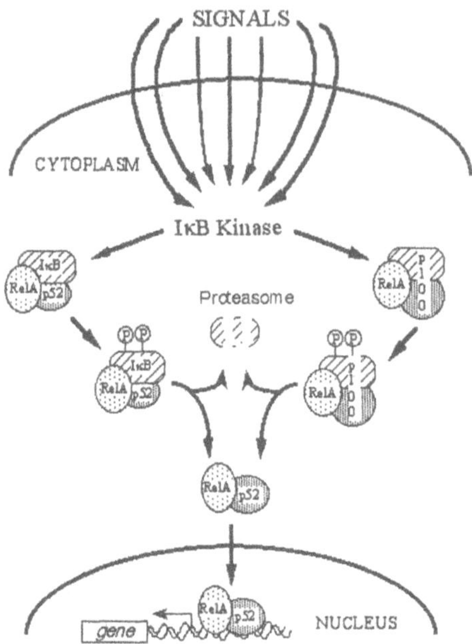

Figure 2. Activation of NF-κB. As discussed in the text, a variety of signals can lead to activation of the Rel/NF-κB pathway. Generally, these signals converge on the activation of the IκB kinase (IKK). Depending on the signal and cell type, active IKK can induce one of two pathways. In one case (to the left), a complex such as p52-RelA is bound by a separate IκB inhibitor; in the second case (to the right), there is a complex such as p100-RelA in which the C-terminal sequences of p100 act as the IκB. In both cases, IKK phosphorylates specific serine residues within the IκB sequences, which targets them for degradation by the proteasome. The liberated complex (p52-RelA) can then accumulate in the nucleus and increase target gene transcription. Although not shown here, the induction of Rel/NF-κB is generally transient: for example, one of the NF-κB target genes encodes IκB, and the newly-synthesized IκB can resequester the active NF-κB complexes in the cytoplasm to terminate the induction.

signal in IκBα that overrides the still exposed nuclear localizing signal of NF-κB. Activation of the IκB kinase results in phosphorylation of IκBα at two N-terminal serine residues (Ser-32 and 36 in human IκBα). Phosphorylated IκBα then undergoes polyubiqutination by a specific ubiquitin ligase complex (β-TRCP-SCF), and ubiquitination targets IκBα for degradation by the proteasome. Degradation of IκBα enables the rapid accumulation of active NF-κB in the nucleus, in that NF-κB is no longer exported from the nucleus by IκBα, and NF-κB is free to bind to promoters/enhancers in DNA to usually increase target gene expression. However, it is now becoming clear that NF-κB activity is also modulated at other points in this simple scheme, such as by phosphorylation of RelA as it enters the nucleus and by acetylation of p50.

One essential feature of activation of NF-κB in most cells is that it is transient, lasting only about 15-45 minutes. Because the gene encoding IκBα contains upstream κB sites, its expression is also increased upon activation of NF-κB. Thus, newly synthesized IκBα protein can shut off the response by removing NF-κB from DNA and causing it to be resequestered in the cytoplasm. In a small number of normal cells, such as B lymphocytes and some neurons, NF-κB is constitutively active, due to chronic degradation of IκBα.

A second Rel/NF-κB pathway activates dimeric complexes that contain p100 (reviewed in Silverman & Maniatis, 2001). As mentioned above, p105 and p100 can act as IκB proteins for complexes such as p105-RelA or p100-RelA, which can then be processed into p50-RelA and p52-RelA, respectively, by selective degradation of the C-terminal ankyrin repeat domains of p105 and p100. Regulated processing is best understood in the case of p100. At least in maturing B cells, processing of p100 to p52 is mediated by NIK-induced activation of IKKα, which then phosphorylates specific residues in the C-terminal half of p100 to lead to its ubiquitination, and processing to p52 (Senftleben et al., 2001; Xiao et al., 2001b). An inactivating mutation in either the gene encoding p52/p100 or NIK results in defects in B-cell development, due at least in part to defects in p100 processing to p52 (Gerondakis et al., 1999; Shinkura et al., 1999; Xiao et al., 2001b).

1.3. Regulation of the IκB Kinase (IKK) Complex

Much attention has focused on the IKK complex because nearly all signals that lead to activation of the Rel/NF-κB pathway pass through IKK (reviewed in Karin & Ben-Neriah, 2000; Silverman & Maniatis, 2001). The IKK complex is a cytoplasmic complex that, in most cells, is comprised of one α, one β, and two γ subunits. IKKα and IKKβ are catalytic kinase subunits, which phosphorylate regulatory serine residues on IκBs. IKKα and β are highly related to one another, and usually exist as a catalytic heterodimer; however, in some cell types homodimers of α or β may serve the catalytic function of the IKK complex. In addition, there are at least two other IKK-like kinases (IKKε and TBK; Peters & Maniatis, 2001). The precise function of IKKγ is a bit unclear; however, under most circumstances IKKγ is required for activation of the NF-κB pathway, and probably acts as a scaffold or sensing molecule for the IKK complex.

IKKα and β are both regulated by a complex series of phosphorylations. In order to be activated, IKKα and β undergo phosphorylation at two closely spaced serine residues within an activation loop. Thus, substitution of glutamic acid residues for these serine residues creates constitutively active kinases. Therefore, IKK is itself regulated by upstream kinases. Here again, there is some controversy, and the simplest resolution is that there are likely to be several IKK regulatory kinases, including the IKKs themselves (which can cross- and auto-phosphorylate), NF-κB-inducing kinase (NIK), and certain MAP kinases, and that these various IKK kinases are involved in transmitting different upstream signals to IKK in different cell types.

Once activated by phosphorylations within the activation loop, the IKK catalytic kinases can, of course, signal to NF-κB by phosphorylating IκBs. However, IKKα and β also undergo extensive trans- or autophosphorylations at clustered serine residues within their C-terminal domains; these C-terminal phosphorylations lead to the return of the IKK complex to its inactive state, shutting off the NF-κB response.

In some cases, activation loop phosphorylation may not be required for activation of IKK. That is, induced or forced clustering of the kinases may be sufficient to activate IKK. Such clustering may occur normally by recruiment of the kinases to the plasma membrane by adaptor proteins (e.g., as by RIP, a TNF receptor adaptor, or by IRAK, an IL-1 signaling adaptor) or upon overexpression in transfection experiments.

The IKK catalytic subunit (i.e., α or β) that is activated in response to different upstream signals can also be distinct. For example, IKKβ (but not α) is required for phosphorylating IκBα in response to proinflammatory stimuli such as TNFα and LPS in liver and lymphoid cells, whereas IKKα leads to activation of NF-κB (p50-RelA) in response to the RANK-ligand in mammary epithelial cells (Cao et al., 2001). Thus, although the general outline of IKK regulation is understood, there are many subtleties that remain to be clarified.

1.4. Inhibition of the Rel/NF-κB Signaling Pathway

The understanding of the regulation of the NF-κB signaling pathway has led to the development of many molecular and pharmacologic inhibitors that act at various points in this pathway (reviewed in Epinat & Gilmore, 1999; Yamamoto & Gaynor, 2001). Perhaps the most commonly used molecular inhibitor of NF-κB activation is the so-called IκBα super-repressor, which is a non-degradable form IκBα that has mutations or deletion of the Ser residues that are phosphorylated by IKK. Similarly, kinase-dead IKKα and β mutants can often act as dominant-negative blockers of NF-κB activation. Other molecular inhibitors include peptides that contain the nuclear targeting sequence of p50 or RelA and thus competitively block nuclear translocation of NF-κB, and κB site oligonucleotides that compete for promoter-enhancer binding by NF-κB. Among pharmacologic inhibitors, one class of commonly-used inhibitors includes ones that inhibit the proteasome and thus block degradation of IκBα. Recent attention has also focused on many chemicals, natural products or small molecules that appear to act as anti-inflammatory agents or anti-tumor agents by inhibiting activation of IKK or DNA binding by NF-κB.

2. THE AVIAN RETROVIRAL ONCOPROTEIN v-Rel AND ONCOGENESIS

The clearest demonstration that Rel/NF-κB transcription factors are involved in cancer is provided by the highly oncogenic avian Rev-T retrovirus, which was originally isolated from a turkey with an extensive malignant reticular disease. Current viral stocks of Rev-T induce a rapidly fatal lymphoma/leukemia in young birds, due to the action of the sole viral gene, v-*rel* (reviewed in Gilmore, 1999b).

Furthermore, transgenic mice in which v-*rel* is expressed under the control of a T cell-specific promoter develop T-cell lymphomas (Carrasco et al., 1996). In vitro, v-Rel can transform and immortalize a variety of chicken hematopoietic cell types, including B- and T-lymphoid cells, myeloid cells, erythroid cells, and dendritic cells. Moreover, retroviral vectors for the overexpression of chicken, mouse, and human c-Rel can transform chicken lymphoid cells in vitro, although these normal c-Rel proteins are less efficient than v-Rel at transforming cells in culture (Gilmore et al., 2001; reviewed in Gilmore, 1999b).

v-Rel is a more effective transforming agent than its avian progenitor c-Rel due to multiple mutations that have arisen during passage of Rev-T in culture. Due to these mutations, v-Rel differs in several structural and functional ways from chicken c-Rel. Most obviously, v-Rel is missing 2 N-terminal amino acids (aa) and 118 C-terminal aa as compared to chicken c-Rel. In place of these c-Rel residues, v-Rel has N-terminal and C-terminal virus-derived Envelope aa. The C-terminal truncation of c-Rel aa confers much of the increased oncogenicity onto v-Rel. That is, a C terminally-truncated chicken c-Rel protein is approximately 10-fold more transforming than wild-type c-Rel in culture (Hrdlicková et al., 1994; Kamens et al., 1990) and deletions in sequences encoding C-terminal sequences often occur in viral vectors containing wild-type c-*rel* that are selected for the ability to transform chicken lymphoid cells (Gilmore et al., 1995; Hrdlicková et al., 1994). The C-terminal deletion removes c-Rel residues that are involved in transactivation and cytoplasmic localization. However, other mutations also contribute to the full oncogenicity of v-Rel, and in some cases the functional consequences of these oncogenic mutations are known. For example, the N-terminal Env aa in v-Rel endow it with a new transactivation domain (Epinat et al., 2000), two mutations decrease the ability of v-Rel to interact with IκBα (Sachdev & Hannnik, 1998), three mutations affect the DNA-binding site specificity of v-Rel (Huang et al., 2001a; Nehyba et al., 1997), and one mutation increases the stability of v-Rel (Mosialos & Gilmore, 1993). Thus, v-Rel is a misregulated version of avian c-Rel.

The ability of v-Rel to transform and immortalize chicken lymphoid cells in culture is dependent on its ability to be expressed at a high level, to form homodimers, to enter the nucleus (in part by escaping regulation by IκBα), to bind to DNA, and to activate transcription (reviewed in Gilmore, 1999b). Genetic studies in mice suggest that v-Rel also transforms mouse T cells by a similar mechanism (Carrasco et al., 1996; Carrasco et al., 1997).

Therefore, it is likely that v-Rel induces oncogenesis in lymphoid cells by increasing the expression of a specific set of genes involved in promoting cell growth and blocking apoptosis (reviewed in Gilmore, 1999b). Consistent with this model, many of the target genes for v-Rel in transformed chicken or mouse cells are involved in cellular growth control or apoptosis. Such v-Rel target genes include proto-oncogenes (c-*jun*, c-*rel*), transcription factors (STAT1), cytokine receptors (IL-2Rα), growth inducing molecules (IRF-4), and anti-apoptotic molecules (IAP1). Nevertheless, it is not precisely known which genes are essential for transformation by v-Rel. Because the altered expression of multiple genes probably contributes to v-Rel-induced oncogenesis, inhibition of only one or a few of these genes may not be sufficient to fully block oncogenesis. In that v-Rel has several mutations that make it a more potent oncoprotein than cellular Rel/NF-κB proteins, all of the molecular details of how v-Rel causes avian lymphoid cell oncogenesis may not be analogous to how misregulated Rel/NF-κB proteins are involved in human oncogenesis. Nevertheless, as discussed below, the general mechanism by which v-Rel is likely to promote avian lymphoid cell oncogenesis--by increasing the expression of cell proliferation and survival genes--is no doubt similar to what occurs in human cancers with misregulated cellular Rel/NF-κB proteins.

3. GENETIC ALTERATIONS OF Rel/NF-κB/IκB IN HUMAN CANCERS

Genetic alterations in Rel/NF-κB and IκB genes have been identified in several human cancers, especially ones of lymphoid origin (reviewed also in Gilmore et al., 2002) (Table 1). These alterations include amplifications, chromosomal rearrangements, and point mutations. The genes in this pathway that appear to be most consistently altered in human cancers are those encoding REL, p52/p100, IκBα, and BCL-3.

Table 1. Genetic alterations in Rel/NF-κB/IκB signaling in human cancers

Alterations	Gene
Rearrangements	*REL, NFKB2, BCL-3*
Amplifications	*REL*
Point mutations	*RELA, IKBA*

3.1. REL *Gene Amplification and Rearrangement in Human B-Cell Malignancies*

The human *REL* gene is located at chromosomal position 2p16.1-15. *REL* gene amplification is seen in perhaps as many as 10-20% of non-Hodgkin's B-cell lymphomas, including diffuse large B-cell lymphomas (DBCLs), follicular lymphomas, and mediastinal thymic B-cell lymphomas (Barth et al., 1998; Barth et al., 2001; Goff et al., 2000; Houldsworth et al., 1996; Joos et al., 1996; Lu et al., 1991; Neat et al., 2001; Palanisamy et al., 2002; Rao et al., 1998). In these cancers, *REL* has been found to be amplified from 4- to 75-fold.

Three lines of evidence indicate that overexpression of REL contributes to proliferation and cell survival in these human B-cell malignancies. First, as mentioned above, overexpression of human REL can malignantly transform and immortalize primary chicken lymphoid cells in culture (Gilmore et al., 2001). Second, several Rel/NF-κB target genes, including genes encoding cytokines, chemokines, and anti-apoptotic factors, are overexpressed in one type of DBCL, classified as an activated B cell-like DBCL based on cDNA microarray expression data (Alizadeh et al., 2000; Davis et al., 2001). Moreover, expression of the super-repressor form of IκBα blocks the growth of DBCL cells with the activated B cell-like expression pattern, but not DBCLs with an expression pattern like germinal center B cells (Davis et al., 2001). Third, the primary defect in c-*rel* knockout mice is found in their B cells, which fail to proliferate in response to many mitogens and show increased apoptosis, indicating that c-Rel is required for normal proliferation and survival pathways of B cells (reviewed in Gerondakis et al., 1999).

Based on the obvious similarities to v-Rel-induced oncogenesis, it is likely that the gene amplification of *REL* seen in human B-cell cancers results in an increased level of active REL homodimers that affects the expression of a set of genes that promotes cell growth and survival. Notably, REL appears to be the only transactivating Rel/NF-κB family member that can contribute directly to human lymphoid cell oncogenesis. That is, there have been no consistent reports of gene amplification or chromosomal alterations of *RELA* or *RELB* in any human lymphoid cell malignancies, nor have RELA or RELB been shown to transform lymphoid cells in any cell or animal model system. Interestingly, c-Rel dimers also appear to have a greater ability than RelA dimers to recognize different κB target sites (Huang et al., 2001a; Kunsch et al., 1992). These results suggest that c-Rel, as compared to RelA, can also affect the expression of a broader array of genes, which may be required for the oncogenic conversion of normal B cells.

In one human B-cell lymphoma, a chromosomal rearrangement has led to the production of an altered REL protein. Namely, the RC-K8 B-cell lymphoma cell line has a deletion on one copy of chromosome 2 that creates a hybrid gene in which 3' exons of *REL* have been replaced by those of a non-*REL* gene (termed *NRG*) of unknown function (Kalaitzidis & Gilmore, 2002; Lu et al., 1991). The resulting REL-NRG protein retains most of the residues of the REL DNA-binding domain, but does not have a C-terminal transactivation domain (Gilmore et al., 1995). RC-K8 cells have constitutively active nuclear DNA-binding complexes containing both wild-type REL and REL-NRG homodimers (D. Kalaitzidis & T. D. Gilmore, unpubl. results), and RC-K8 cells show increased expression of several Rel/NF-κB target genes (L. M. Staudt, pers. commun.). However, it is not known whether REL-NRG contributes to the transformed state of RC-K8 cells, and REL-NRG has not been demonstrated to have transforming activity in vitro.

3.2. Rearrangements at the 3' End of NFKB2 *Result in C Terminally-truncated p100 Proteins in Human B- and T-cell Cancers*

The human *NFKB2* gene, encoding the p52/p100 proteins, is located at chromosome 10q24, and *NFKB2* is structurally altered due to chromosomal rearrangements in several human B- and T-cell lymphomas (reviewed in Gilmore et al., 1996). These rearrangments invariably result in the loss of sequences encoding portions of the ankyrin repeat domain of p100, but leave the DNA-binding/dimerization sequences of the RH domain intact. In one B-cell lymphoma, the aberrant *NFBK2* locus encodes a protein containing residues from the constant region of the immunoglobulin heavy chain fused to the C-terminal ankyrin repeat region of p100; thus, this rearrangement may have accidentally occurred during a normal process of gene rearrangement occurring at the heavy chain locus (Neri et al., 1991).

There is still much debate about how these C terminally-truncated p100 proteins contribute to human lymphoid cell oncogenesis. Moreover, although some of these truncated p100 proteins are weakly oncogenic in mouse 3T3 fibroblasts (Ciano et al., 1997), none has been shown to be oncogenic in any lymphoid cell in transgenic mice or in tissue culture. Whereas the normal p100 protein is a cytoplasmic inhibitor of Rel/NF-κB, one model proposes that these altered p100 proteins contribute to oncogenesis by becoming constitutive activators of transcription. Consistent with this model, 1) the C terminally-truncated p100 proteins from tumor cells are largely nuclear proteins when overexpressed in tissue culture cells (Migliazza et al., 1994; Zhang et al., 1994), 2) homodimers of the truncated p100 proteins can bind to DNA (Chang et al., 1995; Thakur et al., 1994; Zhang et al., 1994), and 3) homodimers of the tumor-specific p100 proteins can activate transcription in reporter gene assays (Chang et al., 1995; Epinat et al., 2000; Kim et al., 2000). A second model proposes that the C-terminal deletion results in the loss of the IκB inhibitory activity of p100. However, this model is unlikely to be correct in that mice with a complete knockout of the *nfkb2* gene do not develop tumors (Caamano et al., 1997). Finally, because the deletions invariably remove residues important for the regulated processing of p100 to p52 (Xiao et al., 2001b), the C-terminal truncations could result in increased production of p52-containing dimers. Supporting the increased processing model, 1) mice that have a knockout of *nfkb2* sequences encoding C-terminal sequences of p100 and thus constitutively express p52, have increased numbers of T lymphocytes, enlarged lymph nodes and gastric hyperplasia (Ishikawa et al., 1998), 2) overexpression of p52-v-Rel heterodimers can malignantly transform avian lymphoid cells (White et al., 1996), and 3) p52 is overexpressed in several other human non-lymphoid cancers (Bours et al., 1994; Cogswell et al., 2000; Dejardin et al., 1995). By whatever mechanism p100 truncation may contribute to oncogenesis, it appears to be specific in that similar 3' deletions have not been identified in *NFKB1* in any human cancers.

3.3. Mutations in Hodgkin's Lymphoma That Inactivate the IκBα Protein and Induce Chronic NF-κB Signaling

Hodgkin's disease (HD) is a common, mixed cell lymphoma that is likely to arise from the malignant conversion of a germinal center B cell, and HD is emerging as a one of the clearest examples of a cancer that is dependent on constitutive activation of NF-κB (reviewed in Staudt, 2000). Both HD cell lines and primary disease tissues have constitutively active p50-RELA and p50-REL complexes, and little or no IκBα protein can be detected in these cells (Bargou et al., 1996; Cabannes et al., 1999). Importantly, overexpression of the super-repressor form of IκBα can lead to apoptosis in these cells (Bargou et al., 1997; Hinz et al., 2001).

In several of these HD cells, the lack of IκBα is the result of loss-of-function mutations in one allele of the *IKBA* gene and probably of the deletion of the second allele (Cabannes et al., 1999; Emmerich et al., 1999; Jungnickel et al., 2000). In other HD cases, the constitutive NF-κB activity is due to chronic degradation of IκBα, which occurs either because of autocrine secretion of an NF-κB-inducing factor by these cells (Emmerich et al., 1999; Krappmann et al., 1999) or because of as yet unknown mutations at another step in NF-κB signaling. As a consequence of the constitutive NF-κB signaling, several NF-κB target genes are overexpressed in HD cells, including ones encoding anti-apoptotic genes (such as A1, c-IAP2, TRAF1, and Bcl-X_L) and growth promoting genes (including cyclin D2, CD86 and CD40) (Hinz et al., 2001). Thus, chronic NF-κB activity is almost certainly the cause of the enhanced survival and proliferation of HD cells.

3.4. Rearrangements at the 5' End of BCL-3 *Result in Elevated Expression in Chronic Lymphocytic Leukemia*

Many patients with B-cell chronic lymphocytic leukemia have a characteristic chromosomal translocation between chromosomes 14 and 19 [i.e., t(14:19)] involving the *BCL-3* gene (McKeithan et al., 1997). These t(14:19) translocations generally position the switch region of the immunoglobulin heavy chain gene (from chromosome 14) 5' to the *BCL-3* gene (chromosome 19), and result in increased expression of *BCL-3* mRNA and protein. Support for the hypothesis that inappropriate expression of BCL-3 contributes to human B-cell cancers comes from the finding that transgenic mice in which Bcl-3 is specifically overexpressed in B cells develop splenomegaly and accumulate excess mature B cells in their bone marrow and lymph nodes (Ong et al., 1998).

Although structurally related to the IκB proteins, Bcl-3 is unique in that it is constitutively a nuclear protein, has transcriptional activation domains, and can associate with p50 and p52 homodimers without blocking their ability to bind to DNA (reviewed in Lenardo & Siebenlist, 1994). Thus, Bcl-3 appears to function as a transcriptional co-activator for p50 and p52 homodimers (Dechend et al., 1999). As such, overexpression of Bcl-3 would result in increased transcription of genes normally regulated by p52 or p50 homodimers. BCL-3 has also been found to be overexpressed in other human cancers, which do not have chromosomal translocations involving BCL-3. For example, some breast cancer cells have increased levels of p52 and BCL-3 (Cogswell et al., 2000), which may contribute to accelerated cell cycle progression through direct activation of the cyclin D1 gene by p52-BCL-3 complexes (Westerheide et al., 2001; see also Section 6, below).

4. CONSTITUTIVE ACTIVATION OF Rel/NF-κB IN HUMAN CANCERS

In addition to the genetic alterations that occur to activate the Rel/NF-κB pathway primarily in hematopoeitic cell cancers (described in Section 3, above), many recent reports have shown that a variety of human tumors and tumor cell lines have constitutively nuclear and active NF-κB DNA-binding activity (Table 2), even in the absence of direct mutations in genes in this pathway. These tumors include carcinomas, neural tumors, and many hematopoietic cell malignancies. In addition, several oncogenes activate NF-κB in in vitro transformation assays (Table 2).

Table 2. Constitutive activation of NF-κB in human cancer cells

Cancer type	Reference
Primary tumors and tumor cell lines	
Breast	Nakshatri et al., 1997; Sovak et al., 1997
Ovary	Dejardin et al., 1999; Huang et al., 2000
Vulva	Seppanen & Vihko, 2000
Prostate	Huang et al., 2001b; Palayoor et al., 1999
Kidney	Oya et al., 2001
Liver	Tai et al., 2000
Pancreas	Wang et al., 1999
Stomach	Sasaki et al., 2001
Colon	Lind et al., 2001
Thyroid	Visconti et al., 1997
Melanoma	Yang & Richmond, 2001
Head and neck	Ondrey et al., 1999
Oral carcinoma	Nakayama et al., 2001
Astrocytoma/glioblastoma	Hayahsi et al., 2001
Hodgkin's lymphoma	Bargou et al., 1997
Acute lymphoblastic leukemia	Kordes et al., 2000
Acute myelogenous leukemia	Guzman et al., 2001
Multiple myeloma	Berenson et al., 2001
Diffuse large B-cell lymphoma	Davis et al., 2001
In vitro transformation	
BCR-ABL	Reuther et al., 1999
DBL/DBS	Whitehead et al., 1999
RAF	Baumann et al., 2000
RAS	Finco et al., 1997
TEL-JAK2	Santos et al., 2001
TEL-PDGFR	Besancon et al., 1998

Tumor cell-specific, active NF-κB is usually demonstrated by using electrophoretic mobility shift assays to compare the level of nuclear κB site DNA-binding activity of the tumor cell to its corresponding normal cell type. Generally, these experiments reveal that the elevated nuclear κB site-binding complex consists of p50-RELA heterodimers, and in many cases, there is also constitutive IKK activity.

In several model systems, constitutive NF-κB activity has been shown to be relevant to some aspect of the tumor cell phenotype by overexpression of a super-repressor form of IκBα to inhibit all cellular Rel/NF-κB activity. From such experiments, it appears that the constitutive NF-κB activity can sometimes contribute to the growth and survival of the tumor cells in vitro and in vivo, and other times only affect the in vivo tumorigenicity of the cells. In the latter cases, tumor cells expressing the IκBα super-repressor often regress or develop quite slowly, even in immunodeficient mice. This indicates that NF-κB has a role in controlling aspects of tumor cell growth or viability that are unique to in vivo tumor formation, i.e., processes such as tumor invasion (Huang et al., 2001b), metastases (Huang et al., 2001b), angiogenesis (Huang et al., 2000; Huang et al., 2001b), or the susceptibility of the tumor cells to anti-tumor effects that are mediated by natural killer cells or cytokines such as TNFα.

5. SOME ONCOGENIC HUMAN VIRUSES ENCODE PROTEINS THAT PERSISTENTLY ACTIVATE Rel/NF-κB SIGNALING

Several human viruses that have been associated with oncogenesis can specifically activate the Rel/NF-κB pathway (Table 3). In all cases, these viruses encode proteins that are involved in both their oncogenic effects and activation of NF-κB. However, each virus has intervened in the Rel/NF-κB signaling pathway at a different point.

Table 3. Oncogenic human viruses that encode proteins that constitutively activate NF-κB

Virus (Reference)	*Viral Protein*	*Protein Activity*
Epstein-Barr virus Cahir McFarland et al., 1999	LMP-1	Plasma membrane receptor
Hepatitis B virus Diao et al., 2001	HBx	Adaptor
Human Herpesvirus-8 Pati et al., 2001	ORF74	Plasma membrane receptor
Human T-cell leukemia virus-1 Jeang, 2001	Tax	Adaptor

5.1. The Tax Oncoprotein of Human T-cell Leukemia Virus Type -1 (HTLV-1) Activates Multiple Components of the NF-κB Signaling Pathway

HTLV-1 is a human retrovirus that induces a fatal adult T-cell leukemia in a subpopulation of infected individuals after a long latency. The HTLV-1-encoded Tax protein is essential for the oncogenic effect, and Tax can transform certain cell types in vitro (reviewed in Sun & Ballard, 1999; Jeang, 2001). Moreover, Tax can chronically activate a variety of cellular signaling pathways including AP-1 and NF-κB, consequently activating an array of cellular genes. Certain Tax mutants that are defective in activation of NF-κB are also defective in their malignant transforming ability. Activation of the Rel/NF-κB pathway in Tax-expressing cells involves interaction of Tax with various components of the signaling pathway, and induction of both nuclear p50-RelA complexes and increased processing of p100 to p52.

One clue to the molecular target for Tax-induced activation of p50-RelA was unveiled in a clever genetic experiment in which Yamaoka et al. (1998) used a rat fibroblast cell line to isolate mutant cells that were defective in Tax-induced activation of NF-κB. These mutant cells were shown to be deficient in the production of a cellular protein originally termed NEMO (NF-κB Essential Modulator), which is now known to be the IKKγ component of the IKK complex. Further studies have shown that Tax can interact directly with IKKγ (reviewed in Sun & Ballard, 1999), and mutations in Tax that abrograte its interaction with IKKγ also abolish its ability to activate NF-κB (Xiao et al., 2000). The Tax-IKKγ interaction leads to activation of the β catalytic subunit of IKK, probably because Tax-IKKγ facilitates clustering of the IKK complex and this induced proximity leads to persistent phosphorylation of the activation loop in IKKβ (Carter et al., 2001). Active IKKβ then targets IκBα and IκBβ for degradation, leading to chronic induction of p50-RelA.

Less is known about the mechanism by which Tax induces processing of p100 to p52. However, Tax can directly bind to p100, and this results in the recruitment of an active IKK complex to p100-Tax (Xiao et al., 2001a). Thus, the Tax-p100 interaction promotes enhanced IKKα-mediated processing of p100 to p52 (as described above in Section 2); however, unlike normal processing of p100, Tax-induced processing of p100 does not require NIK (Xiao et al., 2001b).

5.2. Latent Membrane Protein-1 (LMP-1) of Epstein-Barr Virus Is a Constitutively Active Plasma Membrane Receptor That Activates NF-κB Through a Pathway That Mimics Natural Receptor Signaling

Epstein-Barr virus (EBV) is a human herpesvirus that causes a variety of immune cell disorders, and has been implicated in the development of lymphomas in immunocompromised individuals, nasopharyngeal carcinomas, Hodgkin's disease, and gastric carcinomas. EBV can transform human B cells into continuously proliferating cultures in vitro, which has been a widely used model for EBV-mediated lymphomagenesis (reviewed in Cahir McFarland et al., 1999). Viral protein LMP-1 is essential for this transformation, and LMP-1 can by itself transform some cell types in vitro. Relevant to this review, LMP-1 is also a strong activator of NF-κB.

LMP-1 is a membrane-bound receptor-like protein with six transmembrane domains and a C-terminal cytoplasmic tail. Key to understanding how LMP-1 activates NF-κB was the finding that the cytoplasmic domain of LMP-1 can interact with a variety of cellular adaptors, called TRAFs (TNF receptor-associated factors) and TRADD (TNF receptor-associated death domain), which mediate activation of NF-κB by the cellular TNF receptor (reviewed in Cahir McFarland et al., 1999). Mutations in the cytoplasmic signaling domain that affect the ability of LMP-1 to activate NF-κB, correspondingly affect its ability to transform B cells. Moreover, inhibition of NF-κB by overexpression of an IκBα super-repressor leads to apoptosis in EBV-transformed B cells and suppresses LMP-1-induced transformation and tumorigenicity in rat fibroblasts (Cahir McFarland et al., 2000; Feuillard et al., 2000; He et al., 2000).

Thus, LMP-1 is a constitutively active receptor-like molecule that induces NF-κB (p50-RelA) through a normal pathway of IKKβ-induced degradation of IκBα, and constitutive activation of NF-kB contributes to the survival and perhaps proliferation of EBV-transformed cells. However, it is important to point out that LMP-1 activates additional cellular signaling pathways (including p38, JNK, and STAT pathways) that are almost certain to contribute to its transforming activity; moreover, activation of NF-κB is not by itself sufficient to transform any cell type in culture.

5.3. The Hepatitis Virus Type C Encodes the X Protein (Hbx) that Activates NF-κB

Chronic infection with human hepatitis B virus (HBV) is associated with severe liver disease, including hepatocarcinogenesis (reviewed in Diao et al., 2001). The non-structural X protein (HBx) of HBV appears to play a role in supporting persistent infection by HBV, and high level expression of HBx is seen in many HBV-associated liver cancers. Furthermore, HBx can transform certain liver cell lines in vitro and causes liver cancer in some transgenic mouse model systems. HBx is a 154 aa protein, which can be found in both the cytoplasm and nucleus of infected cells. Like Tax of HTLV-1, HBx may be a multifunctional adaptor-like protein that can activate a number of signal transduction pathways, including STAT, PI3-kinase, MAP kinase, AP-1, and NF-κB.

Overexpression of HBx induces the degradation of IκBα, with the resultant nuclear translocation and transactivation of genes by NF-κB. Two reports have recently suggested that activation of NF-κB by HBx proceeds through a novel pathway that does not require IKK: 1) HBx can directly interact with IκBα, possibly to prevent its association with NF-κB (Weil et al., 1999), and 2) HBx-induced degradation of IκBα requires JAK kinase, but does not require IKK activity (Purcell et al., 2001). In any case, chronic activation of NF-κB by HBx likely contributes to abnormal survival of hepatocytes, perhaps through activation of a set of genes similar to those induced by RelA to maintain the survival of liver cells in the developing embryo (Beg et al., 1995).

5.4. Human Herpesvirus 8 (HHV-8) Encodes a Constitutively Active Chemokine Receptor-like Protein (ORF74) That Activates NF-κB

HHV-8 (also called Karposi-sarcoma-associated herpesvirus, KSHV) is a human herpesvirus that is associated with the development of Kaposi's sarcoma, a skin malignancy containing endothelial cells and immune cells, in immunocompromised individuals, and with the development of some non-Hodgkin's lymphomas called primary effusion lymphomas (reviewed in Cannon & Cesarman, 2000). The virally-encoded protein ORF74 is related to a family of G protein-coupled chemokine receptors. Overexpression of ORF74 has recently been shown to convert primary human endothelial cells to a spindled morphology (Pati et al., 2001). Moreover, ORF74 expression activates NF-κB, resulting in the increased expression of several NF-κB target genes, including ones encoding inflammatory cytokines, angiogenesis factors (i.e, VEGF), and adhesion molecules (e.g., ICAM, VCAM) (Bais et al., 1998; Pati et al., 2001). It is not known precisely how ORF74 activates NF-κB or whether activation direcly contributes to the development of Kaposi's sarcoma; however, inhibition of NF-κB can induce apoptosis in some HHV-8-infected lymphoma cells (Keller et al., 2000).

6. GENES AFFECTED BY ABERRANT Rel/NF-κB ACTIVITY IN HUMAN CANCERS

Whether activated by mutation or a constitutive signaling mechanism, persistent Rel/NF-κB activity no doubt contributes to the oncogenic state by altering the expression of a variety of target genes. Although over 200 Rel/NF-κB target genes have been identified (reviewed in Pahl, 1999), those relevant to the human oncogenesis are likely to be involved in the following broad processes: cell growth or cell cycle; apoptosis; adhesion; metastasis; and angiogenesis (Table 4). As it would be impractical to review all of the literature on Rel/NF-κB target genes whose expression is affected in tumor cells, only two recent and provocative examples are discussed below.

Table 4. Some Rel/NF-κB target genes that may be involved in human malignancies

Cellular Process	Gene
Proliferation/cell cycle	Myc, Rel, IRF-4, Cyclins (D1,D2,D3)
Cytokines, growth factors	Interleukins (1,2,6,8,9,11,12,15), IL-2R, RANTES, GM-CSF
Apoptosis (survival)	Bcl-2, Bcl-Xl, A1/Bfl-1, IAPs, TRAFs, IEX, c-FLIP
Adhesion	ICAM-1, VCAM-1, E-selectin
Metastasis	Urokinase plasminogen activator
Angiogenesis	VEGF

6.1. cDNA Expression Microarrays Have Identified a Subclass of Diffuse Large B-cell Lymphomas That Express Rel/NF-κB-dependent Genes

In a powerful series of experiments, cDNA microarray expression profiles have been used to classify diffuse large B-cell lymphomas (DBCLs) into two distinct subtypes: one with an expression profile similar to normally activated B cells (ABC) and one with a pattern of gene expression similar to germinal center B cells (GCB) (Alizadeh et al., 2000; Shipp et al., 2002). A comprehensive analysis of these complex profiles revealed that ABC DBCLs show the selective induction of a number of NF-κB target genes, including ones involved in proliferation (cyclin D2, IRF-4) and anti-apoptosis (BCL-2, c-FLIP), which are not consistently activated in GCB DBCLs (Davis et al., 2001). More importantly, the growth of certain ABC

DBCLs can be inhibited by the IκBα super-repressor, whereas GCB DBCLs are not affected (Davis et al., 2001). More recently, cDNA expression profiling of DBCLs has also been shown to be useful in predicting clinical outcome in response to chemotherapy (Shipp et al., 2002). Taken together, these studies pay tribute to the diagnostic and predictive power of cDNA microarray analyses, and identify NF-κB signaling as an apt target for some cases of DBCL.

6.2. Cyclin D1 Is an Important Target Gene for NF-κB in Breast Cancer

Activated Rel/NF-κB is seen both during normal mammary gland development and proliferation (Brantley et al., 2001; Clarkson et al., 2000; Geymayer & Doppler, 2000) and in many human breast cancer cell lines and primary disease tissues, particularly ones that are estrogen receptor negative (Biswas et al., 2000; Cogswell et al., 2000; Nakshatri et al., 1997; Sovak et al., 1997). Moreover, inhibition of this activated Rel/NF-κB can reduce the growth and tumorigenicity of breast cancer cell lines (Sovak et al., 1997; Biswas et al., 2001). Although active p50-RELA is generally found in breast cancer cell lines, there is evidence that p52, REL and BCL-3 may be more commonly activated in primary breast cancer tissue (Cogswell et al., 2000; Nakshatri et al., 1997; Sovak et al., 1997).

Cyclin D1 is an important regulator of G1-to-S phase cell cycle progression, and has upstream regulatory κB binding sites (Gutrdige et al., 1999; Hinz et al., 1999). Several lines of evidence suggest that Rel/NF-κB-mediated induction of expression of cyclin D1 is key for the control of both normal and malignant breast cancer cell proliferation. First, transgenic mice in which either cyclin D1 has been knocked out (Fantl et al., 1995; Sicinski et al., 1995) or IKKα has been rendered non-inducible (by Ser to Ala mutations at its critical active loop Ser residues) (Cao et al., 2001) show impaired mammary epithelial cell proliferation, and the mammary cell defect in IKKα-defective mice can be corrected by re-expression of cyclin D1 (Cao et al., 2001). Second, cyclin D1 knockout mice are resistant to the induction of breast cancers by oncogenic *neu* or *ras* (Yu et al., 2001). Furthermore, mammary tumors from transgenic mice overexpressing *neu* or from human breast cancer cell lines overexpressing *neu* show elevated NF-κB activity and increased expression of cyclin D1 (Biswas et al., 2000; Pianetti et al., 2000). That cyclin D1 expression is generally important in the development of breast cancer is further supported by the finding that the cyclin D1 gene is amplified in approximately 15% of human breast cancers and is overexpressed in about 50% of human breast cancers (reviewed in Musgrove et al., 1996). Thus, it is likely that there are certain cancers in which cyclin D1 expression is increased by persistent activation of Rel/NF-κB, others in which cyclin D1 expression is increased by other mechanisms, and some which do not have increased Rel/NF-κB activity or cyclin D1 expression. Therefore, as with the DBCLs discussed above, molecular characterization of breast cancers is likely to identify ones that may respond to anti-Rel/NF-κB therapy, anti-cyclin D1 therapy, or neither.

7. TARGETING Rel/NF-κB ACTIVITY IN THE PREVENTION AND TREATMENT OF HUMAN CANCER

Inhibitors of Rel/NF-κB signaling may have uses in both the prevention and treatment of cancer. In terms of cancer prevention, such inhibitors may exert their effects as anti-inflammatory agents. That is, there is much evidence that chronic immune activation and/or inflammation can lead to human cancers (O'Byrne & Dalgleish, 2001), and that consistent use of certain anti-inflammatory agents can have cancer preventive effects. Given the role of Rel/NF-κB signaling in inflammation and immune function, chronic NF-κB signaling might be one of the primary molecular irritants of persistent inflammation that leads to cancer. As such, it is perhaps significant that some anti-inflammatory agents, such as aspirin and green tea polyphenols, that are thought to have cancer preventative effects can also inhibit activation of NF-κB (Lin & Lin, 1997; Yin et al., 1998). Indeed, Kavanaugh et al. (2001) have recently shown that the green tea polyphenol epigallacatechin-3-gallate, which can also inhibit NF-κB (Lin & Lin, 1997), has preventive effects against chemically-induced tumors in a rat model.

In terms of cancer treatment, Rel/NF-κB inhibitors may have uses either as primary treatment agents or as adjuvant therapeutics. Anti-NF-κB inhibitors will most likely act as adjuvant therapeutics for cancers where constitutive NF-κB activity is contributing an anti-apoptotic (survival) function for the tumor cells. Several experiments have shown that active Rel/NF-κB protects normal cells from apoptosis induced by a variety of natural and synthetic agents (reviewed in Barkett & Gilmore, 1999). Thus, anti-NF-κB inhibitors can sensitize cells to the apoptosis-inducing effects of such agents. For example, Baldwin and colleagues have shown that expression of the IκBα super-repressor can sensitize tumor cells to cell killing by TNFα, ionizing radiation, or certain chemotherapeutic drugs (reviewed in Baldwin, 2001), and my laboratory has recently found that transformed mouse fibroblasts lacking RelA form tumors that spontaneously regress in immunodeficient mice (Gapuzan et al., 2002). Anti-NF-κB inhibitors will likely have direct effects on tumors where constitutive Rel/NF-κB activity is contributing to some aspect of the tumor cells' growth, e.g., proliferation or cell cycle, invasion, or angiogenesis. Indeed, one proteasome inhibitor (PS-341), which is a potent inhibitor of NF-κB activation, is showing promise in clinical trials for the treatment of myelomas (reviewed in Adams, 2001). However, it is not clear that all of PS-341's anti-cancer activity is mediated through its effects on NF-κB.

Unfortunately, all of the current Rel/NF-κB inhibitors are general inhibitors of this signaling pathway. There are no inhibitors that are specific for an individual Rel/NF-κB transcription factor. The *REL* gene or protein may be a suitable first target for such directed inhibitors for three reasons: 1) the *REL* gene is amplified in many human lymphomas (see Section 3.1, above); 2) REL is the only Rel/NF-κB family member that has been shown to have direct oncogenic activity in vitro (Gilmore et al., 2001); and 3) c-*rel* knockout mice show only B-cell defects (reviewed in Gerondakis et al., 1999), indicating that a specific REL inhibitor would not be generally toxic.

8. CONCLUSIONS AND PERSPECTIVES

As outlined herein, there is now much evidence that increased Rel/NF-κB signaling contributes to human cancer, and that this pathway will continue to receive attention as a promising molecular target for cancer therapy and prevention. However, there remain many molecular details to resolve. Moreover, at least in some cases, constitutive p50-RELA activity may be an adaptation of certain tumor cell lines to growth in tissue culture or may be a symptom of an abnormal, tumor-induced differentiation program. For example, Cogswell et al. (2000) found that primary human breast cancer tumor cells have active p52, REL, and BCL-3, whereas breast cancer cell lines have constitutively active RELA. Consistent with that finding, over-expression of RELA *reduces* the tumorigenicity of one breast cancer cell line in vivo (Ricca et al., 2001). Finally, given that the Rel/NF-κB pathway can have opposite effects on growth and apoptosis in different cell types, all cancers may not respond in the same way to inhibition of the NF-κB pathway. Indeed, overexpression of the IκBα super-repressor promotes skin carcinomas in one transgenic mouse model system (van Hogerlinden et al., 1999). Thus, the growth and survival of a given tumor cell type is likely to depend on a balance between the activity of the Rel/NF-κB pathway and the activity of many other signaling pathways in ways that are not always easy to predict. In addition, as documented in this collection of articles, it is likely that the Rel/NF-κB pathway is only one of several signaling pathways that are commonly activated in human cancers.

9. NOTES

I thank D. Ballard, G. Mosialos, S.-C. Sun, and members of my lab for useful comments on the manuscript. Research in the author's laboratory on Rel/NF-κB and cancer is supported by a grant from the National Institutes of Health (CA47763). More information on this topic can be obtained at http://www.nf-kb.org.

Thomas D. Gilmore
Biology Department
Boston University
Boston, MA

10. REFERENCES

Adams, J. (2001). Proteasome inhibition in cancer: development of PS-341. *Seminars in Oncology, 28*, 613-619.

Alizadeh, A. A., Eisen, M. B., Davis, R. E., Ma., C., Lossos, I.S., Rosenwald, A., et al. (2000). Distinct types of diffuse large B-cell lymphoma identified by gene expression profiling. *Nature, 403*, 503-511.

Bais, C. Santomasso, B., Coso, O., Arvanitakis, L, Raaka, E. G., Gutkind, J. S., et al. (1998). G-protein-coupled receptor of Kaposi's sarcoma-associated herpesvirus is a viral oncogene and angiogenesis activator. *Nature, 391*, 86-89.

Baldwin, A. S. (2001). Control of oncogenesis and cancer therapy resistance by the transcription factor NF-κB. *Journal of Clinical Investigation, 107*, 241-246.

Bargou, R. C., Emmerich, F., Krappmann, D., Bommert, K., Mapara, M. Y., Arnold, W., et al. (1997). Constitutive NF-κB-RelA activation is required for proliferation and survival of Hodgkin's disease tumor cells. *Journal of Clinical Investigation, 100*, 2961-2969.

Bargou, R. C., Leng, C., Krappmann, D., Emmerich, F., Mapara, M. Y., Bommert, K., et al. (1996). High-level nuclear NF-κB and Oct-2 is a common feature of cultured Hodgkin/Reed-Sternberg cells. *Blood, 87*, 4340-4347.

Barkett, M., & Gilmore T. D. (1999). Control of apoptosis by Rel/NF-κB transcription factors. *Oncogene, 18*, -6924.

Barth, T. F., Bentz, M., Leithauser, F., Stilgenbauer, S., Siebert, R., Scholtter, M., et al. (2001). Molecular-cytogenetic comparison of mucosa-associated marginal zone B-cell lymphoma and large B-cell lymphoma arising in the gastro-intestinal tract. *Genes, Chromosomes & Cancer, 31*, 316-325.

Barth, T. F. E., Döhner, H., Werner, C. A., Stilgenbauer, S., Schlotter, M., Pawlita, M., et al. (1998). Characteristic pattern of chromosomal gains and losses in primary large B-cell lymphomas of the gastrointestinal tract. *Blood, 91*, 4321-4330.

Baumann, B., Weber, C. K., Troppmair, J., Whiteside, S., Israël, A., Rapp, U. R., et al. (2000). Raf induces NF-κB by membrane shuttle kinase MEKK1, a signaling pathway critical for transformation. *Proceedings of the National Academy of Sciences USA, 97*, 4615-4620.

Beg, A. A., Sha, W. C., Bronson, R. T., Ghosh, S., & Baltimore, D. (1995). Embryonic lethality and liver degeneration in mice lacking the RelA component of NF-κB. Nature, 376, 167-170.

Berenson, J. R., Ma, H. M., & Vascio, R. (2001). The role of nuclear factor-κB in the biology and treatment of multiple myeloma. *Seminars in Oncology,* 28, *626-633.*

Besancon, F., Atfi, A., Gespach, C., Cayre, Y. E., & Bourgeade, M. F. (1998). Evidence for a role of NF-κB in the survival of hematopoietic cells mediated by interleukin-3 and the oncogenic TEL/platelet-derived growth factor β fusion protein. *Proceedings of the National Academy of Sciences USA, 95*, 8081-8086.

Biswas, D. K., Cruz, A. P, Gansberger, E., & Pardee, A. B. (2000). Epidermal growth factor-induced nuclear factor κB activation: a major pathway of cell-cycle progression in estrogen-receptor negative breast cancer cells. *Proceedings of the National Academy of Sciences USA, 97*, 8542-8547.

Biswas, D. K., Dai, S.-C., Cruz, A., Weiser, B., Graner, E., & Pardee, A. B. (2000). The nuclear factor κB (NF-κB): a potential therapeutic target for estrogen receptor breast cancers. *Proceedings of the National Academy of Sciences USA, 98*, 10386-10391.

Bours, V., Dejardin, E., Goujon-Letawe, F., Merville, M.-P., & Castronovo, V. (1994). The NF-κB transcription factor and cancer: high expression of NF-κB- and IκB-related proteins in tumor cell lines. *Biochemical Pharmacology, 47*, 145-149.

Brantley, D. M., Chen, C.-L., Muraoka, R. S., Bushdid, P. B., Bradberry, J. L., Kitterell, F., et al. (2001). Nuclear factor-κB (NF-κB) regulates proliferation and branching in mouse mammary epithelium. *Molecular Biology of the Cell, 12*, 1445-1455.

Caamaño, J.H., Rizzo, C. A., Durham, S. K., Barton, D.S., Raventós-Suárez, C., Snapper, C. M., et al. (1997). NF-κB2 (p100/p52) is required for normal splenic microarchitecture and B cell-mediated immune responses. *Journal of Experimental Medicine, 187*, 185-196.

Cabannes, E., Khan, G., Aillet, F., Jarret, R. F., & Hay, R. T. (1999). Mutations in the IκBα gene in Hodgkin's disease suggest a tumour suppressor role for IκBα. *Oncogene, 18*, 3063-3070.

Cahir McFarland, E. D., Davidson, D. M., Schauer, S. L., Duong, J., & Kieff, E. (2000). NF-κB inhibition causes spontaneous apoptosis in Epstein-Barr virus-transformed lymphoblastoid cells. *Proceedings of the National Academy of Sciences USA, 97*, 6055-6060.

Cahir McFarland, E. D., Izumi, K. M., & Mosialos, G. (1999). Epstein-Barr virus transformation: involvement of latent membrane protein 1-mediated activation of NF-κB. *Oncogene, 18*, 6959-6964.

Cannon, M., & Cesarman, E. (2000). Kaposi's sarcoma-associated herpes virus and acquired immunodeficiency syndrome-related malignancy. *Seminars in Oncology, 27*, 409-419.

Cao, Y., Bonizzi, G., Seagroves, T. N., Greten, F. R., Johnson, R., Schmidt, E.V., et al. (2001). IKKα provides an essential link between RANK signaling and cyclin D1 expression during mammary gland development. *Cell, 107*, 763-775.

Carrasco, D., Rizzo, C. A., Dorfman, K., & Bravo, R. (1996). The v-*rel* oncogene promotes malignant T-cell leukemia/lymphoma in transgenic mice. *EMBO Journal, 15*, 3640-3650.

Carrasco, D., Perez, P., Lewin, A., & Bravo, R. (1997). IκBα overexpression delays tumor formation in v-*rel* transgenic mice. *Journal of Experimental Medicine, 186*, 279-288.

Carter, R. A., Geyer, B. C., Xie, M., Acevedo-Suarez, C. A., & Ballard, D. W. (2001). Persistent activation of NF-κB by the Tax transforming protein involves chronic phosphorylation of IκB kinase subunits IKKβ and IKKγ. *Journal of Biological Chemistry, 276*, 24445-24448.

Chang, C.-C., Zhang, J., Lombardi, L., Neri, A., & Dalla-Favera, R. (1995). Rearranged *NFKB-2* genes in lymphoid neoplasms code for constitutively active nuclear transactivators. *Molecular and Cellular Biology, 15,* 5180-5187.
Chen, F. E., & Ghosh, G. (1999). Regulation of DNA binding by Rel/NF-κB transcription factors: structural views. *Oncogene, 18,* 6845-6852.
Ciana, P., Neri, A., Cappellini, C., Cavallo, F., Pomati, M., Chang, C.-C., et al. (1997). Constitutive expression of lymphoma-associated NFKB-2/Lyt-10 proteins is tumorigenic in murine fibroblasts. *Oncogene, 14,* 1805-1810.
Clarkson, R. W., Heeley, J. L., Chapman, R., Aillet, F., Hay, R. T., Wyllie, A., et al. (2000). NF-kB inhibits apoptosis in murine mammary epithelia. Journal of Biological Chemistry, 275, 12737-12742.
Cogswell, P. C., Guttridge, D. C., Funkhouser, W. K., & Baldwin Jr., A. S. (2000). Selective activation of NF-kB subunits in human breast cancer: potential roles for NF-κB2/p52 and for Bcl-3. Oncogene, 19, 1123-1131.
Davis, R. E., Brown, K. D., Siebenlist, U., & Staudt, L. M. (2001). Constitutive nuclear factor kB activity is required for survival of activated B cell-like diffuse large B cell lymphoma cells. Journal of Experimental Medicine, 194, 1861-1874.
Dechend, R., Hirano, F., Lehmann, K., Heissmeyer, V., Ansieau, S., Wulczyn, F. G., et al. (1999). The Bcl-3 oncoprotein acts as a bridging factor between NF-κB/Rel and nuclear co-regulators. Oncogene, 18, 3316-3323.
Dejardin, E., Bonizzi, G., Bellahcène, A., Castronovo, V., Merville, M.-P., & Bours, V. (1995). Highly-expressed p100/p52 (NFKB2) sequesters other NF-κB-related proteins in the cytoplasm of human breast cancer cells. *Oncogene, 11,* 1835-1841.
Dejardin, E., Deregowski, V., Chapelier, M., Jacobs, N., Gielen, J., Merville, M.-P., et al. (1999). Regulation of NF-κB activity by IκB-related proteins in adenocarcinoma cells. *Oncogene, 18,* 2567-2577.
Diao, J., Garces, R., & Richardson, C. D. (2001). X protein of hepatitis B virus modulates cytokine and growth factor related signal transduction pathways during the course of viral infections and hepatocarcinogenesis. *Cytokine & Growth Factor Reviews, 12,* 189-205.
Emmerich, F., Meiser, M., Hummel, M., Demel, G., Foss, H.-D., Jundt, F., et al. (1999). Overexpression of IκBα without inhibition of NF-κB activity and mutations in the IκBα gene in Reed-Sternberg cells. *Blood, 94,* 3129-3134.
Epinat, J.-C., & Gilmore, T. D. (1999). Diverse agents act at multiple levels to inhibit the Rel/NF-κB signal transduction pathway. *Oncogene, 18,* 6896-6909.
Epinat, J.-C., Kazandjian, D., Harkness, D. D., Petros, S., Dave, J., White, D. W., et al. (2000). Mutant envelope residues confer a transactivation function onto N-terminal sequences of the v-Rel oncoprotein. *Oncogene, 19,* 599-607.
Fantl, V., Stamp, G., Andrews, A., Rosewell, I., & Dickson, C. (1995). Mice lacking cyclin D1 are small and show defects in eye and mammary gland development. *Genes & Development, 9,* 2364-2372.
Feuillard, J., Schuhmacher, M., Kohanna, S. Asso-Bonnet, M., Ledeur, F., Joubert-Caron, R., et al. (2000). Inducible loss of NF-κB activity is associated with apoptosis and Bcl-2 down-regulation in Epstein-Barr virus-transformed B lymphocytes. *Blood, 95,* 2068-2075.
Finco, T.S., Westwick, J. K., Norris, J. L., Beg, A. A.., Der, C. J., & Baldwin Jr., A. S. (1997). Oncogenic Ha-Ras-induced signaling activates NF-κB transcriptional activity, which is required for cellular transformation. *Journal of Biological Chemistry, 272,* 24113-24116.
Gapuzan, M.-E., Yufit, P., & Gilmore, T. D. (2002). Immortalized embryonic mouse fibroblasts lacking the RelA subunit of transcription factor NF-κB have a malignantly transformed phenotype. *Oncogene,* in press.
Gerondakis, S., Grossmann, M., Nakamura, Y., Pohl, T., & Grumont, R. (1999). Genetic approaches in mice to understand Rel/NF-κB and IκB function: transgenics and knockouts. Oncogene, 19, 6888-6895.
Geymayer, S., & Doppler, W. (2000). Activation of NF-kB p50/p65 is regulated in the developing mammary gland and inhibits STAT5-mediated b-casein gene expression. FASEB Journal, 14, 1159-1170.
Ghosh, S., May, M. J., & Kopp, E. B. (1998). NF-kB and Rel proteins: evolutionary conserved mediators of immune responses. Annual Review of Immunology, 16, 225-260.
Gilmore, T. D. (1999). The Rel/NF-kB signal transduction pathway: introduction. Oncogene, 18, 6842-6844.
Gilmore, T. D. (1999). Multiple mutations contribute to the oncogenicity of the retroviral oncoprotein v-Rel. Oncogene, 18, 6925-6937.
Gilmore, T. D., Cormier, C., Jean-Jacques, J., & Gapuzan, M.-E. (2001). Malignant transformation of primary chicken spleen cells by human transcription factor c-Rel. Oncogene, 20, 7098-7103.
Gilmore, T. D., Gapuzan, M.-E., Kalaitzidis, D., & Starczynowski, D. (2002). Rel/NF-kB/IkB signal transduction in the generation and treatment of human cancer. Cancer Letters, in press.
Gilmore, T. D., Koedood, M., Piffat, K. A., & White, D. W. (1996). Rel/NF-κB/IκB proteins and cancer. Oncogene, 13, 1367-1378.

Gilmore, T. D., White, D. W., Sarkar, S., & Sif, S. (1995). Malignant transformation of cells by the v-Rel oncoprotein. In G. M. Cooper, R. Greenberg Temin & B. Sugden (Eds.), The DNA provirus: Howard Temin's scientific legacy (pp. 109-128). Washington DC: ASM Press.

Goff, L. K., Neat, M. J., Crawley, C. R., Jones, L., Jones, E., Lister, T. A., et al. (2000). The use of real-time quantitative polymerase chain reaction and comparative genomic hybridization to identify amplification of the REL gene in follicular lymphoma. *British Journal of Haematology, 111, 618-625.*

Guttridge, D. C., Albanese, C., Reuther, J. Y., Pestell, R. G., & Baldwin Jr., A. S. (1999). NFκB controls cell growth and differentiation through transcriptional regulation of cyclin D1. Molecular and Cellular Biology, 19, 5785-5799.

Guzman, M. L., Neering, S. J., Upchurch, D., Grimes, B., Howard, D. S., Rizzieri, D. A., et al. (2001). Nuclear factor-κB is constitutively activated in primitive human acute myelogenous leukemia cells. Blood, 98, 2301-2307.

Hayashi, S., Yamamoto, M., Ueno, Y., Ikeda, K., Ohshima, K., Soma, G., et al. (2001). Expression of nuclear factor-κB, tumor necrosis factor receptor type 1, and c-Myc in human astrocytomas. Neurologia Medico-Chirufica, 41, 187-195.

He, Z., Xin, B., Yang, X., Chan, C., & Cao, L. (2000). Nuclear factor-κB activation is involved in LMP1-mediated transformation and tumorigenesis of rat-1 fibroblasts. Cancer Research, 60, 1845-1848.

Hinz, M., Krappmann, D., Eichten, A., Heder, A., Scheidereit, C., & Strauss, M. (1999). NF-κB function in growth control: regulation of cyclin D1 expression and G0/G1 to S phase transition. Molecular and Cellular Biology, 19, 2690-2698.

Hinz, M., Loser, P., Mathas, S., Krappmann, D., Dörken, B., & Scheidereit, C. (2001). Constitutive NF-κB maintains high expression of a characteristic gene network, including CD40, CD86, and a set of antiapoptotic genes in Hodgkin/Reed-Sternberg cells. Blood, 97, 2798-2807.

Houldsworth, J., Mathew, S., Rao, P. H., Dyomina, K., Louie, D. C., Parsa, N., et al. (1996). *REL* proto-oncogene is frequently amplified in extranodal diffuse large cell lymphoma. *Blood, 87,* 25-29.

Hrdlicková, R., Nehyba, J., & Humphries, E. H. (1994). In vivo evolution of c-*rel* oncogenic potential. *Journal of Virology, 68,* 2371-2382.

Huang, D. B., Chen, Y. Q., Ruetsche, M., Phelps, C. B., & Ghosh, G. (2001a). X-ray crystal structure of proto-oncogene product c-Rel bound ot the CD28 response element of IL-2. *Structure, 9,* 669-678.

Huang, S., Pettaway, C. A., Uehara, H., Bucana, C. D., & Fidler, I. J. (2001b). Blockade of NF-κB activity in human prostate cancer cells is associated with suppression of angiogenesis, invasion, and metastasis. *Oncogene, 20,* 4188-4197.

Huxford, T., Huang, D.-B., Malek, S., & Ghosh, G. (1998). The crystal structure of the IκBα/NF-κB complex reveals mechanisms of NF-κB inactivation. *Cell, 95,* 759-770.

Ishikawa, H., Carrasco, D. Claudio, E., Ryseck, R.-P., & Bravo, R. (1998). Gastric hyperplasia and increased proliferative responses of lymphocytes in mice lacking the COOH-terminal ankyrin domain of NF-κB2. *Journal of Experimental Medicine, 186,* 999-1014.

Jacobs, M. D., & Harrison, S. (1998). Structure of an IκBα/NF-κB complex. *Cell, 95,* 749-758.

Jeang, K. T. (2001). Functional activities of the human T-cell leukemia virus type I Tax oncoprotein: cellular signaling through NF-κB. *Cytokine and Growth Factor Reviews, 12,* 207-217.

Joos, S., Otaño-Joos, J. I., Ziegler, S., Brüderlein, S., du Manoir, S., Bentz, M., et al. (1996).Primary mediastinal (thymic) B-cell lymphoma is characterized by gains of chromosomal material including 9p and amplification of the *REL* gene. *Blood, 87,* 1571-1578.

Jungnickel, B., Staratscheck-Jox, A., Braunninger, A., Speiker, T., Wolf, J., Diehl, V., et al. (1999). Clonal deleterious mutations in the IκBα gene in the malignant cells in Hodgkin's lymphoma. *Journal of Experimental Medicine, 191,* 395-402.

Kalaitzidis, D., & Gilmore, T. D. (2002). Genomic organization and expression of the rearranged *REL* proto-oncogene in human B-cell lymphoma cell line RC-K8. *Genes, Chromsomes & Cancer,* in press.

Kamens, J., Richardson, P., Mosialos, G., Brent, R., & Gilmore, T. D. (1990). Oncogenic transformation by v-Rel requires an amino-terminal activation domain. *Molecular and Cellular Biology, 10,* 2840-2847.

Karin, M. (1999). How NF-κB is activated: the role of the IκB kinase (IKK) complex. *Oncogene, 18,* 6867-6874.

Karin, M. & Ben-Neriah, Y. (2000). Phosphorylation meets ubiquitination: the control of NF-κB activity. *Annual Review of Immunology, 18,* 621-663.

Kavanagh, K. T., Hafer, L. J., Kim, D. W., Mann, K. K., Sherr, D. H., Rogers, A. E., et al. (2001). Green tea extracts decrease carcinogen-induced mammary tumor burden in rats and rate of breast cancer cell proliferation in culture. *Journal of Cell Biochemistry, 82,* 387-398.

Keller, S. A., Schattner, E. J., & Cesarman, E. (2000). Inhibition of NF-κB induces apoptosis of KSHV-infected primary effusion lymphoma cells. *Blood, 96,* 2537-2542.

Kim, K. E., Gu, C., Thakur, S., Viera, E., Lin, J. C., & Rabson, A. B. (2000). Transcriptional regulatory effects of lymphoma-associated *NFKB2/lyt10* protooncogenes. *Oncogene, 19,* 1334-1345.

Kordes, U., Krappmann, D., Heissmeyer, V., Ludwig, W. D., & Scheidereit, C. (2000). Transcription factor NF-κB is constitutively active in acute lymphoblastic leukemia cells. *Leukemia, 14,* 399-402.

Krappmann, D., Emmerich, F., Kordes, U., Scharschmidt, E., Dörken, B., & Scheidereit, C. (1999). Molecular mechanisms of constitutive NF-κB/Rel activation in Hodgkin/Reed Sternberg cells. *Oncogene, 18,* 943-953.

Kunsch, C., Ruben, S. M., & Rosen, C. A. (1992). Selection of optimal κB/Rel DNA-binding motifs: interaction of both subunits of NF-κB with DNA is required for transcriptional activation. *Molecular and Cellular Biology, 12,* 4412-4421.

Lenardo, M., & Siebenlist, U. (1994). Bcl-3-mediated nuclear regulation of the NF-κB *trans*-activating factor. Immunology Today, 15, 145-147.

Lin, Y.-L., & Lin, J.-K. (1997). (-)-epigallacatechin-3-gallate blocks the induction of nitric oxide synthase by down-regulating lipopolysaccharide-induced activity of transcription factor nuclear factor-κB. MolecularPharmacology, 52, 465-472.

Lind, D. S., Hochwald, S. N., Malaty, J., Rekkas, S., Hebig, P., Mishra, G., et al. (2001). Nuclear factor-κB is upregulated in colorectal cancer. Surgery, 130, 363-369.

Lu, D., Thompson, J. D., Gorski, G. K., Rice, N. R., Mayer, M. G., & Yunis, J. J. (1991).Alterations at the rel locus in human lymphoma. Oncogene, 6, 1235-1241.

McKeithan, T. W., Takimoto, G. S., Ohno, H., Bjorling, V. S., Morgan, R., Hecht, B. K., et al. (1997). BCL3 rearrangements and t(14;19) in chronic lymphocytic leukemia and other B-cell malignancies: a molecular and cytogenetic study. Genes, Chromosomes & Cancer, 20, 64-72.

Migliazza, A., Lombardi, L., Rocchi, M., Trecca, D., Chang, C.-C., Antonacci, R., et al. (1994). Heterogeneous chromosomal aberrations generate 3' truncations of the NFKB2/lyt-10 gene in lymphoid malignancies. Blood, 84, 3850-3860.

Mosialos, G., & Gilmore, T. D. (1993). v-Rel and c-Rel are differentially affected by mutations at a consensus protein kinase recognition sequence. Oncogene, 8, 721-730.

Musgrove, E. A., Hui, R., Sweeney, K. J., Watts, C. K., & Sutherland, R. L. (1996). Cyclins and breast cancer. Journal of Mammary Gland Biology and Neoplasia, 1, 153-162.

Nakayama, H., Ikebe, T., Beppu, M., & Shirasuma, K. (2001). High expression levels of nuclear factor κB, IκB kinase α and Akt kinase in squamous cell carcinoma of the oral cavity. Cancer, 92, 3037-3044.

Nakshatri, H., Bhat-Nakshatri, P., Martin, D. A., Goulet Jr., R. J., & Sledge Jr., G. W. (1997). Constitutive activation of NF-κB during progression of breast cancer to hormone-independent growth. Molecular and Cellular Biology, 17, 3629-3639.

Neat, M. J., Foot, N., Jenner, M., Goff, L., Ashcroft, K., Burford, D., et al. (2001). Localisation of a novel region of recurrent amplification in follicular lymphoma to an ~6.8 Mb region of 13q32-33. Genes, Chromosomes & Cancer, 32, 236-243.

Nehyba, J., Hrdlicková, R., & Bose Jr., H. R. (1997). Differences in κB DNA-binding properties of v-Rel and c-Rel are the result of oncogenic mutations in three distinct functional regions of the Rel protein. Oncogene, 14, 2881-2897.

Neri, A., Chang, C.-C., Lombardi, L., Salina, M., Malolo, A. T., Chaganti, R. S. K., et al. (1991). B cell lymphoma-associated chromosomal translocation involves candidate oncogene lyt-10, homologous to NF-κB p50. Cell, 67, 1075-1087.

O'Byrne, K. J., & Dalgleish, A. G. (2001). Chronic immune activation and inflammation as the cause of malignancy. British Journal of Cancer, 85, 473-483.

Ondrey, F. G., Dong, G., Sunwoo, J., Chen, Z., Wolf, J. S., Crowl-Bancroft, C. V., et al. (1999). Constitutive activation of transcription factors NF-κB, AP-1, and NF-IL6 in human head and neck squamous cell carcinoma cell lines that express pro-inflammatory and pro-angiogenic cytokines. *Molecular Carcinogenesis, 26,* 119-129.

Ong, S. T., Hackbarth, M. L., Degenstein, L. C., Baunoch, D. A., Anastasi, J., & McKeithan, T. W. (1998). Lymphadenopathy, splenomegaly, and altered immunoglobulin production in BCL3 transgenic mice. *Oncogene, 16,* 2333-2343.

Oya, M., Ohtsubo, M., Takayanagi, A., Tachibana, M., Shimizu, N., & Murai, M. (2001). Constitutive activation of NF-κB prevents TRAIL-induced apoptosis in renal cancer cells. *Oncogene, 20,* 3888-3896.

Pahl, H. L. (1999). Activators and target genes of Rel/NF-κB transcription factors. *Oncogene, 18,* 6853-6866.

Palanisamy, N., Abou-Elella, A. A., Chaganti, S. R., Houldsworth, J., Offit, K., Louie, D. C., et al. (2002). Similar patterns of genomic alterations characterize primary mediastinal large B-cell lymphoma and diffuse large B-cell lymphoma. *Genes, Chromosomes & Cancer, 33,*114-122.

Palayoor, S. T., Yourmell, M. Y., Calderwood, S. K., Coleman, C. N., & Price, B. D. (1999). Constitutive activation of IκB kinase α and NF-κB in prostate cancer cells is inhibited by ibuprofen. *Oncogene, 18,* 7389-7394.

Pati, S., Cavrois, M., Guo, H. G., Foulke Jr., J. S., Kim, J., Feldman, R. A., et al. (2001).Activation of NF-κB by the human herpesvirus 8 chemokine receptor ORF74: evidence for a paracrine model of Kaposi's sarcoma pathogenesis. *Journal of Virology, 75,* 8660-8673.

Peters, R. T., & Maniatis, T. (2001). A new family of IKK-related kinases may function as IκB kinase kinases. *Biochimica et Biophysica Acta, 2,* M57-M62.

Pianetti, S., Arsura, M., Romieu-Mourez, R., Coffey, R. J., & Sonenshein, G. E. (2000). Her-2/neu overexpression induces NF-κB via a PI3-kinase/Akt pathway involving calpain-mediated degradation of IκB-α that can be inhibited by the tumor suppressor PTEN. Oncogene, 20, 1287-1299.

Purcell, N. H, Yu, C., He, D., Xiang, J., Paran, N., DiDonato, J. A., et al. (2001). Activation of NF-κB by hepatitis B virus X protein through an I_B kinase-independent mechanism. American Journal of Physiology - Gastrointestinal and Liver Physiology, 280, G669-G677.

Rao, P. H., Houldsworth, J., Dyomina, K., Parsa, N. Z., Cigudosa, J. C., & Louie, D. C. (1998). Chromosomal and gene amplification in diffuse large B-cell lymphoma. Blood, 92, 234-240.

Reuther, J. Y., Reuther, G. W., Cortez, D., Pendergast, A. M., & Baldwin Jr., A. S. (1998). A requirement for NF-κB activation in Bcr-Abl mediated transformation. Genes & Development, 12, 968-981.

Ricca, A., Biroccio, A., Trisciuoglio, D., Cippitelli, M., Zupi, G., & Bufalo, D. D. (2001). rela over-expression reduces tumorigenicity and activates apoptosis in human cancer cells. British Journal of Cancer, 85, 1914-1921.

Sachdev, S., & Hannink, M. (1998). Loss of I_B_-mediated control over nuclear import and DNA-binding enables oncogenic activation of c-Rel. Molecular and Cellular Biology, 18, 5445-5456.

Santos, S. C., Monni, R., Bouchaert, I., Bernard, O., Gisselbrecht, S., Gouilleux, F., et al. (2001). Involvement of the NF-κB pathway in the transforming properties of the TEL-Jak2 leukemogenic fusion protein. FEBS Letters, 497, 148-152.

Sasaki, N., Morisaki, T. Hashizume, K., Yao, T., Tsuneyoshi, M., Noshiro, H., et al. (2001). Nuclear factor-κB p65 (RelA) transcription factor is constitutively activated in human gastric carcimoma tissue. Clinical Cancer Research, 7, 4136-4142.

Senftleben, U., Cao, Y., Xiao, G., Greten, F. R., Krahn, G., Bonizzi, G., et al. (2001). Activation by IKKα of a second, evolutionarily conserved, NF-_B signaling pathway. Science, 293, 1495-1499.

Seppanen, M. & Vihko, K.K. (2000). Activation of transcription factor NF-κB by growth inhibitory cytokines in vulvar carcinoma cells. Immunology Letters, 74, 103-109.

Shinkura, R, Kitada, K., Matsuda, F., Tashiro, K., Ikuda, K., Suzuki, M., et al. (1999). Alymphoplasia is caused by a point mutation in the mouse gene encoding the NF-κB-inducing kinase. *Nature Genetics, 22,* 74-77.

Shipp, M. A., Ross, K. N., Tamayo, P., Weng, A. P., Kutor, J. L., Aguiar, R. C. T., et al. (2002). Diffuse large B-cell lymphoma outcome prediction by gene-expression profiling and supervised machine learning. *Nature Medicine, 8,* 68-74.

Sicinksi, P., Donaher, J. L., Parker, S. B., Li, T., Fazeli, A., Gardner, H., et al. (1995). Cyclin D1 provides a link between development and oncogenesis in the retina and the breast. *Cell, 82,* 621-630.

Silverman, N., & Maniatis, T. (2001). NF-κB signaling pathways in mammalian and insect innate immunity. *Genes & Development, 15,* 2321-2342.

Sovak, M. A., Bellas, R. E., Kim, D. W., Zanieski, G. J., Rogers, A. E., Traish, A. M., et al. (1997). Aberrant nuclear factor-κB/Rel expression and the pathogenesis of breast cancer. *Journal of Clinical Investigation, 100,* 2952-2960.

Staudt, L. M. (2000). The molecular and cellular origins of Hodgkin's disease. *Journal of Experimental Medicine, 191,* 207-212.

Sun, S.-C., & Ballard, D. W. (1999). Peristent activation of NF-κB by the Tax transforming protein of HTLV-1: hijacking cellular IκB kinases. *Oncogene, 18,* 6948-6958.

Tai, D. L., Tsai, S. L., Chang, Y. H., Huang, S. N., Chen, T. C., Chang, K. S., et al. (2000). Constitutive activation of nuclear factor κB in hepatocellular carcinoma. *Cancer, 89,* 2274-2281.

Thakur, S., Lin, H.-C., Tseng, W.-T., Kumar, S., Bravo, R., Foss, F., et al. (1994).Rearrangement and altered expression of the *NFKB-2* gene in human cutaneous T-lymphoma cells. *Oncogene, 9,* 2335-2344.

van Hogerlinden, M., Rozell, B. L., Ährlund-Richter, L., & Toftgård, R. (1999). Squamous cell carcinomas and increased apoptosis in skin with inhibited Rel/nuclear factor-κB signaling. *Cancer Research, 59,* 3299-3303.

Visconti, R., Cerutti, J., Battista, S., Fedele, M., Trapasso, F., Zeki, K., et al. (1997). Expression of the neoplastic phenotype by human thyroid carcinoma cell lines requires NFκB p65 protein expression. *Oncogene, 15,* 1987-1994.

Wang, W., Abbruzzese, J. L., Evans, D. B., Larry, L., Cleary, K., & Chiao, P. J. (1999). The NF-κB RelA transcription factor is constiutively activated in human pancreatic adenocarcinoma cells. *Clinical Cancer Research, 5,* 119-127.

Weil, R., Sirma, H., Giannini, C., Kremsdoft, D., Bessia, C., Dargemont, C., et al. (1999). Direct association and nuclear import of the hepatitits B virus X protein with the NF-κB inhibitor IκBα. *Molecular and Cellular Biology, 19,* 6345-6354.

Westerheide S. D., Mayo M. W., Anest, V., Hanson, J. L., & Baldwin Jr., A. S. (2001). The putative oncoprotein Bcl-3 induces cyclin D1 to stimulate G_1 transition. *Mole*cular and Cellular Biology, 21, 8428-8436.

White, D. W., Pitoc, G. A., & Gilmore, T. D. (1996). Interaction of the v-Rel oncoprotein with NF-κB and IκB proteins: heterodimers of a transformation-defective v-Rel mutant and NF-κB p52 are functional in vitro and in vivo. *Molecular and Cellular Biology, 16,* 1169-1178.

Whitehead, I. P., Lambert, Q. T., Glaven, J. A., Abe, K., Rossman, K. L., Mahon, G. M., et al. (1999).Dependence of Dbl and Dbs transformation on MEK and NF-κB activation. *Molecular and Cellular Biology, 19,* 7759-7770.

Xiao, G. Cvijic, M. E., Fong, A., Warhaj, E. W., Uhik, M. T., Waterfield, M., et al. (2001a).Retroviral oncoprotein Tax induces processing of NF-κB2/p100 in T cells: evidence for the involvement of IKKα. *EMBO Journal, 20,* 6805-6815.

Xiao, G., Harhaj, E. W., & Sun, S.-C. (2000). Domain-specific interaction with IκB kinase (IKK) regulatory subunit IKKγ is an essential step in Tax-mediated activation of IKK. *Journal of Biological Chemistry, 275,* 34060-34067.

Xiao, G., Harhaj, E. W., & Sun, S.-C. (2001b). NF-κB-inducing kinase regulates the processing of NF-κB2 p100. *Molecular Cell, 7,* 401-409.

Yamamoto, Y., & Gaynor, R.B. (2001). Therapeutic potential of inhibition of the NF-κB pathway in the treatment of inflammation and cancer. *Journal of Clinical Investigation, 107,* 135-142.

Yamaoka, S., Courtois, G., Bessia, C., Whiteside, S. T., Weil, R., Agou, F., et al. (1998). Complementation cloning of NEMO, a component of the IκB kinase complex essential for NF-κB activation. *Cell, 93,* 1231-1240.

Yang, J., & Richmond, A. (2001). Constitutive IκB kinase activity correlates with nuclear factor-κB activation in human melanoma cells. Cancer Research, 61, 4901-4909.

Yin, M.-J., Yamamoto, Y., & Gaynor, R. B. (1998). The anti-inflammatory agents aspirin and salicylate inhibit the activity of IκB kinase-α. Nature, 396, 77-80.

Yu, Q., Geng, Y., & Sicinski, P. (2001). Specific protection against breast cancers by cyclin D1 ablation. Nature, 411, 1017-1021.

Zhang, J., Chang, C.-C., Lombardi, L., & Dalla-Favera, R. (1994). Rearranged NFKB2 gene in the HUT78 T-lymphoma cell line codes for a constitutively nuclear factor lacking transcriptional repressor functions. Oncogene, 9, 1931-1937.

STAT SIGNALING IN CANCER: INSIGHTS INTO PATHOGENESIS AND TREATMENT STRATEGIES

DAVID A. FRANK

1. INTRODUCTION

The inappropriate survival and proliferation of cancer cells often arises from the activation of signaling pathways normally under the control of physiologic stimuli. The genetic alterations which occur in a tumor cell lead to the inappropriate activation of these signaling pathways, resulting in the persistent survival or growth of cells independent of the appropriate cues. A pathway which has been found to be important in mediating the effects of many physiologic stimuli is the STAT pathway. Originally identified as playing a key role in hematologic and immune cells, STATs are now recognized to play a prominent role in transducing signals from a wide variety of stimuli, in perhaps every tissue in the body. Given this prominent role in normal homeostasis, it is not surprising that STATs have been found to be activated inappropriately in a wide array of human cancers. This has provided important information about the molecular pathogenesis of cancer, and presents possible strategies for the development of more effective, less toxic treatments.

2. THE STAT FAMILY OF TRANSCRIPTION FACTORS

Interferons are a group of proteins which mediate anti-viral effects in mammals. Although it was known that they produced their effects through the activation of specific target genes, it was not until the late 1980s that the mediators of this effect began to be elucidated. Two complementary strategies, one starting from a mutational analysis of interferon resistance and the other analyzing the promoter regions of genes known to be induced by interferons, led to the discovery of a family of latent transcription factors called *s*ignal *t*ransducers and *a*ctivators of *t*ranscription (STATs) (Darnell, 1997; Ihle, 1996). The seven members of the STAT family encode highly homologous proteins which reside in the cytoplasm under basal conditions. They share a unique tyrosine residue towards their carboxy terminus which can be phosphorylated by a number of tyrosine kinases (Shuai, Stark, Kerr, & Darnell, 1993). The activation of STATs in response to cytokines involves tyrosine phosphorylation mediated by Janus family (Jak) kinases.

Consequently, this signaling cascade is sometimes referred to as the "Jak-STAT" pathway. However, it is now clear that STATs can be phosphorylated by a variety of cellular tyrosine kinases including polypeptide growth factor receptors and src family members. Phosphorylation on this unique tyrosine residue leads to the formation of STAT dimers through reciprocal phosphotyrosine-src homology (SH)-2 interactions (Shuai et al., 1994). These STAT dimers then translocate to the nucleus where they are able to bind to a canonical nine to ten base pair sequence in the reporter region of target genes, thereby activating transcription (Figure 1). It has also been suggested that STATs can modulate transcription through other means, not involving tyrosine phosphorylation, though this area of STAT functioning continues to be elucidated (Kumar, Commane, Flickinger, Horvath, & Stark, 1997).

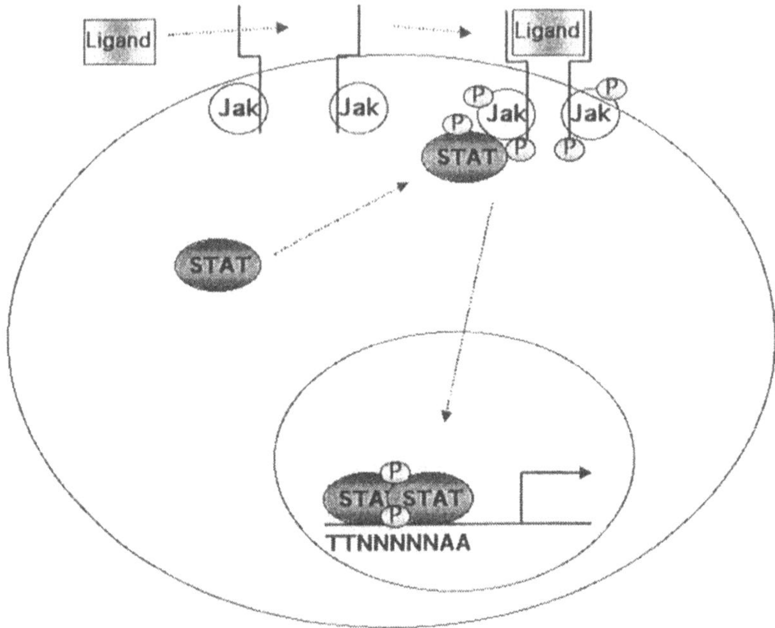

Figure 1. STAT activation. In classical Jak-STAT signaling, a ligand binding to its cell surface receptor induces dimerization of receptor chains. This brings the associated Jak family kinases into juxtaposition thereby activating these kinases, leading to tyrosine phosphorylation of the receptor-kinase complex. STATs are recruited to this complex through their Src homology (SH) 2 domains where they become tyrosine phosphorylated as well. STATs then form dimers through phosphotyrosine-SH2 interactions, translocate to the nucleus, and bind to specific nine base pair sequences in the promoter region of target genes, thereby activating transcription.

While tyrosine phosphorylation is essential for classical STAT activation, it is also clear that STATs can be phosphorylated on serine residues as well.

STAT1, STAT3, and STAT4 have well-conserved carboxy-terminal serine residues located in a pro-met-ser-pro motif. Phosphorylation of this serine residue may have several roles, one of which is the enhancement of transcriptional activation of target genes (Wen, Zhong, & Darnell, 1995; Zhang, Blenis, Li, Schindler, & Chen-Kiang, 1995; Wen & Darnell, 1997). It is likely that a variety of serine, threonine kinases can phosphorylate these sites (Frank, Mahajan, & Ritz, 1997; Turkson et al., 1999; Gollob, Schnipper, Murphy, Ritz, & Frank, 1999). Thus STATs sit at a convergence point of a number of kinase cascades, and serve to integrate a variety of signals emanating from the extracellular milieu.

3. PHYSIOLOGIC FUNCTIONS OF STATS

The seven STAT family members can be divided into three functional categories. Two, STAT4 and STAT6, play roles largely confined to lymphocyte differentiation and function (Kaplan, Schindler, Smiley, & Grusby, 1996; Kaplan, Sun, Hoey, & Grusby, 1996; Thierfelder et al., 1996). STAT2 appears to be a mediator solely of IFN-α function. The third category consists of STAT1, STAT3, and STAT5a and b, two genes which apparently arose from a duplication event, and have highly similar, though not completely redundant function (Liu, Robinson, Gouilleux, Groner, & Hennighausen, 1995). STAT1, STAT3, and the STAT5 isoforms (grouped together as "STAT5") are widely expressed and are activated in response to a variety of stimuli. Although they mediate a variety of effects, many of the stimuli which activate these STATs, particularly STAT3 and STAT5, support cell growth and survival. Many approaches have indicated that the activation of these STATs is necessary for growth and survival, and not a consequence of these processes. One such approach has been the generation of constitutive forms of these proteins. By introducing two carboxy terminal cysteines into STAT3, a variant of this protein which can dimerize spontaneously through disulfide linkages was derived (Bromberg et al., 1999). This so-called STAT3-C can activate target genes which can promote cell cycle progression, such as cyclin D1 and c-myc, as well as those which can promote survival, such as Bcl-xL. Perhaps more dramatically reflecting the importance of genes downstream of STAT3 in mediating events related to tumorigenesis, introduction of STAT3-C into fibroblasts can lead to tumor formation in nude mice. A constitutively activated form of STAT5 has also been generated, in this case using PCR-driven random mutagenesis coupled with an expression screening system (Onishi et al., 1998). This activated form of STAT5 ameliorated the requirement of IL-3 for cell growth in the hematopoietic cell line Ba/F3. Given that these STATs clearly promote growth and survival, it is not surprising that their inappropriate activation occurs commonly in a multitude of human malignancies.

However, the physiological role of STATs is complicated by the fact that these proteins also participate in processes of cellular differentiation. This is particularly true for myeloid differentiation, where the cytokine granulocyte colony-stimulating factor (G-CSF) activates STAT3 during the induction of myeloid maturation (Shimozaki, Nakajima, Hirano, & Nagata, 1997). The introduction of dominant inhibitory forms of STAT3 block this granulocytic differentiation without affecting cellular proliferation. A role in the promotion of myeloid differentiation is not restricted to STAT3. Dominant inhibitory forms of STAT5 have also displayed the ability to inhibit myeloid differentiation in model systems (Ilaria, Hawly, & Van Etten, 1999). Interestingly, these constructs inhibited the proliferation of IL-3 dependent cell lines, indicating that the biological effects of the STATs likely vary with the physiologic system. Nonetheless, the observation that STATs can play an essential role in differentiation raises the possibility that inhibition of STAT function may have the capacity to promote oncogenesis in certain settings.

4. STAT ACTIVATION IN HEMATOLOGIC CANCERS

4.1 Chronic myelogenous leukemia (CML)

After finding that STATs were involved in mediating the effects of IFNs, it soon became clear that STAT activation was a key event induced by the binding of many of cytokines and growth factors to their receptors. Much of this early work was performed in hematopoietic cell lines, whose growth in vitro is characterized by a requirement for the supplementation of the media with soluble factors. For example the murine pro-lymphocytic cell line Ba/F3 requires supplementation of the medium with interleukin (IL)-3 for viability and growth. IL-3 induces phosphorylation of STAT5 and, to a lesser extent, STAT1. Ba/F3 cells can be rendered growth factor-independent by introduction of the Bcr-Abl oncoprotein, the result of a translocation between chromosomes 9 and 22 which leads to the formation of this chimeric tyrosine kinase (Konopka, Watanabe, & Witte, 1984; Daley & Baltimore, 1988). This particular translocation occurs in essentially every patient with chronic myeloid leukemia (CML; Rowley, 1973; Nowell & Hungerford, 1960), as well as in a subset of patients with acute lymphocytic leukemia (ALL). If activation of STAT5 is a critical event for the survival and growth of Ba/F3 cells in response to IL-3, then it could be conjectured that Bcr-Abl leads to factor-independent growth by subverting this signaling pathway and inducing constitutive activation of STAT5. In fact, this was found to be the case, and established the model that ectopic tyrosine kinase activity could lead to constitutive STAT activation (Frank & Varticovski, 1996; Ilaria & Van Etten, 1996; Carlesso, Frank, & Griffin, 1996). Bcr-Abl is a potent tyrosine kinase, with many cellular substrates. Thus, the possibility was considered that STAT5 activation was not critical to the biological actions of Bcr-Abl. However, introduction of a dominant negative form of STAT5 into Bcr-Abl-transformed cells led to an inhibition of growth, and a lowered threshold to undergo apoptosis (Nieborowska-Skorska, et al., 1998; Sillaber, Gesbert, Frank, Sattler, & Griffin, 2000), confirming that STAT5 is a key mediator of the malignant transformation of these cells. Extending the observation that Bcr-Abl transformation of hematopoietic cell lines leads to STAT5 activation, primary cells from patients with CML were examined as well. These also showed constitutive activation of STAT5 suggesting that this is an intrinsic event in cellular transformation, and not an artifact of cell culture (Chai, Nichols, & Rothman, 1997).

4.2 Acute myeloid leukemia (AML) and acute lymphoblastic leukemia (ALL)

Although CML has been an invaluable model for studying the molecular pathogenesis of leukemia, it is a relatively rare tumor both in its frequency and in the fact that essentially every patient has the same underlying molecular abnormality. To determine whether inappropriate STAT activation was common to other forms of leukemia, which arise from a diversity of molecular events, studies were undertaken in samples from patients with acute leukemias. Since a hallmark of STAT activation is translocation from the cytoplasm to the nucleus and binding to DNA, nuclear extracts were prepared from leukemic blasts from patients with ALL and AML and assessed for the presence of STATs which could bind to radiolabeled oligonucleotides containing a canonical STAT binding site. The vast majority of patients examined displayed activation of STAT1, STAT3, and STAT5, alone or in combination, in their leukemia cells (Gouilleux-Gruart et al., 1996; Weber-Nordt et al., 1996). These studies made it clear that inappropriate activation of STATs, manifested by tyrosine phosphorylation and nuclear localization, is a common event in rapidly progressing human leukemias.

An additional level of complexity has arisen from the realization that several STAT family members, particularly STAT1, STAT3, and STAT5, can exist as two forms, a full length α form and a truncated β form. The β form can be generated by alternative splicing of the full length transcript (Yan, Qureshi, Zhong, Wen, & Darnell, 1995), or by proteolytic degradation of full length protein (Azam, Lee, Strehlow, & Schindler, 1997). In either case, this truncated form lacks carboxy terminal sequences including the transcriptional activation domain. Not only is the β form insufficient to support transcription by itself, but it may also display dominant inhibitory activity (Wang, Straopodis, Teglund, Kitazawa, & Ihle, 1996; Mui, Wakao, Kinoshita, Kitamura, & Miyajima, 1996; Moriggl et al., 1996). Wetzler and colleagues have found constitutive activation of STAT3 and STAT5 in a majority of patients with newly diagnosed AML (Xia, Baer, Block, Baumann, & Wetzler, 1998). However, most of these patients expressed β forms of these proteins, generated perhaps through a proteolytic process (Xia, Salzler et al., 2001). Furthermore, at the time of relapse, nearly all of the patients expressed β forms (Xia, Sait et al., 2001). Confirming that activation of β isoforms may portend a worse outcome in patients with AML, it was found that among newly diagnosed patients, activated STAT3 was a negative prognostic factor for disease-free survival. However, those with activated STAT3β had the worse outcome of all in terms of disease-free as well as overall survival (Benekli et al., 2002).

These data on the potential importance of β isoforms in AML raise several interesting issues. An underlying premise in interpreting the activation of STATs in leukemias and other cancers has been that they recapitulate the signaling processes normally activated by cytokines which promote the survival and/or growth of hematopoietic cells. If the β forms of STAT3 and STAT5 function in a dominant inhibitory mode, then this would suggest that, if they do in fact play a role in the pathogenesis of these malignancies, then they are blocking a physiologic process which counters tumorigenesis. Although the critical target genes modulated by STATs in cancer remain largely unknown, most of the candidates have been those which promote cell cycle progression such as c-myc and cyclin D1, or those which promote survival, such as Bcl-xL. However, as noted previously, both STAT3 and STAT5 have also been associated with the process of cellular differentiation. Thus, it may be that the constitutive activation of these STATs in leukemic cells serves to block the normal differentiation process, which may be an important control point in the genesis of leukemias. Alternatively these β forms may have a positive function in transcription or other cellular processes, or they may not interfere with the transcription mediated by full length α forms of STATs. Further experimental work will be necessary to clarify this important point.

4.3 Chronic lymphocytic leukemia

Since STAT tyrosine phosphorylation occurs in response to cytokines which induce the proliferation of hematologic cells in vitro, it is not surprising that this pathway is activated ectopically in rapidly proliferating hematologic malignancies. However, the most common leukemia in western societies, chronic lymphocytic leukemia (CLL), is characterized by lymphocytes with a very low growth fraction. These malignant cells accumulate due to a lack of apoptosis rather than unrestrained proliferation. Not surprisingly, perhaps, it was found that CLL cells do not display constitutive tyrosine phosphorylation of any STATs (Frank, Mahajan, & Ritz, 1997). However, STATs can also be phosphorylated on serine residues. While this does not induce the transcriptional activation mediated by tyrosine phosphorylated STATs, serine phosphorylation is increasingly being recognized as an important modulator of STAT function. Phosphorylation of a conserved carboxy terminal serine residue can increase the transcriptional induction mediated by several STATs (Wen & Darnell, 1997; Wen, Zhong, & Darnell, 1995; Zhang, Blenis, Li, Schindler, & Chen-Kiang, 1995). In addition, for STAT1 in particular, there is evidence that phosphorylation on serine 727 can mediate effects independent of tyrosine phosphorylation (Kumar, Commane, Flickinger, Horvath, & Stark, 1997). While CLL cells lack tyrosine phosphorylated STATs, STAT1 and STAT3 have been found to be phosphorylated on serine residues in primary cells from patients with CLL (Frank et al., 1997). This raises the possibility that serine phosphorylation, even independent of tyrosine phosphorylation, may play an important role in the genesis of common human malignancies.

4.4 Hodgkin's disease and non-Hodgkin's (B cell) lymphoma

Hodgkin's disease is a B cell neoplasm characterized by prominent lymph node enlargement. However, study of this tumor is complicated by the fact that the true malignant B cell, the Hodgkin or Reed-Sternberg cell, represents a small minority of the lymphocytes which populate these lymph nodes. As such, rigorous studies of the unique molecular features of Hodgkin cells require micro-dissection or other specialized techniques which have become available only relatively recently. Using such dissection techniques, and comparative genomic hybridization, it was shown that Jak2 is amplified frequently in Hodgkin cells (Joos et al., 2000). Thus, it was perhaps not surprising to find that STAT3 is activated constitutively in 5 of 7 Hodgkin's disease cell lines (Kube et al., 2001). A more recent report confirmed the presence of activated STAT3 in Hodgkin's disease cell lines (Skinnider et al., 2002). Furthermore, using immunohistochemistry to identify activated STATs in primary tumor samples (Lin, Mahajan, & Frank, 2000), these authors were also able to directly demonstrate STAT3 activation in Hodgkin cells. Even more intriguing, using these same techniques, these authors were able to detect activated STAT6 in both Hodgkin cells and Hodgkin's disease cell lines. This particular STAT family member, which is involved in T helper cell differentiation, has generally not been implicated in the genesis of tumors. It will be interesting to see whether it may play a greater role in cancer, perhaps in lymphocytic malignancies.

Non-Hodgkin's lymphoma (NHL), the most commonly diagnosed hematologic malignancy in the United States, is comprised of a number of different subtypes reflecting the malignant transformation of B and T lymphocytes at any point in the differentiation process. Perhaps reflecting this heterogeneity, there are conflicting data regarding the particular STAT family members activated in this disease. In anaplastic large B cell lymphoma, it has been reported that STAT5 is constitutively activated (Nieborowska-Skorska et al., 2001). In other forms of NHL activation of STAT3 and occasionally STAT6 has been reported (Skinnider et al., 2002).

The role of STAT5, specifically STAT5b, in the pathobiology of NHL has been suggested by an entirely independent line of experimentation. Patients with the common NHL subtype diffuse large B cell lymphoma (DLCL) are generally treated with a four drug combination chemotherapy regimen known by the acronym CHOP. However, even among patients with similar clinical characteristics, there is variability in the tumor response of DLCL patients. Some patients experience prompt and complete eradication of the tumor, whereas other tumors display chemotherapy resistance and progress unabated. To try to determine the molecular events underlying these varied responses, a genetic approach was taken. Using gene expression profiling, genes were identified which correlated with each response. Among the genes associated with a poor outcome was STAT5b (Shipp et al., 2002). The significance of this observation is unknown at this time. It could reflect the activation of a signaling pathway which leads to STAT5b expression, but which may not involve STAT5b itself in the biology of the tumor. Alternatively, the elevated expression of this STAT may be causally related to the poor outcome experienced by these patients. This observation is also intriguing in that STAT5a, which shares 95% amino acid identity with STAT5b, was not detected by this approach. Further work in this area is likely to be informative about many of the roles played by the STAT5 isoforms in the biology of cancer.

4.5 T cell lymphomas

While most lymphoid malignancies arise from B cells, transformation of T cells can occur as well. One manifestation of this is the development of lymphomas which home largely to the skin. The general category of cutaneous T cell lymphomas (CTCL), which are distinct from the rare cutaneous B cell lymphoma, includes diseases such as mycosis fungoides and Sezary syndrome. Like their B cell counterparts, stimuli which activate T cells signal through STAT family transcription factors, and their malignant forms have been found to show constitutive activation of these pathways. Among the cytokines which can activate T cells is IL-2, which is known to induce the tyrosine phosphorylation of STAT1, STAT3, and STAT5 (Frank, Robertson, Bonni, Ritz, & Greenberg, 1995). Despite this diversity of STATs activated by IL-2, only STAT3 has been reported to be activated constitutively in CTCL cells (Nielsen et al., 1997). STAT3 activation appears to be functionally important to the development of this tumor, as pharmacologic inhibition of STAT3 tyrosine phosphorylation and DNA binding alters the expression of proteins regulating cellular survival to favor the induction of apoptosis (Nielsen et al., 1999). Furthermore, CTCL cells may retain responsiveness to IL-2. Inhibition of STAT3 function leads to a loss of expression of the IL-2 receptor α chain, and a loss of mitogenesis in response to IL-2 (Eriksen et al., 2001). Thus, STAT3 may play a role in promoting both the survival and the proliferation of CTCL cells.

Another form of T cell malignancy is adult T cell leukemia/lymphoma (ATL). This is one of the few human cancers directly caused by an oncogenic virus, in this case human T cell lymphotropic virus I (HTLV-I; Kawano, Yamaguchi, Nishimura, Tsuda, & Takatsuki, 1985)As with CTCL, ATL cells are initially dependent on IL-2 for growth, though they eventually become independent of this cytokine. Beginning with cell culture studies, it was found that HTLV-I transformation of T cells led to activation of STAT3 and STAT5 (Migone et al., 1995). T cell lines generated independent of HTLV-I did not display this finding. The activation of STAT3 and STAT5 could also be detected in leukemic cells harvested directly from patients with ATL, indicating that the tissue culture models seemed to accurately recapitulate the molecular events occurring in vivo (Takemoto et al., 1997)

In CML and many other forms of human leukemia, a chimeric tyrosine kinase, arising from a chromosomal translocation, catalyzes phosphorylation of STATs and other cellular substrates. HTLV-I-induced STAT phosphorylation appears to involve the activation of Jak kinases. In model systems in which cellular transformation is induced by tax, a transcriptional activator encoded in the HTLV-I genome, Jak family members become activated (Xu et al., 1995). This may be due to the production of cytokines such as IL-6 which may activate Jaks through an autocrine mechanism, or due to direct activation of the Jaks by other mechanisms (Migone et al., 1995; Takemoto et al., 1997; Xu et al., 1995).

4.6 Multiple myeloma

After non-Hodgkin's lymphomas, multiple myeloma is the most common hematologic cancer in the Unites States (Jemal, Thomas, Murray, & Thun, 2002). This malignancy is characterized by the neoplastic transformation of the most differentiated form of B lymphocyte, the plasma cell. One of the first clues regarding the molecular pathogenesis of myeloma was the finding that these cells secrete IL-6, and also express the IL-6 receptor. Abundant evidence has demonstrated that IL-6 supports both survival and mitogenesis of these cells (Kawano et al., 1988; Anderson, Jones, Morimoto, Leavitt, & Barut, 1989; Klein, Zhang, Yang, & Bataille, 1995; Levy, Tsapis, & Brouet, 1991). Elegant genetic proof of the importance of this relationship was provided by the finding that mice in which the gene for IL-6 had been disrupted were resistant to the development of these kinds of B cell tumors (Hilbert, Kopf, Mock, Kohler, & Rudikoff, 1995). It is often difficult to dissect the critical mechanism by which an autocrine pathway leads to promotion of a malignant cell type. Although IL-6 activates a number of intracellular signaling pathways, several lines of evidence indicate that activation of STATs, in particular STAT3, is critical for myeloma cell propagation. Myeloma cells often become independent of IL-6, though this generally occurs concomitant with the constitutive activation of STAT3, presumably through other pathways (Catlett-Falcone et al., 1999; Hilbert, Migone, Kopf, Leonard, & Rudikoff, 1996; Rawat et al., 2000). Furthermore, inhibition of STAT3 function sensitizes cells to undergoing apoptosis, both spontaneous and Fas-induced (Catlett-Falcone et al., 1999). Thus, STAT3 appears to be a central mediator of the pathogenesis of plasma cell tumors such as myeloma.

5. MECHANISMS OF STAT TYROSINE PHOSPHORYLATION IN HEMATOLOGIC CANCERS

5.1 Autocrine and paracrine activation

Perhaps the simplest mechanism whereby STAT family members can become activated constitutively in cancer is through alteration of a physiologic cytokine or growth factor signaling pathway leading to chronic activation. For example, autocrine or paracrine activation of a receptor can induce inappropriate survival and proliferation promoting tumor development. The tumor system in which this has been explored most fully is multiple myeloma. Early in the disease, the myeloma cells are generally dependent on IL-6, produced either in an autocrine fashion or deriving from associated cells such as bone marrow stroma (Kawano et al., 1988). The resultant activation of STAT3 appears to be a key event in the maintenance of survival of the malignant cells (Catlett-Falcone et al., 1999). As a result, antagonists of the IL-6 receptor, or inhibitors of Jak family tyrosine kinases can have a therapeutic effect, at least in model systems. With continued evolution of the myeloma, the malignant cells may develop alternate mechanisms to activate STAT3 independent of autocrine activation.

Other cytokines may also contribute to autocrine activation of STATs in tumor systems. In Hodgkin's disease, STAT6 has been reported to be activated constitutively (Skinnider et al., 2002). This particular STAT family member is involved in T_H2 differentiation programs, and is phosphorylated primarily in response to IL-4 and related cytokines (Kaplan, Schindler, Smiley, & Grusby, 1996; Shimoda et al., 1996; Takeda et al., 1996). STAT 6 activation in Hodgkin's cell lines could largely be suppressed by a neutralizing antibody to IL-13, suggesting that autocrine production of this cytokine is leading to activation of STAT6 in this model system.

An additional level of complexity arises from the observation that activated STATs can drive the expression and secretion of cytokines. For example, HTLV-1 associated transformation of T cells is associated with Jak activation as well as phosphorylation of STAT3 and STAT5, which may reflect secretion of IL-2, a physiologic stimulus for T cells. Introduction of the transforming protein tax into fibroblasts leads to the secretion of IL-6, another stimulator of STAT activation (Xu et al., 1995). In some patients with cutaneous T cell lymphoma (CTCL), the immune system seems to display features of a T_H2 response, with eosinophilia and elevated IgE levels. Cell lines derived from CTCL cells show enhanced secretion of IL-5 and IL-13 which can be largely suppressed by inhibiting the function of the constitutively activated STAT3 in these cells (Nielsen et al., 2002). Thus it is clear that autocrine and paracrine processes can drive STAT activation, and STAT activation itself may lead to the production of cytokines from tumor cells.

5.2 Chimeric fusion tyrosine kinases arising from chromosomal translocations

Although Jak family tyrosine kinases are critical for STAT phosphorylation in response to cytokines, it is clear that many other kinases can phosphorylate STATs as well. These include polypeptide growth factor receptors and non-receptor kinases such as src. One of the most intriguing aspects of the study of STAT activation in hematologic cancers has been the revelation that previously described chromosomal translocations associated with leukemia were directly leading to the generation of chimeric kinases which could phosphorylate STATs. The prototype of this mechanism is Bcr-Abl, the transforming oncoprotein found in essentially every patient with CML and a fraction of other leukemias such as ALL (Konopka, Watanabe, & Witte, 1984). C-abl is normally present in the nucleus, where its relatively weak tyrosine kinase activity is triggered in response to DNA damage. After its fusion to Bcr, as a result of a translocation between chromosomes 9 and 22, it becomes localized to the cytoplasm and is highly active. As noted above, among its many substrates is STAT5, which appears to be necessary for its transforming ability.

Subsequently, a whole panel of chimeric tyrosine kinases have been found in a variety of leukemias, nearly all of which can lead to the phosphorylation of STATs. Most receptor-associated tyrosine kinases become activated when brought into juxtaposition by ligand-induced receptor oligomerization. A common hallmark of these fusion tyrosine kinases is the association of the catalytic domain of the kinase with a protein that dimerizes constitutively. Often the dimerizing moiety of the fusion kinase derives from a transcription factor which forms dimers in order to bind to DNA. One such transcription factor is the ets-family member Tel. In an number of forms of leukemia, Tel becomes fused to Jak2 as a result of a translocation between chromosomes 9 and 12 (Lacronique et al., 1997; Peeters et al., 1997). This constitutively active kinase can induce cytokine-independent growth of hematopoietic cells in vitro, and depends both on the kinase activity of Jak2, and the dimerization ability of Tel. In Ba/F3 cells, introduction of Tel-Jak2 is associated with the activation of STAT1, STAT3, and STAT5. One concern with these in vitro studies, and the use of factor-independence as a marker, is the question of its relevance to the development of leukemia. To address this concern, Tel-Jak2 was introduced into bone marrow cells by retroviral infection. This led to the development of a fatal myeloproliferative and lymphoproliferative disorder in these animals, reflecting the physiologic importance of this molecular abnormality (Schwaller et al., 1998). Furthermore, introduction of this fusion kinase into mice in which STAT5 has been functionally deleted by gene targeting led to protection from the development of this leukemia-like syndrome (Schwaller et al., 2000), providing in vivo evidence of the physiologic importance of STAT5 in mediating this neoplastic transformation.

Tel can function as a fusion partner with other cellular kinases such as abl and the β chain of the PDGF receptor (Lacronique et al., 2000). Both of these chimeric tyrosine kinases can lead to STAT5 activation. A dominant inhibitory form of STAT5 ameliorates the growth factor independence induced by Tel-Jak2, further reinforcing the importance of this particular pathway in hematopoietic growth control. A number of additional permutations of this process have been described including activation of the PDGFβR by fusion with Huntington interacting protein 1 (Ross, Bernard, Berger, & Gilliland, 1998) and CEV14 (Abe et al., 1997).

The activation of STAT-phosphorylating tyrosine kinases following chromosomal translocations is not restricted to leukemias. Among anaplastic large cell lymphomas, a frequent translocation involves chromosomes 2 and 5 (Morris et al., 1994). The resulting NPM/ALK fusion protein leads to the activation of the ALK receptor tyrosine kinase which can phosphorylate STAT5. Inhibition of STAT5 through the use of dominant inhibitory mutants blocks proliferation of NPM/ALK transformed cells both in vitro and in mouse models (Nieborowska-Skorska et al., 2001). Thus it is likely that analysis of the products of the myriad of chromosomal abnormalities detected in leukemias and lymphomas will continue to reveal the activation of tyrosine kinases with resultant STAT phosphorylation. Furthermore, the recurrent findings that inhibition of STAT function causes a reversion of the cellular phenotype lends weight to the notion that STAT phosphorylation is a critical event in the neoplastic transformation of these cells, and not merely an irrelevant substrate of an activated kinase.

5.3 Src family tyrosine kinases

Many members of the src family of non-receptor tyrosine kinases play a role in normal signal transduction to STATs. When activated inappropriately, they can also lead to constitutive STAT activation and neoplastic transformation. In at least one model system, c-src appears to be more important than Jak family members in catalyzing STAT3 phosphorylation in response to IL-3 (Chaturvedi, Reddy, & Reddy, 1998). C-src can also participate in signaling induce by polypeptide growth factors. Activation of src, as occurs in the mutant v-src, can lead to STAT3-dependent transformation of fibroblasts (Garcia et al., 1997). Other proteins related to src can also participate in tumorigenesis. The Lck tyrosine kinase is important to the development and function of T lymphocytes. Lck-mediated phosphorylation of STAT3 and STAT5 is important in the pathogenesis of a murine T cell lymphoma, as well as in neoplastic transformation induced by the oncogenic herpes Saimiri virus (Yu, Jove, & Burakoff, 1997; Lund, Garcia, Medveczky, Jove, & Medveczky, 1997; Lund, Prator, Medveczky, & Medveczky, 1999). Thus, even in the absence of activation by fusion to another protein, non-receptor tyrosine kinases can play an important role in transformation through STATs.

5.4 Activation of the Flt3 receptor tyrosine kinase in AML

With the exception of Bcr-Abl, each of the fusion tyrosine kinases described above occur infrequently in spontaneous human leukemias. However, in aggregate it may be that these type of events are important in the pathogenesis of these cancers. The leukemia with the greatest incidence in the United States is AML, and among AML patients, a single molecular abnormality appears to activate a tyrosine kinase most frequently. The kinase involved is the receptor tyrosine kinase Flt3. Flt3, which is structurally related to the PDGF receptor, can bind to the Flt3 ligand (FL) and stimulates survival and self renewal of hematopoietic progenitor cells (Mackarehtschain et al., 1995). In model systems, stimulation of Flt3 leads to activation of STAT5, suggesting a role for STATs in this important pathway (Zhang et al., 2000). In approximately one quarter of patients with AML, a mutation occurs in Flt3 leading to constitutive phosphorylation and activation of the kinase. Most commonly, this is the result of an internal tandem duplication of the juxtamembrane domain of the protein (Yokota et al., 1997). In model systems, these mutations of Flt3 confers growth factor independence on hematologic cells in a STAT5-dependent manner (Hayakawa et al., 2000; Mizuki et al., 2000). Mutations of other receptor tyrosine kinases, such as Eyk can also lead to transformation of cells in a STAT-dependent manner (Zong, Yan, August, Darnell, & Hanafusa, 1996; Besser, Bromberg, Darnell, & Hanafusa, 1999). Thus subtle mutations in polypeptide growth factor receptors, may be an important, and perhaps under-appreciated, mechanism for STAT activation in the pathogenesis of cancer.

Thus, the activation of tyrosine kinases through a variety of mechanisms is a recurring theme in the pathogenesis of leukemias and lymphomas. While there are a panoply of events which can underlie this process, it is perhaps telling that they all appear to converge in the activation of STAT family members, particularly STAT3 and STAT5. This raises important issues regarding the molecular events which underlie these tumors, and has implications for the development of targeted molecular therapies to treat these diseases.

6. STAT ACTIVATION IN NON-HEMATOLOGIC CANCERS

Although much of the initial work on STAT signal transduction was performed in hematopoietic cells, it is clear that this signal transduction pathway plays a prominent role in the biology of epithelial and mesenchymal cells as well. This reflects the fact that cytokine receptors are present on non-hematopoietic cells, as well as the fact that kinases other than Jaks can phosphorylate STATs. Kinases such as src family members and polypeptide growth factor receptors can mediate phosphorylation of STAT1, STAT3, and STAT5 during normal physiologic signaling, and inappropriate activation of each of these STAT family members has been observed in human cancers as well. Given the many pathways which converge on STATs, it is not surprising that activation of these pathways occurs in a variety of tumors.

6.1 Breast cancer

The most frequently diagnosed cancer in the United States is breast cancer (Jemal, Thomas, Murray, & Thun, 2002). Two lines of evidence suggest that particular STAT isoforms might be important in the biology of this disease. First, STAT5 was initially identified as "mammary gland factor" for its role in mediating the effects of prolactin on sheep mammary tissue (Wakao, Gouilleux, & Groner, 1994). STAT5 is actually comprised of two isoforms, STAT5a and STAT5b, products of distinct though highly homologous genes (Liu et al., 1995). Mice deficient for STAT5a display defects in expansion of lobuloalveolar mammary tissue during pregnancy, reflecting the physiologic importance of STAT5a in mammary growth (Liu et al., 1997). STAT5b-deficient mice also have defects in lactation, though they exhibit other abnormalities consistent with resistance to growth hormone (Udy et al., 1997). The second clue that STATs might play a prominent role in breast cancer derives from the importance of epidermal growth factor (EGF) receptor family members in the biology of this disease (Slamon et al., 1987), and the fact that these tyrosine kinases can mediate phosphorylation of STAT1, STAT3, and

STAT5 (Ruff-Jamison, Chen, & Cohen, 1993; Ruff-Jamison et al., 1994; Ruff-Jamison, Chen, & Cohen, 1995).

Given this, it was not surprising to find activated STAT3, and to a lesser extent, STAT1 in nuclear extracts from breast cancer specimens (Watson & Miller, 1995). Furthermore, a majority of cell lines derived from human breast cancer also displayed constitutive activation of STAT3 (Garcia et al., 1997). A variety of mechanisms may underlie the activation of these transcription factors, including over-expression of EGF receptor family members (Slamon et al., 1987), autocrine activation of these receptors (Sartor, Dziubinski, Yu, Jove, & Ethier, 1997), or activation of other kinases.

Although STATs may a play a role in tumorigenesis through promotion of survival or proliferation, STATs may also play a role in breast cancer through promotion of expression of mucin-like glycoproteins (Gaemers, Vos, Volders, van der Valk, & Hilkens, 2001). These proteins may aid in tumor invasion and metastasis, and may contribute to the worse prognosis of tumors which over-express them.

6.2 Prostate cancer

Prostate cancer, the most common tumor in men, shares some biological parallels with breast cancer, particularly the interplay of polypeptide growth factor receptor and steroid hormone receptor signaling. Like breast cancer, human and animal models of prostate cancer have been found to contain constitutively activated STAT3 (Ni, Lou, Leman, & Gao, 2000; Chen, Wang, & Farrar, 2000). Furthermore, STAT3 may interact with the androgen receptor and promote its transcriptional activity (Chen, Wang, & Farrar, 2000). Given the clear importance of androgen signaling in the development and progression of prostate cancer, this may be an important aspect of the contribution of STAT3 to prostate cancer biology. In addition, an important molecular epidemiological marker for risk of developing prostate cancer is the serum level of the growth factor IGF-1 (Chan et al., 1997). IGF-1 has also been reported to activate STAT3, and this is an additional mechanism by which STAT3 may contribute to the genesis of prostate cancer (Zong et al., 2000).

6.3 Melanoma

One of the most rapidly increasing tumors in the United States is melanoma. As opposed to hematologic and epithelial cells, the growth factors which control the physiologic proliferation of melanocytes are less well understood. Nonetheless, in common with other cancers, melanoma precursor lesions have been shown to contain activated STAT1 and STAT3 (Kirkwood et al., 1999). A common mouse model of melanoma, the B16 cell line, has also been shown to contain activated STAT3 (Niu et al., 1999). Reflecting the physiologic importance of STAT3 in this system, introduction of a dominant inhibitory form of this transcription factor led to widespread apoptosis.

6.4 Head and neck cancer

The genesis of squamous cell carcinomas of the head and neck, which includes sites such as the tongue and the larynx, is clearly related to exposure to alcohol and cigarette smoke. However, like breast cancer, these tumors are frequently driven by abnormalities of growth factor receptors such as those of the EGF receptor family. Thus, it is not surprising that constitutive activation of STAT3 has been found in tumor cells and cell lines derived from patients with these tumors (Endo et al., 1999; Grandis, Drenning et al., 2000; Grandis, Zeng, & Drenning, 2000). Although STAT1 is also activated by these receptors, it appears that STAT3 is more important in these systems in promoting proliferation and protecting from apoptosis (Grandis et al., 1998). In particular, interfering with STAT3 function blocks the proliferation and survival of these cells.

6.5 Lung cancer

Although lung cancer is the leading cause of cancer death for both women and men in the United States (Jemal et al., 2002), its molecular pathogenesis may be somewhat more pleiotropic than most tumors. Nonetheless, increased expression or activation of EGF receptor family members may play an important role in many cases of non-small cell lung cancer, the most common variant of this tumor. Consistent with other tumors in which this pathway may be involved, STAT3 is reported to be activated in some models of this disease (Fernandes, Hamburger, & Gerwin, 1999).

6.6 Ovarian cancer

Although evidence suggesting a role for inappropriate activation of STAT3 in ovarian cancer is not as well developed as for other cancers, several pieces of data support this possibility. Preliminary evidence in human ovarian cancer cell lines indicates that STAT3 is constitutively activated, and that this contributes to the growth and survival of these cells (Reddy, Chaturvedi, & Reddy, 1999; Huang et al., 2002). Furthermore, in a study of invasive behavior of ovarian epithelial cells in *Drosophila*, a potentially new role for STATs in cellular function was observed (Silver & Montell, 2001). An assay was used to screen for genetic mutations which converted ovarian border cells from their basal stationary state to invasive migratory cells. The genes which were identified were all involved in *Drosophila* STAT signaling. It is unclear whether this is relevant to the biology of normal or neoplastic human ovarian cells. However, it raises the possibility that in addition to the likely roles of STATs in survival, proliferation, and differentiation, they may also play a role in migration and invasion, processes particularly relevant to tumor spread and metastases.

6.7 Colorectal cancer

After lung cancer, colorectal cancer is the leading cause of cancer death in the United States (Jemal et al., 2002). Although definitive evidence for a role of STAT signal transduction in colorectal cancer is not as strong as for other tumors, several pieces of evidence suggests that this pathway may be important in these cancers as well. One of the first clues that STAT signaling was important in the pathogenesis of multiple myeloma came from the observation that myeloma cells could produce IL-6 and also respond to this cytokine. Using in situ hybridization on resected specimens from patients with primary colorectal cancer, it was found that the tumor cells contained significantly increased mRNA for both IL-6 and the IL-6 receptor, when compared to normal adjacent epithelium (Shirota, LeDuy, Yuan, & Jothy, 1990). Similar to what is seen in myeloma, IL-6 appears to prevent Fas-induced apoptosis in colorectal carcinoma cells (Frank, Mahajan, & Yuan, 1999). This may also have relevance to genesis of colorectal carcinomas in humans, as agents known to decrease the risk of these cancers in epidemiological studies also decrease IL-6-induced signaling events. It remains to be determined whether the IL-6 effects seen in colorectal carcinoma cells are mediated by STATs or by another cascade activated by this cytokine.

An interesting consideration which arises from the data derived from colorectal cells concerns the relative role of various STAT family members in transducing signals related to cellular growth and survival. Cytokines such as IL-6, oncostatin M, ciliary neurotrophic factor (CNTF), and leukemia inhibitory factor (LIF) signal through receptor complexes in which the associated Jak family members are coupled to gp130 (Frank & Greenberg, 1996), and all of these cytokines activate both STAT1 and STAT3. The ratios of phosphorylated STAT1 to STAT3 vary among the different cytokines in a given cell type, and among a single cytokine in multiple cell types, although the mechanism for this is not fully understood. In the case of colorectal carcinoma cells, STAT1 is the STAT which is activated predominantly. Much of the evidence concerning the role of STAT1 in malignancy would suggest that this STAT functions primarily to restrain cellular growth, and to function perhaps as a tumor suppressor gene (Levy & Gilliland, 2000). However, much of this evidence arises from mice lacking STAT1, which have an increase in tumor following exposure to carcinogens (Kaplan et al., 1998). This has been interpreted to reflect a role for STAT1 in mediating interferon-γ-dependent immune surveillance. While this may be important in mice, there is much less evidence to suggest such a mechanism in humans. STAT1 activation has been seen in many human tumors, albeit largely in conjunction with other activated STATs. Thus, it remains an important unanswered question to determine the role of this protein in the physiology of a malignant cell.

7. STAT FEEDBACK LOOPS IN CANCER

Although much attention has been given to the mechanisms by which STATs can be activated, the processes by which STAT signal transduction is turned off is also of great importance. In the classical model of "Jak-STAT" signaling, a cytokine binding to its receptor leads to the induction of STAT tyrosine phosphorylation, nuclear translocation, and transcriptional activation. However, for most cytokines, STATs reach peak tyrosine phosphorylation within 15 to 30 minutes, and STAT phosphorylation returns to basal levels in a period of one to two hours. Thus it is clear that negative feedback loops must be quite active to shut off STAT activation. STAT inactivation appears to be dependent on events at the cell membrane which prevent the phosphorylation of additional STAT molecules, and processes targeting the STATs themselves to render them inactive (Figure 2). Two principal mechanisms have been described to inhibit STAT kinases. Receptors can be internalized, leading to degradation or inactivation, and this may curtail the period during which STAT phosphorylation can occur. In addition, inhibitors of Jak family kinases can bind to the receptor-kinase complex, thereby preventing further STAT phosphorylation. This group of proteins, generally termed "suppressors of cytokine signaling" (SOCS), are encoded by genes whose transcription is induced by STATs, generating a negative feedback loop (Endo et al., 1997; Naka et al., 1997; Starr et al., 1997).

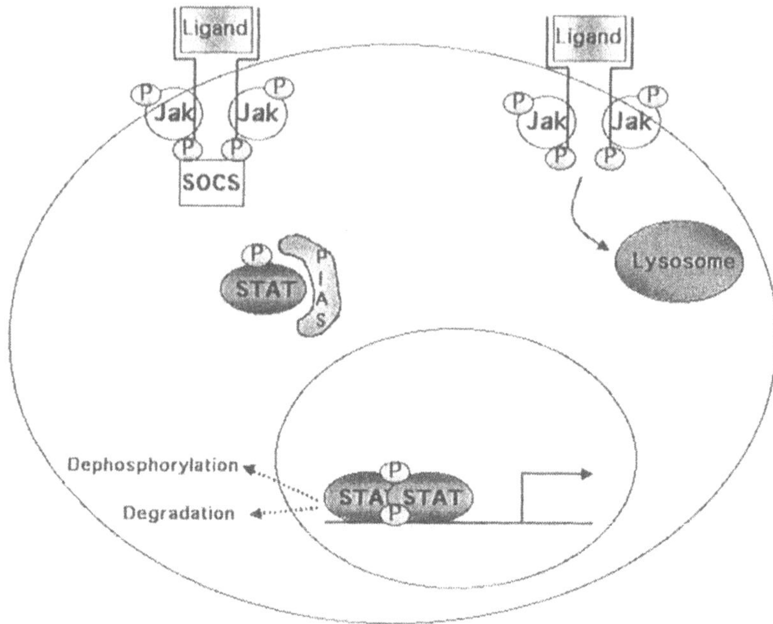

Figure 2. Negative regulatory feedback loops. Activation of the Jak-STAT pathway is down-modulated by several mechanisms directed both at the Jak and the STAT component. The kinase activity of Jaks is inhibited by SOCS proteins induced by STATs. In addition, the receptor-kinase complex can be internalized and degraded. STATs can be inhibited by direct interaction with proteins such as PIAS (which may aid in sumoylation). Activated STATs can also be directly de-phosphorylated and/or degraded, the latter often in a ubiquitin-dependent process

The STATs themselves can be inactivated by three broad mechanisms: they may be dephosphorylated, they can be degraded (often in a ubiquitin-dependent manner), or they can interact with other cellular proteins which can inactivate them (Jackson, 2001). The relative role of each of these mechanisms in a given system remains unclear. Nonetheless, the complexity of the systems down-regulating

STAT activation raises the question of whether defects in the negative regulation of STAT signaling may be an important component of the development of malignancies in which activated STATs appear to play an important role. Since many of these negative regulatory proteins are themselves STAT targets, it would be expected in a malignancy in which STATs are constitutively activated through a receptor-associated process that one or more of these proteins would inhibit further STAT phosphorylation. It has been suggested that in certain cancers the SOCS locus is hypermethylated, thereby blocking transcriptional activation of these genes. Alternatively, it may be that mutations in receptor-kinase complexes render them resistant to suppression by SOCS family proteins. It may well be that non-receptor kinases which become activate in cancer are resistant to SOCS-mediated suppression. Additional work will be necessary to evaluate these possibilities.

8. STATS AS TARGETS FOR ANTI-CANCER THERAPY

8.1 General considerations

An extensive body of data has indicated that STAT family members, particularly STAT3 and STAT5, are activated commonly in primary human cancers. Furthermore, inactivation of these STATs in model systems is generally associated with a cessation of growth and/or a propensity of the cells to undergo apoptosis. These features would make STATs a particularly attractive target for anti-cancer therapies. However, the field of oncology is replete with potential targets, and agents which can disrupt them. A critical point is whether inhibition of such a pathway is more likely to cause damage to cancer cells than the wide variety of normal cells which may also employ this pathway.

Two principal lines of evidence suggests that STAT inhibitors may have modest effects in normal tissue and thus may have a significant therapeutic index. The first argument is based on genetic studies in which STATs have been deleted from mice through gene targeting. With the exception of disruption of STAT3, mice which lack individual STAT members as well as certain combinations of STATs, are viable and fertile (O'Shea, Gadina, & Schreiber, 2002). STAT3 null mice display lethality during embryonic development. However, tissue-specific conditional knockouts of STAT3 have been made, and these animals show more subtle findings. These data suggest that normal tissue in adult animals can tolerate complete inactivation of STATs with manageable consequences. The second line of evidence derives from studies in various in vitro systems. These have repeatedly shown that while malignant cells displaying chronic STAT activation are markedly inhibited by inactivation of STATs, normal cells tolerate this with little measurable effect (Garcia et al., 1997). This is generally thought to reflect the fact that in the unbalanced intracellular environment of a tumor cell, survival and proliferation are dependent on continued STAT activation. Furthermore, the level of STAT activation in a malignant cell is often far in excess of what is seen under physiologic circumstances (Frank & Varticovski, 1996), again perhaps reflecting the requirement for maximal activation of this signaling pathway to maintain neoplasia.

8.2 Strategies to inhibit STAT function

Innumerable approaches can be taken to inhibit STAT function as a potential treatment for cancer. However, they can be divided into several broad areas. The first dichotomy is between approaches which target the STATs directly and those which inhibit upstream activating signals.

8.2.1 Tyrosine kinase inhibitors

The development of tyrosine kinase inhibitors is an area of great interest in developmental therapeutics for cancer. While drugs such as STI-571, an inhibitor of the Bcr-Abl tyrosine kinase, clearly lead to the rapid loss of tyrosine phosphorylation of STAT5, they also exert effects on the many other signaling pathways activated by these kinases. Thus, as they are not uniquely inhibiting STAT activation, their potential for side effects may be greater. On the other hand, since the kinases they inhibit may not be active in normal cells, or may not phosphorylate STATs in normal cells, their toxicity might be significantly different from a "pure" STAT inhibitor. Nonetheless, tyrosine kinase inhibitors which inactivate STATs may be the approach to STAT inhibition whose clinical development is furthest along. In addition to STI-571, the Jak2 inhibitor AG-490 has been shown to have anti-leukemic effects in animal models of human leukemias (Meydan et al., 1996).

8.2.2 Approaches requiring gene therapy

In considering approaches to STAT inhibition, a second dichotomy can be considered, that between approaches which require the expression of newly introduced genes, and those which can be achieved with small organic molecules. In the former category, one could consider the expression of dominant inhibitory forms of STATs. Abundant experimental evidence has indicated that this approach can be effective in vitro, and even in animal models of cancer (Niu et al., 1999). A second approach would be to express genes coding for STAT inhibitors, such as members of the SOCS family (which could potentially inhibit JAK family kinases upstream of STATs), or PIAS families proteins which could inactivate STATs directly, perhaps through the process of sumoylation (Jackson, 2001). While these approaches have attractive features, they require the expression of exogenous genes in human tumors, a process which remains technically quite challenging. As the field of human gene therapy advances, these strategies may become more feasible.

8.2.3 Pharmacologic inhibition of STATs

An attractive strategy would be the use of targeted molecules, preferably orally active, which could inhibit STAT function specifically and potently. While one can consider a number of strategies to achieve this goal, three broad approaches show the potential for clinical utility in the near future (Figure 3).

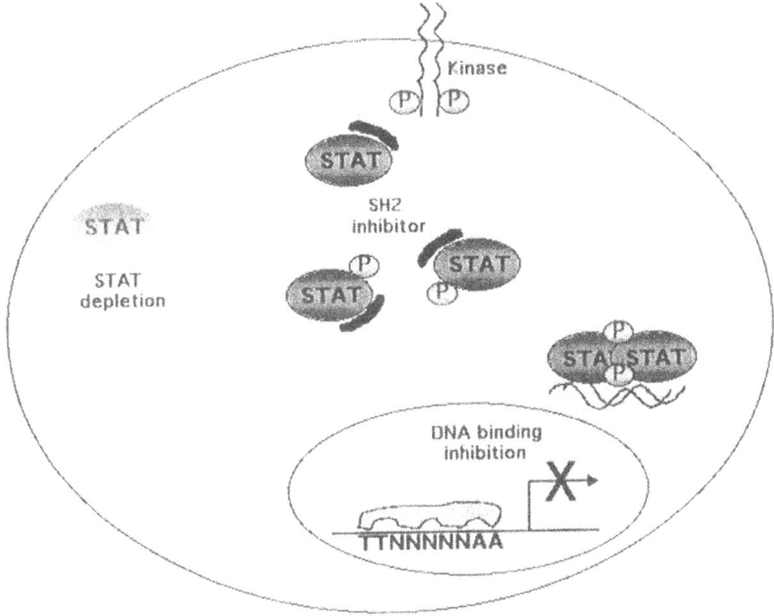

Figure 3. Mechanisms for therapeutic STAT inhibition. Among the many approaches which could be envisioned, clinically feasible strategies include direct depletion of STATs such as by antisense strategies; SH2 inhibitors, which could block STAT recruitment to activated kinases and also prevent the dimerization of tyrosine phosphorylated STATs; and DNA binding inhibitors which can target STATs (as with decoy oligonucleotides) or the DNA sequence to which they bind (as with site directed polyamides).

Antisense molecules. The first is the depletion of a specific STAT through the use of antisense oligonucleotides. Although these molecules are not "small" in a pharmacologic sense, and they are not orally bioavailable, antisense oligonucleotides have demonstrated the ability to deplete STATs in in vitro systems, thereby altering cellular behavior. Antisense molecules targeting other gene products have begun clinical trials in humans, and these molecules have proven to be generally safe when given systemically. Whether this will be an effective way to target activated STATs in tumors is unknown, but the possibility clearly exists.

SH2 inhibitors. As the structure and function of the various domains comprising a STAT molecule have been elucidated, two specific targets have emerged for pharmacologic inhibition. The first is the SH2 domain, which allows STATs to bind to phosphorylated tyrosine residues in receptor-kinase complexes. The SH2 domain confers specificity to an activated kinase which can phosphorylate a given STAT molecule. Blocking a STAT SH2 domain could thereby prevent STAT recruitment to an activated kinase and block its tyrosine phosphorylation. The SH2 domain is also critical for the ability of a STAT to form a dimer, which involves the formation of reciprocal interactions between the SH2 domain of one STAT monomer and the phosphorylated tyrosine of its partner. Thus blocking a STAT SH2 domain has the added feature of blocking two separate steps in the pathway to STAT activation, and this may enhance its efficacy. Initial studies have suggested that small phosphopeptides can be developed which mimic the physiologic binding sequence of STAT SH2 domains, thereby interfering with their function (Turkson et al., 2001). While phosphopeptides themselves are generally not cell permeable, coupling to protein translocation domains such as that encoded by the *antennapedia* gene can allow these molecules to penetrate cells. Alternatively, the development of peptidomimetic compounds may allow the issue of cell permeability to be overcome. In any case, this is an attractive strategy which may have clinical utility not only in STAT inhibition, but in the modulation of other SH2-containing protein as well.

DNA binding inhibitors. The second domain on a STAT molecule which may be susceptible to inhibition is the DNA binding domain. Similar to the strategy of using the sequence of peptides known to bind to the STAT SH2 domain, double-stranded oligonucleotides mimicking the nine base pair STAT consensus binding sequence can also be employed. These so-called "decoy oligonucleotides" can be introduced into cells by diffusion, lipid carriers, or other strategies (Wang, Yang, Kirken, Resau, & Farrar, 2000). Activated STATs would then bind these "decoys," which would be present in molar excess greater than that of the physiologic targets in the promoters of target genes. By competition, they would attenuate STAT-dependent gene activation. Such an approach has been shown to be effective in cell culture systems. Although non-specific effects from oligonucleotides are always possible, the delivery means are similar to those which have already been devised for antisense molecules. Thus, such a strategy is likely to be feasible in human clinical trials.

One final approach is to inhibit STAT-DNA binding from the other half of the interaction, the DNA surface. Small molecules of the polyamide class have been generated which can bind to the minor groove of DNA in a sequence-specific manner (Wemmer, 2000; White, Szewczyk, Turner, Baird, & Dervan, 1998). Thus, one can conceive of an approach where such molecules are synthesized to bind to the consensus sequence for STAT3 or STAT5, or for the specific sequence in the target genes of specific promoters involved in cell cycle progression or cell survival. As these agents can be orally active, this might be a particularly useful approach for long term therapy.

8.3 STAT inhibition as a component of anti-cancer therapy

As much as we wish for a single agent to be effective at eradicating tumor cells, the history of cancer therapy has shown that combination approaches are almost always necessary. In cell culture systems, and some animal models, STAT inhibition alone has been effective in stopping tumor growth or inducing apoptosis. However, in human tumors, it may well be the case that STAT inhibitors will be one component of a multi-pronged approach. Potentially, a combination of approaches to STAT inhibition, such as the use of a tyrosine kinase inhibitor and a STAT SH2 domain inhibitor may be particularly effective. More likely, it may be necessary to combine STAT inhibition with the inhibition of other signal transduction pathways, or processes such as angiogenesis, to optimize the benefits of this approach. Finally, it may also be advantageous to combine a STAT inhibitor with a cytotoxic agent to induce maximal levels of apoptosis. Nonetheless, it is likely that the next generation of anti-cancer therapy will be built upon inhibitors of signaling pathways, and STAT proteins may be excellent targets for this approach.

David A. Frank
Department of Adult Oncology
Dana-Farber Cancer Institute
Departments of Medicine
Harvard Medical School and
Brigham and Women's Hospital
Boston, MA

8. REFERENCES

Abe, A., Emi, N., Tanimoto, M., Terasaki, H., Marunouchi, T., & Saito, H. (1997). Fusion of the platelet-derived growth factor receptor b to a novel gene CEV14 in acute myelogenous leukemia after clonal evolution. *Blood, 90*, 4271-4277.

Anderson, K. C., Jones, R. M., Morimoto, C., Leavitt, P., & Barut, B. A. (1989). Response patterns of purified myeloma cells to hematopoietic growth factors. *Blood, 73*, 1915 1924.

Azam, M., Lee, C. K., Strehlow, I., & Schindler, C. (1997). Functionally distinct isoforms of STAT5 are generated by protein processing. *Immunity, 6*, 691-701.

Benekli, M., Xia, Z., Donohue, K. A., Ford, L. A., Pixley, L. A., Baer, M. R., Baumann, H., & Wetzler, M. (2002). Constitutive activity of signal transducer and activator of transcription 3 protein in acute myeloid leukemia blasts is associated with short disease-free survival. *Blood, 99*, 252-257.

Besser, D., Bromberg, J. F., Darnell, J. E., Jr., & Hanafusa, H. (1999). A single amino acid substitution in the v-Eyk intracellular domain results in activation of Stat3 and enhances cellular transformation. *Mol. Cell. Biol., 19*, 1401-1409.

Bromberg, J. F., Wrzeszczynska, M. H., Devgan, G., Zhao, Y., Pestell, R. G., Albanese, C., & Darnell, J. E., Jr. (1999). *Stat3* as an oncogene. *Cell, 98*, 295-303.

Catlett-Falcone, R., Landowski, T. H., Oshiro, M. M., Turkson, J., Levitzki, A., Savino, R., Ciliberto, G., Moscinski, L., Fernandez-Luna, J. L., Nunez, G., Dalton, W. S., & Jove, R. (1999). Constitutive activation of Stat3 signaling confers resistance to apoptosis in human U266 myeloma cells. *Immunity, 10*, 105-115.

Chai, S. K., Nichols, G. L., & Rothman, P. (1997). Constitutive activation of JAKs and STATs in BCR-Abl-expressing cell lines and peripheral blood cells derived from leukemic patients. *J. Immunol., 159*, 4720-4728.

Chan, J. M., Stampfer, M. J., Giovannucci, E., Gann, P. H., Ma, J., Wilkinson, P., Hennekens, C. H., & Pollak, M. (1997). Plasma insulin-like growth factor-I and prostate cancer risk: a prospective study. *Science, 279*, 563-566.

Chaturvedi, P., Reddy, M. V., & Reddy, E. P. (1998). Src kinases and not JAKs activate STATs during IL-3 induced myeloid cell proliferation. *Oncogene, 16*, 1749-1758.

Chen, T., Wang, L. H., & Farrar, W. L. (2000). Interleukin 6 activates androgen receptor-mediated gene expression through a signal transducer and activator of transcription 3-dependent pathway in LNCaP prostate cancer cells. *Cancer Res., 60*, 2132-2135.

Endo, S., Zeng, Q., He, Y., Drenning, S. D., Watkins, S. L., Huang, L., & Rubin Grandis, J. (1999). Increased Stat3 activation in head and neck tumors in vivo. *Proc. Amer. Assoc. Cancer Res., 40*, 336.

Endo, T. A., Masuhara, M., Yokouchi, M., Suzuki, R., Sakamoto, H., Mitsui, K., Matsumoto, A., Tanimura, S., Ohtsubo, M., Misawa, H., Miyazaki, T., Leonor, N., Taniguchi, T., Fujita, T.,

Kanakura, Y., Komiya, S., & Yoshimura, A. (1997). A new protein containing an SH2 domain that inhibits JAK kinases. *Nature, 387*, 921-924.

Eriksen, K. W., Kaltoft, K., Mikkelsen, G., Nielsen, M., Zhang, Q., Geisler, C., Nissen, M. H., Ropke, C., Wasik, M. A., & Odum, N. (2001). Constitutive STAT3-activation in Sezary syndrome: tyrphostin AG490 inhibits STAT3-activation, interleukin-2 receptor expression and growth of leukemic Sezary cells. *Leukemia, 15*(5), 787-793.

Fernandes, A., Hamburger, A. W., & Gerwin, B. I. (1999). ErbB-2 kinase is required for constitutive stat 3 activation in malignant human lung epithelial cells. *Int. J. Cancer, 83*, 564-570.

Frank, D. A., Robertson, M., Bonni, A., Ritz, J., & Greenberg, M. E. (1995). IL-2 signaling involves the phosphorylation of novel Stat proteins. *Proc. Natl. Acad. Sci., 92*, 7779 7783.

Frank, D. A., & Varticovski, L. (1996). BCR/abl leads to the constitutive activation of Stat proteins, and shares an epitope with tyrosine phosphorylated Stats. *Leukemia, 10*, 1724 1730.

Frank, D. A., Mahajan, S., & Ritz, J. (1997). B lymphocytes from patients with chronic lymphocytic leukemia contain STAT1 and STAT3 constitutively phosphorylated on serine residues. *J. Clin. Invest., 100*, 3140-3148.

Gaemers, I. C., Vos, H. L., Volders, H. H., van der Valk, S. W., & Hilkens, J. (2001). A STAT-responsive element in the promoter of the episialin/*MUC1* gene is involved in its overexpression in carcinoma cells. *J. Biol. Chem., 276*, 6191-6199.

Garcia, R., Yu, C.-L., Hudnall, A., Catlett, R., Nelson, K. L., Smithgall, T., Fujita, D. J., Ethier, S. P., & Jove, R. (1997). Constitutive activation of Stat3 in fibroblasts transformed by diverse oncoproteins and in breast carcinoma cells. *Cell Growth Diff., 8*, 1267-1276.

Gouilleux-Gruart, V., Gouilleux, F., Desaint, C., Claisse, J.-F., Capiod, J.-C., Delobel, J., Weber-Nordt, R., Dusanter-Fourt, I., Dreyfus, F., Groner, B., & Prin, L. (1996). STAT-related transcription factors are constitutively activated in peripheral blood cells from acute leukemia patients. *Blood, 87*, 1692-1697.

Grandis, J. R., Drenning, S. D., Chakraborty, A., Zhou, M.-Y., Zeng, Q., Pitt, A. S., & Tweardy, D. J. (1998). Requirement of Stat3 but not Stat1 activation for epidermal growth factor-mediated cell growth in vitro. *J. Clin. Inv., 102*, 1385-1392.

Grandis, J. R., Drenning, S. D., Zeng, Q., Watkins, S. C., Melhem, M. F., Endo, S., Johnson, D. E., Huang, L., He, Y., & Kim, J. D. (2000). Constitutive activation of Stat3 signaling abrogates apoptosis in squamous cell carcinogenesis in vivo. *Proc Natl Acad Sci U S A, 97*(8), 4227-4232.

Grandis, J. R., Zeng, Q., & Drenning, S. D. (2000). Epidermal growth factor receptor--mediated stat3 signaling blocks apoptosis in head and neck cancer. *Laryngoscope, 110*(5 Pt 1), 868-874.

Hayakawa, F., Towatari, M., Kiyoi, H., Tanimoto, M., Kitamura, T., Saito, H., & Naoe, T. (2000). Tandem-duplicated Flt3 constitutively activates STAT5 and MAP kinase and introduces autonomous cell growth in IL-3-dependent cell lines. *Oncogene, 19*, 624-631.

Hilbert, D. M., Kopf, M., Mock, B. A., Kohler, G., & Rudikoff, S. (1995). Interleukin 6 is essential for in vivo development of B lineage neoplasms. *J. Exp. Med., 182*, 243-248.

Hilbert, D. M., Migone, T.-S., Kopf, M., Leonard, W. J., & Rudikoff, S. (1996). Distinct tumorigenic potential of *abl* and *raf* in B cell neoplasia: *abl* activates the IL-6 signaling pathway. *Immunity, 5*, 81-89.

Ilaria, R. L. J., Hawly, R. G., & Van Etten, R. A. (1999). Dominant negative mutants implicate STAT5 in myeloid cell proliferation and neutrophil differentiation. *Blood, 93*, 4154-4166.

Jackson, P. K. (2001). A new RING for SUMO: wrestling transcription responses into nuclear bodies with PIAS family E3 SUMO ligases. *Genes Dev., 15*, 3053-3058.

Jemal, A., Thomas, A., Murray, T., & Thun, M. (2002). Cancer statistics, 2002. *CA Cancer J. Clin., 52*, 23-47.

Joos, S., Kupper, M., Ohl, S., Von Bonin, F., Mechtersheimer, G., Bentz, M., Marynen, P., Moller, P., Pfreundschuh, M., Trumper, L., & Lichter, P. (2000). Genomic imbalances including amplification of the tyrosine kinase gene *JAK2* in CD30^{+} Hodgkin cells. *Cancer Res., 60*, 549-552.

Kawano, F., Yamaguchi, K., Nishimura, H., Tsuda, H., & Takatsuki, K. (1985). Variation in the clinical courses of adult T-cell leukemia. *Cancer Res, 55*, 851-856.

Kawano, M., Hirano, T., Matsuda, T., Taga, T., Horii, Y., Iwato, K., Asaoku, H., Tang, B., Tanabe, O., Tanaka, H., & Kishimoto, T. (1988). Autocrine generation and requirement of BSF-2/IL-6 for human multiple myelomas. *Nature, 332*, 83-85.

Kirkwood, J. M., Farkas, D. L., Chakraborty, A., Dyer, K. F., Tweardy, D. J., Abernethy, J. L., Edington, H. D., Donnelly, S. S., & Becker, D. (1999). Systemic interferon-a (IFN a) treatment leads to Stat3 inactivation in melanoma precursor lesions. *Mol. Med., 5*, 11-20.

Klein, B., Zhang, X. G., Yang, L. Z., & Bataille, R. (1995). Interleukin-6 in human multiple myeloma. *Blood, 85*, 863-874.
Konopka, J. B., Watanabe, S. M., & Witte, O. N. (1984). An alteration of the human c-abl protein in K562 unmasks associated tyrosine kinase activity. *Cell, 37*, 1035-1042.
Kube, D., Hotlick, U., Vockerodt, M., Ahmadi, T., Haier, B., Behrmann, I., Heinrich, P., Diehl, V., & Tesch, H. (2001). STAT3 is constitutively activated in Hodgkin cell lines. *Blood, 98*, 762-770.
Lacronique, V., Boreux, A., Monni, R., Dumon, S., Mauchauffe, M., Mayeux, P., Gouilleux, F., Berger, R., Gisselbrecht, S., Ghysdael, J., & Bernard, O. A. (2000). Transforming properties of chimeric TEL-JAK proteins in Ba/F3 cells. *Blood, 95*, 2076-2083.
Lacronique, V., Boureux, A., Della Valle, V., Poirel, H., Quang, C. T., Mauchaufee, M., Berthou, C., Lessard, M., Berger, R., Ghysdael, J., & Bernard, O. A. (1997). A TEL-JAK2 fusion protein with constitutive kinase activity in human leukemia. *Science, 278*, 1309-1312.
Levy, Y., Tsapis, A., & Brouet, J. C. (1991). Interleukin-6 antisense oligonucleotides inhibit the growth of human myeloma cell lines. *J. Clin. Invest., 88*, 696-699.
Lin, T. S., Mahajan, S., & Frank, D. A. (2000). STAT signaling in the pathogenesis and treatment of leukemias. *Oncogene, 19*, 2496-2504.
Liu, X., Robinson, G. W., Gouilleux, F., Groner, B., & Hennighausen, L. (1995). Cloning and expression of stat5 and an additional homologue (stat5b) involved in prolactin signal transduction in mouse mammary tissue. *Proc. Natl. Acad. Sci., 92*, 8831-8835.
Liu, X., Robinson, G. W., Wagner, K.-U., Garrett, L., Wynshaw-Boris, A., & Hennighausen, L. (1997). Stat5a is mandatory for adult mammary gland development and lactogenesis. *Genes Dev., 11*, 179-186.
Lund, T. C., Garcia, R., Medveczky, M. M., Jove, R., & Medveczky, P. G. (1997). Activation of STAT transcription factors by herpesvirus Saimiri Tip-484 requires p56lck. *J. Virol., 71*, 6677-6682.
Lund, T. C., Prator, P. C., Medveczky, M. M., & Medveczky, P. G. (1999). The Lck binding domain of herpesvirus saimiri tip-484 constitutively activates Lck and STAT3 in T cells. *J. Virol., 73*, 1689-1694.
Mackarehtschain, K., Hardin, J. D., Moore, K. A., Boast, S., Goff, S. P., & Lemischka, I. R. (1995). Targeted disruption of the flk2/flt3 gene leads to deficiencies in primitive hematopoietic progenitors. *Immunity, 3*, 147-161.
Meydan, N., Grunberger, T., Dadi, H., Shahar, M., Arpaia, E., Lapidot, Z., Leeder, J. S., Freedman, M., Cohen, A., Gazit, A., Levitzki, A., & Roifman, C. M. (1996). Inhibition of acute lymphoblastic leukaemia by a Jak-2 inhibitor. *Nature, 379*, 645-648.
Migone, T.-S., Lin, J.-X., Cereseto, A., Mulloy, J. C., O'Shea, J. J., Franchini, G., & Leonard, W. J. (1995). Constitutively activated Jak-STAT pathway in T cells transformed with HTLV-I. *Science, 269*, 79-81.
Mizuki, M., Fenski, R., Halfter, H., Matsumura, I., Schmidt, R., Muller, C., Gruning, W., Kratz Albers, K., Serve, S., Steyr, C., Buchner, T., Kienast, J., Kanakura, Y., Berdel, W. E., & Serve, H. (2000). Flt3 mutations from patients with acute myeloid leukemia induce transformation of 32D cells mediated by the Ras and STAT5 pathways. *Blood, 96*, 3907 3914.
Morris, S. W., Kirstein, M. N., Valentine, M. B., Dittmer, K. G., Shapiro, D. N., Saltman, D. L., & Look, A. T. (1994). Fusion of a kinase gene, *ALK*, to a nucleolar protein gene, *NPM*, in non-Hodgkin's lymphoma. *Science, 263*, 1281-1284.
Naka, T., Narazaki, M., Hirata, M., Matsumoto, T., Minamoto, S., Aono, A., Nishimoto, N., Kajita, T., Taga, T., Yoshizaki, K., Akira, S., & Kishimoto, T. (1997). Structure and function of a new STAT-induced STAT inhibitor. *Nature, 387*, 924-928.
Nieborowska-Skorska, M., Slupianek, A., Xue, L., Zhang, Q., Raghunath, P. N., Hoser, G., Wasik, M. A., Morris, S. W., & Skorski, T. (2001). Role of signal transducer and activator of transcription 5 in nucleophosmin/ anaplastic lymphoma kinase-mediated malignant transformation of lymphoid cells. *Cancer Res, 61*(17), 6517-6523.
Nielsen, M., Kaestel, C. G., Eriksen, K. W., Woetmann, A., Stokkedal, T., Kaltoft, K., Geisler, C., Ropke, C., & Odum, N. (1999). Inhibition of constitutively activated Stat3 correlates with altered Bcl-2/Bax expression and induction of apoptosis in mycosis fungoides tumor cells. *Leukemia, 13*, 735-738.
Nielsen, M., Kaltoft, K., Nordahl, M., Ropke, C., Geisler, C., Mustelin, T., Dobson, P., Svejgaard, A., & Odum, N. (1997). Constitutive activation of a slowly migrating isoform of Stat3 in mycosis fungoides: Tyrphostin AG490 inhibits Stat3 activation and growth of mycosis fungoides tumor cell lines. *Proc. Natl. Acad. Sci., 94*, 6764-6769.

Nielsen, M., Nissen, M. H., Gerwien, J., Zocca, M.-B., Rasmussen, H. M., Nakajima, K., Ropke, C., Geisler, C., Kaltoft, K., & Odum, N. (2002). Spontaneous interleukin-5 production in cutaneous T-cell lymphoma lines is mediated by constitutively activated Stat3. *Blood, 99*, 973-977.

Niu, G., Heller, R., Catlett-Falcone, R., Coppola, D., Jaroszeski, M., Dalton, W., Jove, R., & Yu, H. (1999). Gene therapy with dominant-negative Stat3 suppresses growth of the murine melanoma B16 tumor in vivo. *Cancer Res, 59*(20), 5059-5063.

Onishi, M., Nosaka, T., Misawa, K., Mui, A. L.-F., Gorman, D., McMahon, M., Miyajima, A., & Kitamura, T. (1998). Identification and characterization of a constitutively active STAT5 mutant that promotes cell proliferation. *Mol Cell Biol, 18*, 3871-3879.

O'Shea, J. J., Gadina, M., & Schreiber, R. D. (2002). Cytokine signaling in 2002: New surprises in the Jak/Stat pathway. *Cell, 109*, S121-S131.

Peeters, P., Raynaud, S. D., Cools, J., Wlodarska, I., Grosgeorge, J., Philip, P., Monpoux, F., Van Rompaey, L., Baens, M., Van den Berghe, H., & Marynen, P. (1997). Fusion of *Tel*, the ETS-variant gene 6 (*ETV6*), to the receptor-associated kinase *Jak2* as a result of t(9;12) in a lymphoid and t(9;15;12) in a myeloid leukemia. *Blood, 90*, 2535-2540.

Rawat, R., Rainey, G. J., Thompson, C. D., Frazier-Jessen, M. R., Brown, R. T., & Nordan, R. P. (2000). Constitutive activation of STAT3 is associated with the acquisition of an interleukin 6-independent phenotype by murine plasmacytomas and hybridomas. *Blood, 96*, 3514-3521.

Ross, T., Bernard, O., Berger, R., & Gilliland, D. G. (1998). Fusion of the Huntington interacting protein 1 to platelet-derived growth factor b receptor (PDGFbR) in chronic myelomonocytic leukemia with t(5;7)(q33;q11.2). *Blood, 91*, 4419-4426.

Sartor, C. I., Dziubinski, M. L., Yu, C. L., Jove, R., & Ethier, S. P. (1997). Role of epidermal growth factor receptor and STAT-3 activation in autonomous proliferation of SUM-102PT human breast cancer cells. *Cancer Res., 57*, 978-987.

Schwaller, J., Frantsve, J., Aster, J., Williams, I. R., Tomasson, M. H., Ross, T. S., Peeters, P., Van Rompaey, L., Van Etten, R. A., Ilaria, R. J., Marynen, P., & Gilliland, D. G. (1998). Transformation of hematopoietic cell lines to growth-factor independence and induction of a fatal myelo- and lymphoproliferative disease in mice by retrovirally transduced TEL/JAK2 fusion genes. *EMBO J., 17*, 5321-5333.

Schwaller, J., Parganas, E., Wang, D., Cain, D., Aster, J. C., Williams, I. R., Lee, C.-K., Gerthner, R., Kitamura, T., Frantsve, J., Anastasiadou, E., Loh, M. L., Levy, D. E., Ihle, J. N., & Gilliland, D. G. (2000). Stat5 is essential for the myelo- and lymphoproliferative disease induced by TEL/JAK2. *Mol. Cell, 6*, 693-704.

Shimoda, K., van Deursen, J., Sangster, M. Y., Sarawar, S. R., Carson, R. T., Tripp, R. A., Chu, C., Quelle, F. W., Nosaka, T., Vignali, D. A., Doherty, P. C., Grosveld, G., Paul, W. E., & Ihle, J. N. (1996). Lack of IL-4-induced Th2 response and IgE class switching in mice with disrupted Stat6 gene. *Nature, 380*, 630-633.

Shimozaki, K., Nakajima, K., Hirano, T., & Nagata, S. (1997). Involvement of STAT3 in the granulocyte colony-stimulating factor-induced differentiation of myeloid cells. *J. Biol. Chem., 272*, 25184-25189.

Skinnider, B. F., Elia, A. J., Gascoyne, R. D., Patterson, B., Trumper, L., Kapp, U., & Mak, T. M. (2002). Signal transducer and activator of transcription 6 is frequently activated in Hodgkin and Reed-Sternberg cells of Hodgkin lymphoma. *Blood, 99*, 618-626.

Slamon, D. J., Clark, G. M., Wong, S. G., Levin, W. J., Ullrich, A., & McGuire, W. L. (1987). Human breast cancer: correlation of relapse and survival with amplification of the HER-2/neu oncogene. *Science, 235*, 177-182.

Starr, R., Willson, T. A., Viney, E. M., Murray, L. J. L., Rayner, J. R., Jenkins, B. J., Gonda, T. J., Alexander, W. S., Metcalf, D., Nicola, N. A., & Hilton, D. J. (1997). A family of cytokine-inducible inhibitors of signaling. *Nature, 387*, 917-921.

Takeda, K., Tanaka, T., Shi, W., Matsumoto, M., Minami, M., Kashiwamura, S., Nakanishi, K., Yoshida, N., Kishimoto, T., & Akira, S. (1996). Essential role of Stat6 in IL-4 signalling. *Nature, 380*, 627-630.

Takemoto, S., Mulloy, J. C., Cereseto, A., Migone, T.-S., Patel, B. K. R., Matsuoka, M., Yamaguchi, K., Takatsuki, K., Kamihira, S., White, J. D., Leonard, W. J., Waldmann, T., & Franchini, G. (1997). Proliferation of adult T cell leukemia/lymphoma cells is associated with the constitutive activation of JAK/STAT proteins. *Proc. Natl. Acad. Sci., 94*, 13897-13902.

Turkson, J., Ryan, D., Kim, J. S., Zhang, Y., Chen, Z., Haura, E., Laudano, A., Sebti, S., Hamilton, A. D., & Jove, R. (2001). Phosphotyrosyl peptides block Stat3-mediated DNA binding activity, gene regulation, and cell transformation. *J Biol Chem, 276*(48), 45443-45455.

Udy, G. B., Towers, R. P., Snell, R. G., Wilkins, R. J., Park, S.-H., Ram, P. A., Waxman, D. J., & Davey, H. W. (1997). Requirement of STAT5b for sexual dimorphism of body growth rates and liver gene expression. *Proc. Natl. Acad. Sci., 94*, 7239-7244.

Wakao, H., Gouilleux, F., & Groner, B. (1994). Mammary gland factor (MGF) is a novel member of the cytokine regulated transcription factor gene family and confers the prolactin response. *EMBO J., 13*, 2182-2191.

Wang, L. H., Yang, X. Y., Kirken, R. A., Resau, J. H., & Farrar, W. L. (2000). Targeted disruption of Stat6 DNA binding activity by an oligonucleotide decoy blocks IL-4-driven TH2 cell response. *Blood, 95*, 1249-1257.

Watson, C. J., & Miller, W. R. (1995). Elevated levels of members of the STAT family of transcription factors in breast carcinoma nuclear extracts. *Br. J. Cancer, 71*, 840-844.

Weber-Nordt, R. M., Egen, C., Wehinger, J., Ludwig, W., Gouilleux-Gruart, V., Mertelsmann, R., & Finke, J. (1996). Constitutive activation of STAT proteins in primary lymphoid and myeloid leukemia cells and in Epstein-Barr virus (EBV)-related lymphoma cell lines. *Blood, 88*, 809-816.

Wemmer, D. E. (2000). Designed sequence-specific minor groove ligands. *Annu. Rev. Biophys. Biomol. Struct., 29*, 439-461.

White, S., Szewczyk, J. W., Turner, J. M., Baird, E. E., & Dervan, P. B. (1998). Recognition of the four Watson-Crick base pairs in the DNA minor groove by synthetic ligands. *Nature, 391*, 468-471.

Xia, Z., Baer, M. R., Block, A. W., Baumann, H., & Wetzler, M. (1998). Expression of signal transducers and activators of transcription proteins in acute myeloid leukemia blasts. *Cancer Res., 58*, 3173-3180.

Xia, Z., Sait, S. N. J., Baer, M. R., Barcos, M., Donohue, K. A., Lawrence, D., Ford, L. A., Block, A. M. W., Baumann, H., & Wetzler, M. (2001). Truncated STAT proteins are prevalent at relapse of acute myeloid leukemia. *Leuk. Res., 25*, 473-482.

Xia, Z., Salzler, R. R., Kunz, D. P., Baer, M. R., Kazim, L., Baumann, H., & Wetzler, M. (2001). A novel serine-dependent proteolytic activity is responsible for truncated signal transducer and activator of transcription proteins in acute myeloid leukemia blasts. *Cancer Res., 61*, 1747-1753.

Xu, X., Kang, S. H., Heidenreich, O., Okerholm, M., O'Shea, J. J., & Nerenberg, M. I. (1995). Constitutive activation of different Jak kinases in human T cell leukemia virus type 1 (HTLV-1) tax protein or virus-transformed cells. *J. Clin. Inv., 96*, 1548-1555.

Yan, R., Qureshi, S., Zhong, Z., Wen, Z., & Darnell, J. E., Jr. (1995). *Nucleic Acids Res., 23*, 459-463.

Yokota, S., Kiyoi, H., Nakao, M., Iwai, T., Misawa, S., Okuda, T., Sonoda, Y., Abe, T., Kahsima, K., Matsuo, Y., & Naoe, T. (1997). Internal tandem duplication of the FLT3 gene is preferentially seen in acute myeloid leukemia and myelodysplastic syndrome among various hematological malignancies. A study on large series of patients and cell lines. *Leukemia, 11*, 1605-1609.

Yu, C. L., Jove, R., & Burakoff, S. J. (1997). Constitutive activation of the Janus kinase-STAT pathway in T lymphoma overexpressing the Lck protein tyrosine kinase. *J. Immunol., 159*, 5206-5210.

Zhang, S., Fukuda, S., Lee, Y., Hangoc, G., Cooper, S., Spolski, R., Leonard, W. J., & Broxmeyer, H. E. (2000). Essential role of signal transducer and activator of transcription (Stat)5a but not Stat5b for Flt3-dependent signaling. *J. Exp. Med., 192*, 719-728.

Zong, C., Yan, R., August, A., Darnell, J. E., Jr., & Hanafusa, H. (1996). Unique signal transduction of Eyk: constitutive stimulation of the JAK-STAT pathway by an oncogenic receptor-type tyrosine kinase. *EMBO J., 15*, 4515-4525.

Zong, C. S., Chan, J., Levy, D. E., Horvath, C., Sadowski, H. B., & Wang, L. H. (2000). Mechanism of STAT3 activation by insulin-like growth factor I receptor. *J. Biol. Chem., 275*, 15099-15105.

STEROID HORMONE RECEPTOR SIGNALING IN CANCER

SHINTA CHENG AND STEVEN P. BALK

1. INTRODUCTION

Steroid hormone receptors (SHRs) are a family of closely related steroid activated sequence specific transcription factors, and are part of the larger nuclear receptor superfamily (Mangelsdorf et al., 1995). The SHR family includes glucocorticoid, progesterone, mineralocorticoid, androgen, and estrogen receptors. The most recent addition to this family is estrogen receptorα (ERα) which may mediate some of the functions previously attributed to the "classical" ER, now termed ERα. The link between SHRs and cancer has been well established for many years with respect to prostate and breast cancers. The large majority of prostate cancers express high levels of androgen receptor (AR) and respond to androgen deprivation therapies, which include castration and AR antagonists. Expression of both ERα and the progesterone receptor (PR) (the latter being ERα regulated) are increased in breast cancers and in precursor lesions relative to normal mammary epithelium, and a large fraction of these ER$^+$ breast cancers similarly respond to ERα antagonists. Moreover, current clinical trials indicate that treatment with ERα antagonists can prevent (or at least delay) breast cancer development.

Early studies of SHRs provided a straightforward model in which hormone binding to cytoplasmic SHRs resulted in a conformational change, nuclear translocation, binding to specific DNA sequences (steroid responsive elements, SREs) and transcriptional activation of steroid regulated genes. The basic mechanisms underlying this classical model by which SHRs function as sequence specific transcription factors are now becoming established, and they involve interactions with many other proteins and diverse signal transduction pathways. As a consequence of these multiple interactions, the functions of SHRs can vary markedly in different tissues and cell types. SHRs may also modulate the activities of other sequence specific transcription factors through protein-protein interactions that do not necessarily involve DNA binding to specific SREs. Moreover, SHRs appear to have nongenomic effects, possibly mediated through plasma membrane associated receptors, and can activate other signal transduction proteins and pathways, including phosphotidylinositol 3-kinase (PI3 kinase) and mitogen activated protein kinase (MAP kinase) pathways.

A further major advance has been the identification of drugs that function as selective modulators, or partial agonists, of SHR action. Studies done primarily with the ERα demonstrate that these drugs, termed selective ER modulators (SERMs), induce unique conformational changes in the ligand binding domain (LBD) that alter interactions with transcriptional coactivator and corepressor proteins. These drugs can stimulate distinct responses in different tissues and cell types and provide tools to understand the mechanisms mediating particular responses. Moreover, as demonstrated by the use of SERMs in breast cancer prevention and treatment, these drugs offer the opportunity to selectively antagonize SHR functions mediating disease (neoplastic and non-neoplastic).

Unfortunately, despite the advances in understanding basic mechanisms of SHR action over the past decade, the specific functions of SHRs that contribute to cancer development and progression remain to be determined. In contrast to other established oncogenes and tumor suppressor genes, SHR mutations, amplification, or other alterations in SHR expression have yet to be established as playing direct roles in cancer development. Moreover, specific SHR regulated genes whose expression (normal or aberrant) contribute to cancer development remain to be identified. This review will focus on the ERα in breast cancer and AR in prostate cancer and how these receptors or interacting proteins may contribute to cancer development and progression.

2. ERα EXPRESSION IN NORMAL BREAST AND BREAST CANCER

SHR are widely expressed, but their levels of expression and contribution to the biology of particular tissues and cells vary widely. The ERα is highly expressed in female reproductive tissues including breast, uterus, cervix and vagina, but it is also expressed and has important functions in many other organs and in males (Lubahn et al., 1993; Smith et al., 1994). ERα appears to be more limited, with highest expression in ovary, prostate, lung and hypothalamus (Couse, Lindzey, Grandien, Gustafsson, & Korach, 1997). ERα in the breast is expressed by ductal epithelial cells (which give rise to breast cancer), but the majority of ductal epithelial cells are ERα negative. In particular, even during puberty and estrous cycles, the majority of the proliferating ductal and acinar cells express low or undetectable levels of ERα (Clarke, Howell, Potten, & Anderson, 1997).

ERα is also expressed by scattered cells in breast stroma, and the estradiol induced proliferative response in mammary epithelium appears to be due primarily to estrogen stimulated growth factor production in the stroma (Wiesen, Young, Werb, & Cunha, 1999). Consistent with this conclusion, reconstitution experiments using stroma and epithelium from ERα knockout versus wildtype mice have shown that ERα expression in the stroma, but not the epithelium, is required for estradiol stimulated ductal epithelium development and growth (Cunha et al., 1997). These and related studies have similarly shown that ERα does not mediate epithelial growth. Finally, ectopic expression of ERα in cells that are ERα negative consistently results in cell cycle arrest and cell death. Taken together, these findings are most consistent with ERα expression in mammary epithelium mediating cell cycle arrest and differentiation.

In contrast to ERα expression by a minority of cells in normal mammary duct epithelium, ERα is expressed by the majority of ductal epithelial cells in breast cancer precursor lesions and in breast cancers. Moreover, estradiol has a direct mitogenic effect on breast cancer cells, with their growth being inhibited by ERα antagonists. These findings indicate that there are changes in ERα function at an early stage in the development of breast cancer. As outlined below, similar changes in AR function appear to occur during prostate cancer development.

3. ANDROGEN RECEPTOR EXPRESSION IN NORMAL PROSTATE AND PROSTATE CANCER

The AR is widely expressed in male and female tissues, but is most highly expressed in testes and prostate. Prostatic acini and ducts are lined with secretory epithelial cells that express high levels of AR. Beneath these secretory cells is a basal cell layer, with weak or absent AR expression (Leav, McNeal, Kwan, Komminoth, & Merk, 1996). AR is also expressed by scattered myoepithelial cells in the prostate stroma. The major direct targets of AR in the epithelium are genes encoding seminal fluid proteins such as prostate specific antigen (PSA), a serine protease that functions to liquefy semen. Similarly to the function of ERα in normal breast epithelium, the AR does not appear to deliver a strong direct mitogenic signal to secretory epithelial cells. In particular, the secretory epithelial cells in normal prostate have an extremely low proliferation rate *in vivo* and do not respond to androgen when freshly isolated *in vitro* (Peehl & Stamey, 1986; Grant, Batchelor, & Habib, 1996; Berthon et al., 1997). Indeed, cells that grow from normal prostate epithelium *in vitro* generally express low or undetectable levels of AR, and reintroduction of AR into prostate cells that have lost AR expression results in cell cycle arrest or apoptosis (Heisler et al., 1997).

Proliferative effects of androgen in prostate appear to be mediated largely by growth factors produced in the stroma in response to androgen, such as keratinocyte growth factor (Yan, Fukabori, Nikolaropoulos, Wang, & McKeehan, 1992; Byrne, Leung, & Neal, 1996). Moreover, reconstitution experiments using cells from wildtype versus AR deficient (testicular feminization mice with a mutant AR) have shown that expression of a functional AR in stroma is necessary for the initial development of prostate epithelium (Cunha, 1984). Nonetheless, increased epithelial proliferation is observed in transgenic mice overexpressing AR in prostate epithelium, indicating that the AR in epithelium can (directly or indirectly) drive the proliferation of prostate epithelium (Stanbrough, Leav, Kwan, Bubley, & Balk, 2001).

Prostate secretory epithelial cells appear to be derived from AR negative stem cells (located either in the basal cell layer or scattered amongst the secretory epithelium), with the induction of AR contributing to (or mediating) G_0 arrest and differentiation (Evans & Chandler, 1987; English, Santen, & Isaacs, 1987). Prostate cancer cells express many AR regulated proteins typical of secretory epithelium, such as PSA. However, they also express multiple genes typical of basal cells, including a basal cell cytokeratin profile. These results suggest a model in which prostate cancer derives from a transitional cell that fails to undergo G_0 arrest subsequent to induction of AR expression. In conjunction with other data showing that ectopically expressed AR can induce cell cycle arrest, these findings indicate fundamental alterations in AR function as an early step in prostate cancer development. Similarly to the ERα in breast cancer, the nature of these functional changes remain to be determined. As outlined below, they may be due to mutations in the ER or AR genes, but more likely reflect posttranslational modifications or alterations in ERα and AR interacting proteins.

4. STEROID HORMONE RECEPTOR STRUCTURE

The overall structure of SHRs is highly conserved and similar to the larger nuclear receptor family (Tsai & O'Malley, 1994; Mangelsdorf et al., 1995; Figure 1). The most conserved region of SHRs is the central DNA binding domain (DBD), which is composed of two zinc finger DNA binding motifs (Zilliacus, Wright, Carlstedt-Duke, & Gustafsson, 1995). The SHRs bind as homodimers to SREs that are imperfect palindromes separated by three bases. The AR, glucocorticoid receptor (GR), mineralocorticoid receptor (MR), and PR can recognize the same optimal consensus sequence (GGAACAnnnTGTTCT). However, many SREs *in vivo* vary from this optimal strong site, and additional protein-DNA and protein-protein interactions mediate specific binding *in vivo*. The C-terminus encodes the ligand binding domain (LBD), which also contains a transcriptional activation function (termed AF-2) (Danielian, White, Lees, & Parker, 1992). This domain is very similar in overall structure between the SHRs with 10-13 α-helices (see below), although it has lower homology at the amino acid level.

The N-terminus has an autonomous transactivation function (termed activation function 1, AF-1) and is the most variable. The AR has a long N-terminal domain with a very active transactivation function, which represents the major transactivation function in the AR(Quigley et al., 1995; Brinkmann et al., 1999). In contrast, the ERα has a shorter N-terminal AF-1 and the relative contribution of this AF-1 versus the AF-2 function in the LBD depends on the cell type and ligand (Tora et al., 1989; McInerney & Katzenellenbogen, 1996; Nilsson et al., 2001). The region between the DBD and LBD, termed the hinge region, contributes to a number of functions including dimerization, nuclear localization, and binding to coactivator proteins.

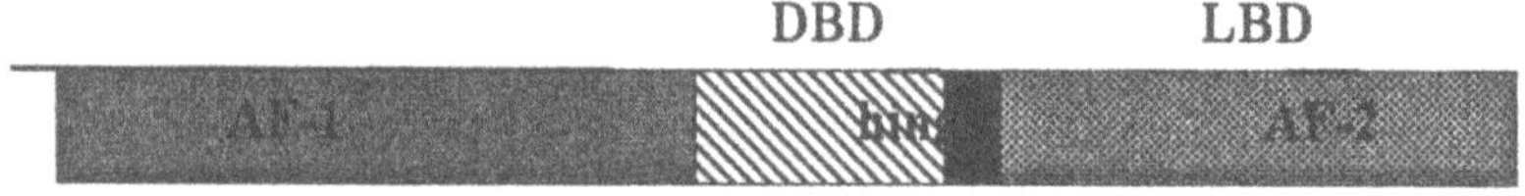

Figure 1. Outline of steroid hormone receptor structure.

5. STEROID HORMONE RECEPTOR TRANSCRIPTIONAL ACTIVATION BY STEROID HORMONES

SHRs associate with a heat shock protein 90 (HSP90) chaperone complex that helps to fold the protein in a ligand binding conformation (Pratt & Toft, 1997). Significantly, HSP90 complexes also catalyze the folding of multiple signaling kinases, suggesting the potential for SHR and kinase interactions at this stage. Nuclear translocation is not strictly ligand dependent, but ligand generally enhances nuclear association. Most significantly, steroid binding induces conformational changes in the LBD that result in homodimerization and recruitment of multiple coactivator proteins (Wurtz et al., 1996; Brzozowski et al., 1997; Heery, Kalkhoven, Hoare, & Parker, 1997; Torchia et al., 1997; Feng et al., 1998; Ding et al., 1998; Shiau et al., 1998). The major conformational change is movement of a conserved C-terminal helix in the LBD (helix 12) so that it packs against helices 3 and 5. This repositioning of helix 12 generates a small hydrophobic cleft that serves as a binding site for multiple proteins containing leucine-x-x-leucine-leucine (LXXLL) motifs, and this binding site is responsible for the transcriptional activity (AF-2) of the LBD (Figure 2).

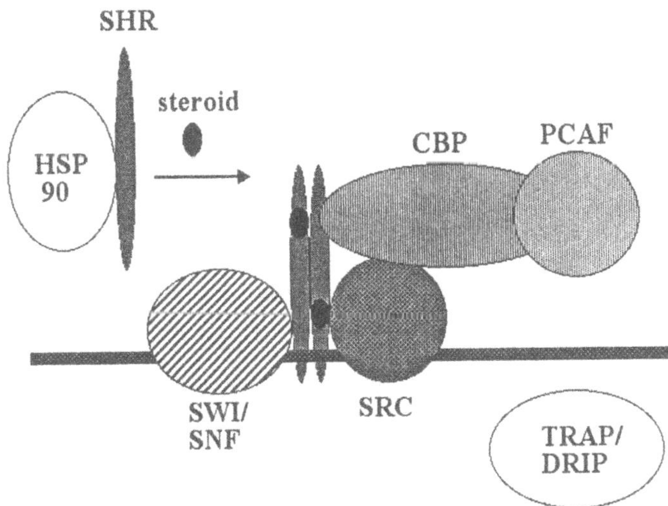

Figure 2. Steps in transcriptional activation by steroid hormone receptors. Unliganded SHR associates with an HSP90 complex, with steroid binding inducing dimerization, DNA binding, and coactivator association. Although not indicated in the figure, SRC-1 and -2 contact both the N- and C-termini of SHRs and may interact with both molecules in the dimer. PCAF protein complex may also directly bind to SHRs. The TRAP/DRIP complex may displace SRC binding the LBD.

Major proteins containing LXXLL motifs and binding to this hydrophobic cleft are the p160 family of transcriptional coactivators, which include steroid receptor coactivator-1 (SRC-1), SRC-2 (human TIF2 or murine GRIP1), and the more divergent SRC-3 (also termed AIB1, ACTR, RAC3, pCIP) (Onate, Tsai, Tsai, & O'Malley, 1995; Voegel, Heine, Zechel, Chambon, & Gronemeyer, 1996; Hong, Kohli, Garabedian, & Stallcup, 1997; Anzick et al., 1997; Chen et al., 1997). Studies in SRC-1 knockout mice have confirmed decreased ligand responses by SHRs, as well as other nuclear receptors that bind SRC-1 (Xu et al., 1998). Expression of SRC-2 is increased SRC-1 knockout mice, likely compensating for the loss of SRC-1 function in target tissues. In contrast, SRC-3 knockout mice have marked defects, indicating distinct functions for this coactivator (Xu et al., 2000).

These SRC proteins contain multiple LXXLL motifs that can contribute to receptor multimerization, but also bind through another distinct glutamine rich site to the N-terminus of AR and ERα (Ding et al., 1998; Berrevoets, Doesburg, Steketee, Trapman, & Brinkmann, 1998; Webb et al., 1998; Alen, Claessens, Verhoeven, Rombauts, & Peeters, 1999; Bevan, Hoare, Claessens, Heery, & Parker, 1999). In the case of AR, the N-terminal is the major site for SRC-1 binding as the AR LBD binds the SRC-1 LXXLL motifs very weakly. The AR and ERα N-termini have also been shown to bind directly in a ligand dependent manner to the C-terminal LBD (Wong, Zhou, Sar, & Wilson, 1993; Zhou, Lane, Kemppainen, French, & Wilson, 1995; Kraus, McInerney, & Katzenellenbogen, 1995). This binding by the AR is via an N-terminal LXXLL-like motif (FXXLF), which appears to compete with SRC LXXLL motifs for binding to the LBD (He, Kemppainen, & Wilson, 2000).
SRC-1 has intrinsic histone acetyltransferase (HAT) activity, and the SRC proteins recruit additional HATs, in particular cAMP response element binding protein (CBP) and the related p300, as well as protein methyltransferases (Glass, Rose, & Rosenfeld, 1997; Kamei et al., 1996; Torchia et al., 1997; Rosenfeld & Glass, 2001; Koh, Chen, Lee, & Stallcup, 2001). CBP and p300 are complex multifunctional transcriptional coactivators that also interact with SHRs through their N-terminal AF-1 domains, and associate with the basal transcriptional machinery. CBP/p300 further recruits P/CAF (p300/CBP associated factor), which also has HAT activity and is part of a large complex containing proteins that associate with basal transcription factors (Blanco et al., 1998; Ogryzko et al., 1998).

A function of these SHR recruited proteins is to remodel chromatin into a more transcriptionally active configuration. Histone acetylation and methylation weaken histone interactions with DNA, which contributes to the chromatin remodeling. Acetylated histones also serve as a binding site for bromodomain containing factors, including the ATP dependent SWI/SNF chromatin remodeling complex (Yoshinaga, Peterson, Herskowitz, & Yamamoto, 1992; Ostlund Farrants, Blomquist, Kwon, & Wrange, 1997; Fryer & Archer, 1998). There are also direct interactions between SHRs and BRG-1, a component of the mammalian SWI/SNF complex (Ichinose, Garnier, Chambon, & Losson, 1997; DiRenzo et al., 2000).

A second class of cofactor recruited by ligand bound SHRs is a large coactivator complex (or group of related complexes) termed the SMCC/TRAP/DRIP/ARC complex (Fondell, Ge, & Roeder, 1996; Rachez et al.,

1998; Ito et al., 1999; Zhu, Qi, Jain, Rao, & Reddy, 1997; Gu et al., 1999). The direct receptor binding component of this complex is TRAP220 (also termed DRIP205 or PBP), which contains LXXLL motifs and binds to the agonist liganded LBD (Yuan, Ito, Fondell, Fu, & Roeder, 1998; Burakov, Wong, Rachez, Cheskis, & Freedman, 2000). This complex shares proteins with the TATA complex, and appears to connect SHRs directly to the RNA polymerase containing basal transcriptional machinery.

It is not clear whether this complex binds at the same time or subsequent to the SRC proteins and other coactivator proteins. The observations that SHRs and SRC proteins become acetylated suggests a sequential model regulated by HAT activity (Chen, Lin, Xie, Wilpitz, & Evans, 1999; Wang et al., 2001; Fu et al., 2000), and recent chromatin immunoprecipitation data support cycles of coactivator binding and release (Shang, Hu, DiRenzo, Lazar, & Brown, 2000). However, as SHRs are dimers and SHR regulated genes typically have multiple SREs, there may be simultaneous binding of HAT and SMCC/TRAP/DRIP/ARC complexes. In any case, binding of these multiple proteins by SHRs supports a two-step model for transcriptional activation by SHR, in which chromatin remodeling (by acetylases, methylases, and helicases) is followed by recruitment of general transcription factors (Archer, Lefebvre, Wolford, & Hager, 1992; Jenster et al., 1997).

A large number of additional candidate transcriptional coactivator or modulator proteins for SHRs have been identified, including many with LXXLL or related motifs, which likely further regulate and integrate SHR responses with other pathways (Jackson et al., 1997; Endoh et al., 1999; Watanabe et al., 2001a; Brady et al., 1999; Boonyaratanakornkit et al., 1998; Lanz et al., 1999; Alen et al., 1999; Moilanen, Karvonen, Poukka, Janne, & Palvimo, 1998b; Moilanen et al., 1999; Moilanen et al., 1998a; Poukka, Aarnisalo, Karvonen, Palvimo, & Janne, 1999; Muller et al., 2000; Poukka, Aarnisalo, Santti, Janne, & Palvimo, 2000; Huang & Stallcup, 2000; Kang, Yeh, Fujimoto, & Chang, 1999; Fujimoto et al., 1999). In addition to coactivator proteins, a number of corepressor proteins binding to SHRs have been identified (Wei, Hu, Chandra, Seto, & Farooqui, 2000; Johansson et al., 2000; Zhang, Thomsen, Johansson, Gustafsson, & Treuter, 2000; Yuan, Lu, Li, & Balk, 2001; Shi et al., 2001; Yu, Li, Roeder, & Wang, 2001). In contrast to recruitment of HATs, these corepressors recruit histone deacetylases (HDACs) that remove acetyl groups from histones and thereby repress transcription. The initially identified corepressor proteins, NCoR and SMRT, were isolated as mediators of transcriptional repression by unliganded nuclear receptors (Horlein et al., 1995; Chen & Evans, 1995; Seol, Mahon, Lee, & Moore, 1996; Sande & Privalsky, 1996), and their role in SHR function remains uncertain (see below).

6. TRANCRIPTIONAL ACTIVATION BY PARTIAL AGONISTS

An important distinction between SHRs and the larger nuclear receptor family (including thyroid hormone and retinoid receptors) is that the latter nuclear receptors do not require HSP90 for folding, are bound to DNA in the absence of ligand, and generally form heterodimers (Mangelsdorf et al., 1995; Mangelsdorf & Evans, 1995). The unliganded LBD of these nuclear receptors is in a distinct conformation, with helix 12 positioned away from helices 3 and 5 (Wagner et al., 1995; Renaud et al., 1995; Bourguet, Ruff, Chambon, Gronemeyer, & Moras, 1995; Brzozowski et al., 1997). This conformation generates a larger hydrophobic surface that can bind to an extended LXXLL related motif in the corepressor proteins NCoR and SMRT (Hu & Lazar, 1999; Perissi et al., 1999; Nagy et al., 1999). In contrast to coactivator proteins that recruit HAT activity, NCoR and SMRT recruit HDACs that deacetylate histones and result in transcriptional repression (Nagy et al., 1997; Alland et al., 1997; Heinzel et al., 1997). Binding of agonist ligands to these nuclear receptors induces a conformational change similar to that seen in SHR, with movement of helix 12 adjacent to helices 3 and 5, occluding the corepressor site and generating the site for coactivator binding via LXXLL motifs.

The selective ER modulators (SERMs) tamoxifen and raloxifene have been shown to induce an alternative conformation of the LBD, with helix 12 positioned away from helices 3 and 5, that allows for binding of these corepressors (Brzozowski et al., 1997; Feng et al., 1998). The failure to recruit SRC coactivators to the LBD, in conjunction with recruitment of corepressors, are mechanisms consistent with the antagonist properties of tamoxifen and raloxifene in breast cancer (although other mechanisms may also contribute). The agonist activities of these drugs in uterus, bone, and other sites may reflect a more dominant role for the N-terminal AF-1 function and decreased levels of corepressors versus coactivators in these tissues.

The physiological role of NCoR and SMRT in ER function is uncertain as these corepressors do not appear to interact with the estradiol liganded ER. However, we have recently shown that NCoR can antagonize androgen stimulated AR transcriptional activity, supporting a physiological role for NCoR in modulating AR activity (Cheng et al., 2002). In any case, the success of SERMs in breast cancer demonstrates the therapeutic potential of selective SHR activation, and intensive efforts are underway to further develop such drugs for other SHRs.

7. PROTEINS AND PATHWAYS THAT MODULATE STEROID HORMONE RECEPTOR ACTIVATION

7.1 SHR regulation by phosphorylation

Although ligand binding is clearly a major determinant of SHR transcriptional activation, the activity of these receptors can be activated or modulated by multiple mechanisms, including posttranslational modifications and direct association with other signaling proteins. The most studied system is ERα activation by peptide growth factors, in particular by epidermal growth factor (EGF). EGF can mimic the mitogenic and other effects of estradiol in the female reproductive tract and EGF blockade can attenuate estradiol responses, while treatment with an ERα antagonist can reduce responses to EGF (Ignar-Trowbridge et al., 1992). Moreover, estrogenic effects of EGF in uterus are blocked in ERα knockout mice, confirming that they are ERα mediated (Curtis et al., 1996).

The mechanisms by which ERα stimulates EGF signaling are not clear, but may be due to receptor upregulation or nongenomic effects of ERα (see below). A mechanism by which EGF can stimulate ERα is through the EGF receptor, with downstream activation of Ras, Raf, and the MAP kinases Erk1 and Erk2 (Kato et al., 1995; Bunone, Briand, Miksicek, & Picard, 1996). Activated MAP kinases then phosphorylate Ser-118 in the human ERα N-terminus, which can enhance binding of the ERα coactivator protein p68 RNA helicase (Watanabe et al., 2001b).

There are also alternative pathways linking growth factor and MAP kinase activation to ERα signaling, including ERα phosphorylation at Ser-167_by the kinase pp90^{rsk1} (a downstream target of Erk) (Joel et al., 1998). Moreover, mechanisms of SHR phosphorylation and activation by growth factors may be cell type specific (Patrone, Gianazza, Santagati, Agrati, & Maggi, 1998). It should be noted that Ser-118 is also phosphorylated in response to ligand binding by a MAP kinase independent mechanism (Joel, Traish, & Lannigan, 1998).

This MAP kinase pathway can mediate ERα activation by other peptide growth factors, including insulin and insulin like growth factor-1 (Aronica & Katzenellenbogen, 1993; Ignar-Trowbridge, Pimentel, Parker, McLachlan, & Korach, 1996). Interestingly, activated MAP kinases can also directly phosphorylate a site the ERα N-terminus, but this results in ligand independent binding of SRC-1 (Tremblay, Tremblay, Labrie, & Giguere, 1999). In contrast to SHR activation, MAP kinase phosphorylation can also increase receptor downregulation (Shen, Horwitz, & Lange, 2001). Finally, MAP kinases can phosphorylate a number of coactivator and corepressor proteins, indirectly affecting SHR activities (Font & Brown, 2000; Rowan, Weigel, & O'Malley, 2000).

Protein kinase A (PKA) has been found to stimulate ligand independent ERα and PR activities, alter responses to antagonists, and enhance ligand stimulated AR transcriptional activity (Denner, Weigel, Maxwell, Schrader, & O'Malley, 1990; Aronica et al., 1993; Sartorius, Tung, Takimoto, & Horwitz, 1993). A direct effect of phosphorylation may be to enhance SHR dimerization (Chen, Pace, Coombes, & Ali, 1999). It has more recently been shown that PKA stimulation results in the phosphorylation and enhanced activity of SRC-1 and CBP, events that may indirectly mediate PKA activation of SHRs (Rowan, Garrison, Weigel, & O'Malley, 2000).

The transcriptional activity of the AR can also be stimulated by PKA, growth factors, and direct MAP kinase activation, and can be modulated by protein kinase C (Culig et al., 1995; Ikonen, Palvimo, Kallio, Reinikainen, & Janne, 1994; de Ruiter, Teuwen, Trapman, Dijkema, & Brinkmann, 1995; Nazareth & Weigel, 1996; Sadar, 1999; Craft, Shostak, Carey, & Sawyers, 1999; Abreu-Martin, Chari, Palladino, Craft, & Sawyers, 1999; Lin, Yeh, Kang, & Chang, 2001; Yeh et al., 1999; Putz et al., 1999). However, whether effects of these pathways reflect direct AR versus coactivator phosphorylation remains unclear (Zhou, Kemppainen, & Wilson, 1995; Brinkmann et al., 1999).

The ERα can be tyrosine phosphorylated at tyr-537 and mutations at this site can activate the ERα and enhance SRC-1 binding, but the role of this site in modulating ERα activity *in vivo* is uncertain (Arnold, Obourn, Jaffe, & Notides, 1995; Weis, Ekena, Thomas, Lazennec, & Katzenellenbogen, 1996). Heregulin, which is a ligand for erbB2 (Her-2/Neu), can enhance ER_ activation through tyrosine phosphorylation (Pietras et al., 1995), and has been reported to enhance ligand independent AR activity (Craft et al., 1999). These findings are of clear interest due to erbB2 amplification in a subset of breast cancers and an association with tamoxifen resistance (Pietras et al., 1995; Borg et al., 1994; Leitzel et al., 1995), and data indicating increased erbB2 expression in advanced androgen independent prostate cancer (Signoretti et al., 2000).

Further proteins shown to phosphorylate ERα include cdk 7 and cyclin A. Cdk7 is a component of the general transcription factor TFIIH complex and plays an activating role by phosphorylating the receptor at ser-118 (Chen et al., 2000).

Cyclin A (a G1 cyclin) complexed to CDK2 can phosphorylate ERα at Ser-104 and Ser-106, which results in activation (Rogatsky, Trowbridge, & Garabedian, 1999). Other potential proteins regulating SHR activity by phosphorylation include Akt (Campbell et al., 2001; Lin et al., 2001) and a number of SHR associated kinases (Moilanen et al., 1998b; Lee et al., 2002).

8. SHR MODULATION BY OTHER POSTTRANSLATIONAL MODIFICATIONS

It is now clear that HATs recruited to activate transcription can also acetylate many transcription factors. ERα and AR can be acetylated by CBP/p300 and/or PCAF on lysines in the hinge regions and acetylation appears to downregulate transcriptional activity (Fu et al., 2000; Wang et al., 2001). Significantly, a point mutation in an ERα hinge region lysine (lysine to arginine in codon 303) that enhances transcriptional activity has been found in premalignant breast lesions (Fuqua et al., 2000) (see below).

SHRs can be modified by addition of ubiquitin, or the ubiquitin related protein SUMO, and ligases for these proteins (E6-AP and UBC9, respectively) have been isolated as SHR interacting proteins (Nawaz et al., 1999; Poukka et al., 1999). While ubiquitin can enhance receptor degradation, there may be additional roles for these modifications in regulating cellular localization and protein interactions.

9. PROTEIN-PROTEIN INTERACTIONS MODULATING SHR ACTIVITY

In addition to proteins that clearly function as transcriptional coactivators or corepressors, many other proteins have been found to interact with one or more SHR. Cyclin D1 binds to ERα and can stimulate ligand independent activation, which appears to reflect increased SRC binding (Neuman et al., 1997; Zwijsen et al., 1997). Cyclin D1 can also bind to the AR, but this interaction inhibits AR activation (Knudsen, Cavenee, & Arden, 1999; Reutens et al., 2001). The AR has been found to interact with β-catenin, a finding that may be relevant to the early loss of E-cadherin expression and to β-catenin mutations in prostate cancer (Voeller, Truica, & Gelmann, 1998; Truica, Byers, & Gelmann, 2000). SHR can interact with other sequence specific transcription factors (see below). Multiple additional SHR interacting proteins have also been reported (see above), but in many cases the biological significance of the interactions remain to be defined.

10. DNA BINDNG INDEPENDENT TRANSCRIPTIONAL ACTIVITIES OF STEROID HORMONE RECEPTORS

SHR can modulate transcription by interaction with other transcription factors at sites that do not contain SREs. Indeed, the results of one study suggest that the many critical functions of the GR may not require DNA binding (Reichardt et al., 1998). Several studies have now shown that SHRs can interact with AP-1 and modulate transcription from AP-1 promoters (Schule et al., 1990; Yang-Yen et al., 1990; Kallio, Poukka, Moilanen, Janne, & Palvimo, 1995). Estradiol or antagonist liganded ERα enhances AP-1 activity and this appears to be mediated by both the AF-1 and AF-2 domains and recruitment of SRC proteins (Webb, Lopez, Uht, & Kushner, 1995; Webb et al., 1999). In contrast, only the antagonist liganded ERα activates AP1 and this can be blocked with estradiol. The ERα interaction is mediated by the DBD and may be due to sequestration of corepressors (Paech et al., 1997). Binding of c-jun to the AR N-terminus can enhance AR activity by augmenting N-terminal interaction with the LBD, and this can be blocked by fos (Bubulya et al., 2001).

GR, AR, and ERα can bind to NFκB (p65), which may suppress inflammatory responses and modulate SHR activities (Galien & Garcia, 1997; McKay & Cidlowski, 1998). The agonist liganded ERα and AR can bind to and enhance Sp1 transcriptional activity (Porter, Saville, Hoivik, & Safe, 1997; Lu, Jenster, & Epner, 2000; Qin, Singh, & Safe, 1999), and this Sp1 interaction has been reported to enhance c-myc expression (Dubik & Shiu, 1992). ERα and ERβ can bind to and potentiate STAT5b transcriptional activity (Bjornstrom, Kilic, Norman, Parker, & Sjoberg, 2001). AR can bind activated STAT3, and this interaction has been reported to mediate IL-6 enhancement of AR transcriptional activity (Chen, Wang, & Farrar, 2000).

In addition to these SRE independent interactions, SHRs complexed to SREs can bind to other sequence specific transcription factors and stabilize their DNA binding (Adler, Danielsen, & Robins, 1992). These cooperative interactions are probably a very general mechanism for regulating tissue specific gene expression, particularly on the frequently identified weak nonconcensus SREs. Indeed, it remains possible that some of the above SRE independent effects of SHRs may actually be mediated *in vivo* through weak SREs. Examples include AR interaction with AML3 and Oct-1 on the murine Slp1 promoter (Ning & Robins, 1999; Gonzalez & Robins, 2001) and AR interaction with PDEF (an ets factor) on the PSA enhancer (Oettgen et al., 2000). Interactions between AR and Sp1, both bound to specific *cis*-elements, can regulate the p21 cyclin dependent kinase inhibitor gene (Lu et al., 2000).

11. NONGENOMIC LIGAND ACTIVATED EFFECTS OF STEROID HORMONE RECEPTORS

In addition to transcriptional effects of SHRs, steroid hormones can elicit rapid activation of intracellular signaling pathways by nongenomic mechanisms (Revelli, Massobrio, & Tesarik, 1998; Coleman & Smith, 2001). Ligation of the ERα or AR in steroid hormone starved cells can trigger rapid MAP kinase (Erk1 and Erk2) activation (Migliaccio, Pagano, & Auricchio, 1993; Castoria et al., 1999; Peterziel et al., 1999), which may be mediated by direct binding of Src and Shc (Migliaccio et al., 1998; Kousteni et al., 2001; Song et al., 2002). ERα can also activate phosphatidylinositol-3-OH kinase (PI3 kinase) and has been reported to interact directly with the p85 PI3 kinase regulatory subunit (Simoncini et al., 2000). This PI3 kinase and subsequent Akt activation mediates ERα σtimulated production of nitric oxide in vascular endothelial cells, which may contribute to the cardioprotective effects of estrogens (Chen et al., 1999; Haynes et al., 2000; Hisamoto et al., 2001).

Some nongenomic effects of estrogen in ERα knockout mice suggest that there may be alternative nonclassical membrane SHRs (Singh, Setalo, Jr., Guan, Frail, & Toran-Allerand, 2000). This is supported by a recent report showing estradiol activation of MAP kinases through a G protein coupled receptor, GPR30, which appears to trigger release of heparin bound EGF and activate the EGF receptor (Filardo, Quinn, Bland, & Frackelton, Jr., 2000). However, other data indicate that many nongenomic effects of steroid hormones are mediated by membrane associated classical SHRs (Razandi, Pedram, & Levin, 2000). Significantly, membrane ERα localizes to caveolae, which are discrete caveolin-1 organized plasma membrane domains that are enriched in signaling molecules including receptor tyrosine kinases and PI3 kinase (Kim et al., 1999; Chambliss et al., 2000). Moreover, additional studies have demonstrated caveolin-1 binding to ERα and AR, and caveolin-1 stimulation of ERα and AR transcriptional activity (Schlegel, Wang, Katzenellenbogen, Pestell, & Lisanti, 1999; Lu, Schneider, Zheng, Zhang, & Richie, 2001). Taken together, these finding support the hypothesis that SHR and other signaling pathways are integrated by multiple protein-protein interactions in caveolae, and suggest that more detailed studies of caveolin-1 knockout mice might reveal defects in these nongenomic SHR signaling pathways (Drab et al., 2001; Razani et al., 2001).

12. CANCER ASSOCIATED ALTERATIONS IN STEROID HORMONE RECEPTOR STRUCTURE AND FUNCTION

12.1 ERα mutations in breast cancer

A number of ERα mutations that can enhance activity have been identified in primary breast cancers (Sommer & Fuqua, 2001). One example is a tyrosine to asparagine mutation in codon 573, which alters a site that is tyrosine phosphorylated and may result in ligand independent SRC-1 binding and activation (Weis et al., 1996; Zhang, Borg, Wolf, Oesterreich, & Fuqua, 1997). However, ERα mutations have been found in only a small fraction of primary breast cancers, with no consistent site or function altered (Roodi et al., 1995). Alternative splicing of the ERα has been found in some breast cancers and breast cancer lines, with deletion of exon 5 (resulting in loss of the LBD) in one such transcript. This exon 5 deletion mutant is constitutively active, and has been suggested to function as a dominant positive receptor. However, the encoded protein is unstable and does not activate transcription of ERE regulated reporter genes (Ohlsson, Lykkesfeldt, Madsen, & Briand, 1998). Taken together, these results suggest a very minor role for ERα mutations or alternative transcripts in breast cancer development.

In contrast to these rare ERα mutations in breast cancer, a lysine to arginine mutation at codon 303 has been reported in premalignant breast lesions from approximately a third of patients (Fuqua et al., 2000). As noted above, this mutation removes an acetylation site in the hinge region and can enhance transcriptional activation (Wang et al., 2001). However, if this mutation does play a frequent early role in breast cancer development, then it is unclear why it has not yet been reported at high frequency in actual breast cancers. Further studies focused in the natural history of premalignant lesions bearing this mutant ERα will be of clear interest. Finally, ERα mutations are infrequent in tamoxifen (or ERα antagonist) resistant breast cancer, indicating that other as yet unclear mechanisms are involved (Sommer et al., 2001).

12.2 AR mutations in prostate cancer

AR mutations appear to be rare in primary androgen dependent prostate cancer, although such mutations may occur in a subset of androgen dependent prostate cancer patients as a higher frequency of AR mutations and association with progression to androgen independence were reported in two studies (Tilley, Buchanan, Hickey, & Bentel, 1996; Marcelli et al., 2000). Two of these mutations in the AR hinge region have been reported to enhance transcriptional activity (Buchanan et al., 2001), but the functional consequences of most of the these diverse mutations remain to be determined. The AR has a highly polymorphic polyglutamine (CAG) repeat in exon 1, and ARs containing shorter CAG repeats are transcriptionally more active *in vivo* (Chamberlain, Driver, & Miesfeld, 1994; Irvine et al., 2000) and/or more highly expressed (Choong, Kemppainen, Zhou, & Wilson, 1996). Prostate cancer risk, or risk of more aggressive prostate cancer, is modestly increased in men with shorter CAG repeats (Hardy et al., 1996; Giovannucci et al., 1997; Stanford et al., 1997; Hakimi, Schoenberg, Rondinelli, Piantadosi, & Barrack, 1997; Nam et al., 2000; Hsing et al., 2000), and a mutant AR with a contracted CAG repeat has been found prostate cancer (Schoenberg et al., 1994).

AR activity might also be increased by receptor upregulation, but most studies indicate that AR expression levels are not increased in primary prostate cancer, or in precursor lesions (prostatic intraepithelial neoplasia, PIN) (Leav et al., 1996; Sweat, Pacelli, Bergstralh, Slezak, & Bostwick, 1999). In contrast to primary androgen dependent prostate cancer, AR gene expression is increased in prostate cancers that relapse after androgen deprivation therapies, and AR gene amplification has been observed in about 30% of these androgen independent prostate cancers (van der Kwast et al., 1991; Ruizeveld de Winter et al., 1994; Visakorpi et al., 1995). This increased AR expression appears to enhance AR activity in the setting of reduced androgen levels after androgen deprivation therapies, and selective pressure for AR upregulation supports a critical role for continued AR signaling even in advanced androgen independent prostate cancer. This is in contrast to tamoxifen resistant breast cancer, although it will be of interest to determine whether ERα expression differs in patients who relapse after treatment with tamoxifen versus treatment with pure ERα antagonists.

AR mutations also occur in relapsed androgen independent prostate cancer, although the frequency varies widely in different studies and may depend on methodologies and patient populations. We have found a relatively high frequency of AR mutations (approximately 35%) in patients who were initially treated with androgen deprivation therapy in conjunction with the AR antagonist flutamide (Taplin et al., 1995; Taplin et al., 1999). Significantly, these mutations were predominantly in codons 874 and 877 and the resulting mutants were strongly activated, rather than inhibited by flutamide. Mutations in these codons (particularly T877A) have been reported in other studies, and also enhance AR activation by estradiol, progesterone, and weak androgens derived from the adrenal gland. Taken together, these results further support the hypothesis that there is strong selective pressure to maintain AR protein and AR transcriptional activity in relapsed androgen independent prostate cancer.

12.3 Alteration in coactivators or corepressors in cancer

SRC-3 (AIB1, amplified in breast cancer 1), was found to be amplified and overexpressed in multiple estrogen receptor-positive breast and ovarian cancer cell lines. In primary breast cancer samples, AIB1 gene amplification found in approximately 10% and high expression in 64% (Anzick et al., 1997). Altered SRC-1 or SRC-2 expression have not been found in primary breast or prostate cancers. However, increased expression of both has been reported in prostate cancers that recur after androgen deprivation therapy, suggesting a role for these coactivators in stimulating AR activity in the setting of castrate androgen levels (Gregory et al., 2001). TRAP220 (DRIP205, PBP) is overexpressed in approximately 50% of breast cancers, and the gene is amplified in approximately 25% (Zhu et al., 1999). These findings are consistent with increased coactivator expression mediating enhanced ERα signaling in breast cancer, although both SRC-3 and TRAP220 can interact with other receptors and enhanced ERα activation has not been directly demonstrated.

12.4 SHR modulation by other mechanisms in cancer

Alterations in multiple signal transduction pathways have been reported in breast and prostate cancer. In particular, increased ErbB2 expression is associated with a subset of aggressive breast cancers (see above). In prostate cancer, complete loss of PTEN is observed in approximately half of advanced tumors (Cairns et al., 1997; Whang et al., 1998; McMenamin et al., 1999), indicating that activation of the PI3 kinase pathway makes a major contribution to prostate carcinogenesis. However, there is limited evidence clearly linking these or other pathways with altered SHR activities in cancer. Nonetheless, the data outlined here clearly demonstrate extensive cross-talk between SHR and other signal transduction pathways in normal cells, and it would be very surprising if these pathways did not contribute to cancer development and progression. Indeed, the data strongly suggest that roles for ER, AR, and coactivator phosphorylation in augmenting activity in recurrent breast and prostate cancer.

13. SUMMARY AND CONCLUSIONS

SHRs function as hormone activated, sequence specific DNA binding transcription factors that recruit multiple coactivator and other proteins to specific genes and generally stimulate transcription of these genes. SHR may have further genomic actions, that do not involve direct DNA binding, through protein-protein interactions with other sequence specific transcription factors, although these may still involve weak binding to nonconsensus steroid responsive elements *in vivo*. SHRs also appear to have nongenomic effects mediated through interactions with cytoplasmic signaling proteins. The major functions of SHRs in normal adult tissues appear to involve stimulation of differentiation, rather than proliferation. In contrast, the ERα and AR directly stimulate the growth of breast and prostate cancers, respectively, indicating a critical change in their functions. The ERα and AR appear to undergo further adaptation in tumor cells in response to hormonal therapies, that render these therapies ineffective. Understanding the molecular basis for these changes in SHR function during cancer development and progression may provide new targets for the generation of drugs to prevent and treat steroid stimulated cancers.

Shinta Cheng and Steven P. Balk
Cancer Biology Program
Hematology-Oncology Division
Beth Israel Deaconess Medical Center
Harvard Medical School
Boston, MA

14. REFERENCES

Abreu-Martin,M.T., Chari,A., Palladino,A.A., Craft,N.A., & Sawyers,C.L. (1999). Mitogen-activated protein kinase kinase kinase 1 activates androgen receptor-dependent transcription and apoptosis in prostate cancer. Mol.Cell Biol., 19(7), 5143-5154.

Adler,A.J., Danielsen,M., & Robins,D.M. (1992). Androgen-specific gene activation via a consensus glucocorticoid response element is determined by interaction with nonreceptor factors. Proc.Natl.Acad.Sci.U.S.A. 89(24), 11660-11663.

Alen,P., Claessens,F., Schoenmakers,E., Swinnen,J.V., Verhoeven,G., Rombauts,W., & Peeters,B. (1999). Interaction of the putative androgen receptor-specific coactivator ARA70/ELE1alpha with multiple steroid receptors and identification of an internally deleted ELE1beta isoform. Mol.Endocrinol., 13(1), 117-128.

Alen,P., Claessens,F., Verhoeven,G., Rombauts,W., & Peeters,B. (1999). The androgen receptor amino-terminal domain plays a key role in p160 coactivator-stimulated gene transcription. Mol.Cell Biol., 19(9), 6085-6097.

Alland,L., Muhle,R., Hou,H., Jr., Potes,J., Chin,L., Schreiber-Agus,N., & DePinho,R.A. (1997). Role for N-CoR and histone deacetylase in Sin3-mediated transcriptional repression. Nature, 387(6628), 49-55.

Anzick,S.L., Kononen,J., Walker,R.L., Azorsa,D.O., Tanner,M.M., Guan,X.Y., Sauter,G., Kallioniemi,O.P., Trent,J.M., & Meltzer,P.S. (1997). AIB1, a steroid receptor coactivator amplified in breast and ovarian cancer. Science, 277(5328), 965-968.

Archer,T.K., Lefebvre,P., Wolford,R.G., & Hager,G.L. (1992). Transcription factor loading on the MMTV promoter: a bimodal mechanism for promoter activation. Science, 255(5051), 1573-1576.

Arnold,S.F., Obourn,J.D., Jaffe,H., & Notides,A.C. (1995). Phosphorylation of the human estrogen receptor on tyrosine 537 in vivo and by src family tyrosine kinases in vitro. Mol.Endocrinol., 9(1), 24-33.

Aronica,S.M., & Katzenellenbogen,B.S. (1993). Stimulation of estrogen receptor-mediated transcription and alteration in the phosphorylation state of the rat uterine estrogen receptor by estrogen, cyclic adenosine monophosphate, and insulin-like growth factor-I. Mol.Endocrinol., 7(6), 743-752.

Berrevoets,C.A., Doesburg,P., Steketee,K., Trapman,J., & Brinkmann,A.O. (1998). Functional interactions of the AF-2 activation domain core region of the human androgen receptor with the amino-terminal domain and with the transcriptional coactivator TIF2 (transcriptional intermediary factor2). Mol.Endocrinol., 12(8), 1172-1183.

Berthon,P., Waller,A.S., Villette,J.M., Loridon,L., Cussenot,O., & Maitland,N.J. (1997). Androgens are not a direct requirement for the proliferation of human prostatic epithelium in vitro. Int.J.Cancer, 73(6), 910-916.

Bevan,C.L., Hoare,S., Claessens,F., Heery,D.M., & Parker,M.G. (1999). The AF1 and AF2 domains of the androgen receptor interact with distinct regions of SRC1. Mol.Cell Biol., 19(12), 8383-8392.

Bjornstrom,L., Kilic,E., Norman,M., Parker,M.G., & Sjoberg,M. (2001). Cross-talk between Stat5b and estrogen receptor-alpha and -beta in mammary epithelial cells. J.Mol.Endocrinol., 27(1), 93-106.

Blanco,J.C., Minucci,S., Lu,J., Yang,X.J., Walker,K.K., Chen,H., Evans,R.M., Nakatani,Y., & Ozato,K. (1998). The histone acetylase PCAF is a nuclear receptor coactivator. Genes Dev., 12(11), 1638-1651.
Boonyaratanakornkit,V., Melvin,V., Prendergast,P., Altmann,M., Ronfani,L., Bianchi,M.E., Taraseviciene,L., Nordeen,S.K., Allegretto,E.A., & Edwards,D.P. (1998). High-mobility group chromatin proteins 1 and 2 functionally interact with steroid hormone receptors to enhance their DNA binding in vitro and transcriptional activity in mammalian cells. Mol.Cell Biol., 18(8), 4471-4487.
Borg,A., Baldetorp,B., Ferno,M., Killander,D., Olsson,H., Ryden,S., & Sigurdsson,H. (1994). ERBB2 amplification is associated with tamoxifen resistance in steroid- receptor positive breast cancer. Cancer Lett., 81(2), 137-144.
Bourguet,W., Ruff,M., Chambon,P., Gronemeyer,H., & Moras,D. (1995). Crystal structure of the ligand-binding domain of the human nuclear receptor RXR-alpha [see comments]. Nature, 375(6530), 377-382.
Brady,M.E., Ozanne,D.M., Gaughan,L., Waite,I., Cook,S., Neal,D.E., & Robson,C.N. (1999). Tip60 is a nuclear hormone receptor coactivator. J.Biol.Chem., 274(25), 17599-17604.
Brinkmann,A.O., Blok,L.J., de Ruiter,P.E., Doesburg,P., Steketee,K., Berrevoets,C.A., & Trapman,J. (1999). Mechanisms of androgen receptor activation and function. J.Steroid Biochem.Mol.Biol., 69 (1-6), 307-313.
Brzozowski,A.M., Pike,A.C., Dauter,Z., Hubbard,R.E., Bonn,T., Engstrom,O., Ohman,L., Greene,G.L., Gustafsson,J.A., & Carlquist,M. (1997). Molecular basis of agonism and antagonism in the oestrogen receptor. Nature, 389(6652), 753-758.
Bubulya,A., Chen,S.Y., Fisher,C.J., Zheng,Z., Shen,X.Q., & Shemshedini,L. (2001). c-Jun potentiates the functional interaction between the amino and carboxyl termini of the androgen receptor. J.Biol.Chem., 276(48), 44704-44711.
Buchanan,G., Yang,M., Harris,J.M., Nahm,H.S., Han,G., Moore,N., Bentel,J.M., Matusik,R.J., Horsfall,D.J., Marshall,V.R., Greenberg,N.M., & Tilley,W.D. (2001). Mutations at the Boundary of the Hinge and Ligand Binding Domain of the Androgen Receptor Confer Increased Transactivation Function. Mol.Endocrinol., 15(1), 46-56.
Bunone,G., Briand,P.A., Miksicek,R.J., & Picard,D. (1996). Activation of the unliganded estrogen receptor by EGF involves the MAP kinase pathway and direct phosphorylation. EMBO J., 15(9), 2174-2183.
Burakov,D., Wong,C.W., Rachez,C., Cheskis,B.J., & Freedman,L.P. (2000). Functional interactions between the estrogen receptor and DRIP205, a subunit of the heteromeric DRIP coactivator complex. J.Biol.Chem., 275(27), 20928-20934.
Byrne,R.L., Leung,H., & Neal,D.E. (1996). Peptide growth factors in the prostate as mediators of stromal epithelial interaction. Br.J.Urol., 77(5), 627-633.
Cairns,P., Okami,K., Halachmi,S., Halachmi,N., Esteller,M., Herman,J.G., Jen,J., Isaacs,W.B., Bova,G.S., & Sidransky,D. (1997). Frequent inactivation of PTEN/MMAC1 in primary prostate cancer. Cancer Res., 57(22), 4997-5000.
Campbell,R.A., Bhat-Nakshatri,P., Patel,N.M., Constantinidou,D., Ali,S., & Nakshatri,H. (2001). Phosphatidylinositol 3-kinase/AKT-mediated activation of estrogen receptor alpha: a new model for anti-estrogen resistance. J.Biol.Chem., 276(13), 9817-9824.
Castoria,G., Barone,M.V., Di Domenico,M., Bilancio,A., Ametrano,D., Migliaccio,A., & Auricchio,F. (1999). Non-transcriptional action of oestradiol and progestin triggers DNA synthesis. EMBO J., 18(9), 2500-2510.
Chamberlain,N.L., Driver,E.D., & Miesfeld,R.L. (1994). The length and location of CAG trinucleotide repeats in the androgen receptor N-terminal domain affect transactivation function. Nucleic Acids Res., 22(15), 3181-3186.
Chambliss,K.L., Yuhanna,I.S., Mineo,C., Liu,P., German,Z., Sherman,T.S., Mendelsohn,M.E., Anderson,R.G., & Shaul,P.W. (2000). Estrogen receptor alpha and endothelial nitric oxide synthase are organized into a functional signaling module in caveolae. Circ.Res., 87(11), E44-E52
Chen,D., Pace,P.E., Coombes,R.C., & Ali,S. (1999). Phosphorylation of human estrogen receptor alpha by protein kinase A regulates dimerization. Mol.Cell Biol., 19(2), 1002-1015.

Chen,D., Riedl,T., Washbrook,E., Pace,P.E., Coombes,R.C., Egly,J.M., & Ali,S. (2000). Activation of estrogen receptor alpha by S118 phosphorylation involves a ligand-dependent interaction with TFIIH and participation of CDK7. Mol.Cell, 6(1), 127-137.

Chen,H., Lin,R.J., Schiltz,R.L., Chakravarti,D., Nash,A., Nagy,L., Privalsky,M.L., Nakatani,Y., & Evans,R.M. (1997). Nuclear receptor coactivator ACTR is a novel histone acetyltransferase and forms a multimeric activation complex with P/CAF and CBP/p300. Cell, 90(3), 569-580.

Chen,H., Lin,R.J., Xie,W., Wilpitz,D., & Evans,R.M. (1999). Regulation of hormone-induced histone hyperacetylation and gene activation via acetylation of an acetylase. Cell, 98(5), 675-686.

Chen,J.D., & Evans,R.M. (1995). A transcriptional co-repressor that interacts with nuclear hormone receptors. Nature, 377(6548), 454-457.

Chen,T., Wang,L.H., & Farrar,W.L. (2000). Interleukin 6 activates androgen receptor-mediated gene expression through a signal transducer and activator of transcription 3-dependent pathway in LNCaP prostate cancer cells. Cancer Res., 60(8), 2132-2135.

Chen,Z., Yuhanna,I.S., Galcheva-Gargova,Z., Karas,R.H., Mendelsohn,M.E., & Shaul,P.W. (1999). Estrogen receptor alpha mediates the nongenomic activation of endothelial nitric oxide synthase by estrogen [published erratum appears in J Clin Invest 1999 May;103(9):1363]. J.Clin.Invest, 103(3), 401-406.

Choong,C.S., Kemppainen,J.A., Zhou,Z.X., & Wilson,E.M. (1996). Reduced androgen receptor gene expression with first exon CAG repeat expansion. Mol.Endocrinol., 10(12), 1527-1535.

Clarke,R.B., Howell,A., Potten,C.S., & Anderson,E. (1997). Dissociation between steroid receptor expression and cell proliferation in the human breast. Cancer Res., 57(22), 4987-4991.

Coleman,K.M., & Smith,C.L. (2001). Intracellular signaling pathways: nongenomic actions of estrogens and ligand-independent activation of estrogen receptors. Front Biosci., 6, D1379-D1391

Couse,J.F., Lindzey,J., Grandien,K., Gustafsson,J.A., & Korach,K.S. (1997). Tissue distribution and quantitative analysis of estrogen receptor- alpha (ERalpha) and estrogen receptor-beta (ERbeta) messenger ribonucleic acid in the wild-type and ERalpha-knockout mouse. Endocrinology, 138(11), 4613-4621.

Craft,N., Shostak,Y., Carey,M., & Sawyers,C.L. (1999). A mechanism for hormone-independent prostate cancer through modulation of androgen receptor signaling by the HER-2/neu tyrosine kinase [see comments]. Nat.Med., 5(3), 280-285.

Culig,Z., Hobisch,A., Cronauer,M.V., Radmayr,C., Trapman,J., Hittmair,A., Bartsch,G., & Klocker,H. (1995). Androgen receptor activation in prostatic tumor cell lines by insulin- like growth factor-I, keratinocyte growth factor and epidermal growth factor. Eur.Urol., 27 Suppl 2, 45-47.

Cunha,G.R. (1984). Androgenic effects upon prostatic epithelium are mediated via trophic influences from stroma. Prog.Clin.Biol.Res., 145, 81-102.

Cunha,G.R., Young,P., Hom,Y.K., Cooke,P.S., Taylor,J.A., & Lubahn,D.B. (1997). Elucidation of a role for stromal steroid hormone receptors in mammary gland growth and development using tissue recombinants. J.Mammary.Gland.Biol.Neoplasia., 2(4), 393-402.

Curtis,S.W., Washburn,T., Sewall,C., DiAugustine,R., Lindzey,J., Couse,J.F., & Korach,K.S. (1996). Physiological coupling of growth factor and steroid receptor signaling pathways: estrogen receptor knockout mice lack estrogen-like response to epidermal growth factor. Proc.Natl.Acad.Sci.U.S.A, 93(22), 12626-12630.

Danielian,P.S., White,R., Lees,J.A., & Parker,M.G. (1992). Identification of a conserved region required for hormone dependent transcriptional activation by steroid hormone receptors. EMBO J., 11 (3), 1025-1033.

de Ruiter,P.E., Teuwen,R., Trapman,J., Dijkema,R., & Brinkmann,A.O. (1995). Synergism between androgens and protein kinase-C on androgen-regulated gene expression. Mol.Cell Endocrinol., 110(1-2), R1-R6

Denner,L.A., Weigel,N.L., Maxwell,B.L., Schrader,W.T., & O'Malley,B.W. (1990). Regulation of progesterone receptor-mediated transcription by phosphorylation. Science, 250(4988), 1740-1743.

Ding,X.F., Anderson,C.M., Ma,H., Hong,H., Uht,R.M., Kushner,P.J., & Stallcup,M.R. (1998). Nuclear receptor-binding sites of coactivators glucocorticoid receptor interacting protein 1 (GRIP1) and steroid receptor coactivator 1 (SRC- 1): multiple motifs with different binding specificities. Mol.Endocrinol., 12(2), 302-313.

DiRenzo,J., Shang,Y., Phelan,M., Sif,S., Myers,M., Kingston,R., & Brown,M. (2000). BRG-1 is recruited to estrogen-responsive promoters and cooperates with factors involved in histone acetylation. Mol.Cell Biol., 20(20), 7541-7549.

Drab,M., Verkade,P., Elger,M., Kasper,M., Lohn,M., Lauterbach,B., Menne,J., Lindschau,C., Mende,F., Luft,F.C., Schedl,A., Haller,H., & Kurzchalia,T.V. (2001). Loss of caveolae, vascular dysfunction, and pulmonary defects in caveolin-1 gene-disrupted mice. Science, 293(5539), 2449-2452.

Dubik,D., & Shiu,R.P. (1992). Mechanism of estrogen activation of c-myc oncogene expression. Oncogene, 7(8), 1587-1594.

Endoh,H., Maruyama,K., Masuhiro,Y., Kobayashi,Y., Goto,M., Tai,H., Yanagisawa,J., Metzger,D., Hashimoto,S., & Kato,S. (1999). Purification and identification of p68 RNA helicase acting as a transcriptional coactivator specific for the activation function 1 of human estrogen receptor alpha. Mol.Cell Biol., 19(8), 5363-5372.

English,H.F., Santen,R.J., & Isaacs,J.T. (1987). Response of glandular versus basal rat ventral prostatic epithelial cells to androgen withdrawal and replacement. Prostate, 11(3), 229-242.

Evans,G.S., & Chandler,J.A. (1987). Cell proliferation studies in rat prostate. I. The proliferative role of basal and secretory epithelial cells during normal growth. Prostate, 10(2), 163-178.

Feng,W., Ribeiro,R.C., Wagner,R.L., Nguyen,H., Apriletti,J.W., Fletterick,R.J., Baxter,J.D., Kushner,P.J., & West,B.L. (1998). Hormone-dependent coactivator binding to a hydrophobic cleft on nuclear receptors. Science, 280(5370), 1747-1749.

Filardo,E.J., Quinn,J.A., Bland,K.I., & Frackelton,A.R., Jr. (2000). Estrogen-induced activation of Erk-1 and Erk-2 requires the G protein- coupled receptor homolog, GPR30, and occurs via trans-activation of the epidermal growth factor receptor through release of HB-EGF. Mol.Endocrinol., 14(10), 1649-1660.

Fondell,J.D., Ge,H., & Roeder,R.G. (1996). Ligand induction of a transcriptionally active thyroid hormone receptor coactivator complex. Proc.Natl.Acad.Sci.U.S.A, 93(16), 8329-8333.

Font,d.M., & Brown,M. (2000). AIB1 is a conduit for kinase-mediated growth factor signaling to the estrogen receptor. Mol.Cell Biol., 20(14), 5041-5047.

Fryer,C.J., & Archer,T.K. (1998). Chromatin remodelling by the glucocorticoid receptor requires the BRG1 complex. Nature, 393(6680), 88-91.

Fu,M., Wang,C., Reutens,A.T., Wang,J., Angeletti,R.H., Siconolfi-Baez,L., Ogryzko,V., Avantaggiati,M.L., & Pestell,R.G. (2000). p300 and p300/cAMP-response element-binding protein-associated factor acetylate the androgen receptor at sites governing hormone-dependent transactivation. J.Biol.Chem., 275(27), 20853-20860.

Fujimoto,N., Yeh,S., Kang,H.Y., Inui,S., Chang,H.C., Mizokami,A., & Chang,C. (1999). Cloning and characterization of androgen receptor coactivator, ARA55, in human prostate. J.Biol.Chem., 274(12), 8316-8321.

Fuqua,S.A., Wiltschke,C., Zhang,Q.X., Borg,A., Castles,C.G., Friedrichs,W.E., Hopp,T., Hilsenbeck,S., Mohsin,S., O'Connell,P., & Allred,D.C. (2000). A hypersensitive estrogen receptor-alpha mutation in premalignant breast lesions. Cancer Res., 60(15), 4026-4029.

Galien,R., & Garcia,T. (1997). Estrogen receptor impairs interleukin-6 expression by preventing protein binding on the NF-kappaB site. Nucleic Acids Res., 25(12), 2424-2429.

Giovannucci,E., Stampfer,M.J., Krithivas,K., Brown,M., Dahl,D., Brufsky,A., Talcott,J., Hennekens,C.H., & Kantoff,P.W. (1997). The CAG repeat within the androgen receptor gene and its relationship to prostate cancer [published erratum appears in Proc Natl Acad Sci U S A 1997 Jul 22;94(15):8272]. Proc.Natl.Acad.Sci.U.S.A, 94(7), 3320-3323.

Glass,C.K., Rose,D.W., & Rosenfeld,M.G. (1997). Nuclear receptor coactivators. Curr.Opin.Cell Biol., 9(2), 222-232.

Gonzalez,M.I., & Robins,D.M. (2001). Oct-1 preferentially interacts with androgen receptor in a DNA- dependent manner that facilitates recruitment of SRC-1. J.Biol.Chem., 276(9), 6420-6428.

Grant,E.S., Batchelor,K.W., & Habib,F.K. (1996). Androgen independence of primary epithelial cultures of the prostate is associated with a down-regulation of androgen receptor gene expression. Prostate, 29(6), 339-349.

Gregory,C.W., He,B., Johnson,R.T., Ford,O.H., Mohler,J.L., French,F.S., & Wilson,E.M. (2001). A mechanism for androgen receptor-mediated prostate cancer recurrence after androgen deprivation therapy. Cancer Res., 61(11), 4315-4319.

Gu,W., Malik,S., Ito,M., Yuan,C.X., Fondell,J.D., Zhang,X., Martinez,E., Qin,J., & Roeder,R.G. (1999). A novel human SRB/MED-containing cofactor complex, SMCC, involved in transcription regulation. Mol.Cell, 3(1), 97-108.

Hakimi,J.M., Schoenberg,M.P., Rondinelli,R.H., Piantadosi,S., & Barrack,E.R. (1997). Androgen receptor variants with short glutamine or glycine repeats may identify unique subpopulations of men with prostate cancer. Clin.Cancer Res., 3(9), 1599-1608.

Hardy,D.O., Scher,H.I., Bogenreider,T., Sabbatini,P., Zhang,Z.F., Nanus,D.M., & Catterall,J.F. (1996). Androgen receptor CAG repeat lengths in prostate cancer: correlation with age of onset. J.Clin.Endocrinol.Metab, 81(12), 4400-4405.

Haynes,M.P., Sinha,D., Russell,K.S., Collinge,M., Fulton,D., Morales-Ruiz,M., Sessa,W.C., & Bender,J.R. (2000). Membrane estrogen receptor engagement activates endothelial nitric oxide synthase via the PI3-kinase-Akt pathway in human endothelial cells. Circ.Res., 87(8), 677-682.

He,B., Kemppainen,J.A., & Wilson,E.M. (2000). FXXLF and WXXLF sequences mediate the NH2-terminal interaction with the ligand binding domain of the androgen receptor. J.Biol.Chem., 275(30), 22986-22994.

Heery,D.M., Kalkhoven,E., Hoare,S., & Parker,M.G. (1997). A signature motif in transcriptional co-activators mediates binding to nuclear receptors [see comments]. Nature, 387(6634), 733-736.

Heinzel,T., Lavinsky,R.M., Mullen,T.M., Soderstrom,M., Laherty,C.D., Torchia,J., Yang,W.M., Brard,G., Ngo,S.D., Davie,J.R., Seto,E., Eisenman,R.N., Rose,D.W., Glass,C.K., & Rosenfeld,M.G. (1997). A complex containing N-CoR, mSin3 and histone deacetylase mediates transcriptional repression. Nature, 387(6628), 43-48.

Heisler,L.E., Evangelou,A., Lew,A.M., Trachtenberg,J., Elsholtz,H.P., & Brown,T.J. (1997). Androgen-dependent cell cycle arrest and apoptotic death in PC-3 prostatic cell cultures expressing a full-length human androgen receptor. Mol.Cell Endocrinol., 126(1), 59-73.

Hisamoto,K., Ohmichi,M., Kurachi,H., Hayakawa,J., Kanda,Y., Nishio,Y., Adachi,K., Tasaka,K., Miyoshi,E., Fujiwara,N., Taniguchi,N., & Murata,Y. (2001). Estrogen induces the Akt-dependent activation of endothelial nitric- oxide synthase in vascular endothelial cells. J.Biol.Chem., 276(5), 3459-3467.

Hong,H., Kohli,K., Garabedian,M.J., & Stallcup,M.R. (1997). GRIP1, a transcriptional coactivator for the AF-2 transactivation domain of steroid, thyroid, retinoid, and vitamin D receptors. Mol.Cell Biol., 17(5), 2735-2744.

Horlein,A.J., Naar,A.M., Heinzel,T., Torchia,J., Gloss,B., Kurokawa,R., Ryan,A., Kamei,Y., Soderstrom,M., & Glass,C.K. (1995). Ligand-independent repression by the thyroid hormone receptor mediated by a nuclear receptor co-repressor [see comments]. Nature, 377(6548), 397-404.

Hsing,A.W., Gao,Y.T., Wu,G., Wang,X., Deng,J., Chen,Y.L., Sesterhenn,I.A., Mostofi,F.K., Benichou,J., & Chang,C. (2000). Polymorphic CAG and GGN repeat lengths in the androgen receptor gene and prostate cancer risk: a population-based case-control study in China. Cancer Res., 60(18), 5111-5116.

Hu,X., & Lazar,M.A. (1999). The CoRNR motif controls the recruitment of corepressors by nuclear hormone receptors. Nature, 402(6757), 93-96.

Huang,S.M., & Stallcup,M.R. (2000). Mouse Zac1, a transcriptional coactivator and repressor for nuclear receptors. Mol.Cell Biol., 20(5), 1855-1867.

Ichinose,H., Garnier,J.M., Chambon,P., & Losson,R. (1997). Ligand-dependent interaction between the estrogen receptor and the human homologues of SWI2/SNF2. Gene, 188(1), 95-100.

Ignar-Trowbridge,D.M., Nelson,K.G., Bidwell,M.C., Curtis,S.W., Washburn,T.F., McLachlan,J.A., & Korach,K.S. (1992). Coupling of dual signaling pathways: epidermal growth factor action involves the estrogen receptor. Proc.Natl.Acad.Sci.U.S.A, 89(10), 4658-4662.

Ignar-Trowbridge,D.M., Pimentel,M., Parker,M.G., McLachlan,J.A., & Korach,K.S. (1996). Peptide growth factor cross-talk with the estrogen receptor requires the A/B domain and occurs independently of protein kinase C or estradiol. Endocrinology, 137(5), 1735-1744.

Ikonen,T., Palvimo,J.J., Kallio,P.J., Reinikainen,P., & Janne,O.A. (1994). Stimulation of androgen-regulated transactivation by modulators of protein phosphorylation. Endocrinology, 135(4), 1359-1366.

Irvine,R.A., Ma,H., Yu,M.C., Ross,R.K., Stallcup,M.R., & Coetzee,G.A. (2000). Inhibition of p160-mediated coactivation with increasing androgen receptor polyglutamine length. Hum.Mol.Genet., 9(2), 267-274.

Ito,M., Yuan,C.X., Malik,S., Gu,W., Fondell,J.D., Yamamura,S., Fu,Z.Y., Zhang,X., Qin,J., & Roeder,R.G. (1999). Identity between TRAP and SMCC complexes indicates novel pathways for the function of nuclear receptors and diverse mammalian activators. Mol.Cell. 3(3), 361-370.

Jackson,T.A., Richer,J.K., Bain,D.L., Takimoto,G.S., Tung,L., & Horwitz,K.B. (1997). The partial agonist activity of antagonist-occupied steroid receptors is controlled by a novel hinge domain-binding coactivator L7/SPA and the corepressors N-CoR or SMRT. Mol.Endocrinol., 11 (6), 693-705.

Jenster,G., Spencer,T.E., Burcin,M.M., Tsai,S.Y., Tsai,M.J., & O'Malley,B.W. (1997). Steroid receptor induction of gene transcription: a two-step model. Proc.Natl.Acad.Sci.U.S.A. 94(15), 7879-7884.

Joel,P.B., Smith,J., Sturgill,T.W., Fisher,T.L., Blenis,J., & Lannigan,D.A. (1998). pp90rsk1 regulates estrogen receptor-mediated transcription through phosphorylation of Ser-167. Mol.Cell Biol., 18(4), 1978-1984.

Joel,P.B., Traish,A.M., & Lannigan,D.A. (1998). Estradiol-induced phosphorylation of serine 118 in the estrogen receptor is independent of p42/p44 mitogen-activated protein kinase. J.Biol.Chem., 273(21), 13317-13323.

Johansson,L., Bavner,A., Thomsen,J.S., Farnegardh,M., Gustafsson,J.A., & Treuter,E. (2000). The orphan nuclear receptor SHP utilizes conserved LXXLL-related motifs for interactions with ligand-activated estrogen receptors. Mol.Cell Biol., 20(4), 1124-1133.

Kallio,P.J., Poukka,H., Moilanen,A., Janne,O.A., & Palvimo,J.J. (1995). Androgen receptor-mediated transcriptional regulation in the absence of direct interaction with a specific DNA element. Mol.Endocrinol., 9(8), 1017-1028.

Kamei,Y., Xu,L., Heinzel,T., Torchia,J., Kurokawa,R., Gloss,B., Lin,S.C., Heyman,R.A., Rose,D.W., Glass,C.K., & Rosenfeld,M.G. (1996). A CBP integrator complex mediates transcriptional activation and AP-1 inhibition by nuclear receptors. Cell, 85(3), 403-414.

Kang,H.Y., Yeh,S., Fujimoto,N., & Chang,C. (1999). Cloning and characterization of human prostate coactivator ARA54, a novel protein that associates with the androgen receptor. J.Biol.Chem., 274(13), 8570-8576.

Kato,S., Endoh,H., Masuhiro,Y., Kitamoto,T., Uchiyama,S., Sasaki,H., Masushige,S., Gotoh,Y., Nishida,E., & Kawashima,H. (1995). Activation of the estrogen receptor through phosphorylation by mitogen- activated protein kinase. Science, 270(5241), 1491-1494.

Kim,H.P., Lee,J.Y., Jeong,J.K., Bae,S.W., Lee,H.K., & Jo,I. (1999). Nongenomic stimulation of nitric oxide release by estrogen is mediated by estrogen receptor alpha localized in caveolae. Biochem.Biophys.Res.Commun., 263(1), 257-262.

Knudsen,K.E., Cavenee,W.K., & Arden,K.C. (1999). D-type cyclins complex with the androgen receptor and inhibit its transcriptional transactivation ability. Cancer Res., 59(10), 2297-2301.

Koh,S.S., Chen,D., Lee,Y.H., & Stallcup,M.R. (2001). Synergistic Enhancement of Nuclear Receptor Function by p160 Coactivators and Two Coactivators with Protein Methyltransferase Activities. J.Biol.Chem., 276(2), 1089-1098.

Kousteni,S., Bellido,T., Plotkin,L.I., O'Brien,C.A., Bodenner,D.L., Han,L., Han,K., DiGregorio,G.B., Katzenellenbogen,J.A., Katzenellenbogen,B.S., Roberson,P.K., Weinstein,R.S., Jilka,R.L., & Manolagas,S.C. (2001). Nongenotropic, sex-nonspecific signaling through the estrogen or androgen receptors: dissociation from transcriptional activity. Cell, 104(5), 719-730.

Kraus,W.L., McInerney,E.M., & Katzenellenbogen,B.S. (1995). Ligand-dependent, transcriptionally productive association of the amino- and carboxyl-terminal regions of a steroid hormone nuclear receptor. Proc.Natl.Acad.Sci.U.S.A. 92(26), 12314-12318.

Lanz,R.B., McKenna,N.J., Onate,S.A., Albrecht,U., Wong,J., Tsai,S.Y., Tsai,M.J., & O'Malley,B.W. (1999). A steroid receptor coactivator, SRA, functions as an RNA and is present in an SRC-1 complex. Cell, 97(1), 17-27.

Leav,I., McNeal,J.E., Kwan,P.W., Komminoth,P., & Merk,F.B. (1996). Androgen receptor expression in prostatic dysplasia (prostatic intraepithelial neoplasia) in the human prostate: an immunohistochemical and in situ hybridization study. Prostate, 29(3), 137-145.

Lee,S.R., Ramos,S.M., Ko,A., Masiello,D., Swanson,K.D., Lu,M.L., & Balk,S.P. (2002). AR and ER Interaction with a p21-Activated Kinase (PAK6). Mol.Endocrinol., 16(1), 85-99.

Leitzel,K., Teramoto,Y., Konrad,K., Chinchilli,V.M., Volas,G., Grossberg,H., Harvey,H., Demers,L., & Lipton,A. (1995). Elevated serum c-erbB-2 antigen levels and decreased response to hormone therapy of breast cancer. J.Clin.Oncol., 13(5), 1129-1135.

Lin,H.K., Yeh,S., Kang,H.Y., & Chang,C. (2001). Akt suppresses androgen-induced apoptosis by phosphorylating and inhibiting androgen receptor. Proc.Natl.Acad.Sci.U.S.A. 98(13), 7200-7205.

Lu,M.L., Schneider,M.C., Zheng,Y., Zhang,X., & Richie,J.P. (2001). Caveolin-1 interacts with androgen receptor. A positive modulator of androgen receptor mediated transactivation. J.Biol.Chem., 276(16), 13442-13451.

Lu,S., Jenster,G., & Epner,D.E. (2000). Androgen induction of cyclin-dependent kinase inhibitor p21 gene: role of androgen receptor and transcription factor Sp1 complex. Mol.Endocrinol., 14(5), 753-760.

Lubahn,D.B., Moyer,J.S., Golding,T.S., Couse,J.F., Korach,K.S., & Smithies,O. (1993). Alteration of reproductive function but not prenatal sexual development after insertional disruption of the mouse estrogen receptor gene. Proc.Natl.Acad.Sci.U.S.A. 90(23), 11162-11166.

Mangelsdorf,D.J., & Evans,R.M. (1995). The RXR heterodimers and orphan receptors. Cell, 83(6), 841-850.

Mangelsdorf,D.J., Thummel,C., Beato,M., Herrlich,P., Schutz,G., Umesono,K., Blumberg,B., Kastner,P., Mark,M., & Chambon,P. (1995). The nuclear receptor superfamily: the second decade. Cell, 83(6), 835-839.

Marcelli,M., Ittmann,M., Mariani,S., Sutherland,R., Nigam,R., Murthy,L., Zhao,Y., DiConcini,D., Puxeddu,E., Esen,A., Eastham,J., Weigel,N.L., & Lamb,D.J. (2000). Androgen receptor mutations in prostate cancer. Cancer Res., 60(4), 944-949.

McInerney,E.M., & Katzenellenbogen,B.S. (1996). Different regions in activation function-1 of the human estrogen receptor required for antiestr. J.Biol.Chem., 271(39), 24172-24178.

McKay,L.I., & Cidlowski,J.A. (1998). Cross-talk between nuclear factor-kappa B and the steroid hormone receptors: mechanisms of mutual antagonism. Mol.Endocrinol., 12(1), 45-56.

McMenamin,M.E., Soung,P., Perera,S., Kaplan,I., Loda,M., & Sellers,W.R. (1999). Loss of PTEN expression in paraffin-embedded primary prostate cancer correlates with high Gleason score and advanced stage. Cancer Res., 59(17), 4291-4296.

Migliaccio,A., Pagano,M., & Auricchio,F. (1993). Immediate and transient stimulation of protein tyrosine phosphorylation by estradiol in MCF-7 cells. Oncogene, 8(8), 2183-2191.

Migliaccio,A., Piccolo,D., Castoria,G., Di Domenico,M., Bilancio,A., Lombardi,M., Gong,W., Beato,M., & Auricchio,F. (1998). Activation of the Src/p21ras/Erk pathway by progesterone receptor via cross-talk with estrogen receptor. EMBO J., 17(7), 2008-2018.

Moilanen,A.M., Karvonen,U., Poukka,H., Janne,O.A., & Palvimo,J.J. (1998b). Activation of androgen receptor function by a novel nuclear protein kinase. Mol.Biol.Cell, 9(9), 2527-2543.

Moilanen,A.M., Karvonen,U., Poukka,H., Yan,W., Toppari,J., Janne,O.A., & Palvimo,J.J. (1999). A testis-specific androgen receptor coregulator that belongs to a novel family of nuclear proteins. J.Biol.Chem., 274(6), 3700-3704.

Moilanen,A.M., Poukka,H., Karvonen,U., Hakli,M., Janne,O.A., & Palvimo,J.J. (1998a). Identification of a novel RING finger protein as a coregulator in steroid receptor-mediated gene transcription. Mol.Cell Biol., 18(9), 5128-5139.

Muller,J.M., Isele,U., Metzger,E., Rempel,A., Moser,M., Pscherer,A., Breyer,T., Holubarsch,C., Buettner,R., & Schule,R. (2000). FHL2, a novel tissue-specific coactivator of the androgen receptor. EMBO J., 19(3), 359-369.

Nagy,L., Kao,H.Y., Chakravarti,D., Lin,R.J., Hassig,C.A., Ayer,D.E., Schreiber,S.L., & Evans,R.M. (1997). Nuclear receptor repression mediated by a complex containing SMRT, mSin3A, and histone deacetylase. Cell, 89(3), 373-380.

Nagy,L., Kao,H.Y., Love,J.D., Li,C., Banayo,E., Gooch,J.T., Krishna,V., Chatterjee,K., Evans,R.M., & Schwabe,J.W. (1999). Mechanism of corepressor binding and release from nuclear hormone receptors. Genes Dev., 13(24), 3209-3216.

Nam,R.K., Elhaji,Y., Krahn,M.D., Hakimi,J., Ho,M., Chu,W., Sweet,J., Trachtenberg,J., Jewett,M.A., & Narod,S.A. (2000). Significance of the CAG repeat polymorphism of the androgen receptor gene in prostate cancer progression. J.Urol., 164(2), 567-572.

Nawaz,Z., Lonard,D.M., Smith,C.L., Lev-Lehman,E., Tsai,S.Y., Tsai,M.J., & O'Malley,B.W. (1999). The Angelman syndrome-associated protein, E6-AP, is a coactivator for the nuclear hormone receptor superfamily. Mol.Cell Biol., 19(2), 1182-1189.

Nazareth,L.V., & Weigel,N.L. (1996). Activation of the human androgen receptor through a protein kinase A signaling pathway. J.Biol.Chem., 271(33), 19900-19907.

Neuman,E., Ladha,M.H., Lin,N., Upton,T.M., Miller,S.J., DiRenzo,J., Pestell,R.G., Hinds,P.W., Dowdy,S.F., Brown,M., & Ewen,M.E. (1997). Cyclin D1 stimulation of estrogen receptor transcriptional activity independent of cdk4. Mol.Cell Biol., 17(9), 5338-5347.

Nilsson,S., Makela,S., Treuter,E., Tujague,M., Thomsen,J., Andersson,G., Enmark,E., Pettersson,K., Warner,M., & Gustafsson,J.A. (2001). Mechanisms of estrogen action. Physiol Rev., 81(4), 1535-1565.

Ning,Y.M., & Robins,D.M. (1999). AML3/CBFalpha1 is required for androgen-specific activation of the enhancer of the mouse sex-limited protein (Slp) gene. J.Biol.Chem., 274(43), 30624-30630.

Oettgen,P., Finger,E., Sun,Z., Akbarali,Y., Thamrongsak,U., Boltax,J., Grall,F., Dube,A., Weiss,A., Brown,L., Quinn,G., Kas,K., Endress,G., Kunsch,C., & Libermann,T.A. (2000). PDEF, a novel prostate epithelium-specific ets transcription factor, interacts with the androgen receptor and activates prostate-specific antigen gene expression. J.Biol.Chem., 275(2), 1216-1225.

Ogryzko,V.V., Kotani,T., Zhang,X., Schiltz,R.L., Howard,T., Yang,X.J., Howard,B.H., Qin,J., & Nakatani,Y. (1998). Histone-like TAFs within the PCAF histone acetylase complex. Cell, 94(1), 35-44.

Ohlsson,H., Lykkesfeldt,A.E., Madsen,M.W., & Briand,P. (1998). The estrogen receptor variant lacking exon 5 has dominant negative activity in the human breast epithelial cell line HMT-3522S1. Cancer Res., 58(19), 4264-4268.

Onate,S.A., Tsai,S.Y., Tsai,M.J., & O'Malley,B.W. (1995). Sequence and characterization of a coactivator for the steroid hormone receptor superfamily. Science, 270(5240), 1354-1357.

Ostlund Farrants,A.K., Blomquist,P., Kwon,H., & Wrange,O. (1997). Glucocorticoid receptor-glucocorticoid response element binding stimulates nucleosome disruption by the SWI/SNF complex. Mol.Cell Biol., 17(2), 895-905.

Paech,K., Webb,P., Kuiper,G.G., Nilsson,S., Gustafsson,J., Kushner,P.J., & Scanlan,T.S. (1997). Differential ligand activation of estrogen receptors ERalpha and ERbeta at AP1 sites. Science, 277(5331), 1508-1510.

Patrone,C., Gianazza,E., Santagati,S., Agrati,P., & Maggi,A. (1998). Divergent pathways regulate ligand-independent activation of ER alpha in SK-N-BE neuroblastoma and COS-1 renal carcinoma cells. Mol.Endocrinol., 12(6), 835-841.

Peehl,D.M., & Stamey,T.A. (1986). Serum-free growth of adult human prostatic epithelial cells. In Vitro Cell Dev.Biol., 22(2), 82-90.

Perissi,V., Staszewski,L.M., McInerney,E.M., Kurokawa,R., Krones,A., Rose,D.W., Lambert,M.H., Milburn,M.V., Glass,C.K., & Rosenfeld,M.G. (1999). Molecular determinants of nuclear receptor-corepressor interaction. Genes Dev., 13(24), 3198-3208.

Peterziel,H., Mink,S., Schonert,A., Becker,M., Klocker,H., & Cato,A.C. (1999). Rapid signalling by androgen receptor in prostate cancer cells. Oncogene, 18(46), 6322-6329.

Pietras,R.J., Arboleda,J., Reese,D.M., Wongvipat,N., Pegram,M.D., Ramos,L., Gorman,C.M., Parker,M.G., Sliwkowski,M.X., & Slamon,D.J. (1995). HER-2 tyrosine kinase pathway targets estrogen receptor and promotes hormone-independent growth in human breast cancer cells. Oncogene, 10(12), 2435-2446.

Porter,W., Saville,B., Hoivik,D., & Safe,S. (1997). Functional synergy between the transcription factor Sp1 and the estrogen receptor. Mol.Endocrinol., 11(11), 1569-1580.

Poukka,H., Aarnisalo,P., Karvonen,U., Palvimo,J.J., & Janne,O.A. (1999). Ubc9 interacts with the androgen receptor and activates receptor- dependent transcription. J.Biol.Chem., 274(27), 19441-19446.

Poukka,H., Aarnisalo,P., Santti,H., Janne,O.A., & Palvimo,J.J. (2000). Coregulator small nuclear RING finger protein (SNURF) enhances Sp1- and steroid receptor-mediated transcription by different mechanisms. J.Biol.Chem., 275(1), 571-579.

Pratt,W.B., & Toft,D.O. (1997). Steroid receptor interactions with heat shock protein and immunophilin chaperones. Endocr.Rev., 18(3), 306-360.

Putz,T., Culig,Z., Eder,I.E., Nessler-Menardi,C., Bartsch,G., Grunicke,H., Uberall,F., & Klocker,H. (1999). Epidermal growth factor (EGF) receptor blockade inhibits the action of EGF, insulin-like growth factor I, and a protein kinase A activator on the mitogen-activated protein kinase pathway in prostate cancer cell lines. Cancer Res., 59(1), 227-233.

Qin,C., Singh,P., & Safe,S. (1999). Transcriptional activation of insulin-like growth factor binding protein-4 by 17beta-estradiol in MCF-7 cells: role of estrogen receptor- Sp1 complexes. Endocrinology, 140(6), 2501-2508.

Quigley,C.A., De Bellis,A., Marschke,K.B., el Awady,M.K., Wilson,E.M., & French,F.S. (1995). Androgen receptor defects: historical, clinical, and molecular perspectives [published erratum appears in Endocr Rev 1995 Aug;16(4):546]. Endocr.Rev., 16(3), 271-321.

Rachez,C., Suldan,Z., Ward,J., Chang,C.P., Burakov,D., Erdjument-Bromage,H., Tempst,P., & Freedman,L.P. (1998). A novel protein complex that interacts with the vitamin D3 receptor in a ligand-dependent manner and enhances VDR transactivation in a cell- free system. Genes Dev., 12(12), 1787-1800.

Razandi,M., Pedram,A., & Levin,E.R. (2000). Plasma membrane estrogen receptors signal to antiapoptosis in breast cancer. Mol.Endocrinol., 14(9), 1434-1447.

Razani,B., Engelman,J.A., Wang,X.B., Schubert,W., Zhang,X.L., Marks,C.B., Macaluso,F., Russell,R.G., Li,M., Pestell,R.G., Di Vizio,D., Hou,H., Jr., Kneitz,B., Lagaud,G., Christ,G.J., Edelmann,W., & Lisanti,M.P. (2001). Caveolin-1 null mice are viable but show evidence of hyperproliferative and vascular abnormalities. J.Biol.Chem., 276(41), 38121-38138.

Reichardt,H.M., Kaestner,K.H., Tuckermann,J., Kretz,O., Wessely,O., Bock,R., Gass,P., Schmid,W., Herrlich,P., Angel,P., & Schutz,G. (1998). DNA binding of the glucocorticoid receptor is not essential for survival. Cell, 93(4), 531-541.

Renaud,J.P., Rochel,N., Ruff,M., Vivat,V., Chambon,P., Gronemeyer,H., & Moras,D. (1995). Crystal structure of the RAR-gamma ligand-binding domain bound to all- trans retinoic acid. Nature, 378(6558), 681-689.

Reutens,A.T., Fu,M., Wang,C., Albanese,C., McPhaul,M.J., Sun,Z., Balk,S.P., Janne,O.A., Palvimo,J.J., & Pestell,R.G. (2001). Cyclin D1 Binds the Androgen Receptor and Regulates Hormone-Dependent Signaling in a p300/CBP-Associated Factor (P/CAF)-Dependent Manner. Mol.Endocrinol., 15(5), 797-811.

Revelli,A., Massobrio,M., & Tesarik,J. (1998). Nongenomic actions of steroid hormones in reproductive tissues. Endocr.Rev., 19(1), 3-17.

Rogatsky,I., Trowbridge,J.M., & Garabedian,M.J. (1999). Potentiation of human estrogen receptor alpha transcriptional activation through phosphorylation of serines 104 and 106 by the cyclin A-CDK2 complex. J.Biol.Chem., 274(32), 22296-22302.

Roodi,N., Bailey,L.R., Kao,W.Y., Verrier,C.S., Yee,C.J., Dupont,W.D., & Parl,F.F. (1995). Estrogen receptor gene analysis in estrogen receptor-positive and receptor-negative primary breast cancer. J.Natl.Cancer Inst., 87(6), 446-451.

Rosenfeld,M.G., & Glass,C.K. (2001). Coregulator codes of transcriptional regulation by nuclear receptors. J.Biol.Chem., 276(40), 36865-36868.

Rowan,B.G., Garrison,N., Weigel,N.L., & O'Malley,B.W. (2000). 8-Bromo-cyclic AMP induces phosphorylation of two sites in SRC-1 that facilitate ligand-independent activation of the chicken progesterone receptor and are critical for functional cooperation between SRC-1 and CREB binding protein [In Process Citation]. Mol.Cell Biol., 20(23), 8720-8730.

Rowan,B.G., Weigel,N.L., & O'Malley,B.W. (2000). Phosphorylation of steroid receptor coactivator-1. Identification of the phosphorylation sites and phosphorylation through the mitogen- activated protein kinase pathway. J.Biol.Chem., 275(6), 4475-4483.

Ruizeveld de Winter,J.A., Janssen,P.J., Sleddens,H.M., Verleun-Mooijman,M.C., Trapman,J., Brinkmann,A.O., Santerse,A.B., Schroder,F.H., & van der Kwast,T.H. (1994). Androgen receptor status in localized and locally progressive hormone refractory human prostate cancer. Am.J.Pathol., 144(4), 735-746.

Sadar,M.D. (1999). Androgen-independent induction of prostate-specific antigen gene expression via cross-talk between the androgen receptor and protein kinase A signal transduction pathways. J.Biol.Chem., 274(12), 7777-7783.

Sande,S., & Privalsky,M.L. (1996). Identification of TRACs (T3 receptor-associating cofactors), a family of cofactors that associate with, and modulate the activity of, nuclear hormone receptors. Mol.Endocrinol., 10(7), 813-825.

Sartorius,C.A., Tung,L., Takimoto,G.S., & Horwitz,K.B. (1993). Antagonist-occupied human progesterone receptors bound to DNA are functionally switched to transcriptional agonists by cAMP. J.Biol.Chem., 268(13), 9262-9266.

Schlegel,A., Wang,C., Katzenellenbogen,B.S., Pestell,R.G., & Lisanti,M.P. (1999). Caveolin-1 potentiates estrogen receptor alpha (ERalpha) signaling. caveolin-1 drives ligand-independent nuclear translocation and activation of ERalpha. J.Biol.Chem., 274(47), 33551-33556.

Schoenberg,M.P., Hakimi,J.M., Wang,S., Bova,G.S., Epstein,J.I., Fischbeck,K.H., Isaacs,W.B., Walsh,P.C., & Barrack,E.R. (1994). Microsatellite mutation (CAG24-->18) in the androgen receptor gene in human prostate cancer. Biochem.Biophys.Res.Commun., 198(1), 74-80.

Schule,R., Rangarajan,P., Kliewer,S., Ransone,L.J., Bolado,J., Yang,N., Verma,I.M., & Evans,R.M. (1990). Functional antagonism between oncoprotein c-Jun and the glucocorticoid receptor. Cell, 62(6), 1217-1226.

Seol,W., Mahon,M.J., Lee,Y.K., & Moore,D.D. (1996). Two receptor interacting domains in the nuclear hormone receptor corepressor RIP13/N-CoR. Mol.Endocrinol., 10(12), 1646-1655.

Shang,Y., Hu,X., DiRenzo,J., Lazar,M.A., & Brown,M. (2000). Cofactor dynamics and sufficiency in estrogen receptor-regulated transcription. Cell, 103(6), 843-852.

Shen,T., Horwitz,K.B., & Lange,C.A. (2001). Transcriptional hyperactivity of human progesterone receptors is coupled to their ligand-dependent down-regulation by mitogen-activated protein kinase-dependent phosphorylation of serine 294. Mol.Cell Biol., 21(18), 6122-6131.

Shi,Y., Downes,M., Xie,W., Kao,H.Y., Ordentlich,P., Tsai,C.C., Hon,M., & Evans,R.M. (2001). Sharp, an inducible cofactor that integrates nuclear receptor repression and activation. Genes Dev., 15 (9), 1140-1151.

Shiau,A.K., Barstad,D., Loria,P.M., Cheng,L., Kushner,P.J., Agard,D.A., & Greene,G.L. (1998). The structural basis of estrogen receptor/coactivator recognition and the antagonism of this interaction by tamoxifen. Cell, 95(7), 927-937.

Signoretti,S., Montironi,R., Manola,J., Altimari,A., Tam,C., Bubley,G., Balk,S., Thomas,G., Kaplan,I., Hlatky,L., Hahnfeldt,P., Kantoff,P., & Loda,M. (2000). Her-2-neu expression and progression toward androgen independence in human prostate cancer. J.Natl.Cancer Inst., 92(23), 1918-1925.

Simoncini,T., Hafezi-Moghadam,A., Brazil,D.P., Ley,K., Chin,W.W., & Liao,J.K. (2000). Interaction of oestrogen receptor with the regulatory subunit of phosphatidylinositol-3-OH kinase [In Process Citation]. Nature, 407(6803), 538-541.

Singh,M., Setalo,G., Jr., Guan,X., Frail,D.E., & Toran-Allerand,C.D. (2000). Estrogen-induced activation of the mitogen-activated protein kinase cascade in the cerebral cortex of estrogen receptor-alpha knock-out mice. J.Neurosci., 20(5), 1694-1700.

Smith,E.P., Boyd,J., Frank,G.R., Takahashi,H., Cohen,R.M., Specker,B., Williams,T.C., Lubahn,D.B., & Korach,K.S. (1994). Estrogen resistance caused by a mutation in the estrogen-receptor gene in a man. N.Engl.J.Med., 331(16), 1056-1061.

Sommer,S., & Fuqua,S.A. (2001). Estrogen receptor and breast cancer. Semin.Cancer Biol., 11(5), 339-352.

Song,R.X., McPherson,R.A., Adam,L., Bao,Y., Shupnik,M., Kumar,R., & Santen,R.J. (2002). Linkage of Rapid Estrogen Action to MAPK Activation by ERalpha-Shc Association and Shc Pathway Activation. Mol.Endocrinol., 16(1), 116-127.

Stanbrough,M., Leav,I., Kwan,P.W., Bubley,G.J., & Balk,S.P. (2001). Prostatic intraepithelial neoplasia in mice expressing an androgen receptor transgene in prostate epithelium. Proc.Natl.Acad.Sci.U.S.A, 98(19), 10823-10828.

Stanford,J.L., Just,J.J., Gibbs,M., Wicklund,K.G., Neal,C.L., Blumenstein,B.A., & Ostrander,E.A. (1997). Polymorphic repeats in the androgen receptor gene: molecular markers of prostate cancer risk [see comments]. Cancer Res., 57(6), 1194-1198.

Sweat,S.D., Pacelli,A., Bergstralh,E.J., Slezak,J.M., & Bostwick,D.G. (1999). Androgen receptor expression in prostatic intraepithelial neoplasia and cancer. J.Urol., 161(4), 1229-1232.

Taplin,M.E., Bubley,G.J., Ko,Y.J., Small,E.J., Upton,M., Rajeshkumar,B., & Balk,S.P. (1999). Selection for androgen receptor mutations in prostate cancers treated with androgen antagonist. Cancer Res., 59(11), 2511-2515.

Taplin,M.E., Bubley,G.J., Shuster,T.D., Frantz,M.E., Spooner,A.E., Ogata,G.K., Keer,H.N., & Balk,S.P. (1995). Mutation of the androgen-receptor gene in metastatic androgen- independent prostate cancer. N.Engl.J.Med., 332(21), 1393-1398.

Tilley,W.D., Buchanan,G., Hickey,T.E., & Bentel,J.M. (1996). Mutations in the androgen receptor gene are associated with progression of human prostate cancer to androgen independence. Clin.Cancer Res., 2(2), 277-285.

Tora,L., White,J., Brou,C., Tasset,D., Webster,N., Scheer,E., & Chambon,P (1989). The human estrogen receptor has two independent nonacidic transcriptional activation functions. Cell, 59(3), 477-487.

Torchia,J., Rose,D.W., Inostroza,J., Kamei,Y., Westin,S., Glass,C.K., & Rosenfeld,M.G. (1997). The transcriptional co-activator p/CIP binds CBP and mediates nuclear- receptor function [see comments]. Nature, 387(6634), 677-684.

Tremblay,A., Tremblay,G.B., Labrie,F., & Giguere,V. (1999). Ligand-independent recruitment of SRC-1 to estrogen receptor beta through phosphorylation of activation function AF-1. Mol.Cell, 3(4), 513-519.

Truica,C.I., Byers,S., & Gelmann,E.P. (2000). Beta-catenin affects androgen receptor transcriptional activity and ligand specificity. Cancer Res., 60(17), 4709-4713.

Tsai,M.J., & O'Malley,B.W. (1994). Molecular mechanisms of action of steroid/thyroid receptor superfamily members. Annu.Rev.Biochem., 63, 451-486.

van der Kwast,T.H., Schalken,J., Ruizeveld de Winter,J.A., van Vroonhoven,C.C., Mulder,E., Boersma,W., & Trapman,J. (1991). Androgen receptors in endocrine-therapy-resistant human prostate cancer. Int.J.Cancer, 48(2), 189-193.

Visakorpi,T., Hyytinen,E., Koivisto,P., Tanner,M., Keinanen,R., Palmberg,C., Palotie,A., Tammela,T., Isola,J., & Kallioniemi,O.P. (1995). In vivo amplification of the androgen receptor gene and progression of human prostate cancer. Nat.Genet., 9(4), 401-406.

Voegel,J.J., Heine,M.J., Zechel,C., Chambon,P., & Gronemeyer,H. (1996). TIF2, a 160 kDa transcriptional mediator for the ligand-dependent activation function AF-2 of nuclear receptors. EMBO J., 15(14), 3667-3675.

Voeller,H.J., Truica,C.I., & Gelmann,E.P. (1998). Beta-catenin mutations in human prostate cancer. Cancer Res., 58(12), 2520-2523.

Wagner,R.L., Apriletti,J.W., McGrath,M.E., West,B.L., Baxter,J.D., & Fletterick,R.J. (1995). A structural role for hormone in the thyroid hormone receptor. Nature, 378(6558), 690-697.

Wang,C., Fu,M., Angeletti,R.H., Siconolfi-Baez,L., Reutens,A.T., Albanese,C., Lisanti,M.P., Katzenellenbogen,B.S., Kato,S., Hopp,T., Fuqua,S.A., Lopez,G.N., Kushner,P.J., & Pestell,R.G. (2001). Direct acetylation of the estrogen receptor alpha hinge region by p300 regulates transactivation and hormone sensitivity. J.Biol.Chem., 276(21), 18375-18383.

Watanabe,M., Yanagisawa,J., Kitagawa,H., Takeyama,K., Ogawa,S., Arao,Y., Suzawa,M., Kobayashi,Y., Yano,T., Yoshikawa,H., Masuhiro,Y., & Kato,S. (2001a). A subfamily of RNA-binding DEAD-box proteins acts as an estrogen receptor alpha coactivator through the N-terminal activation domain (AF- 1) with an RNA coactivator, SRA. EMBO J., 20(6), 1341-1352.

Watanabe,M., Yanagisawa,J., Kitagawa,H., Takeyama,K., Ogawa,S., Arao,Y., Suzawa,M., Kobayashi,Y., Yano,T., Yoshikawa,H., Masuhiro,Y., & Kato,S. (2001b). A subfamily of RNA-binding DEAD-box proteins acts as an estrogen receptor alpha coactivator through the N-terminal activation domain (AF- 1) with an RNA coactivator, SRA. EMBO J., 20(6), 1341-1352.

Webb,P., Lopez,G.N., Uht,R.M., & Kushner,P.J. (1995). Tamoxifen activation of the estrogen receptor/AP-1 pathway: potential origin for the cell-specific estrogen-like effects of antiestrogens. Mol.Endocrinol., 9(4), 443-456.

Webb,P., Nguyen,P., Shinsako,J., Anderson,C., Feng,W., Nguyen,M.P., Chen,D., Huang,S.M., Subramanian,S., McKinerney,E., Katzenellenbogen,B.S., Stallcup,M.R., & Kushner,P.J. (1998). Estrogen receptor activation function 1 works by binding p160 coactivator proteins. Mol.Endocrinol., 12(10), 1605-1618.

Webb,P., Nguyen,P., Valentine,C., Lopez,G.N., Kwok,G.R., McInerney,E., Katzenellenbogen,B.S., Enmark,E., Gustafsson,J.A., Nilsson,S., & Kushner,P.J. (1999). The estrogen receptor enhances AP-1 activity by two distinct mechanisms with different requirements for receptor transactivation functions. Mol.Endocrinol., 13(10), 1672-1685.

Wei,L.N., Hu,X., Chandra,D., Seto,E., & Farooqui,M. (2000). Receptor-interacting protein 140 directly recruits histone deacetylases for gene silencing. J.Biol.Chem., 275(52), 40782-40787.

Weis,K.E., Ekena,K., Thomas,J.A., Lazennec,G., & Katzenellenbogen,B.S. (1996). Constitutively active human estrogen receptors containing amino acid substitutions for tyrosine 537 in the receptor protein. *Mol.Endocrinol., 10*(11), 1388-1398.

Whang,Y.E., Wu,X., Suzuki,H., Reiter,R.E., Tran,C., Vessella,R.L., Said,J.W., Isaacs,W.B., & Sawyers,C.L. (1998). Inactivation of the tumor suppressor PTEN/MMAC1 in advanced human prostate cancer through loss of expression. *Proc.Natl.Acad.Sci.U.S.A, 95*(9), 5246-5250.

Wiesen,J.F., Young,P., Werb,Z., & Cunha,G.R. (1999). Signaling through the stromal epidermal growth factor receptor is necessary for mammary ductal development. *Development, 126*(2), 335-344.

Wong,C.I., Zhou,Z.X., Sar,M., & Wilson,E.M. (1993). Steroid requirement for androgen receptor dimerization and DNA binding. Modulation by intramolecular interactions between the NH2-terminal and steroid-binding domains. *J.Biol.Chem., 268*(25), 19004-19012.

Wurtz,J.M., Bourguet,W., Renaud,J.P., Vivat,V., Chambon,P., Moras,D., & Gronemeyer,H. (1996). A canonical structure for the ligand-binding domain of nuclear receptors. *Nat.Struct.Biol., 3*(1), 87-94.

Xu,J., Liao,L., Ning,G., Yoshida-Komiya,H., Deng,C., & O'Malley,B.W. (2000). The steroid receptor coactivator SRC-3 (p/CIP/RAC3/AIB1/ACTR/TRAM-1) is required for normal growth, puberty, female reproductive function, and mammary gland development. *Proc.Natl.Acad.Sci.U.S.A,*

Xu,J., Qiu,Y., DeMayo,F.J., Tsai,S.Y., Tsai,M.J., & O'Malley,B.W. (1998). Partial hormone resistance in mice with disruption of the steroid receptor coactivator-1 (SRC-1) gene. *Science, 279*(5358), 1922-1925.

Yan,G., Fukabori,Y., Nikolaropoulos,S., Wang,F., & McKeehan,W.L. (1992). Heparin-binding keratinocyte growth factor is a candidate stromal-to- epithelial-cell andromedin. *Mol.Endocrinol., 6*(12), 2123-2128.

Yang-Yen,H.F., Chambard,J.C., Sun,Y.L., Smeal,T., Schmidt,T.J., Drouin,J., & Karin,M. (1990). Transcriptional interference between c-Jun and the glucocorticoid receptor: mutual inhibition of DNA binding due to direct protein- protein interaction. *Cell, 62*(6), 1205-1215.

Yeh,S., Lin,H.K., Kang,H.Y., Thin,T.H., Lin,M.F., & Chang,C. (1999). From HER2/Neu signal cascade to androgen receptor and its coactivators: a novel pathway by induction of androgen target genes through MAP kinase in prostate cancer cells. *Proc.Natl.Acad.Sci.U.S.A, 96*(10), 5458-5463.

Yoshinaga,S.K., Peterson,C.L., Herskowitz,I., & Yamamoto,K.R. (1992). Roles of SWI1, SWI2, and SWI3 proteins for transcriptional enhancement by steroid receptors. *Science, 258*(5088), 1598-1604.

Yu,X., Li,P., Roeder,R.G., & Wang,Z. (2001). Inhibition of androgen receptor-mediated transcription by amino- terminal enhancer of split. *Mol.Cell Biol., 21*(14), 4614-4625.

Yuan,C.X., Ito,M., Fondell,J.D., Fu,Z.Y., & Roeder,R.G. (1998). The TRAP220 component of a thyroid hormone rece. *Proc.Natl.Acad.Sci.U.S.A, 95*(14), 7939-7944.

Yuan,X., Lu,M.L., Li,T., & Balk,S.P. (2001). SRY interacts with and negatively regulates androgen receptor transcriptional activity. *J.Biol.Chem.,*

Zhang,H., Thomsen,J.S., Johansson,L., Gustafsson,J.A., & Treuter,E. (2000). DAX-1 functions as an LXXLL-containing corepressor for activated estrogen receptors. *J.Biol.Chem., 275*(51), 39855-39859.

Zhang,Q.X., Borg,A., Wolf,D.M., Oesterreich,S., & Fuqua,S.A. (1997). An estrogen receptor mutant with strong hormone-independent activity from a metastatic breast cancer. *Cancer Res., 57*(7), 1244-1249.

Zhou,Z.X., Kemppainen,J.A., & Wilson,E.M. (1995). Identification of three proline-directed phosphorylation sites in the human androgen receptor. *Mol.Endocrinol., 9*(5), 605-615.

Zhou,Z.X., Lane,M.V., Kemppainen,J.A., French,F.S., & Wilson,E.M. (1995). Specificity of ligand-dependent androgen receptor stabilization: receptor domain interactions influence ligand dissociation and receptor stability. *Mol.Endocrinol., 9*(2), 208-218.

Zhu,Y., Qi,C., Jain,S., Le Beau,M.M., Espinosa,R., III, Atkins,G.B., Lazar,M.A., Yeldandi,A.V., Rao,M.S., & Reddy,J.K. (1999). Amplification and overexpression of peroxisome proliferator-activated receptor binding protein (PBP/PPARBP) gene in breast cancer. *Proc.Natl.Acad.Sci.U.S.A, 96*(19), 10848-10853.

Zhu,Y., Qi,C., Jain,S., Rao,M.S., & Reddy,J.K. (1997). Isolation and characterization of PBP, a protein that interacts with peroxisome proliferator-activated receptor. *J.Biol.Chem., 272*(41), 25500-25506.

Zilliacus,J., Wright,A.P., Carlstedt-Duke,J., & Gustafsson,J.A. (1995). Structural determinants of DNA-binding specificity by steroid receptors. *Mol.Endocrinol., 9*(4), 389-400.

Zwijsen,R.M., Wientjens,E., Klompmaker,R., van der,S.J., Bernards,R., & Michalides,R.J. (1997). CDK-independent activation of estrogen receptor by cyclin D1. *Cell, 88*(3), 405-415.

CELL DEATH SIGNALING IN MALIGNANCY

TIMOTHY F. BURNS AND WAFIK S. EL-DEIRY

1. INTRODUCTION

Research over the last several decades has established that tumor formation is a clonal multi-step process in which a single normal cell develops into a malignant transformed lesion. This process requires multiple genomic alterations in several key signaling pathways, which control proliferation, apoptosis, metastasis, and angiogenesis. Although in the majority of tumor types it is unclear which exact loci are targeted in a particular tumor, it is clear that several key signaling pathways are always targeted. Disruptions of these key pathways allow for uncontrolled growth and spread of a local lesion throughout the body. Despite the differences in cell origin and morphology, it is becoming clear that all tumors share several essential characteristics that are necessary for malignancy. Hanahan and Weinberg proposed six "Hallmarks of Cancer" that are required in tumorigenesis: growth factor independence, resistance to anti-proliferative signals, protection from apoptosis, unlimited replicative potential, angiogenic potential and invasive/metastatic capabilities (Hanahan & Weinberg, 2000). In this chapter we will examine the role of apoptosis in tumor suppression and therapy and explore current work on various therapies to overcome resistance to apoptosis found in neoplasia.

Apoptosis is a normal cellular process by which multi-cellular organisms eliminate their damage or excess cells during their development and lifetime to maintain tissue homeostasis. Apoptosis is characterized by distinct morphological changes in the cell notably, chromatin condensation, DNA fragmentation, cytoskeletal and nuclear disassembly and cell blebbing. When the normal regulation of this process is disrupted human disease is often the result. Excessive cell death has been implicated in several neurological disorders while reduced cell death leads to malignancy. The concept that tumor progression requires not only uncontrolled proliferation but inhibition of apoptosis was first elucidated in work showing that in follicular B-cell lymphoma, the Bcl-2 gene was fused to the immunoglobulin heavy chain in translocation t(14; 18) (Tsujimoto, Cossman, Jaffe, & Croce, 1985; Vaux, Cory, & Adams, 1988). Since then many studies have demonstrated an absolute requirement for disruption of the apoptotic signaling pathways normally employed by cells to prevent uncontrolled growth. Furthermore the inhibition of apoptosis is essential for many of the other hallmarks of cancer.

2. APOPTOTIC STIMULI DURING TUMORIGENESIS

For a single normal cell to progress to a malignant neoplasm it must survive several critical junctures in which the apoptotic program would normally delete the aberrantly proliferating cell (Figure 1). In order to get a quiescent cell to enter the cell cycle and divide, oncogenes such as c-myc are upregulated to allow cell cycle progression. However, the upregulation of c-myc is a double-edged sword as increased c-myc expression alone results in both proliferation and apoptosis in normal fibroblasts especially in low serum situations (Evan & Vousden, 2001). Furthermore transgenic c-myc models have also demonstrated that c-myc expression results in tumor formation after a long latency period. However, when the cell death was inhibited by overexpression of bcl-2, inhibition of caspase 9 or deletion of p53, c-myc tumor progression was greatly accelerated (Schmitt, 2002). Similar findings have been observed for E2F-1 in central nervous system models of tumor development (Pan et al., 1998).

Abnormally proliferating cells are also in a growth factor deficient environment. Normally, these cells would senesce or die by neglect. In order to survive this environment, there is a strong selection pressure to inhibit cell death. To solve this problem tumors evolve several mechanisms to supply their own growth factors or to inhibit cell death. Several tumor types develop constitutively active growth factor receptors, increase the activity of serine threonine kinase Akt/PKB or directly inhibit the downstream apoptotic cascade by overexpressing the anti-apoptotic molecule, Bcl-2 (Hanahan & Weinberg, 2000). Furthermore, developing tumors must also contend with a hypoxic environment which leads to apoptosis. To overcome this potential roadblock, upregulation of anti-apoptotic genes such IAP2 or inactivation of p53 are often selected for in hypoxic regions of tumors (Harris, 2002).

For a carcinoma in situ to invade and metastasize it must not only develop mechanisms to detach from neighboring cells and from the extracellular matrix, but must also overcome the apoptosis or "anoikis" that normally occurs when cells lose their attachment. Upregulation of some integrin subtypes can provide the necessary survival signals allowing cells to survive detachment. Furthermore, loss of p53 expression or upregulation of Akt/PKB can also provide a protective effect against cell death (Harris, 2002). Finally for a tumor to grow it must overcome the immune surveillance carried out in part by cytotoxic T cells and Natural Killer cells which can induce apoptosis through use of the death receptor or extrinsic apoptotic pathway (Rosen et al., 2000; Takeda et al., 2001). Tumor cells have devised a variety of mechanisms including expressing death ligands to kill invading T lymphocytes (Krammer, 2000). In summary, inhibition of the cell death pathway is required at several steps during the development of a malignant lesion. As shown by some the examples given above many of the same inhibitors and mediators are selected for and against in response to each of these cellular and environmental

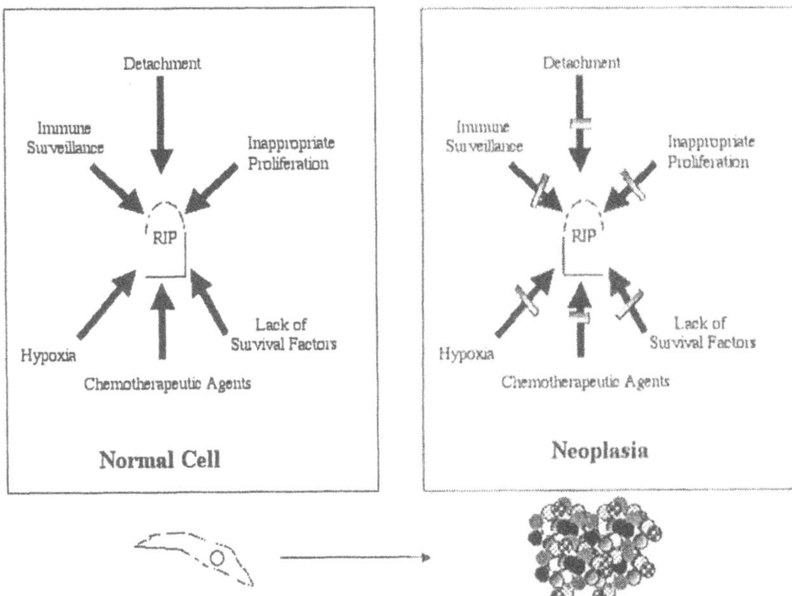

Figure 1: Inactivation of the Apoptotic Response to Cellular and Extracellular Stimuli During Tumorigenesis: For a normal cell to progress to a malignant neoplasm it must survive several critical junctures in which the apoptotic program would normally delete the aberrantly proliferating cell. For transformation to occur, a cell must proliferate and avoid the inherent apoptotic response that is activated during proliferation. Furthermore, it must avoid death by neglect when it begins to proliferate in the absence of growth/survival factors. Developing tumors must also contend with a hypoxic environment that leads to apoptosis. For a carcinoma in situ to invade and metastasize it must not only develop mechanisms to detach from neighboring cells and from the extracellular matrix, but must also overcome the apoptosis or "anoikis" that normally occurs when cells lose attachment. Finally for a tumor to grow it must overcome the immune surveillance carried out in part by cytotoxic T cells and Natural Killer cells which can induce apoptosis through use of the death receptor or extrinsic apoptotic pathway. All of these roads to death must be disrupted or circumvented for tumor formation to occur. After establishment, the neoplasm must overcome the DNA damage induced apoptotic response after treatment with chemotherapeutic agents (See Text for Details).

stresses. Below we will examine the apoptotic signaling pathways which when present eliminate these aberrantly dividing cells thus preventing tumor formation.

3. MAJOR APOPTOTIC SIGNALING PATHWAYS IN CANCER: THE EXTRINSIC AND INTRINSIC PATHWAYS

In response to a variety of environmental and cellular stresses, damaged or abnormal cells are eliminated through programmed cell death or apoptosis. Two major apoptotic pathways have been delineated and both are utilized depending on the stimulus (Hengartner, 2000). The first pathway is known as the death receptor pathway or extrinsic pathway. Binding of an extracellular death ligand to its cell surface results in downstream activation of cysteine aspartate-specific proteases or caspases. The second pathway is known as the intrinsic or mitochondrial pathway. In response to variety of apoptotic stimuli such serum starvation, hypoxia, and DNA damage, members of the Bcl-2 family translocate to the mitochondria resulting in the release of pro-apoptotic factors such cytochrome c, AIF, Smac/DIABLO and subsequent activation of caspases (Figure 2). Although these pathways are presented as distinct signaling cascades they are in fact interconnected and some stimuli which result in activation of the intrinsic pathway (DNA damage) also influence the extrinsic pathway.

The extrinsic pathway plays a key role in tumor immune surviellance and disruption of this pathway results in autoimmune disorders and increased spontaneous and carcinogen-induced tumorigenesis (Cretney et al., 2002; Krammer, 2000; Takeda et al., 2002) Furthermore the extrinsic pathway is involved in mediating c-myc induced apoptosis after serum starvation (Hueber et al., 1997). DNA damage induced apoptosis may also be partially mediated through the extrinsic pathway since several death receptors are p53 target genes that are induced after DNA damage (Vogelstein, Lane, & Levine, 2000). However its role in the DNA damage apoptotic pathway may also be mediated through its link to the intrinsic pathway.

The extrinsic pathway is initiated by members of Tumor Necrosis Factor (TNF) superfamily. Members of the TNF superfamily are type II membrane proteins with conserved C-terminal extracellular domains responsible for trimer formation (Locksley, Killeen, & Lenardo, 2001). Several members of this family (TNF-α, FasL, TRAIL/Apo-2L) have been shown to induce apoptosis through binding of their respective receptors. FasL/CD95 and TRAIL induce apoptosis through binding their respective pro-apoptotic receptors, Fas/APO1 and DR4 (TRAIL-R1) and KILLER/DR5 (TRAIL-R2, TRICK2) respectively. Ligation of FasL or TRAIL to its receptors results in trimerization of the receptors and clustering of the receptor's intracellular death domains (DD) leading to the formation of a death inducing signaling complex (DISC). Trimerization of the death domains leads to the recruitment of an adaptor molecule, FADD and subsequent binding and activation of caspase 8 and caspase 10. Activated caspase 8 and caspase10 then cleave caspase 3 which then leads to cleavage of death substrates (Ashkenazi & Dixit, 1999). Caspase 8 has also been shown to cleave the pro-apoptotic bcl-2 family member, Bid which leads to the activation of intrinsic or mitochondrial pathway (Li, Zhu, Xu, & Yuan, 1998). Cells can be classified by their response to death ligands as either Type I or Type II cells. In Type I cells, activation of caspase 8 at the level of the DISC (Death Inducing Signaling Complex) is sufficient to activate caspase 3 and induce death independent of the intrinsic or mitochondrial pathway. Therefore overexpression of the anti-apoptotic members of the Bcl-2 family does not inhibit death induced by TRAIL or Fas ligand (CD95L) in Type I cells. In Type II cells, activation of caspase 8 at the level of the DISC is insufficient to induce death and requires amplification of the apoptotic signal through cleavage of bid and activation of the mitochondrial apoptotic pathway (Krammer, 2000). Previous studies in cell lines and in vivo have demonstrated the existence of Type I and Type II cell lines in response to Fas ligand (CD95L) and TRAIL (Burns & El-Deiry, 2001; Hinz et al., 2000; Lacronique et al., 1996; Ozoren, Kim et al., 2000; Scaffidi et al., 1998; Strasser, Harris, Huang, Krammer, & Cory, 1995).

The extrinsic pathway is regulated at several levels. At the level of the membrane, the FasL signaling pathway is modulated by two soluble anti-apoptotic receptors, sCD95 and DcR3 which bind FasL/CD95, therefore preventing it from binding to Fas/APO1(Cheng et al., 1994; Pitti et al., 1998). Similarly, the TRAIL signaling pathway is modulated by two anti-apoptotic TRAIL decoy receptors, TRID (DcR1, TRAIL-R3) and TRUNDD (DcR2, TRAIL-R4) (Pan et al., 1997). TRID and TRUNDD do not contain functional death domains and act as extracellular competitors for TRAIL, therefore preventing the binding of TRAIL to DR4 or KILLER/DR5. TRUNDD, which contains a partial death domain, may also transduce anti-apoptotic effects possibly through the NF-κB pathway or other pro-survival pathways (Degli-Esposti et al., 1997; Meng, McDonald, Sheikh, Fornace, & El-Deiry, 2000).

Signaling at the level of the DISC can be inhibited by the cellular FLICE Inhibitory Protein (c-FLIP) (also cloned as Casper, I-FLICE, FLAME-1, CASH, CLARP, MRIT) (Thome et al., 1997). c-FLIP is highly homologous to caspase 8 and 10 and contains a death effector domain (DED) that allows it to interact with FADD and inhibit the binding of caspase 8 and 10. In Type II cells, in which the mitochondrial pathway is required for efficient killing, overexpression of the anti-apoptotic Bcl-2 family members, Bcl-2 and Bcl-X_L or loss of the pro-apoptotic Bcl-2 family members, Bak and Bax have been shown inhibit cell killing (Burns & El-Deiry, 2001; Lindsten et al., 2000; Scaffidi et al., 1998). As indicated by the examples above it clear that the extrinsic pathway is coupled to the intrinsic one and some cases requires this pathway.

The intrinsic or mitochondrial pathway plays an essential role in mediating apoptosis in response to DNA damage, oncogenic stimulation and serum starvation. Knockout and transgenic models have established that key components of the intrinsic pathway are required for DNA damage and c-myc induced apoptosis in several tissue and cell types (Wang, 2001). Furthermore several lines of evidence have suggested that the mitochondrial pathway is required for p53-dependent apoptosis and tumor suppression. Studies using the caspase 9 -/- animals have shown that caspase 9 is required for gamma-irradiation induced p53-dependent apoptosis in the spleen and thymus (Hakem et al., 1998). Furthermore, both Apaf-1 and caspase 9 were shown to be required for p53-dependent apoptosis after oncogene overexpression in mouse embryonic fibroblasts and inhibition of Caspase 9 or overexpression of Bcl-2 can substitute for p53 deficiency in vivo (Schmitt, 2002; Soengas et al., 1999).

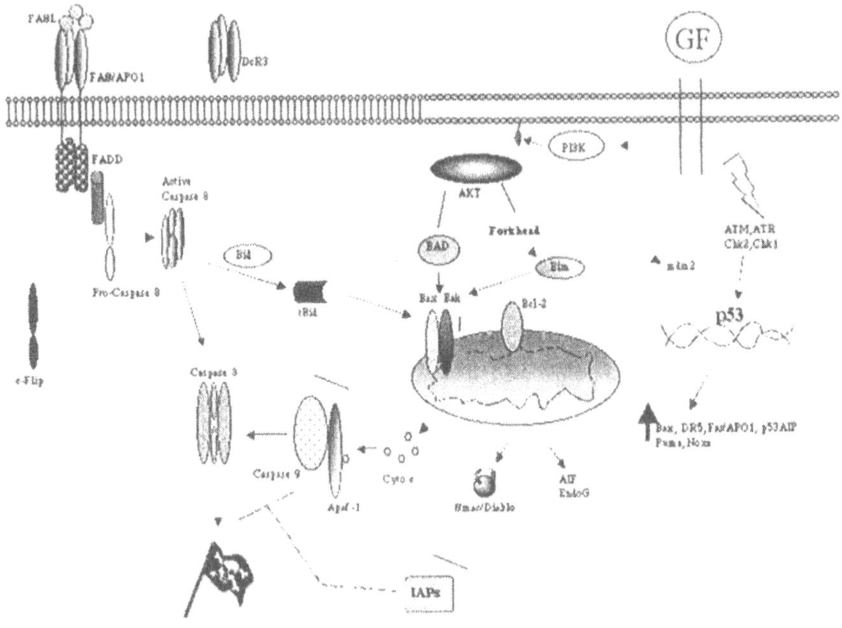

Figure 2: Two Apoptotic Pathways in Cancer: Two major apoptotic pathways have been delineated and both are utilized depending on the stimulus. The first pathway is known as the death receptor pathway or extrinsic pathway. Binding of an extracellular death ligand to its cell surface results in downstream activation of cysteine aspartate-specific proteases or caspases. This pathway can directly induce death through activation of caspase 3 or through activation of the intrinsic pathway through cleavage of Bid. This pathway can be inhibited at the membrane by both membrane bound and soluble Decoy receptors (DcR3). This pathway can also be inhibited at the DISC by c-Flip. The second pathway is known as the intrinsic or mitochondrial pathway. In response to variety of apoptotic stimuli such serum starvation, hypoxia, and DNA damage, members of the Bcl-2 family translocate to the mitochondria resulting in the release of pro-apoptotic factors such cytochrome c, AIF, Smac/DIABLO and subsequent activation of caspases. The release of cytochrome c results in activation of Apaf-1 and subsequent activation of caspase 9. Activated caspase 9 activates caspase 3 resulting in cleavage of death substrates followed by cell death. Upon release, Smac/DIABLO binds and inhibits IAPs further increasing caspase activity. AIF and EndoG can cause a caspase-independent death. Members of the Anti-apoptotic members of the Bcl-2 family can inhibit this pathway at the level of mitochondria. These pathways can be modulated by pro-apoptotic regulators such as p53 and the Forkhead and pro-survival factors such Akt/PKB.

Members of the Bcl-2 family of proteins control activation of the intrinsic pathway. All family members contain at least one of four Bcl-2 homology domains (BH1-4). Initiation of this pathway begins when a pro-apoptotic Bcl-2 family member is activated or upregulated and translocates to the mitochondria. In general these translocating pro-apoptotic Bcl-2 family members contain only a BH3 domain and are known as BH3-only proteins (Wang, 2001). Bid, a BH3-only protein, is cleaved by caspase 8 which results in its activation and translocation (Li et al., 1998). Bad is a BH3 only family member, whose localization is controlled by phosphorylation. In response to survival signals Bad is phosphorylated by Akt/PKB and sequestered in the cytoplasm by 14-3-3 proteins (Datta et al., 1997; del Peso, Gonzalez-Garcia, Page, Herrera, & Nunez, 1997). Bim is associated with microtubules and is released upon apoptotic stimuli (Puthalakath, Huang, O'Reilly, King, & Strasser, 1999). After translocation of these BH3-only proteins to the mitochondria, they bind to two pro-apoptotic Bcl-2 family members, bax and bak. Interaction between the BH3-only proteins and Bax/Bak results in a conformational change and oligomerization of Bax and Bak. Formation of Bax/Bak mitochondrial pores then directly or indirectly lead to the release of apoptotic factors. The exact mechanism by which the pro-apoptotic members of the Bcl-2 family release apoptotic factors is still an area of active research and debate. The net result is the release of cytochrome c, ATP, Smac/Diablo, Apoptosis-inducing factor (AIF), and endonuclease G. This pathway can be inhibited by the anti-apoptotic members of the Bcl-2 family, such as Bcl-2 and Bcl-X_L which prevent Bax and Bak oligomerization (Wang, 2001).

Release of apoptotic factors induces cell death through several mechanisms. After cytochrome c and ATP are released, they bind and oligomerize the CED4 homolog, Apaf-1. The initiator caspase, caspase 9 is then recruited to this complex and is activated. The apoptosome is then able to cleave caspase 3 resulting in the activation of caspase 3, caspase 7, and caspase 6 and cleavage of intracellular death substrates. Mouse knockout studies have demonstrated a key role for Apaf-1 and caspase 9 in mediating DNA damage cell death response, however, several studies have shown that other mitochondria-dependent Apaf-1/caspase 9 independent apoptotic pathways exist in some cell types and in response to some apoptotic stimuli (Johnstone, Ruefli, & Lowe, 2002). Smac/Diablo is released along with cytochrome c, and binds and inhibits an important class of anti-apoptotic proteins know as IAPs (Inhibitors of Apoptosis Proteins) (Du, Fang, Li, Li, & Wang, 2000; Verhagen et al., 2000). All IAPs contain a BIR (Baculovirus IAP repeat) domain that is required for their ability to inhibit apoptosis. IAPs have been shown to bind and inhibit caspase 3, caspase7 and caspase 9. IAPs are conserved throughout evolution and there are several human family members that have been implicated in suppression of apoptosis and tumorigenesis(Deveraux & Reed, 1999). The N-terminus of Smac/Diablo is able to bind to the BIR domain of IAPs preventing their binding to caspases. This inhibition of IAPs is significant since IAPs have been demonstrated to not only block the intrinsic pathway but may also protect against FasL and TRAIL signaling through the extrinsic pathway (Verhagen, Coulson, & Vaux, 2001).

Less is known about the mechanism by which AIF mediates cell death. Upon release, AIF apparently translocates to the nucleus where it is believed to mediate chromatin condensation and large scale DNA fragmentation through an unclear mechanism (Susin et al., 1999). AIF -/- mice die at an early embryonic age with defects in cavitation resulting from defective apoptosis. Furthermore, the AIF -/- ES cells have defective serum starvation induced death (Joza et al., 2001). Endonuclease G is released from the mitochondria and is able to induce nucleosomal DNA fragmentation (Li, Luo, & Wang, 2001). AIF and Endonuclease G do not require cleavage by caspases and may partially explain the caspase-independent cell death that is observed in some cases.

4. MAJOR UPSTREAM MODULATORS OF THE APOPTOTIC SIGNALING PATHWAYS

Activation of cell death is a tightly regulated process that is positively and negatively controlled by many parallel and converging signaling pathways. Many studies have demonstrated that loss or disruption of positive modulators of apoptosis is essential to tumor development. Conversely inappropriate expression or increased activity of negative modulators of apoptosis occurs frequently in most tumor types.

One of the most critical positive regulatory pathways for apoptosis is the p53 signaling pathway. Mutation or loss of p53 has been observed in over 50 % of all tumors and almost every tumor type (Hollstein, Sidransky, Vogelstein, & Harris, 1991). Furthermore, it has been estimated the p53 pathway is disrupted by mutation or inhibition of its function in the vast majority of tumors (Vogelstein & Kinzler, 1992). Hereditary loss of p53 results in Li-Fraumeni syndrome which is characterized by a greater than 50% incidence of neoplasia by the age of thirty (Malkin et al., 1990). Although animals in which the p53 locus has been deleted develop normally, 75 % of the p53-null animals develop tumors by six months of age and all the p53-null animals develop tumors and die by ten months of age (Donehower et al., 1992). Loss of p53 or disruption of the p53 pathway is clearly a critical step in carcinogenesis.

p53 mediates many of its key functions through the transactivation of its target genes. Although p53 can in some situations induce apoptosis in the absence of transactivation (Haupt, Barak, & Oren, 1996; Haupt, Rowan, Shaulian, Vousden, & Oren, 1995) or de novo mRNA or protein synthesis(Caelles, Helmberg, & Karin, 1994), most tumor-derived mutants of p53 are defective in DNA binding and transactivation supporting a critical role for transactivation in p53's ability to suppress neoplasia. p53 has been shown to signal death through both the extrinsic and intrinsic and both pathways may be required for mediating p53-dependent apoptosis depending on the stimulus and tissue type (Burns, Bernhard, & El-Deiry, 2001). p53 induces several members of extrinsic pathway including FAS/APO1, DR4, and DR5. Furthermore, p53 has been shown to regulate several members of the intrinsic pathway including the BH3-only family members, Noxa and Puma and the Bcl-2 family member Bax. Furthermore several other targets that appear to signal through the mitochondrial pathway have been cloned and characterized including EI24/PIG8, PERP and p53AIP1 (Vogelstein et al., 2000). Because of its potent growth inhibitory and apoptotic effects, the level and activity of p53 is tightly regulated.

In response to a variety of genotoxic stresses (DNA damaging agents, UV damage, nucleotide depletion, hypoxia, or hypoglycemia) or inappropriate proliferative signals (c-Myc, E2F-1, E1A, or Ras), p53 protein becomes stabilized and its DNA binding activity increases allowing p53 to mediate cell cycle arrest or apoptosis. In response to DNA damaging agents, p53 becomes phosphorylated and acetylated leading to stabilization and activation. Phosphorylation of p53 at its N-terminus prevents binding of the p53 target gene and E3 ubiquitin ligase, Mdm2. Mdm2 binding inhibits p53 dependent transactivation and leads to p53 degradation (Haupt, Maya, Kazaz, & Oren, 1997; Honda, Tanaka, & Yasuda, 1997; Kubbutat, Jones, & Vousden, 1997; Midgley & Lane, 1997; Momand, Zambetti, Olson, George, & Levine, 1992; Oliner et al., 1993; Thut, Goodrich, & Tjian, 1997). The mdm2 gene was first discovered in a mouse tumor cell line as an amplified gene contained in a murine double minute (Fakharzadeh, Trusko, & George, 1991) and mdm2 has been shown to be amplified in 20%-40% of human sarcomas (Oliner, Kinzler, Meltzer, George, & Vogelstein, 1992). The phosphorylation of p53 in response to ionizing radiation is dependent on the ataxia telangiectasia mutated (ATM) protein, a member of the phosphoinositide-3-kinase-related (PIK) superfamily. Patients suffering from ataxia telangiectasia are highly tumor prone indicating a important role for ATM in suppressing tumor development. Although ATM can directly phosphorylate p53, its ability to stabilize p53 depends on its ability to phosphorylate Chk2 which then phosphorylates p53 (Abraham, 2001). Interestingly, mutations of Chk2 have been found in Li-Fraumeni syndrome suggesting a key role for Chk2 in regulating p53 (Bell et al., 1999). Another member of the phosphoinositide-3-kinase-related (PIK) superfamily, ATR appears to regulate p53 phosphorylation and stabilization in response to UV irradiation or chemotherapeutic agents. Similar to ATM, ATR mediates its effect primarily by phosphorylating another kinase, Chk1 which phosphorylates p53 (Abraham, 2001).

In response to inappropriate proliferative signals (c-Myc, E2F-1, E1A, or Ras), p53 is stabilized by a phosphorylation independent manner through p14ARF. p14ARF was discovered as an alternative open reading frame in the INK4a locus which was previously shown to encode the CDK inhibitor p16INK4a (Quelle, Zindy, Ashmun, & Sherr, 1995). Early studies demonstrated that p14ARF overexpression induce a p16-independent p53-dependent G1 cell cycle arrest(Stott et al., 1998). Several studies have shown that p14ARF is induced by a variety of oncogenes (Zindy et al., 1998). P14ARF then stabilizes p53 by binding Mdm2 and sequestering it in the nucleolus (Vousden & Woude, 2000). Studies performed in p19ARF -/- animals demonstrated that ARF was required for p53 stabilization by a variety of oncogenes (Zindy et al., 1998). Furthermore, the p19ARF -/- animals phenocopied the p53 -/- animals in terms of tumor spectrum and survival (Schmitt, McCurrach, de Stanchina, Wallace-Brodeur, & Lowe, 1999). Mutations of p14ARF have been observed in several tumor types including breast, brain and lung tumors (Sherr, 2001). Although recent studies have found some tissue specific examples where ARF is not required for p53 stabilization after oncogenic stimulation, the p19ARF -/- animals and mutation in human tumors clearly show that ARF is a critical regulator of p53 (Russell et al., 2002; Tolbert, Lu, Yin, Tantama, & Van Dyke, 2002).

In addition to p53, several lines of evidence indicate that the conserved Forkhead family of transcription factors may play an important role in inducing cell death and prevention of tumorigenesis. Each of the three mammalian family members (FKHR, FKHRL1/AF6q21 and AFX) is present at the site of translocations in several human tumor types (Borkhardt et al., 1997; Davis et al., 1995; Hillion, Le Coniat, Jonveaux, Berger, & Bernard, 1997; Sublett, Jeon, &

Shapiro, 1995). Furthermore, the Forkhead family has been demonstrated to play a key role in growth factor withdrawal induced death (Brunet, Datta, & Greenberg, 2001). In the presence of growth factors, Akt/PKB is active and phosphorylates Forkhead family members. Upon phosphorylation, Forkhead proteins are exported from the nucleus and become sequestered in the cytoplasm by 14-3-3 proteins. In the absence of survival factors or if a non-phosphorylable form of Forkhead is expressed, these proteins translocate to the nucleus and induce expression of pro-apoptotic genes leading to cell death (Brunet et al., 2001). Several studies have demonstrated that Forkhead proteins induce FasL/CD95L and the BH3-only Bcl-2 family member, Bim (Brunet et al., 1999; Dijkers, Medema, Lammers, Koenderman, & Coffer, 2000). Both of these targets appear to be required for Forkhead induced cell death as studies that have inhibited FasL signaling or deleted Bim have demonstrated defects in Forkhead mediated apoptosis (Le-Niculescu et al., 1999; Putcha et al., 2001). Although mutations of Forkhead proteins are infrequent, it negative regulator, Akt/PKB is a central mediator of tumorigenesis and its activity is frequently upregulated in cancer.

The serine/threonine kinase Akt/PKB was first discovered as the cellular homologue of the viral oncogene, v-Akt (Bellacosa, Testa, Staal, & Tsichlis, 1991). Akt/PKB has been implicated in several processes that promote tumorigenesis including growth factor independence, resistance to anti-proliferative signals, cell survival, unlimited replication, angiogenesis, invasion and metastasis. Akt clearly plays a key role in preventing cell death as several studies have demonstrated a role for Akt in preventing apoptosis after growth factor withdrawal, matrix detachment, FasL treatment and exposure to DNA damaging agents (Datta, Brunet, & Greenberg, 1999). In mammals, three closely related family members, Akt1, Akt2, and Akt3 exist and appear to play a role in cell survival and metabolism. In response to a variety of signals including growth factors, insulin, IGF-1 or activated Ras, Akt is recruited to the membrane and activated. This occurs through the phosphatidylinositol 3-kinase (PI3K) pathway. In response to growth factor signaling, PI3K is recruited to the plasma membranes where it phosphorylates membrane phosphoinositides generating 3'phosphorylated phosphoinositides primarily PI-3, 4,5-P_3 and PI-3, 4-P_2. Akt then binds these phospholipids and is phosphorylated and activated by PDK1 and a yet unidentified PDK2. Akt then mediates it pro-survival effects through phosphorylation of several known targets resulting in the relocalization of these substrates in the cell (Testa & Bellacosa, 2001). Several pro-apoptotic substrates have been identified for Akt and each may play a role in mediating cell survival depending on the cellular context. The pro-apoptotic BH3-only Bcl-2 family member, Bad is phosphorylated by Akt and then sequestered by 14-3-3 proteins (Datta et al., 1997; del Peso et al., 1997). Akt also appears to phosphorylate and inhibit caspase 9 (Cardone et al., 1998). However, the caspase 9 Akt phosphorylation site is not conserved in mice and it remains unclear whether this is a critical substrate for promoting survival (Fujita et al., 1999). As discussed above, the pro-apoptotic Forkhead family of transcription factors is phosphorylated by Akt resulting in nuclear export and sequestration in the cytoplasm by 14-3-3 proteins. Akt can also disrupt the p53 pathway through phosphorylation of the negative p53 regulator, Mdm2. Upon phosphorylation, Mdm2 translocates into the nucleus where it can bind and degrade p53 (Mayo & Donner, 2001; Zhou et al., 2001). Finally, Akt has been implicated in increasing the pro-survival NF-κB activity (Kane, Shapiro,

Stokoe, & Weiss, 1999; Romashkova & Makarov, 1999). Akt has been shown to phosphorylate IκB kinase (IKK) which leads to degradation of IκB and translocation of NF-κB to the nucleus (Ozes et al., 1999).

Due to its pro-survival and other tumorgenic effects, Akt levels and/or activity are elevated in most human neoplasia by a variety of mechanisms. In some tumor types, upstream growth factors such as PDGF and EGF are produced in an autocrine manner resulting in Akt activation. Furthermore activated Ras mutations which are present in 30 % of all tumors have been demonstrated to activate PI3K and Akt (Kauffmann-Zeh et al., 1997). A key upstream regulator PI3K, is itself amplified in ovarian cancers(Shayesteh et al., 1999). At the membrane level, PTEN, a lipid phosphatase which dephosphorylates PI-3, 4-P_2 and PI-3, 4,5-P_3 is mutated in variety of human neoplasms (Di Cristofano & Pandolfi, 2000). Loss of PTEN leads to widespread resistance to a variety of apoptotic stimuli that can be overcome by inhibiting the PI3K pathway (Stambolic et al., 1998) (Suzuki et al., 1998). Finally amplification of Akt1 in gastric tumors and Akt2 in ovarian and pancreatic cancers has been observed at a significant rate (Testa & Bellacosa, 2001).

The transcription factor NF-κB is another key survival factor in cancer and in addition to its role in inhibiting cell death it has been implicated in controlling cellular proliferation. NFκB can promote or induce apoptosis in some cellular contexts; however, several lines of evidence suggest that inhibition of apoptosis appears to be critical for its tumor promoting properties. Both the TNF receptor pathway and DNA damaging agents induce NFκB rendering the cell resistant to these stimuli. Furthermore, inhibiting NFκB activity sensitizes the tumor cells to a wide variety of apoptotic stimuli. Finally inhibition of NF κB also prevents transformation and leads to apoptosis after expression of oncogenic H-Ras (Baldwin, 2001). NF-κB is not a single protein or complex but rather a small collection of protein dimers. These dimers consist of the five members of the NF-κB family: p50/p105 (NF-κB1), p52/p100 (NF-κB2), c-Rel, RelB, and p65 (RelA). In normal unstressed cells, NF-κB is bound to the IκB family of proteins and remains cytoplasmic and inactive. In response to bacterial LPS, pro-inflammatory cytokines, DNA damaging agents, or oncogenic stimulation (Ras, Akt, Bcr-abl) the IκB family members are phosphorylated by the IκB kinase family and degraded. NF-κB is then released and translocates to the nucleus where it can transactivate its target genes. NF-κB is further activated in the nucleus by phosphorylation of its subunits (Karin, 2002). Several studies have demonstrated that NFκB can inhibit the extrinsic pathway primarily through its induction of c-IAP1 & 2, Traf 1 & Traf2 and c-Flip (Karin, 2002; Kreuz, Siegmund, Scheurich, & Wajant, 2001). NFκB can also inhibit the intrinsic pathway through its regulation of the anti-apoptotic Bcl-2 family members, A1/Bfl-1 and Bcl-X_L (Karin, 2002).

As expected there are many examples in which NFκB is activated in human neoplasia. The NFκB pathway is often a critical target of many viral transforming proteins. Furthermore several cellular oncogenes such as Ras and Her2/Neu through activation of Akt and BCR-ABL fusion protein lead to NFκB activation (Madrid et al., 2000; Reuther, Reuther, Cortez, Pendergast, & Baldwin, 1998; Zhou et al., 2000). Several NFκB subunits, most notably c-Rel, and NF-κB2 are amplified or involved in rearrangements in some lymphomas (Fracchiolla et al., 1993; Gilmore, Koedood, Piffat, & White, 1996; Rayet & Gelinas, 1999). The negative regulator IκBβ is mutated in Hodgkin's Lymphomas (Cabannes, Khan, Aillet, Jarrett, & Hay, 1999). Furthermore a positive regulator of the NF-κB activity, Bcl-3 was identified in t (14,19)(q32; q13.1) chromosomal translocation in B-cell chronic lymphocytic leukemias (McKeithan et al., 1997). Finally, elevated NF-κB activity has been implicated in the development of many solid tumors including breast and gastric carcinomas (Karin, 2002).

5. DISRUPTION OF THE EXTRINSIC AND INTRINSIC SIGNALING PATHWAY IN NEOPLASIA

Inactivation of the extrinsic pathway is observed in many tumors through a variety of resistance mechanisms (Table 1). Mutations of Fas/APO1 are observed in myeloma and T-cell leukemias as well as in solid tumors such as hepatocellular carcinomas, colon carcinomas and melanomas (Muschen, Warskulat, & Beckmann, 2000). Similarly, previous studies have found rare TRAIL receptor mutations in non-small cell lung cancer (Lee et al., 1999) and a nasopharyngeal cancer cell line (Ozoren, Fisher et al., 2000). Several studies have also reported increased levels of sCD95 in various tumors and DcR3 is amplified in several lung and colon carcinomas and overexpressed in several other malignancies (Cheng et al., 1994; Midis, Shen, & Owen-Schaub, 1996; Pitti et al., 1998; Roth et al., 2001). Although TRID and TRUNDD may play some role in protecting normal cells, the expression levels of these decoy receptors does not correlate with the observed resistance to TRAIL of some tumor cell lines (Griffith, Chin, Jackson, Lynch, & Kubin, 1998; Kim, Fisher, Xu, & El-Deiry, 2000). Several observations support a key role for c-FLIP in mediated resistance to both FasL and TRAIL mediated death. Overexpression of c-FLIP is sufficient to block FasL and TRAIL mediated death (Irmler et al., 1997). Furthermore, c-FLIP -/- mouse embryonic fibroblasts are extremely sensitive to FasL or TRAIL while wild-type mouse embryonic fibroblasts are resistant(Bin, Li, Xu, & Shu, 2002). Furthermore c-FLIP protein levels correlate with TRAIL resistance in some but not all tumor cell types (Griffith et al., 1998; Kim et al., 2000). Furthermore, viral forms of cellular FLIP are present in HHV8 and other tumorigenic viruses and inhibit FasL and TRAIL induced death (Bertin et al., 1997; Thome et al., 1997). Finally studies have demonstrated that overexpression of c-Flip allowed tumors to escape immune surveillance in vivo(Djerbi et al., 1999; Medema, de Jong, van Hall, Melief, & Offringa, 1999). c-Flip mRNA and protein are positively regulated by the pro-survival factors, Akt/PKB and NF-κB and this regulation may also contribute to their pro-survival effects (Panka, Mano, Suhara, Walsh, & Mier, 2001) (Kreuz et al., 2001). In addition to increased c-FLIP levels, several mechanisms can contribute to intracellular resistance to death ligands. In neuroblastoma cell lines, deletion or methylation of the caspase 8 locus has been observed and this correlated with TRAIL resistance (Eggert et al., 2001; Hopkins-Donaldson et al., 2000). In type II cells, several studies have demonstrated that overexpression of the anti-apoptotic Bcl-2 family members, Bcl-2 and Bcl-X_L or loss of the pro-apoptotic Bcl-2 family members, Bid, Bak and Bax have been shown inhibit cell killing (Burns & El-Deiry, 2001; Hinz et al., 2000; Lindsten et al., 2000; Scaffidi et al., 1998; Yin et al., 1999). Finally recent studies demonstrating the methylation of Apaf-1 in malignant melanoma may be an additional mechanism of TRAIL and FasL resistance in this tumor type (Soengas et al., 2001).

Table 1: Disruption of the Apoptotic Pathway in Human Neoplasia

	Genomic Alterations	*Tumor Types/syndromes*	*References*
Extrinsic Pathway			
Fas/APO1	Point mutations	Myeloma, T-cell leukemias, hepatocellular and colon carcinoma, melanoma	(Muschen et al., 2000)
sFasL	Elevated expression levels	Bladder, ovary, lung, melanoma, leukemia	(Cheng et al., 1994; Midis et al., 1996; Ugurel, Rappl, Tilgen, & Reinhold, 2001)
DcR3	Amplified (lung and colon); overexpressed	Lung, colon, stomach, esophagus, rectum, gliomas	(Bai et al., 2000; Pitti et al., 1998; Roth et al., 2001)
DR4/DR5	Deletion, Point mutations	Nasopharyngeal, lung, breast, gastric	(Lee et al., 1999; Ozoren, Fisher et al., 2000; Park et al., 2001; Shin et al., 2001)
Caspase 8	Deletion, Methylation	Neuroblastoma	(Eggert et al., 2000; Hopkins-Donaldson et al., 2000)
c-Flip	Elevated expression levels, viral Flip isoforms	Melanoma, Burkitt's Lymphoma (EBV), Kaposi's sarcoma	(Krueger, Baumann, Krammer, & Kirchhoff, 2001)

Intrinsic Pathway			
Bax	Frameshift mutations; loss of expression	Colon, breast, ALL	(Ionov, Yamamoto, Krajewski, Reed, & Perucho, 2000; Krajewski et al., 1995; Meijerink et al., 1998; Rampino et al., 1997)
Bcl-2/Bcl-X_L	Translocation, Overexpression	Follicular lymphomas; multiple other tumor types	(Reed, 1999)
Apaf-1	Methylation	melanoma	(Soengas et al., 2001)
IAPs	Overexpression, Translocations	Non-Hodgkin's lymphoma, Marginal cell lymphoma, lung, breast, colon, prostate	(Deveraux & Reed, 1999)

Positive Regulators of Apoptosis			
P53 pathway:			
p53	Point mutations, deletion, viral inactivation	Majority of tumor types, Li-Fraumeni syndrome	(Hollstein et al., 1991; Malkin et al., 1990; Vogelstein & Kinzler, 1992; Vogelstein et al., 2000)
p19ARF	Deletion, methylation	Breast, Brain, Lung	(Sherr, 2001)
Mdm2	Amplification	Sarcomas, Brain	(Michael & Oren, 2002; Oliner et al., 1992)

Positive Regulators(Cont.)			
Chk2	Point mutations	Li-Fraumeni syndrome	(Bell et al., 1999) (Wu, Webster, & Chen, 2001)
ATM	Deletions; point mutations	Lymphoma; ataxia telangiectasia	(Abraham, 2001)
Forkhead Proteins	Translocations	Acute leukemia, alveolar rhabdomyosarcoma	(Davis et al., 1995) (Sublett et al., 1995) (Borkhardt et al., 1997) (Hillion et al., 1997)
Negative Regulators of Apoptosis			
AKT pathway:			
AKT(1,2,3)	Overexpression, Increased Activity	Ovarian, pancreatic, gastric, breast	(Testa & Bellacosa, 2001)
Ras proteins	Overexpression, Increased Activity	Pancreatic adenocarcinomas, myeloid leukemia, lung, colon	(Bar-Sagi, 2001)
PI3K	Amplification	ovarian	(Shayesteh et al., 1999)
PTEN	Deletion, Point mutations,	glioblastomas, ovarian, endometrial, advanced prostate cancers	(Di Cristofano & Pandolfi, 2000)
NF-κB	Elevated expression	Lymphomas, Leukemias, breast, gastric	(Baldwin, 2001) (Karin, 2002)

Inactivation of the intrinsic pathway is observed in many tumor types and may be required for tumor formation. Mutation or loss of BH3 only proteins in tumors is not frequently observed however; transcription factors (p53, Forkhead) that control their induction in response to apoptotic stimuli are frequently mutated or inactivated. Furthermore, some BH3-only family members are inhibited post-translationally, for example Bad is sequestered in the cytoplasm after phosphorylation by the pro-survival factor, Akt/PKB. At the level of the mitochondria, mutation of Bax and Bak mutations are observed in some tumor types. Loss of Bax expression has been correlated with chemoresistance and decreased survival rates in some tumor types (Krajewski et al., 1995). Frequently, Bcl-2 and Bcl-X_L are overexpressed in many tumors and correlate with chemoresistance (Johnstone et al., 2002). Inactivation of the intrinsic pathway can occur downstream of the mitochondria as Apaf-1 is methylated in malignant melanoma (Soengas et al., 2001). Furthermore, nine mammalian IAPs have been discovered and a strong link to tumorigenesis has been established for at least two family members. Elevated levels of one IAP family member, Survivin have been detected in non-Hodgkin's lymphomas and many solid tumors types including lung, colon, breast and prostate cancer and its expression correlates with unfavorable clinical outcome (Deveraux & Reed, 1999). Moreover, inhibition of its function has suppressed tumor growth (Grossman, Kim, Schechner, & Altieri, 2001). cIAP2 is overexpressed in 50 % of marginal cell lymphomas due to its presence in a translocation t (11; 18)(q21; q21) (Deveraux & Reed, 1999). It is likely that disruption of the intrinsic pathway occurs at some level in every tumor type.

6. APOPTOSIS-BASED THERAPEUTIC APPROACHES TO CANCER

Although chemotherapy has been tremendously successful against childhood acute leukemia and testicular carcinoma, its effectiveness against adult carcinomas of the breast, lung, prostate and colon has been disappointing. Although chemotherapeutic agents can be both cytostatic and as well as cytotoxic it is clear that induction of apoptosis is essential for their mechanism of action. Several studies using transgenic animals overexpressing Bcl-2 or Bcl-XL or knockout animals deficient for both bax and bak or apaf-1 have demonstrated that apoptosis is critical for chemosensitivity (Johnstone et al., 2002). Furthermore several studies of primary tumors and tumor cell lines have correlated increased Bcl-2 expression and loss of p53 with chemoresistance (Reed, 1999; Wallace-Brodeur & Lowe, 1999). Since induction of apoptosis is critical to chemosensitivity and tumor regression, much work has focused on new therapies that could induce apoptosis in a more tumor specific manner and/or resensitize the chemoresistant tumors to chemotherapeutic agents. Ideally the reactivation of tumor suppressors such as p53 or the inhibition of survival factors such Akt or Bcl-2 could target tumor cells for destruction while preserving the surrounding normal tissue. Below we will highlight several strategies currently being developed to access the cell death pathway in malignant cells through induction of apoptosis through the extrinsic pathway, inhibition of survival factors or reactivation of tumor suppressors.

Activation of the extrinsic pathway may be one potential mechanism for activating tumor specific apoptosis as demonstrated by studies with recombinant TRAIL. The TNF-related apoptosis-inducing ligand (TRAIL), also cloned as Apo-

2L, is a pro-apoptotic cytokine and is a member of the Tumor Necrosis Factor (TNF) superfamily (Pitti et al., 1996; Wiley et al., 1995). Several members of this family (TNF-α, FasL, TRAIL) have been shown to induce apoptosis through binding of their respective receptors. TRAIL has cytotoxic effects against a wide range of tumor cell types whereas most normal cell lines examined are resistant to TRAIL treatment (Ashkenazi et al., 1999; Walczak et al., 1999). Unlike FasL and TNF-α whose severe systemic side effects have precluded their clinical use, no systemic side effects in murine or non-human primates have been observed with TRAIL (Ashkenazi et al., 1999). Recent studies had raised questions of whether normal cell types were truly protected from TRAIL as human hepatocytes and keratinocytes were found to be sensitive to TRAIL (Jo et al., 2000; Leverkus et al., 2000; Ozoren, Kim et al., 2000). However, these cytotoxic effects may depend on the particular preparation of TRAIL used, as the TRAIL currently being developed for clinical trials has been reported to apparently not cause death in human hepatocytes and keratinocytes despite its ability to signal death in a manner otherwise identical to other TRAIL preparations (Lawrence et al., 2001; Qin, Chaturvedi, Bonish, & Nickoloff, 2001). Therefore TRAIL remains a promising therapeutic agent for a wide range of human tumors. Although TRAIL can kill cells independent of the mitochondria or intrinsic pathway in some cell types it is clear that that TRAIL mediated cell death can be inhibited by Bcl-2 family members in some cell types. Therefore the expression levels of Bcl-2 family members and inhibitors of the extrinsic pathway such as c-Flip should be considered when using this as a potential therapeutic agent. Several studies have also seen synergy between TRAIL and chemotherapeutic agents and TRAIL may also find a role as an adjuvant therapeutic (El-Deiry, 2001; Keane, Ettenberg, Nau, Russell, & Lipkowitz, 1999).

Another potentially fruitful strategy is to inhibit pro-survival factors through anti-sense strategies and small molecule inhibitors. Although several groups have designed anti-sense strategies to target Bcl-2, Bcl-X_L, Ras, mdm2, survivin, and c-Flip, this strategy is furthest along for Bcl-2 (Nicholson, 2000). An 18-mer all-phophorothioate Bcl-2 antisense oligonucleotide, G-3139 (Genta) has been developed and has undergone both pre-clinical studies and phase I and II clinical trials. Pre-clinical data demonstrated that the this oligonucleotide alone was superior to standard chemotherapy for Merkel cell carcinomas and enhanced apoptosis in other tumor models when used in combination with chemotherapy (Banerjee, 2001; Jansen et al., 1998). Phase I and II trials have found promising results for this treatment in malignant melanoma and non-Hodgkin's lymphoma. Studies are currently underway to examine the effectiveness of co-administration of this oligonucleotide with standard chemotherapy and to examine its effectiveness for other tumor types (Banerjee, 2001). In addition to anti-sense strategies, small inhibitors are which block homo- and heterodimerization of Bcl-2 and result in apoptosis have been developed (Wang, 2001). Inhibitors of the PI3K/Akt pathway currently exist and the development of Akt specific inhibitors is an active area of research.

The NFκB pathway has been implicated in tumorigenesis and chemoresistance and previous studies have shown that inhibition of this pathway resulted in tumor regression and sensitization of tumors to chemotherapeutic agents (Baldwin, 2001). Recent pre-clinical and clinical studies have suggested that the NFκB can be inhibited through the use of proteasome inhibitors and that the inhibition of NFκB is at least partially responsible for the therapeutic effects observed with this class of drugs (Adams, 2002). In most tumors, IκB is phosphorylated and degraded allowing for the active NFκB complexes in the nucleus, however, in the presence of a non-degradable IκB or proteasome inhibitors, IκB is not degraded and NFκB is inactive leading to chemosensitization and cell death. One proteasome inhibitor, PS-341 has been used in clinical Phase I trials with promising results and is currently being studied in several phase II trials (Adams, 2002). Since PS-341 appears to have a high therapeutic index with tolerable side effects, this strategy could be another effective way to inhibit pro-survival factors in tumor cells.

The strategies discussed above have focused on inhibiting survival factors that allow tumor cells to evade apoptosis. Although it may be more difficult to achieve from a practical standpoint, it may also be possible to reactivated tumor suppressors that are important to the apoptotic response associated with cancer therapy. The p53 tumor suppressor plays a key role in mediating apoptosis in response to a variety of cellular and therapeutic stresses. p53 is more often mutated than deleted in primary tumors, and the majority of these point mutations cluster in the DNA binding domain of p53, which suggested it may be possible for p53 at least theoretically to be reactivated in these malignant cells (Bullock & Fersht, 2001). A recent small molecule screen has identified several potential drugs that may bind and stabilize the wild type conformation of p53 (Foster, Coffey, Morin, & Rastinejad, 1999). Two compounds, CP-257042 and CP-31398 appeared to stabilize p53 in its wild type conformation and CP-31398 has been demonstrated to induce apoptosis or growth arrest. CP-31398 also exhibited tumor suppressive effects in human xenographs model systems without significant toxicity (Foster, Coffey, Morin, & Rastinejad, 1999). CP-313398 is not currently being actively pursued in clinical trials because of some difficulties in maintaining CP-31398 at therapeutic levels (Bullock & Fersht, 2001). None-the-less the animal data would suggest there is hope that therapeutic levels of CP-31398 can be achieved in vivo(Foster, Coffey, Morin, & Rastinejad, 1999). Moreover, CP-31398 studies are proof of principle that that reactivation of p53 is possible and can have anti-tumor effects alone(Foster, Coffey, Morin, & Rastinejad, 1999; Takimoto et al., 2002). These studies may serve as a model other modulators of p53 function or other tumor suppressor such as Rb (Bykov et al., 2002).

Several gene therapy approaches are currently being undertaken to target tumor cells specifically. One approach is the design of adenovirus (ONYX-015) that only divides in cells lacking functional p53, therefore limiting the toxicity to normal tissue. Similar adenoviruses have also been designed that can only divide in Rb negative cells. These viruses appear to target tumor cells specifically and the clinical trial data for ONYX-015 is somewhat encouraging (McCormick, 2001). Another gene therapy strategy to specifically target tumor cells is to express so called "suicide genes" such as herpes simplex virus thymine kinase under the control of tumor specific promoters (E2F-1) (McCormick, 2001). Although these are potentially promising therapies, they depend on efficient infection of the tumor and avoidance of immune clearance to be effective. Therefore the current generation of adenoviral vectors appears to be limited to local therapy (McCormick, 2001).

These are just a few examples of the therapeutic strategies currently being developed. Current therapeutic agent development will focus on increasing tumor specific toxicity by targeting the molecules involved in mediating or inhibiting cell death. As our knowledge increases about the resistance mechanisms used by tumors to evade apoptosis and our ability to circumvent these defects present in malignant lesions, newer agents should become more specific and effective. The inhibition of apoptosis is critical for tumor development at several stages and thus represents a critical target. Therefore agents that aim to restore the apoptosis pathway in tumor cells (Bcl-2 or Bcl-XL anti-sense) as well as those agents that induce death directly (rTRAIL) continue to have great therapeutic potential.

7. ACKNOWLEDGEMENTS

W.S.E.-D. is an Assistant Investigator of the Howard Hughes Medical Institute.

Timothy F. Burns and Wafik S. El-Deiry
Howard Hughes Medical Institute
University of Pennsylvania School of Medicine
Philadelphia, PA 19104

8. REFERENCES

Abraham, R. T. (2001). Cell cycle checkpoint signaling through the ATM and ATR kinases. *Genes Dev, 15*(17), 2177-2196.
Adams, J. (2002). Proteasome inhibition: a novel approach to cancer therapy. *Trends Mol Med, 8*(4), S49-54.
Ashkenazi, A., & Dixit, V. M. (1999). Apoptosis control by death and decoy receptors. *Curr Opin Cell Biol, 11*(2), 255-260.
Ashkenazi, A., Pai, R. C., Fong, S., Leung, S., Lawrence, D. A., Marsters, S. A., Blackie, C., Chang, L., McMurtrey, A. E., Hebert, A., DeForge, L., Koumenis, I. L., Lewis, D., Harris, L., Bussiere, J., Koeppen, H., Shahrokh, Z., & Schwall, R. H. (1999). Safety and antitumor activity of recombinant soluble Apo2 ligand. *J Clin Invest, 104*(2), 155-162.
Bai, C., Connolly, B., Metzker, M. L., Hilliard, C. A., Liu, X., Sandig, V., Soderman, A., Galloway, S. M., Liu, Q., Austin, C. P., & Caskey, C. T. (2000). Overexpression of M68/DcR3 in human gastrointestinal tract tumors independent of gene amplification and its location in a four-gene cluster. *Proc Natl Acad Sci U S A, 97*(3), 1230-1235.
Baldwin, A. S. (2001). Control of oncogenesis and cancer therapy resistance by the transcription factor NF-kappaB. *J Clin Invest, 107*(3), 241-246.
Banerjee, D. (2001). Genasense (Genta Inc). *Curr Opin Investig Drugs, 2*(4), 574-580.
Bar-Sagi, D. (2001). A Ras by any other name. *Mol Cell Biol, 21*(5), 1441-1443.
Bell, D. W., Varley, J. M., Szydlo, T. E., Kang, D. H., Wahrer, D. C., Shannon, K. E., Lubratovich, M., Verselis, S. J., Isselbacher, K. J., Fraumeni, J. F., Birch, J. M., Li, F. P., Garber, J. E., & Haber, D. A. (1999). Heterozygous germ line hCHK2 mutations in Li-Fraumeni syndrome. *Science, 286*(5449), 2528-2531.
Bellacosa, A., Testa, J. R., Staal, S. P., & Tsichlis, P. N. (1991). A retroviral oncogene, akt, encoding a serine-threonine kinase containing an SH2-like region. *Science, 254*(5029), 274-277.
Bertin, J., Armstrong, R. C., Ottilie, S., Martin, D. A., Wang, Y., Banks, S., Wang, G. H., Senkevich, T. G., Alnemri, E. S., Moss, B., Lenardo, M. J., Tomaselli, K. J., & Cohen, J. I. (1997). Death effector domain-containing herpesvirus and poxvirus proteins inhibit both Fas- and TNFR1-induced apoptosis. *Proc Natl Acad Sci U S A, 94*(4), 1172-1176.
Bin, L., Li, X., Xu, L. G., & Shu, H. B. (2002). The short splice form of Casper/c-FLIP is a major cellular inhibitor of TRAIL-induced apoptosis. *FEBS Lett, 510*(1-2), 37-40.
Borkhardt, A., Repp, R., Haas, O. A., Leis, T., Harbott, J., Kreuder, J., Hammermann, J., Henn, T., & Lampert, F. (1997). Cloning and characterization of AFX, the gene that fuses to MLL in acute leukemias with a t(X;11)(q13;q23). *Oncogene, 14*(2), 195-202.
Brunet, A., Bonni, A., Zigmond, M. J., Lin, M. Z., Juo, P., Hu, L. S., Anderson, M. J., Arden, K. C., Blenis, J., & Greenberg, M. E. (1999). Akt promotes cell survival by phosphorylating and inhibiting a Forkhead transcription factor. *Cell, 96*(6), 857-868.

Brunet, A., Datta, S. R., & Greenberg, M. E. (2001). Transcription-dependent and -independent control of neuronal survival by the PI3K-Akt signaling pathway. *Curr Opin Neurobiol, 11*(3), 297-305.
Bullock, A. N., & Fersht, A. R. (2001). Rescuing the function of mutant p53. *Nature Rev Cancer, 1*(1), 68-76.
Burns, T. F., Bernhard, E. J., & El-Deiry, W. S. (2001). Tissue specific expression of p53 target genes suggests a key role for KILLER/DR5 in p53-dependent apoptosis in vivo. *Oncogene, 20*(34), 4601-4612.
Burns, T. F., & El-Deiry, W. S. (2001). Identification of inhibitors of TRAIL-induced death (ITIDs) in the TRAIL-sensitive colon carcinoma cell line SW480 using a genetic approach. *J Biol Chem, 276*(41), 37879-37886.
Bykov, V.J.N., Issaeva, N., Shilov, A., Hultcrantz, M., Pugacheva, E., Chumakov, P., Bergman, J., Wiman, K.G. & Selivanova, G. (2002). Restoration of the tumor suppressor function to mutant p53 by a low-molecular-weight compound. *Nature Med.* 8, 282-288.
Cabannes, E., Khan, G., Aillet, F., Jarrett, R. F., & Hay, R. T. (1999). Mutations in the IkBa gene in Hodgkin's disease suggest a tumour suppressor role for IkappaBalpha. *Oncogene, 18*(20), 3063-3070.
Caelles, C., Helmberg, A., & Karin, M. (1994). p53-dependent apoptosis in the absence of transcriptional activation of p53-target genes. *Nature, 370*(6486), 220-223.
Cardone, M. H., Roy, N., Stennicke, H. R., Salvesen, G. S., Franke, T. F., Stanbridge, E., Frisch, S., & Reed, J. C. (1998). Regulation of cell death protease caspase-9 by phosphorylation. *Science, 282*(5392), 1318-1321.
Cheng, J., Zhou, T., Liu, C., Shapiro, J. P., Brauer, M. J., Kiefer, M. C., Barr, P. J., & Mountz, J. D. (1994). Protection from Fas-mediated apoptosis by a soluble form of the Fas molecule. *Science, 263*(5154), 1759-1762.
Cretney, E., Takeda, K., Yagita, H., Glaccum, M., Peschon, J. J., & Smyth, M. J. (2002). Increased susceptibility to tumor initiation and metastasis in TNF-related apoptosis-inducing ligand-deficient mice. *J Immunol, 168*(3), 1356-1361.
Datta, S. R., Brunet, A., & Greenberg, M. E. (1999). Cellular survival: a play in three Akts. *Genes Dev, 13*(22), 2905-2927.
Datta, S. R., Dudek, H., Tao, X., Masters, S., Fu, H., Gotoh, Y., & Greenberg, M. E. (1997). Akt phosphorylation of BAD couples survival signals to the cell-intrinsic death machinery. *Cell, 91*(2), 231-241.
Davis, R. J., Bennicelli, J. L., Macina, R. A., Nycum, L. M., Biegel, J. A., & Barr, F. G. (1995). Structural characterization of the FKHR gene and its rearrangement in alveolar rhabdomyosarcoma. *Hum Mol Genet, 4*(12), 2355-2362.
Degli-Esposti, M. A., Dougall, W. C., Smolak, P. J., Waugh, J. Y., Smith, C. A., & Goodwin, R. G. (1997). The novel receptor TRAIL-R4 induces NF-kappaB and protects against TRAIL-mediated apoptosis, yet retains an incomplete death domain. *Immunity, 7*(6), 813-820.
del Peso, L., Gonzalez-Garcia, M., Page, C., Herrera, R., & Nunez, G. (1997). Interleukin-3-induced phosphorylation of BAD through the protein kinase Akt. *Science, 278*(5338), 687-689.
Deveraux, Q. L., & Reed, J. C. (1999). IAP family proteins--suppressors of apoptosis. *Genes Dev, 13*(3), 239-252.
Di Cristofano, A., & Pandolfi, P. P. (2000). The multiple roles of PTEN in tumor suppression. *Cell, 100*(4), 387-390.
Dijkers, P. F., Medema, R. H., Lammers, J. W., Koenderman, L., & Coffer, P. J. (2000). Expression of the pro-apoptotic Bcl-2 family member Bim is regulated by the forkhead transcription factor FKHR-L1. *Curr Biol, 10*(19), 1201-1204.
Djerbi, M., Screpanti, V., Catrina, A. I., Bogen, B., Biberfeld, P., & Grandien, A. (1999). The inhibitor of death receptor signaling, FLICE-inhibitory protein defines a new class of tumor progression factors. *J Exp Med, 190*(7), 1025-1032.
Donehower, L. A., Harvey, M., Slagle, B. L., McArthur, M. J., Montgomery, C. A., Jr., Butel, J. S., & Bradley, A. (1992). Mice deficient for p53 are developmentally normal but susceptible to spontaneous tumours. *Nature, 356*(6366), 215-221.
Du, C., Fang, M., Li, Y., Li, L., & Wang, X. (2000). Smac, a mitochondrial protein that promotes cytochrome c-dependent caspase activation by eliminating IAP inhibition. *Cell, 102*(1), 33-42.
Eggert, A., Grotzer, M. A., Zuzak, T. J., Wiewrodt, B. R., Ho, R., Ikegaki, N., & Brodeur, G. M. (2001). Resistance to tumor necrosis factor-related apoptosis-inducing ligand (TRAIL)-induced apoptosis in neuroblastoma cells correlates with a loss of caspase-8 expression. *Cancer Res, 61*(4), 1314-1319.
Eggert, A., Grotzer, M. A., Zuzak, T. J., Wiewrodt, B. R., Ikegaki, N., & Brodeur, G. M. (2000). Resistance to TRAIL-induced apoptosis in neuroblastoma cells correlates with a loss of caspase-8 expression. *Med Pediatr Oncol, 35*(6), 603-607.
El-Deiry, W. S. (2001). Insights into cancer therapeutic design based on p53 and TRAIL receptor signaling. *Cell Death Differ, 8*(11), 1066-1075.
Evan, G. I., & Vousden, K. H. (2001). Proliferation, cell cycle and apoptosis in cancer. *Nature, 411*(6835), 342-348.

Fakharzadeh, S. S., Trusko, S. P., & George, D. L. (1991). Tumorigenic potential associated with enhanced expression of a gene that is amplified in a mouse tumor cell line. *Embo J, 10*(6), 1565-1569.

Foster, B. A., Coffey, H. A., Morin, M. J., & Rastinejad, F. (1999). Pharmacological rescue of mutant p53 conformation and function. *Science, 286*(5449), 2507-2510.

Fracchiolla, N. S., Lombardi, L., Salina, M., Migliazza, A., Baldini, L., Berti, E., Cro, L., Polli, E., Maiolo, A. T., & Neri, A. (1993). Structural alterations of the NF-kappa B transcription factor lyt-10 in lymphoid malignancies. *Oncogene, 8*(10), 2839-2845.

Fujita, E., Jinbo, A., Matuzaki, H., Konishi, H., Kikkawa, U., & Momoi, T. (1999). Akt phosphorylation site found in human caspase-9 is absent in mouse caspase-9. *Biochem Biophys Res Commun, 264*(2), 550-555.

Gilmore, T. D., Koedood, M., Piffat, K. A., & White, D. W. (1996). Rel/NF-kappaB/IkappaB proteins and cancer. *Oncogene, 13*(7), 1367-1378.

Griffith, T. S., Chin, W. A., Jackson, G. C., Lynch, D. H., & Kubin, M. Z. (1998). Intracellular regulation of TRAIL-induced apoptosis in human melanoma cells. *J Immunol, 161*(6), 2833-2840.

Grossman, D., Kim, P. J., Schechner, J. S., & Altieri, D. C. (2001). Inhibition of melanoma tumor growth in vivo by survivin targeting. *Proc Natl Acad Sci U S A, 98*(2), 635-640.

Hakem, R., Hakem, A., Duncan, G. S., Henderson, J. T., Woo, M., Soengas, M. S., Elia, A., de la Pompa, J. L., Kagi, D., Khoo, W., Potter, J., Yoshida, R., Kaufman, S. A., Lowe, S. W., Penninger, J. M., & Mak, T. W. (1998). Differential requirement for caspase 9 in apoptotic pathways in vivo. *Cell, 94*(3), 339-352.

Hanahan, D., & Weinberg, R. A. (2000). The hallmarks of cancer. *Cell, 100*(1), 57-70.

Harris, A. L. (2002). Hypoxia--a key regulatory factor in tumour growth. *Nature Rev Cancer, 2*(1), 38-47.

Haupt, Y., Barak, Y., & Oren, M. (1996). Cell type-specific inhibition of p53-mediated apoptosis by mdm2. *Embo J, 15*(7), 1596-1606.

Haupt, Y., Maya, R., Kazaz, A., & Oren, M. (1997). Mdm2 promotes the rapid degradation of p53. *Nature, 387*(6630), 296-299.

Haupt, Y., Rowan, S., Shaulian, E., Vousden, K. H., & Oren, M. (1995). Induction of apoptosis in HeLa cells by trans-activation-deficient p53. *Genes Dev, 9*(17), 2170-2183.

Hengartner, M. O. (2000). The biochemistry of apoptosis. *Nature, 407*(6805), 770-776.

Hillion, J., Le Coniat, M., Jonveaux, P., Berger, R., & Bernard, O. A. (1997). AF6q21, a novel partner of the MLL gene in t(6;11)(q21;q23), defines a forkhead transcriptional factor subfamily. *Blood, 90*(9), 3714-3719.

Hinz, S., Trauzold, A., Boenicke, L., Sandberg, C., Beckmann, S., Bayer, E., Walczak, H., Kalthoff, H., & Ungefroren, H. (2000). Bcl-XL protects pancreatic adenocarcinoma cells against CD95- and TRAIL-receptor-mediated apoptosis. *Oncogene, 19*(48), 5477-5486.

Hollstein, M., Sidransky, D., Vogelstein, B., & Harris, C. C. (1991). p53 mutations in human cancers. *Science, 253*(5015), 49-53.

Honda, R., Tanaka, H., & Yasuda, H. (1997). Oncoprotein MDM2 is a ubiquitin ligase E3 for tumor suppressor p53. *FEBS Lett, 420*(1), 25-27.

Hopkins-Donaldson, S., Bodmer, J. L., Bourloud, K. B., Brognara, C. B., Tschopp, J., & Gross, N. (2000). Loss of caspase-8 expression in highly malignant human neuroblastoma cells correlates with resistance to tumor necrosis factor-related apoptosis-inducing ligand-induced apoptosis. *Cancer Res, 60*(16), 4315-4319.

Hueber, A. O., Zornig, M., Lyon, D., Suda, T., Nagata, S., & Evan, G. I. (1997). Requirement for the CD95 receptor-ligand pathway in c-Myc-induced apoptosis. *Science, 278*(5341), 1305-1309.

Ionov, Y., Yamamoto, H., Krajewski, S., Reed, J. C., & Perucho, M. (2000). Mutational inactivation of the proapoptotic gene BAX confers selective advantage during tumor clonal evolution. *Proc Natl Acad Sci U S A, 97*(20), 10872-10877.

Irmler, M., Thome, M., Hahne, M., Schneider, P., Hofmann, K., Steiner, V., Bodmer, J. L., Schroter, M., Burns, K., Mattmann, C., Rimoldi, D., French, L. E., & Tschopp, J. (1997). Inhibition of death receptor signals by cellular FLIP. *Nature, 388*(6638), 190-195.

Jansen, B., Schlagbauer-Wadl, H., Brown, B. D., Bryan, R. N., van Elsas, A., Muller, M., Wolff, K., Eichler, H. G., & Pehamberger, H. (1998). bcl-2 antisense therapy chemosensitizes human melanoma in SCID mice. *Nat Med, 4*(2), 232-234.

Jo, M., Kim, T. H., Seol, D. W., Esplen, J. E., Dorko, K., Billiar, T. R., & Strom, S. C. (2000). Apoptosis induced in normal human hepatocytes by tumor necrosis factor-related apoptosis-inducing ligand. *Nat Med, 6*(5), 564-567.

Johnstone, R. W., Ruefli, A. A., & Lowe, S. W. (2002). Apoptosis: a link between cancer genetics and chemotherapy. *Cell, 108*(2), 153-164.

Joza, N., Susin, S. A., Daugas, E., Stanford, W. L., Cho, S. K., Li, C. Y., Sasaki, T., Elia, A. J., Cheng, H. Y., Ravagnan, L., Ferri, K. F., Zamzami, N., Wakeham, A., Hakem, R., Yoshida, H., Kong, Y. Y., Mak, T. W., Zuniga-Pflucker, J. C., Kroemer, G., & Penninger, J. M. (2001). Essential role of the mitochondrial apoptosis-inducing factor in programmed cell death. *Nature, 410*(6828), 549-554.

Kane, L. P., Shapiro, V. S., Stokoe, D., & Weiss, A. (1999). Induction of NF-kappaB by the Akt/PKB kinase. *Curr Biol, 9*(11), 601-604.

Karin, M., Cao, Y., Greten, F.R., and Li, Z.-W. (2002). NF-κB IN CANCER: FROM INNOCENT BYSTANDER TO MAJOR CULPRIT. *Nature Rev Cancer, 2*, 301-310.

Kauffmann-Zeh, A., Rodriguez-Viciana, P., Ulrich, E., Gilbert, C., Coffer, P., Downward, J., & Evan, G. (1997). Suppression of c-Myc-induced apoptosis by Ras signalling through PI(3)K and PKB. *Nature, 385*(6616), 544-548.

Keane, M. M., Ettenberg, S. A., Nau, M. M., Russell, E. K., & Lipkowitz, S. (1999). Chemotherapy augments TRAIL-induced apoptosis in breast cell lines. *Cancer Res, 59*(3), 734-741.

Kim, K., Fisher, M. J., Xu, S. Q., & el-Deiry, W. S. (2000). Molecular determinants of response to TRAIL in killing of normal and cancer cells. *Clin Cancer Res, 6*(2), 335-346.

Krajewski, S., Blomqvist, C., Franssila, K., Krajewska, M., Wasenius, V. M., Niskanen, E., Nordling, S., & Reed, J. C. (1995). Reduced expression of proapoptotic gene BAX is associated with poor response rates to combination chemotherapy and shorter survival in women with metastatic breast adenocarcinoma. *Cancer Res, 55*(19), 4471-4478.

Krammer, P. H. (2000). CD95's deadly mission in the immune system. *Nature, 407*(6805), 789-795.

Kreuz, S., Siegmund, D., Scheurich, P., & Wajant, H. (2001). NF-kappaB inducers upregulate cFLIP, a cycloheximide-sensitive inhibitor of death receptor signaling. *Mol Cell Biol, 21*(12), 3964-3973.

Krueger, A., Baumann, S., Krammer, P. H., & Kirchhoff, S. (2001). FLICE-inhibitory proteins: regulators of death receptor-mediated apoptosis. *Mol Cell Biol, 21*(24), 8247-8254.

Kubbutat, M. H., Jones, S. N., & Vousden, K. H. (1997). Regulation of p53 stability by Mdm2. *Nature, 387*(6630), 299-303.

Lacronique, V., Mignon, A., Fabre, M., Viollet, B., Rouquet, N., Molina, T., Porteu, A., Henrion, A., Bouscary, D., Varlet, P., Joulin, V., & Kahn, A. (1996). Bcl-2 protects from lethal hepatic apoptosis induced by an anti-Fas antibody in mice. *Nat Med, 2*(1), 80-86.

Lawrence, D., Shahrokh, Z., Marsters, S., Achilles, K., Shih, D., Mounho, B., Hillan, K., Totpal, K., DeForge, L., Schow, P., Hooley, J., Sherwood, S., Pai, R., Leung, S., Khan, L., Gliniak, B., Bussiere, J., Smith, C. A., Strom, S. S., Kelley, S., Fox, J. A., Thomas, D., & Ashkenazi, A. (2001). Differential hepatocyte toxicity of recombinant Apo2L/TRAIL versions. *Nat Med, 7*(4), 383-385.

Le-Niculescu, H., Bonfoco, E., Kasuya, Y., Claret, F. X., Green, D. R., & Karin, M. (1999). Withdrawal of survival factors results in activation of the JNK pathway in neuronal cells leading to Fas ligand induction and cell death. *Mol Cell Biol, 19*(1), 751-763.

Lee, S. H., Shin, M. S., Kim, H. S., Lee, H. K., Park, W. S., Kim, S. Y., Lee, J. H., Han, S. Y., Park, J. Y., Oh, R. R., Jang, J. J., Han, J. Y., Lee, J. Y., & Yoo, N. J. (1999). Alterations of the DR5/TRAIL receptor 2 gene in non-small cell lung cancers. *Cancer Res, 59*(22), 5683-5686.

Leverkus, M., Neumann, M., Mengling, T., Rauch, C. T., Brocker, E. B., Krammer, P. H., & Walczak, H. (2000). Regulation of tumor necrosis factor-related apoptosis-inducing ligand sensitivity in primary and transformed human keratinocytes. *Cancer Res, 60*(3), 553-559.

Li, H., Zhu, H., Xu, C. J., & Yuan, J. (1998). Cleavage of BID by caspase 8 mediates the mitochondrial damage in the Fas pathway of apoptosis. *Cell, 94*(4), 491-501.

Li, L. Y., Luo, X., & Wang, X. (2001). Endonuclease G is an apoptotic DNase when released from mitochondria. *Nature, 412*(6842), 95-99.

Lindsten, T., Ross, A. J., King, A., Zong, W. X., Rathmell, J. C., Shiels, H. A., Ulrich, E., Waymire, K. G., Mahar, P., Frauwirth, K., Chen, Y., Wei, M., Eng, V. M., Adelman, D. M., Simon, M. C., Ma, A., Golden, J. A., Evan, G., Korsmeyer, S. J., MacGregor, G. R., & Thompson, C. B. (2000). The combined functions of proapoptotic Bcl-2 family members bak and bax are essential for normal development of multiple tissues. *Mol Cell, 6*(6), 1389-1399.

Locksley, R. M., Killeen, N., & Lenardo, M. J. (2001). The TNF and TNF receptor superfamilies: integrating mammalian biology. *Cell, 104*(4), 487-501.

Madrid, L. V., Wang, C. Y., Guttridge, D. C., Schottelius, A. J., Baldwin, A. S., Jr., & Mayo, M. W. (2000). Akt suppresses apoptosis by stimulating the transactivation potential of the RelA/p65 subunit of NF-kappaB. *Mol Cell Biol, 20*(5), 1626-1638.

Malkin, D., Li, F. P., Strong, L. C., Fraumeni, J. F., Jr., Nelson, C. E., Kim, D. H., Kassel, J., Gryka, M. A., Bischoff, F. Z., Tainsky, M. A., & et al. (1990). Germ line p53 mutations in a familial syndrome of breast cancer, sarcomas, and other neoplasms. *Science, 250*(4985), 1233-1238.

Mayo, L. D., & Donner, D. B. (2001). A phosphatidylinositol 3-kinase/Akt pathway promotes translocation of Mdm2 from the cytoplasm to the nucleus. *Proc Natl Acad Sci U S A, 98*(20), 11598-11603.

McCormick, F. (2001). Cancer gene therapy: fringe or cutting edge? *Nature Rev Cancer, 1*(2), 130-141.

McKeithan, T. W., Takimoto, G. S., Ohno, H., Bjorling, V. S., Morgan, R., Hecht, B. K., Dube, I., Sandberg, A. A., & Rowley, J. D. (1997). BCL3 rearrangements and t(14;19) in chronic lymphocytic leukemia and other B-cell malignancies: a molecular and cytogenetic study. *Genes Chromosomes Cancer, 20*(1), 64-72.

Medema, J. P., de Jong, J., van Hall, T., Melief, C. J., & Offringa, R. (1999). Immune escape of tumors in vivo by expression of cellular FLICE-inhibitory protein. *J Exp Med, 190*(7), 1033-1038.

Meijerink, J. P., Mensink, E. J., Wang, K., Sedlak, T. W., Sloetjes, A. W., de Witte, T., Waksman, G., & Korsmeyer, S. J. (1998). Hematopoietic malignancies demonstrate loss-of-function mutations of BAX. *Blood, 91*(8), 2991-2997.

Meng, R. D., McDonald, E. R., 3rd, Sheikh, M. S., Fornace, A. J., Jr., & El-Deiry, W. S. (2000). The TRAIL decoy receptor TRUNDD (DcR2, TRAIL-R4) is induced by adenovirus-p53 overexpression and can delay TRAIL-, p53-, and KILLER/DR5-dependent colon cancer apoptosis. *Mol Ther, 1*(2), 130-144.

Michael, D., & Oren, M. (2002). The p53 and Mdm2 families in cancer. *Curr Opin Genet Dev, 12*(1), 53-59.

Midgley, C. A., & Lane, D. P. (1997). p53 protein stability in tumour cells is not determined by mutation but is dependent on Mdm2 binding. *Oncogene, 15*(10), 1179-1189.

Midis, G. P., Shen, Y., & Owen-Schaub, L. B. (1996). Elevated soluble Fas (sFas) levels in nonhematopoietic human malignancy. *Cancer Res, 56*(17), 3870-3874.

Momand, J., Zambetti, G. P., Olson, D. C., George, D., & Levine, A. J. (1992). The mdm-2 oncogene product forms a complex with the p53 protein and inhibits p53-mediated transactivation. *Cell, 69*(7), 1237-1245.

Muschen, M., Warskulat, U., & Beckmann, M. W. (2000). Defining CD95 as a tumor suppressor gene. *J Mol Med, 78*(6), 312-325.

Nicholson, D. W. (2000). From bench to clinic with apoptosis-based therapeutic agents. *Nature, 407*(6805), 810-816.

Oliner, J. D., Kinzler, K. W., Meltzer, P. S., George, D. L., & Vogelstein, B. (1992). Amplification of a gene encoding a p53-associated protein in human sarcomas. *Nature, 358*(6381), 80-83.

Oliner, J. D., Pietenpol, J. A., Thiagalingam, S., Gyuris, J., Kinzler, K. W., & Vogelstein, B. (1993). Oncoprotein MDM2 conceals the activation domain of tumour suppressor p53. *Nature, 362*(6423), 857-860.

Ozes, O. N., Mayo, L. D., Gustin, J. A., Pfeffer, S. R., Pfeffer, L. M., & Donner, D. B. (1999). NF-kappaB activation by tumour necrosis factor requires the Akt serine-threonine kinase. *Nature, 401*(6748), 82-85.

Ozoren, N., Fisher, M. J., Kim, K., Liu, C. X., Genin, A., Shifman, Y., Dicker, D. T., Spinner, N. B., Lisitsyn, N. A., & El-Deiry, W. S. (2000). Homozygous deletion of the death receptor DR4 gene in a nasopharyngeal cancer cell line is associated with TRAIL resistance. *Int J Oncol, 16*(5), 917-925.

Ozoren, N., Kim, K., Burns, T. F., Dicker, D. T., Moscioni, A. D., & El-Deiry, W. S. (2000). The caspase 9 inhibitor Z-LEHD-FMK protects human liver cells while permitting death of cancer cells exposed to tumor necrosis factor-related apoptosis-inducing ligand. *Cancer Res, 60*(22), 6259-6265.

Pan, G., Ni, J., Wei, Y. F., Yu, G., Gentz, R., & Dixit, V. M. (1997). An antagonist decoy receptor and a death domain-containing receptor for TRAIL. *Science, 277*(5327), 815-818.

Pan, H., Yin, C., Dyson, N. J., Harlow, E., Yamasaki, L., & Van Dyke, T. (1998). Key roles for E2F1 in signaling p53-dependent apoptosis and in cell division within developing tumors. *Mol Cell, 2*(3), 283-292.

Panka, D. J., Mano, T., Suhara, T., Walsh, K., & Mier, J. W. (2001). Phosphatidylinositol 3-Kinase/Akt Activity Regulates c-FLIP Expression in Tumor Cells. *J Biol Chem, 276*(10), 6893-6896.

Park, W. S., Lee, J. H., Shin, M. S., Park, J. Y., Kim, H. S., Kim, Y. S., Park, C. H., Lee, S. K., Lee, S. H., Lee, S. N., Kim, H., Yoo, N. J., & Lee, J. Y. (2001). Inactivating mutations of KILLER/DR5 gene in gastric cancers. *Gastroenterology, 121*(5), 1219-1225.

Pitti, R. M., Marsters, S. A., Lawrence, D. A., Roy, M., Kischkel, F. C., Dowd, P., Huang, A., Donahue, C. J., Sherwood, S. W., Baldwin, D. T., Godowski, P. J., Wood, W. I., Gurney, A. L., Hillan, K. J., Cohen, R. L., Goddard, A. D., Botstein, D., & Ashkenazi, A. (1998). Genomic amplification of a decoy receptor for Fas ligand in lung and colon cancer. *Nature, 396*(6712), 699-703.

Pitti, R. M., Marsters, S. A., Ruppert, S., Donahue, C. J., Moore, A., & Ashkenazi, A. (1996). Induction of apoptosis by Apo-2 ligand, a new member of the tumor necrosis factor cytokine family. *J Biol Chem, 271*(22), 12687-12690.

Putcha, G. V., Moulder, K. L., Golden, J. P., Bouillet, P., Adams, J. A., Strasser, A., & Johnson, E. M. (2001). Induction of BIM, a proapoptotic BH3-only BCL-2 family member, is critical for neuronal apoptosis. *Neuron, 29*(3), 615-628.

Puthalakath, H., Huang, D. C., O'Reilly, L. A., King, S. M., & Strasser, A. (1999). The proapoptotic activity of the Bcl-2 family member Bim is regulated by interaction with the dynein motor complex. *Mol Cell, 3*(3), 287-296.

Qin, J., Chaturvedi, V., Bonish, B., & Nickoloff, B. J. (2001). Avoiding premature apoptosis of normal epidermal cells. *Nat Med, 7*(4), 385-386.

Quelle, D. E., Zindy, F., Ashmun, R. A., & Sherr, C. J. (1995). Alternative reading frames of the INK4a tumor suppressor gene encode two unrelated proteins capable of inducing cell cycle arrest. *Cell, 83*(6), 993-1000.

Rampino, N., Yamamoto, H., Ionov, Y., Li, Y., Sawai, H., Reed, J. C., & Perucho, M. (1997). Somatic frameshift mutations in the BAX gene in colon cancers of the microsatellite mutator phenotype. *Science, 275*(5302), 967-969.

Rayet, B., & Gelinas, C. (1999). Aberrant rel/nfkb genes and activity in human cancer. *Oncogene, 18*(49), 6938-6947.
Reed, J. C. (1999). Dysregulation of apoptosis in cancer. *J Clin Oncol, 17*(9), 2941-2953.
Reuther, J. Y., Reuther, G. W., Cortez, D., Pendergast, A. M., & Baldwin, A. S., Jr. (1998). A requirement for NF-kappaB activation in Bcr-Abl-mediated transformation. *Genes Dev, 12*(7), 968-981.
Romashkova, J. A., & Makarov, S. S. (1999). NF-kappaB is a target of AKT in anti-apoptotic PDGF signalling. *Nature, 401*(6748), 86-90.
Rosen, D., Li, J. H., Keidar, S., Markon, I., Orda, R., & Berke, G. (2000). Tumor immunity in perforin-deficient mice: a role for CD95 (Fas/APO-1). *J Immunol, 164*(6), 3229-3235.
Roth, W., Isenmann, S., Nakamura, M., Platten, M., Wick, W., Kleihues, P., Bahr, M., Ohgaki, H., Ashkenazi, A., & Weller, M. (2001). Soluble decoy receptor 3 is expressed by malignant gliomas and suppresses CD95 ligand-induced apoptosis and chemotaxis. *Cancer Res, 61*(6), 2759-2765.
Russell, J. L., Powers, J. T., Rounbehler, R. J., Rogers, P. M., Conti, C. J., & Johnson, D. G. (2002). ARF differentially modulates apoptosis induced by E2F1 and Myc. *Mol Cell Biol, 22*(5), 1360-1368.
Scaffidi, C., Fulda, S., Srinivasan, A., Friesen, C., Li, F., Tomaselli, K. J., Debatin, K. M., Krammer, P. H., & Peter, M. E. (1998). Two CD95 (APO-1/Fas) signaling pathways. *Embo J, 17*(6), 1675-1687.
Schmitt, C. A., Fridman, J.S., Yang M., Baranov, E., Hoffman, R.M., and Lowe, S.W. (2002). Dissecting p53 tumor suppressor functions in vivo. *Cancer Cell, 1*, 289-298.
Schmitt, C. A., McCurrach, M. E., de Stanchina, E., Wallace-Brodeur, R. R., & Lowe, S. W. (1999). INK4a/ARF mutations accelerate lymphomagenesis and promote chemoresistance by disabling p53. *Genes Dev, 13*(20), 2670-2677.
Shayesteh, L., Lu, Y., Kuo, W. L., Baldocchi, R., Godfrey, T., Collins, C., Pinkel, D., Powell, B., Mills, G. B., & Gray, J. W. (1999). PIK3CA is implicated as an oncogene in ovarian cancer. *Nat Genet, 21*(1), 99-102.
Sherr, C. J. (2001). The INK4a/ARF network in tumour suppression. *Nat Rev Mol Cell Biol, 2*(10), 731-737.
Shin, M. S., Kim, H. S., Lee, S. H., Park, W. S., Kim, S. Y., Park, J. Y., Lee, J. H., Lee, S. K., Lee, S. N., Jung, S. S., Han, J. Y., Kim, H., Lee, J. Y., & Yoo, N. J. (2001). Mutations of tumor necrosis factor-related apoptosis-inducing ligand receptor 1 (TRAIL-R1) and receptor 2 (TRAIL-R2) genes in metastatic breast cancers. *Cancer Res, 61*(13), 4942-4946.
Soengas, M. S., Alarcon, R. M., Yoshida, H., Giaccia, A. J., Hakem, R., Mak, T. W., & Lowe, S. W. (1999). Apaf-1 and caspase-9 in p53-dependent apoptosis and tumor inhibition. *Science, 284*(5411), 156-159.
Soengas, M. S., Capodieci, P., Polsky, D., Mora, J., Esteller, M., Opitz-Araya, X., McCombie, R., Herman, J. G., Gerald, W. L., Lazebnik, Y. A., Cordon-Cardo, C., & Lowe, S. W. (2001). Inactivation of the apoptosis effector Apaf-1 in malignant melanoma. *Nature, 409*(6817), 207-211.
Stambolic, V., Suzuki, A., de la Pompa, J. L., Brothers, G. M., Mirtsos, C., Sasaki, T., Ruland, J., Penninger, J. M., Siderovski, D. P., & Mak, T. W. (1998). Negative regulation of PKB/Akt-dependent cell survival by the tumor suppressor PTEN. *Cell, 95*(1), 29-39.
Stott, F. J., Bates, S., James, M. C., McConnell, B. B., Starborg, M., Brookes, S., Palmero, I., Ryan, K., Hara, E., Vousden, K. H., & Peters, G. (1998). The alternative product from the human CDKN2A locus, p14(ARF), participates in a regulatory feedback loop with p53 and MDM2. *Embo J, 17*(17), 5001-5014.
Strasser, A., Harris, A. W., Huang, D. C., Krammer, P. H., & Cory, S. (1995). Bcl-2 and Fas/APO-1 regulate distinct pathways to lymphocyte apoptosis. *Embo J, 14*(24), 6136-6147.
Sublett, J. E., Jeon, I. S., & Shapiro, D. N. (1995). The alveolar rhabdomyosarcoma PAX3/FKHR fusion protein is a transcriptional activator. *Oncogene, 11*(3), 545-552.
Susin, S. A., Lorenzo, H. K., Zamzami, N., Marzo, I., Snow, B. E., Brothers, G. M., Mangion, J., Jacotot, E., Costantini, P., Loeffler, M., Larochette, N., Goodlett, D. R., Aebersold, R., Siderovski, D. P., Penninger, J. M., & Kroemer, G. (1999). Molecular characterization of mitochondrial apoptosis-inducing factor. *Nature, 397*(6718), 441-446.
Suzuki, A., de la Pompa, J. L., Stambolic, V., Elia, A. J., Sasaki, T., del Barco Barrantes, I., Ho, A., Wakeham, A., Itie, A., Khoo, W., Fukumoto, M., & Mak, T. W. (1998). High cancer susceptibility and embryonic lethality associated with mutation of the PTEN tumor suppressor gene in mice. *Curr Biol, 8*(21), 1169-1178.
Takimoto, R., Wang, W., Dicker, D.T., Rastinejad, F., Lyssikatos, J. & El-Deiry, W.S. (2002). The mutant p53-conformation modifying drug, CP-31398, can induce apoptosis of human cancer cells and can stabilize wild-type p53 protein. *Cancer Biol. Ther.* 1, 47-55.
Takeda, K., Hayakawa, Y., Smyth, M. J., Kayagaki, N., Yamaguchi, N., Kakuta, S., Iwakura, Y., Yagita, H., & Okumura, K. (2001). Involvement of tumor necrosis factor-related apoptosis-inducing ligand in surveillance of tumor metastasis by liver natural killer cells. *Nat Med, 7*(1), 94-100.

Takeda, K., Smyth, M. J., Cretney, E., Hayakawa, Y., Kayagaki, N., Yagita, H., & Okumura, K. (2002). Critical role for tumor necrosis factor-related apoptosis-inducing ligand in immune surveillance against tumor development. *J Exp Med, 195*(2), 161-169.
Testa, J. R., & Bellacosa, A. (2001). AKT plays a central role in tumorigenesis. *Proc Natl Acad Sci U S A, 98*(20), 10983-10985.
Thome, M., Schneider, P., Hofmann, K., Fickenscher, H., Meinl, E., Neipel, F., Mattmann, C., Burns, K., Bodmer, J. L., Schroter, M., Scaffidi, C., Krammer, P. H., Peter, M. E., & Tschopp, J. (1997). Viral FLICE-inhibitory proteins (FLIPs) prevent apoptosis induced by death receptors. *Nature, 386*(6624), 517-521.
Thut, C. J., Goodrich, J. A., & Tjian, R. (1997). Repression of p53-mediated transcription by MDM2: a dual mechanism. *Genes Dev, 11*(15), 1974-1986.
Tolbert, D., Lu, X., Yin, C., Tantama, M., & Van Dyke, T. (2002). p19(ARF) is dispensable for oncogenic stress-induced p53-mediated apoptosis and tumor suppression in vivo. *Mol Cell Biol, 22*(1), 370-377.
Tsujimoto, Y., Cossman, J., Jaffe, E., & Croce, C. M. (1985). Involvement of the bcl-2 gene in human follicular lymphoma. *Science, 228*(4706), 1440-1443.
Ugurel, S., Rappl, G., Tilgen, W., & Reinhold, U. (2001). Increased soluble CD95 (sFas/CD95) serum level correlates with poor prognosis in melanoma patients. *Clin Cancer Res, 7*(5), 1282-1286.
Vaux, D. L., Cory, S., & Adams, J. M. (1988). Bcl-2 gene promotes haemopoietic cell survival and cooperates with c-myc to immortalize pre-B cells. *Nature, 335*(6189), 440-442.
Verhagen, A. M., Coulson, E. J., & Vaux, D. L. (2001). Inhibitor of apoptosis proteins and their relatives: IAPs and other BIRPs. *Genome Biol, 2*(7), REVIEWS3009.
Verhagen, A. M., Ekert, P. G., Pakusch, M., Silke, J., Connolly, L. M., Reid, G. E., Moritz, R. L., Simpson, R. J., & Vaux, D. L. (2000). Identification of DIABLO, a mammalian protein that promotes apoptosis by binding to and antagonizing IAP proteins. *Cell, 102*(1), 43-53.
Vogelstein, B., & Kinzler, K. W. (1992). p53 function and dysfunction. *Cell, 70*(4), 523-526.
Vogelstein, B., Lane, D., & Levine, A. J. (2000). Surfing the p53 network. *Nature, 408*(6810), 307-310.
Vousden, K. H., & Woude, G. F. (2000). The ins and outs of p53. *Nat Cell Biol, 2*(10), E178-180.
Walczak, H., Miller, R. E., Ariail, K., Gliniak, B., Griffith, T. S., Kubin, M., Chin, W., Jones, J., Woodward, A., Le, T., Smith, C., Smolak, P., Goodwin, R. G., Rauch, C. T., Schuh, J. C., & Lynch, D. H. (1999). Tumoricidal activity of tumor necrosis factor-related apoptosis-inducing ligand in vivo. *Nat Med, 5*(2), 157-163.
Wallace-Brodeur, R. R., & Lowe, S. W. (1999). Clinical implications of p53 mutations. *Cell Mol Life Sci, 55*(1), 64-75.
Wang, X. (2001). The expanding role of mitochondria in apoptosis. *Genes Dev, 15*(22), 2922-2933.
Wiley, S. R., Schooley, K., Smolak, P. J., Din, W. S., Huang, C. P., Nicholl, J. K., Sutherland, G. R., Smith, T. D., Rauch, C., Smith, C. A., & et al. (1995). Identification and characterization of a new member of the TNF family that induces apoptosis. *Immunity, 3*(6), 673-682.
Wu, X., Webster, S. R., & Chen, J. (2001). Characterization of tumor-associated Chk2 mutations. *J Biol Chem, 276*(4), 2971-2974.
Yin, X. M., Wang, K., Gross, A., Zhao, Y., Zinkel, S., Klocke, B., Roth, K. A., & Korsmeyer, S. J. (1999). Bid-deficient mice are resistant to Fas-induced hepatocellular apoptosis. *Nature, 400*(6747), 886-891.
Zhou, B. P., Hu, M. C., Miller, S. A., Yu, Z., Xia, W., Lin, S. Y., & Hung, M. C. (2000). HER-2/neu blocks tumor necrosis factor-induced apoptosis via the Akt/NF-kappaB pathway. *J Biol Chem, 275*(11), 8027-8031.
Zhou, B. P., Liao, Y., Xia, W., Zou, Y., Spohn, B., & Hung, M. C. (2001). HER-2/neu induces p53 ubiquitination via Akt-mediated MDM2 phosphorylation. *Nat Cell Biol, 3*(11), 973-982.
Zindy, F., Eischen, C. M., Randle, D. H., Kamijo, T., Cleveland, J. L., Sherr, C. J., & Roussel, M. F. (1998). Myc signaling via the ARF tumor suppressor regulates p53-dependent apoptosis and immortalization. *Genes Dev, 12*(15), 2424-2433.

CERAMIDE AND SPHINGOSINE 1-PHOSPHATE IN ANTI-CANCER THERAPIES

DAVID K. PERRY AND RICHARD N. KOLESNICK

1. INTRODUCTION

The body of research amassed over the last ten years in the field of sphingolipid signal transduction has provided a biochemical basis to explore new therapeutic modalities in the treatment of cancer. Importantly, two signaling molecules, ceramide and sphingosine 1-phosphate, have emerged as sphingolipid regulators of apoptosis and mitosis, respectively. As such, a successful implementation of sphingolipid-based therapies is largely dependent on the modulation of these molecules, either by direct addition or by pharmacological modification of the enzymes involved in their metabolism.

Ceramide is generated and eliminated through multiple pathways that provide several targets for therapeutic intervention (Figure 1). Generation occurs primarily through activation of one or more agonist-regulated sphingomyelinases or by a multi-step pathway that generates ceramide de novo from serine and palmitoyl CoA. The intracellular locations of the enzymes involved in ceramide generation include the plasma membrane (Linardic & Hannun, 1994) (neutral pH-optimum sphingomyelinase), sphingolipid-rich rafts within the plasma membrane (Grassme, Jekle, Riehle, Schwarz, Berger, Sandhoff, Kolesnick & Gulbins, 2001) (acid pH-optimum sphingomyelinase), and endoplasmic reticulum (Mandon, Ehses, Rother, van Echten & Sandhoff, 1992) and mitochondria (Lee & Kolesnick, 2002) (de novo pathway). Whereas the manner in which these enzymes are activated is poorly understood, studies on the mechanism of action of current cancer therapeutics are demonstrating their integral role in the modulation of signaling pathways necessary for apoptosis.

Elimination of ceramide, conversely, can occur through the action of a ceramidase, a glucosylceramide synthase, or a sphingomyelin synthase (figure 1). Ceramidase cleaves the amide bond of ceramide resulting in a fatty acid and sphingosine, a substrate for synthesis of sphingosine 1-phosphate, an antagonist of ceramide action. The glucosylceramide synthase attenuates ceramide levels by glycosylating the primary hydroxyl group, the site that also serves as the acceptor for a phosphocholine moiety in the reaction catalyzed by sphingomyelin synthase. Inhibitors of these enzymes are being developed for potential use in the next generation of chemotherapeutics.

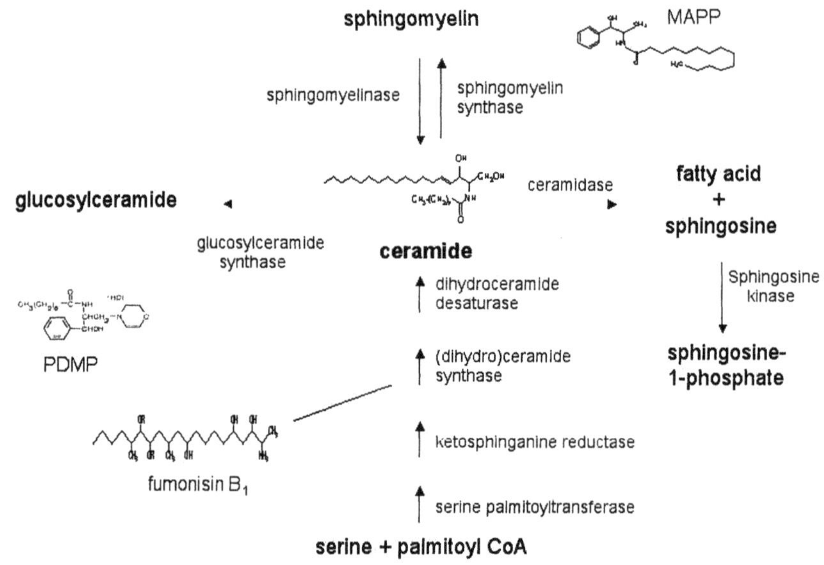

Figure 1. Ceramide Metabolism

1.1 Tissue culture models

The biochemical basis for ceramide-based cancer therapies has largely been determined in tissue culture models of apoptotic cell death. In investigating the molecular mechanisms of apoptosis induced by the common cancer treatments of chemotherapy or radiation, it was found that ceramide elevation occurred through activation of sphingomyelinases (Cabot, Han & Giuliano, 1998; Laethem, Hannun, Jayadev, Sexton, Strum, Sundseth & Smith, 1998; Haimovitz-Friedman, Kan, Ehleiter, Persaud, McLoughlin, Fuks & Kolesnick, 1994; Chmura, Mauceri, Advani, Heimann, Beckett, Nodzenksi, Quintans, Kufe & Weichselbaum, 1997) and/or the de novo pathway in a cell-type specific manner (Bose, Verheij, Haimovitz-Friedman, Scotto, Fuks & Kolesnick, 1995; Suzuki, Iwasaki, Kato & Wagai, 1997; Cabot, Giuliano, Han & Liu, 1999; Liao, Haimovitz-Friedman, Persaud, McLoughlin, Ehleiter, Zhang, Gatei, Lavin, Kolesnick & Fuks, 1999; Perry, Carton, Shah, Meredith, Uhlinger & Hannun, 2000; Wang, Maurer, Reynolds & Cabot, 2001). To understand whether ceramide was a consequence of the ensuing apoptosis or an integral signaling component of apoptotic cascades, studies have been undertaken using either genetic or pharmacological approaches to modulate ceramide-metabolizing enzymes.

The genetic studies have primarily involved utilization of cells from patients with Niemann-Pick disease. This inherited disorder is characterized by the lack of acid sphingomyelinase activity and has provided an elegant model to study the role of the enzyme in signal transduction. Lymphoblasts from these patients, as opposed to a control population, fail to produce ceramide in response to radiation and are resistant to apoptosis. However, sensitivity and ceramide generation were restored when the cells were transfected with a vector containing the functional acid sphingomyelinase gene (Santana, Pena, Haimovitz-Friedman, Martin, Green, McLoughlin, Cordon-Cardo, Schuchman, Fuks & Kolesnick, 1996). To understand further the cell specificity of this response, an acid sphingomyelinase knockout mouse was generated and submitted to whole body radiation. Examination of mouse tissues revealed that the apoptotic response was not uniform in that various endothelial cell populations were more dependent on acid sphingomyelinase function and other tissues including thymus and spleen were less dependent (Santana, Pena, Haimovitz-Friedman, Martin, Green, McLoughlin, Cordon-Cardo, Schuchman, Fuks & Kolesnick, 1996).

Acid sphingomyelinase as well as neutral sphingomyelinase have also been implicated in cancer therapy-induced apoptotic responses on the basis of enzyme activity assays. Several fold increases in the activity of these enzymes have been observed in response to radiation and various chemotherapy agents (Haimovitz-Friedman, Kan, Ehleiter, Persaud, McLoughlin, Fuks & Kolesnick, 1994; Cabot, Han & Giuliano, 1998; Laethem, Hannun, Jayadev, Sexton, Strum, Sundseth & Smith, 1998; Jaffrezou, Bruno, Moisand, Levade & Laurent, 2001; Chmura, Mauceri, Advani, Heimann, Beckett, Nodzenksi, Quintans, Kufe & Weichselbaum, 1997). Whereas the production of ceramide in these studies is consistent with an important role in that it precedes or coincides with the onset of apoptosis, its necessity is less clear due to the fact that specific inhibitors of the two enzymes have yet to be discovered.

Specific inhibitors have, however, been identified for enzymes in the de novo pathway and have allowed for pharmacological intervention. De novo ceramide generation is inhibited by fungal compounds known as fumonisins that share structural similarity to the sphingoid base backbone (Wang, Norred, Bacon, Riley & Merrill, 1991; Merrill, van Echten, Wang & Sandhoff, 1993). In those cell culture models where the anti-cancer agent is activating de novo synthesis, the fumonisins have provided partial to complete protection from apoptosis (Bose, Verheij, Haimovitz-Friedman, Scotto, Fuks & Kolesnick, 1995; Cabot, Giuliano, Han & Liu, 1999; Suzuki, Iwasaki, Kato & Wagai, 1997; Wieder, Orfanos & Geilen, 1998; Perry, Carton, Shah, Meredith, Uhlinger & Hannun, 2000).

Neither radiation nor the chemotherapy agents now in use are known to directly activate any of the enzymes involved in ceramide generation. However, small molecules that directly inhibit enzymes in ceramide elimination are being explored as novel chemotherapy treatments. One of these routes of elimination is through glycosylation of ceramide by glucosylceramide synthase (GCS). This enzyme has long been of interest in cancer studies due to the role of glycosphingolipids in the proliferation and metastasis of cancer cells (Inokuchi, Mason & Radin, 1987;

Inokuchi, Jimbo, Momosaki, Shimeno, Nagamatsu & Radin, 1990), and it's been proposed as a site of intervention for chemotherapy on that basis (Radin, 1994). A ceramide analog, PDMP (1-phenyl-2-decanoylamino-3-morpholino-1-propanol), that acts as an inhibitor of the enzyme results in the growth arrest of NIH3T3 cells. This response was mimicked by the addition of short-chain ceramides, and it suggested that elevation of substrate (ceramide) through inhibition of GCS is as significant to the reduction of product (glycosylated sphingolipids) in attenuating cell growth (Rani, Abe, Chang, Rosenzweig, Saltiel, Radin & Shayman, 1995).

Cabot and co-workers have further explored the dual potential of GCS inhibition and inquired whether its elimination of ceramide may play a role in resistance to traditional chemotherapeutics. These studies were prompted by the observation that many multidrug resistant (MDR) cell lines contain elevated levels of glucosylceramide that are due to synthetic rather than degradative abnormalities (Lavie, Cao, Bursten, Giuliano & Cabot, 1996). Moreover, the investigators were able to confer resistance to both adriamycin- and short-chain ceramide-induced death by over-expressing GCS in a wild-type MCF-7 breast cancer cell line. This conferred drug resistance was independent of P-glycoprotein and Bcl-2 status (Liu, Han, Giuliano & Cabot, 1999). Further confirmation of their hypothesis was obtained by showing that attenuation of GCS with antisense methodology resulted in a restoration of chemotherapy sensitivity in MDR overexpressors (Liu, Han, Giuliano, Hansen & Cabot, 2000).

Some of the common agents used to reverse multidrug resistance, such as verapamil and cyclosporine A, do so through varying degrees of inhibition of GCS (Lavie, Cao, Volner, Lucci, Han, Geffen, Giuliano & Cabot, 1997). Alternatively, other MDR inhibitors such as the cyclosporine analog, PSC 833, exert part of their influence by enhancing ceramide synthesis through the de novo pathway (Cabot, Han & Giuliano, 1998; Cabot, Giuliano, Han & Liu, 1999). This ability of increased de novo ceramide synthesis to overcome the MDR phenotype is apparently dependent on the GCS level or topography in a particular cell type. In Jurkat cells, for example, GCS, presumably due to its Golgi location and proximity to de novo synthesis, attenuates de novo ceramide and its apoptotic function. In contrast, GCS was unable to attenuate the levels of sphingomyelinase-derived ceramide (Tepper, Diks, van Blitterswijk & Borst, 2000). These results provide a basis for designing therapeutic protocols based upon tumoral GCS levels and the ceramide pathway(s) activated by a particular chemotherapeutic.

In addition to the work performed in MDR cells with elevated levels of GCS activity and in the acid sphingomyelinase knockout models, a failure in apoptosis resulting from deficient ceramide production has been observed in several other systems of radiation- and chemotherapy-induced apoptosis (Gottschalk, McShan, Kilkus, Dawson & Quintans, 1995; Chmura, Nodzenski, Beckett, Kufe, Quintans & Weichselbaum, 1997; Wang, Beebe, Pwiti, Bielawska & Smyth, 1999; Chmura, Nodzenski, Kharbanda, Pandey, Quintans, Kufe & Weichselbaum, 2000).

A second, but equally important route of ceramide elimination is through the action of a family of ceramidases. An interesting aspect of the ceramidases is that they not only degrade ceramide but in doing so provide a product, sphingosine, that can be phosphorylated to sphingosine 1-phosphate, an antagonist of ceramide-mediated apoptosis (Cuvillier, Pirianov, Kleuser, Vanek, Coso, Gutkind & Spiegel, 1996). Therefore, chemotherapeutics that target ceramidase such as D-*erythro*-N-myristoylamino-1-phenyl-1-propanol, (D-MAPP) would have the dual effect of not only elevating ceramide, but also perhaps of inhibiting the pathway for synthesis of a natural ceramide antagonist. The attractiveness of this approach is complicated by the fact that at least two isoenzymes of ceramidase exist. Small molecule inhibitors of the alkaline pH optimum form are able to induce growth arrest (Bielawska, Greenberg, Perry, Jayadev, Shayman, McKay & Hannun, 1996) and over-expression of the acid pH optimum enzyme can attenuate apoptotic responses (Strelow, Bernardo, Adam-Klages, Linke, Sandhoff, Kronke & Adam, 2000; Jan, Chatterjee & Griffin, 2000).

Finally, a third mechanism for ceramide reduction is through a sphingomyelin synthase activity that transfers the phosphocholine headgroup from phosphatidylcholine to ceramide, generating sphingomyelin and diacylglycerol in the process. This enzyme is up-regulated in SV40-transformed cells, and it may be involved in the progression to or maintenance of the transformed state (Luberto & Hannun, 1998). Moreover, the enzyme is activated in astrocytes treated with bFGF and its elimination of ceramide is involved in bFGF-induced proliferation (Riboni, Viani, Bassi, Giussani & Tettamanti, 2001). The elevated activity and involvement of sphingomyelin synthase in these mitogenic responses makes it an attractive target for the development of chemotherapeutics.

2. APOPTOTIC MODULATORS AFFECTING CERAMIDE FUNCTION OR GENERATION

Elevation of ceramide in a cell is generally considered a signal of stress rather than an event sufficient for induction of apoptosis. Whether ceramide induces apoptosis or other non-proliferative biologies, such as growth arrest or differentiation, is dependent on downstream regulators. For instance, the anti-apoptotic protein, Bcl-2, prevents apoptotic signaling of short-chain ceramides added exogenously to cells (Fang, Rivard, Ganser, LeBien, Nath, Mueller & Behrens, 1995; Zhang, Alter, Reed, Borner, Obeid & Hannun, 1996; Smyth, Perry, Zhang, Poirier, Hannun & Obeid, 1996). However, Bcl-2 neither inhibits the generation of ceramide from the sphingomyelin pathway (Dbaibo, Perry, Gamard, Platt, Poirier, Obeid & Hannun, 1997) nor does it prevent the role of ceramide in signaling growth arrest through dephosphorylation of the retinoblastoma gene product (Zhang, Alter, Reed, Borner, Obeid & Hannun, 1996). The fact that ceramide generation is unimpeded in apoptosis-resistant, Bcl-2 over-expressing cells refutes the notion that it's an innocent byproduct of the apoptotic process.

Several studies have also elucidated the role of p53 in ceramide-mediated apoptosis. What is the most consistent finding is that p53 is not a downstream mediator of ceramide action. While radiation-induced endothelial apoptosis was blocked in the acid sphingomyelinase-deficient mice, it was unaffected by lack of p53 (Santana, Pena, Haimovitz-Friedman, Martin, Green, McLoughlin, Cordon-Cardo, Schuchman, Fuks & Kolesnick, 1996). This result was consistent with earlier findings that suggested radiation-induced ceramide generation was independent of nuclear events (Haimovitz-Friedman, Kan, Ehleiter, Persaud, McLoughlin, Fuks & Kolesnick, 1994). However, the upstream involvement of p53 appears to be agonist- and cell type-specific in that leukemic T cells required functional p53 to induce ceramide generation and apoptosis in response to actinomycin D or radiation (Dbaibo, Pushkareva, Rachid, Alter, Smyth, Obeid & Hannun, 1998).

2.1 Small animal in vivo models

From a therapeutic standpoint, some of the earliest *in vivo* work interested in the role of sphingolipids in modulation of cancer investigated the ability of diets enriched in sphingolipids to modulate colon carcinogenesis. Using a mouse model of chemical-induced colon cancer, sphingomyelin or glycosphingolipid-enriched diets resulted in over a 50% reduction in the incidence of tumor formation (Dillehay, Webb, Schmelz & Merrill, 1994; Schmelz, Sullards, Dillehay & Merrill, 2000) as well as a reduction in the proportion of adenocarcinomas *vs.* adenomas (Schmelz, Dillehay, Webb, Reiter, Adams & Merrill, 1996). A possible mechanism by which the sphingolipids suppress colon tumor formation is by correcting defects associated with the adenomatous polyposis coli (APC) regulatory system (Schmelz, Roberts, Kustin, Lemonnier, Sullards, Dillehay & Merrill, 2001). The causal protective agent in these studies is unknown but metabolism studies of radiolabeled sphingolipid substrates are most consistent with sphingosine and/or ceramide being the effector molecule (Schmelz, Crall, Larocque, Dillehay & Merrill, 1994).

The work of Kester and colleagues, though not yet directly applied to cancer therapy, has provided proof in principle for the efficacy of direct delivery *in vivo* of short-chain ceramides. These investigators demonstrated that ceramide arrested the growth of smooth muscle cells *in vitro* (Coroneus, Wang, Panuska, Templeton & Kester, 1996) and hypothesized that it could be applied to treat the proliferation of vascular smooth muscle cells - an event responsible for lumenal narrowing that often follows angioplasty-associated stretch injury. Using rabbit carotid arteries as a model system, they demonstrated that short fatty acyl chain ceramide delivered on the tip of balloon catheters was taken up by the target cells, growth factor-stimulated ERK and PKB pathways were down-regulated, and smooth muscle cell growth was arrested (Charles, Sandirasegarane, Yun, Bourbon, Wilson, Rothstein, Levison & Kester, 2000). This resulted in marked reduction in neointimal hyperplasia and patent blood vessels.

Ceramidase has been exploited as a target using a model of human colon cancer cells metastatic to the nude mouse liver. In tissue culture, both primary and metastatic colon cancer cells had less than half the baseline ceramide of normal colon mucosa but underwent apoptotic cell death with treatment of short-chain ceramides or ceramidase inhibitors. The tumor cell lines were injected into the mouse portal vein and the liver examined 5 weeks later in animals treated with or without the ceramidase inhibitor, B13, post-injection. Large hepatic tumor masses were observed in all animals receiving injection without ceramidase inhibitor therapy as opposed to the tumor-free livers of animals with B13 treatment (Selzner, Bielawska, Morse, Rudiger, Sindram, Hannun & Clavien, 2001). Whether B13 resulted in tumor cell apoptosis in the hepatic sinusoids or whether it prevented tumor cell adhesion is unknown, but it had the important quality of being non-toxic to normal hepatocytes.

Tilly and co-workers have considered the detrimental effects that chemotherapy and radiation have upon female germ cells. Using anthracylines, whose mechanism of death is known to involve ceramide formation (Bose, Verheij, Haimovitz-Friedman, Scotto, Fuks & Kolesnick, 1995; Jaffrezou, Levade, Bettaieb, Andrieu, Bezombes, Maestre, Vermeersch, Rousse & Laurent, 1996), mouse oocytes could be rescued from apoptosis with sphingosine 1-phosphate (Perez, Kunuson, Leykin, Korsmeyer & Tilly, 1997), an antagonist of ceramide-mediated apoptosis (Cuvillier, Pirianov, Kleuser, Vanek, Coso, Gutkind & Spiegel, 1996). Similar results were found *in vivo* mouse models where radiation-induced oocyte apoptosis was rescued by sphingosine 1-phosphate therapy (Morita, Perez, Paris, Miranda, Ehleiter, Haimovitz-Friedman, Fuks, Xie, Reed, Schuchman, Kolesnick & Tilly, 2000). Importantly, either disruption of the acid sphingomyelinase gene or sphingosine 1-phosphate therapy was also able to reduce the normal, age-related depletion of oocytes (Morita, Perez, Paris, Miranda, Ehleiter, Haimovitz-Friedman, Fuks, Xie, Reed, Schuchman, Kolesnick & Tilly, 2000). The antagonizing of ceramide-mediated apoptosis with sphingosine 1-phosphate may provide promising results in extending the lifetime of ovulation as well as in providing oocyte protection during standard cancer therapeutic regimens.

Similarly, in a continuation of the studies of the role of acid sphingomyelinase in radiation-induced death of endothelial cells, Kolesnick and colleagues have considered the mechanism of damage incurred by the gastrointestinal (GI) tract with common treatments of chemotherapy or radiation. It was believed that GI syndrome was due to radiation-induced damage of epithelial stem cells. Their results demonstrated, however, that stem cell damage was secondary to that incurred by microvascular endothelial cells and that the effect could be reversed by endothelial cell growth factors including basic fibroblast growth factor (bFGF) or by deletion of the acid sphingomyelinase gene (Paris, Fuks, Kang, Capodieci, Juan, Ehleiter, Haimovitz-Friedman, Cordon-Cardo & Kolesnick, 2001). As in the work of Tilly et al., sphingosine 1-phosphate therapy might also be expected to spare radiation-induced damage of microvascular endothelial cells. It is noted, however, that in both of these studies, maximum therapeutic benefit would only be obtained if the tumors being treated were refractory to the mitogens used in sparing non-target cells.

In summary, the biochemical understanding of the metabolism and role of ceramide in apoptosis has provided novel targets for therapeutic intervention. The translation of this research into efficacious treatment is being borne out in small animal models. Depending on the whether the goal is to enhance ceramide generation in cancer tissue or to antagonize its function in non-target tissue, the results thus far demonstrate the feasibility of such an approach and predict future success for implementation of similar strategies in clinical trials.

David K. Perry
Department of Biochemistry and Molecular Biology
Medical University of South Carolina
Charleston, SC 29425

Richard N. Kolesnick
Laboratory of Signal Transduction
Memorial Sloan-Kettering Cancer Center
New York, NY 10021

3. REFERENCES

Bielawska, A., Greenberg, M. S., Perry, D., Jayadev, S., Shayman, J. A., McKay, C. & Hannun, Y. A. (1996). (1*S*,2*R*)-D-*erythro*-2-(*N*-myristoylamino)-1-phenyl-1-propano l as an inhibitor of ceramidase. *Journal of Biological Chemistry*, *271*, 12646-12654.

Bose, R., Verheij, M., Haimovitz-Friedman, A., Scotto, K., Fuks, Z. & Kolesnick, R. (1995). Ceramide synthase mediates daunorubicin-induced apoptosis: an alternative mechanism for generating death signals. *Cell*, *82*, 405-414.

Cabot, M. C., Giuliano, A. E., Han, T. -Y. & Liu, Y. -Y. (1999). SDZ PSC 833, the cyclosporine A analogue and multidrug resistance modulator, activates ceramide synthesis and increases vinblastine sensitivity in drug-sensitive and drug-resistant cancer cells. *Cancer Research*, *59*, 880-885.

Cabot, M. C., Han, T. -Y. & Giuliano, A. E. (1998). The multidrug resistance modulator SDZ PSC 833 is a potent activator of cellular ceramide formation. *FEBS Letters*, *431*, 185-188.

Charles, R., Sandirasegarane, L., Yun, J., Bourbon, N., Wilson, R., Rothstein, R. P., Levison, S. W. & Kester, M. (2000). Ceramide-coated balloon catheters limit neointimal hyperplasia after stretch injury in carotid arteries. *Circulation Research*, *87*, 282-288.

Chmura, S. J., Mauceri, H. J., Advani, S., Heimann, R., Beckett, M. A., Nodzenksi, E., Quintans, J., Kufe, D. W. & Weichselbaum, R. R. (1997). Decreasing the apoptotic threshold of tumor cells through protein kinase C inhibition and sphingomyelinase activation increases tumor killing by ionizing radiation. *Cancer Research*, *57*, 4340-4347.

Chmura, S. J., Nodzenski, E., Beckett, M. A., Kufe, D. W., Quintans, J. & Weichselbaum, R. R. (1997). Loss of ceramide production confers resistance to radiation-induced apoptosis. *Cancer Research*, *57*, 1270-1275.

Chmura, S. J., Nodzenski, E., Kharbanda, S., Pandey, P., Quintans, J., Kufe, D. W. & Weichselbaum, R. R. (2000). Down-regulation of ceramide production abrogates ionizing radiation-induced cytochrome c release and apoptosis. *Molecular Pharmacology*, *57*, 792-796.

Coroneus, E., Wang, Y., Panuska, J. R., Templeton, D. J. & Kester, M. (1996). Sphingolipid metabolites differentially regulate extracellular signal-regulated kinase and stress-activated protein kinase cascades. *Biochemical Journal*, *316*, 13-17.

Cuvillier, O., Pirianov, G., Kleuser, B., Vanek, P. G., Coso, O. A., Gutkind, J. S. & Spiegel, S. (1996). Suppression of ceramide-mediated programmed cell death by sphingosine-1-phosphate. *Nature*, *381*, 800-803.

Dbaibo, G. S., Perry, D. K., Gamard, C. J., Platt, R., Poirier, G. G., Obeid, L. M. & Hannun, Y. A. (1997). Cytokine response modifier A (CrmA) inhibits ceramide formation in response to tumor necrosis factor (TNF-_): CrmA and Bcl-2 target distinct components in the apoptotic pathway. *Journal of Experimental Medicine*, *185*, 481-490.

Dbaibo, G. S., Pushkareva, M. Y., Rachid, R. A., Alter, N., Smyth, M. J., Obeid, L. M. & Hannun, Y. A. (1998). p53-dependent ceramide response to genotoxic stress. *Journal of Clinical Investigation*, *102*, 329-339.

Dillehay, D. L., Webb, S. K., Schmelz, E. M. & Merrill, A. H. Jr. (1994). Dietary sphingomyelin inhibits 1,2-dimethylhydrazine-induced colon cancer in CF1 mice. *Journal of Nutrition*, *124*, 615-620.

Fang, W., Rivard, J. J., Ganser, J. A., LeBien, T. W., Nath, K. A., Mueller, D. L. & Behrens, T. W. (1995). Bcl-x_L rescues WEHI 231 B lymphocytes from oxidant-mediated death following diverse apoptotic stimuli. *Journal of Immunology*, *155*, 66-75.

Gottschalk, A. R., McShan, C. L., Kilkus, J., Dawson, G. & Quintans, J. (1995). Resistance to anti-IgM-induced apoptosis in a WEHI-231 subline is due to insufficient production of ceramide. *European Journal of Immunology*, *25*, 1032-1038.

Grassme, H., Jekle, A., Riehle, A., Schwarz, H., Berger, J., Sandhoff, K., Kolesnick, R. & Gulbins, E. (2001). CD95 signaling via ceramide-rich membrane rafts. *Journal of Biological Chemistry*, *276*, 20589-20596.

Haimovitz-Friedman, A., Kan, C. -C., Ehleiter, D., Persaud, R. S., McLoughlin, M., Fuks, Z. & Kolesnick, R. N. (1994). Ionizing radiation acts on cellular membranes to generate ceramide and initiate apoptosis. *Journal of Experimental Medicine*, *180*, 525-535.

Inokuchi, J., Jimbo, M., Momosaki, K., Shimeno, H., Nagamatsu, A. & Radin, N. S. (1990). Inhibition of experimental metastasis of murine lewis lung carcinoma by an inhibitor of glucosylceramide synthase and its possible mechanism of action. *Cancer Research*, *50*, 6731-6737.

Inokuchi, J. -I., Mason, I. & Radin, N. S. (1987). Antitumor activity via inhibition of glycosphingolipid biosynthesis. *Cancer Letters*, *38*, 23-30.

Jaffrezou, J. P., Bruno, A. P., Moisand, A., Levade, T. & Laurent, G. (2001). Activation of nuclear sphingomyelinase in radiation-induced apoptosis. *FASEB Journal*, *15*, 123-133.

Jaffrezou, J. P., Levade, T., Bettaieb, A., Andrieu, N., Bezombes, C., Maestre, N., Vermeersch, S., Rousse, A. & Laurent, G. (1996). Daunorubicin-induced apoptosis: triggering of ceramide generation through sphingomyelin hydrolysis. *EMBO Journal*, *15*, 2417-2424.

Jan, J. -T., Chatterjee, S. & Griffin, D. E. (2000). Sindbis virus entry into cells triggers apoptosis by activating sphingomyelinase, leading to the release of ceramide. *Journal of Virology*, *74*, 6425-6432.

Laethem, R. M., Hannun, Y. A., Jayadev, S., Sexton, C. J., Strum, J. C., Sundseth, R. & Smith, G. K. (1998). Increases in neutral, Mg^{2+}-dependent and acidic, Mg^{2+}-independent sphingomyelinase activities precede commitment to apoptosis and are not a consequence of caspase 3-like activity in Molt-4 cells in responses to thymidylate synthase inhibition by GW1843. *Blood*, *91*, 4350-4360.

Lavie, Y., Cao, h., Bursten, s. l., Giuliano, A. E. & Cabot, M. C. (1996). Accumulation of glucosylceramides in multidrug-resistant cancer cells. *Journal of Biological Chemistry*, *271*, 19530-19536.

Lavie, Y., Cao, h., Volner, A., Lucci, A., Han, T. Y., Geffen, V., Giuliano, A. E. & Cabot, M. C. (1997). Agents that reverse multidrug resistance, tamoxifen, verapamil, and cyclosporine A, block glycosphingolipid metabolism by inhibiting ceramide glycosylation in human cancer cells. *Journal of Biological Chemistry*, *272*, 1682-1687.

Lee, & Kolesnick, R.N. (manuscript submitted)

Liao, W. -C., Haimovitz-Friedman, A., Persaud, R. S., McLoughlin, M., Ehleiter, D., Zhang, N., Gatei, M., Lavin, M., Kolesnick, R. & Fuks, Z. (1999). Ataxia telangiectasia-mutated gene product inhibits DNA damage-induced apoptosis via ceramide synthase. *Journal of Biological Chemistry*, *274*, 17908-17917.

Linardic, C. M. & Hannun, Y. A. (1994). Identification of a distinct pool of sphingomyelin involved in the sphingomyelin cycle. *Journal of Biological Chemistry*, *269*, 23530-23537.

Liu, Y. -Y., Han, T. -Y., Giuliano, A. E. & Cabot, M. C. (1999). Expression of glucosylceramide synthase, converting ceramide to glucosylceramide, confers adriamycin resistance in human breast cancer cells. *Journal of Biological Chemistry*, *274*, 1140-1146.

Liu, Y. -Y., Han, T. -Y., Giuliano, A. E., Hansen, N. & Cabot, M. C. (2000). Uncoupling ceramide glycosylation by transfection of glucosylceramide synthase antisense reverses adriamycin resistance. *Journal of Biological Chemistry*, *275*, 7138-7143.

Luberto, C. & Hannun, Y. A. (1998). Sphingomyelin synthase, a potential regulator of intracellular levels of ceramide and diacylglycerol during SV40 transformation. *Journal of Biological Chemistry*, *273*, 14550-14559.

Mandon, E. C., Ehses, I., Rother, J., van Echten, G. & Sandhoff, K. (1992). Subcellular localization and membrane topology of serine palmitoyltransferase, 3-dehydrosphinganine reductase, and sphinganine *N*-acyltransferase in mouse liver. *Journal of Biological Chemistry*, *267*, 11144-11148.

Merrill, A. H. Jr., van Echten, G., Wang, E. & Sandhoff, K. (1993). Fumonisin B_1 inhibits sphingosine (sphinganine) N-acyltransferase and *de novo* sphingolipid biosynthesis in cultured neurons *in situ*. *Journal of Biological Chemistry*, *268*, 27299-27306.

Morita, Y., Perez, G. I., Paris, F., Miranda, S. R., Ehleiter, D., Haimovitz-Friedman, A., Fuks, Z., Xie, Z., Reed, J. C., Schuchman, E. H., Kolesnick, R. N. & Tilly, J. L. (2000). Oocyte apoptosis is suppressed by disruption of the acid sphingomyelinase gene or by sphingosine-1-phosphate therapy. *Nature Medicine*, *10*, 1109-1114.

Paris, F., Fuks, Z., Kang, A., Capodieci, P., Juan, G., Ehleiter, D., Haimovitz-Friedman, A., Cordon-Cardo, C. & Kolesnick, R. (2001). Endothelial apoptosis as the primary lesion initiating intestinal radiation damage in mice. *Science*, *293*, 293-297.

Perez, G. I., Kunuson, M., Leykin, L., Korsmeyer, S. J. & Tilly, J. L. (1997). Apoptosis-associated signaling pathways are required for chemotherapy-mediated female germ cell destruction. *Nature Medicine*, *3*, 1228-1232.

Perry, D. K., Carton, J., Shah, A. K., Meredith, F., Uhlinger, D. J. & Hannun, Y. A. (2000). Serine palmitoyltransferase regulates de nove ceramide generation during etoposide-induced apoptosis. *Journal of Biological Chemistry, 275*, 9078-9084.
Radin, N. S. (1994). Rationales for cancer chemotherapy with PDMP, a specific inhibitor of glucosylceramide synthase. *Molecular and Chemical Neuropathology, 21*, 111-127.
Rani, C. S. S., Abe, A., Chang, Y., Rosenzweig, N., Saltiel, A. R., Radin, N. S. & Shayman, J. A. (1995). Cell cycle arrest induced by an inhibitor of glucosylceramide synthase. *Journal of Biological Chemistry, 270*, 2859-2867.
Riboni, L., Viani, P., Bassi, R., Giussani, P. & Tettamanti, G. (2001). Basic fibroblast growth factor-induced proliferation of primary astrocytes. *Journal of Biological Chemistry, 276*, 12797-12804.
Santana, P., Pena, L. A., Haimovitz-Friedman, A., Martin, S., Green, D., McLoughlin, M., Cordon-Cardo, C., Schuchman, E. H., Fuks, Z. & Kolesnick, R. (1996). Acid sphingomyelinase-deficient human lymphoblasts and mice are defective in radiation-induced apoptosis. *Cell, 86*, 189-799.
Schmelz, E. M., Crall, K. J., Larocque, R., Dillehay, D. L. & Merrill, A. H. Jr. (1994). Uptake and metabolism of sphingolipids in isolated intestinal loops of mice. *Journal of Nutrition, 124*, 702-712.
Schmelz, E. M., Dillehay, D. L., Webb, S. K., Reiter, A., Adams, J. & Merrill, A. H. Jr. (1996). Sphingomyelin consumption suppresses aberrant colonic crypt foci and increases the proportion of adenomas versus adenocarcinomas in CF1 mice treated with 1,2-dimethylhydrazine: Implications for dietary sphingolipids and colon carcinogenesis. *Cancer Research, 56*, 4936-4941.
Schmelz, E. M., Roberts, P. C., Kustin, E. M., Lemonnier, L. A., Sullards, M. C., Dillehay, D. L. & Merrill, A. H. Jr. (2001). Modulation of intracellular beta-catenin localization and intestinal tumorigenesis in vivo and in vitro by sphingolipids. *Cancer Research, 61*, 6723-6729.
Schmelz, E. M., Sullards, M. C., Dillehay, D. L. & Merrill, A. H. Jr. (2000). Colonic cell proliferation and aberrant crypt foci formation are inhibited by dairy glycosphingolipids in 1,2-dimethylhydrazine-treated CF1 mice. *Journal of Nutrition, 130*, 522-527.
Selzner, M., Bielawska, A., Morse, M. A., Rudiger, H. A., Sindram, D., Hannun, Y. A. & Clavien, P. A. (2001). Induction of apoptotic cell death and prevention of tumor growth by ceramide analogues in metastatic human colon cancer. *Cancer Research, 61*, 1233-1240.
Smyth, M. J., Perry, D. K., Zhang, J., Poirier, G. G., Hannun, Y. A. & Obeid, L. M. (1996). prICE: a downstream target for ceramide-induced apoptosis and for the inhibitory action of bcl-2. *Biochemical Journal, 316*, 25-28.
Strelow, A., Bernardo, K., Adam-Klages, S., Linke, T., Sandhoff, K., Kronke, M. & Adam, D. (2000). Overexpression of acid ceramidase protects from tumor necrosis factor-induced cell death. *Journal of Experimental Medicine, 192*, 601-612.
Suzuki, A., Iwasaki, M., Kato, M. & Wagai, N. (1997). Sequential operation of ceramide synthesis and ICE cascade in CPT-11-initiated apoptotic death signaling. *Experimental Cell Research, 233*, 41-47.
Tepper, A. D., Diks, S. H., van Blitterswijk, W. J. & Borst, J. (2000). Glucosylceramide synthase does not attenuate the ceramide pool accumulating during apoptosis induced by CD95 or anti-cancer agents. *Journal of Biological Chemistry, 275*, 34810-34817.
Wang, E., Norred, W. P., Bacon, C. W., Riley, R. T. & Merrill, A. H. Jr. (1991). Inhibition of sphingolipid biosynthesis by fumonisins. *Journal of Biological Chemistry, 266*, 14486-14490.
Wang, H., Maurer, B. J., Reynolds, C. P. & Cabot, M. C. (2001). N-(4-hydroxyphenyl) retinamide elevates ceramide in neuroblastoma cell lines by coordinate activation of serine palmitoyltransferase and ceramide synthase. *Cancer Research, 61*, 5102-5105.
Wang, X. Z., Beebe, J. R., Pwiti, L., Bielawska, A. & Smyth, M. J. (1999). Aberrant sphingolipid signaling is involved in the resistance of prostate cancer cell lines to chemotherapy. *Cancer Research, 59*, 5842-5848.
Wieder, T., Orfanos, C. E. & Geilen, C. C. (1998). Induction of ceramide-mediated apoptosis by the anticancer phospholipid analog, hexadecylphosphocholine. *Journal of Biological Chemistry, 273*, 11025-11031.
Zhang, J., Alter, N., Reed, J. C., Borner, C., Obeid, L. M. & Hannun, Y. A. (1996). Bcl-2 interrupts the ceramide-mediated pathway of cell death. *Proceedings of the National Academy of Science USA, 93*, 5325-5328.

GPSR Compliance
The European Union's (EU) General Product Safety Regulation (GPSR) is a set of rules that requires consumer products to be safe and our obligations to ensure this.

If you have any concerns about our products, you can contact us on

ProductSafety@springernature.com

In case Publisher is established outside the EU, the EU authorized representative is:

Springer Nature Customer Service Center GmbH
Europaplatz 3
69115 Heidelberg, Germany

www.ingramcontent.com/pod-product-compliance
Ingram Content Group UK Ltd.
Pitfield, Milton Keynes, MK11 3LW, UK
UKHW012153240726
13966UKWH00002B/300

* 9 7 8 1 4 7 5 7 7 8 2 0 5 *